Immunology Immunopathology and Immunity

Fourth Edition

Immunology Immunopathology and Immunity

Stewart Sell, M.D.

Professor and Chairman
Department of Pathology and Laboratory Medicine
Medical School
University of Texas Health Science Center at Houston

Elsevier

New York • Amsterdam • London

The author and publisher have made every effort to ensure that drug selection and dosage set forth in this text are in accord with current recommendations and practice at the time of publication. However, in view of ongoing research, changes in government regulations, and the constant flow of information concerning drug therapy and drug reactions, the reader is urged to check the package insert for each drug for any change in indications and dosage and for added warnings and precautions. This is particularly important when the recommended agent is a new and/or infrequently employed drug.

Elsevier Science Publishing Company, Inc.
52 Vanderbilt Avenue, New York, New York 10017

Sole distributors outside the United States and Canada:
Elsevier Applied Science Publishers Ltd.
Crown House, Linton Road, Barking, Essex IG11 8JU, England

Library of Congress Cataloging-in-Publication Data

Sell, Stewart, 1935–
  Immunology, immunopathology, and immunity.

  Includes bibliographies and index.
  1. Immunology. 2. Immunopathology 3. Immunity.
I. Title. [DNLM: 1. Immunity 2. Immunologic Diseases.
QW 504 S465i]
QR181.S39 1987   616.07′9   86-29336
ISBN 0-444-01137-4

Current printing (last digit)
10 9 8 7 6 5 4 3 2 1

Manufactured in the United States of America

To the late Edward S. Smuckler, M.D., Ph.D.
A friend
A colleague
A mensch
We will miss your wisdom, enthusiasm, and humor!

Contents

vii

Preface

In the seven years since the third edition of *Immunology, Immunopathology, and Immunity* there has been exponential growth of the understanding of basic immunology as well as appreciation of the inflammatory mechanisms activated by immune reactions that lead to tissue damage and disease. This has required a complete revision of every chapter of this book as well as addition of several new chapters. Emphasis has been placed on aspects of immunology that are related to the relationship of humans to their environment and, in particular, to the contribution of immune mechanisms to human disease.

The book is divided into three parts, Immunology, Immunopathology, and Immunity. Part 1, Immunology, covers the fundamentals of basic immunology that are needed to begin the study of the role of immunology in human physiology and disease; it includes sufficient information to be meaningful for the student of the health sciences, without the details required of working scientists in molecular biology or immunobiology. The second section, Immunopathology, thoroughly describes the immunopathologic mechanisms that cause tissue lesions that lead to human disease as well as the manifestations of these lesions, without the clinical detail required of a diagnostician or therapist. The third section deals with the immunologic mechanisms that protect us against infectious disease and cancer, as well as what happens when the immune system doesn't work (immune deficiency diseases) or goes out of control (lymphoproliferative diseases).

I would like to thank the many reviewers who have made critical suggestions for improvement of this text:

Frank Arnett
Ira Berkower
Nicholas Cohen
Stanley Cohen

xv

Joseph C. Fantone
Agnes B. Kane
Paul M. Knopf
D. Scott Linthicum
Scott Rodkey
Noel R. Rose
Thomas G. Wegmann

Also a very special thanks to Ann Rose for interpreting my handwriting and typing the manuscript.

Preface to First Edition

Frequently I have been asked by medical and biology students to recommend a text that covers both basic immunology and immunopathology. At best, I could recommend a basic text for immunology and individual chapters in several books for immunopathology—admitting that still, certain fundamental areas would remain uncovered. I could not identify a single text that encompasses the material that I thought important in a manner palatable to a beginner in the field.

In general, medical or pathology texts present immune reactions according to individual diseases or organ systems: they therefore lack a coherent mechanistic organization. Other texts, usually multiauthored, provide excellent reference sources but are too large and detailed and lack the organization necessary to be of general use for students unfamiliar with immunologic principles. My goal in writing this book is to give an organized, concise, yet meaningful presentation of immunology, immunopathology, and immunity, stressing their interrelationships. This book is intended for biology and medical students, house officers, and faculty who wish an introduction to the role played by immune mechanisms in disease.

In order to present both the protective and destructive mechanisms of the mammalian immune system, the text is divided into three parts: Immunology, Immunopathology, and Immunity. The first part, Immunology, presents the basic principles of the induction and expression of specific immune reactions. Aspects of immunology important for the understanding of immunopathologic mechanisms are emphasized. This provides an introduction for the second and major part of the book, Immunopathology. In this section, I have organized the fundamentals of how immune reactions cause tissue damage and disease in order to stress a classification based on immune mechanisms. The last part, Immunity, covers the role of immune reactions in protecting against infection and cancer. Detailed coverage is provided in areas of current interest, such as tissue transplantation and tumor immunity; the more classical topics receive a simplified treatment.

xvii

PART 1
IMMUNOLOGY

1 | Introduction to Immunology

The human organism, from the time of conception, must maintain its integrity in the face of a changing and often threatening environment. Our bodies have many physiological mechanisms that permit us to adjust to basic variables such as temperature, supply of food and water, and physical injury. In addition, we must defend ourselves against invasion and colonization by foreign organisms. This defensive ability is called *immunity*.

Immunity

Immunity comes from the Latin word *immunitas* and means "protection from." In legal terms, immunity means that an immune person is not subject to certain laws (e.g., diplomatic immunity) or is exempt from certain duties (e.g., not required to serve in the armed forces). In medical terms immunity means protection from certain diseases, particularly infectious disease. For instance, the commonly used statement "She is immune to measles" implies that the person indicated has had measles once and will not get measles again. Immunology (*-ology*, study of) is the study of immunity.

The protective mechanisms of the body may be divided into two major groups: innate and adaptive (Table 1-1). Innate

Table 1-1. Comparison of Innate and Adaptive Immunity

Characteristic	Innate Resistance	Adaptive Resistance
Specificity	Nonspecific, indiscriminate	Specific, discriminating
Mechanical	Epithelium	Immune induced reactive fibrosis (granuloma)
Humoral	pH, lysozyme, serum proteins	Antibody
Cellular	White blood cells	Specifically sensitized lymphocytes
Induction	Does not require immunization; constitutive	Requires immunization

3

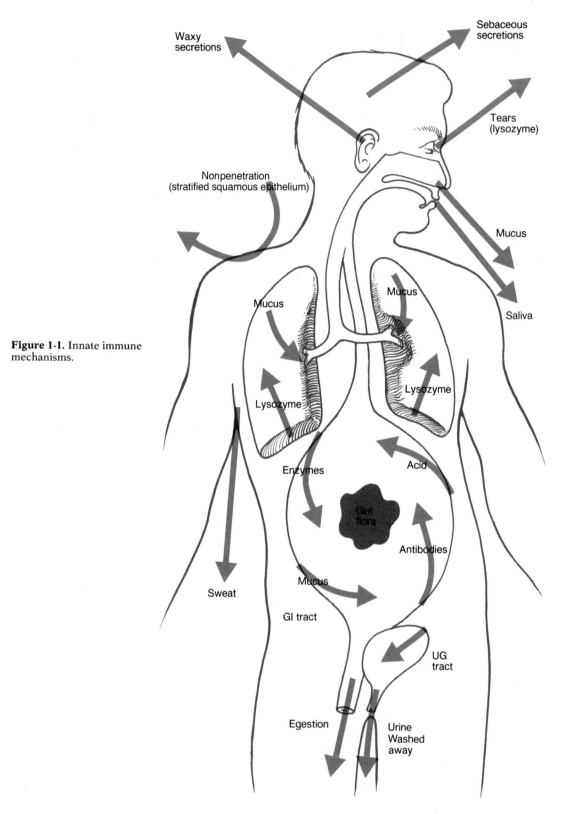

Figure 1-1. Innate immune
mechanisms.

resistance is present in all normal individuals and operates on different infectious agents in the same way every time the individual is exposed to the agent. The adaptive, specific immune defense system is not actively present in all individuals. It requires stimulation or *immunization* to become activated, and is mediated by products that specifically recognize one organism and do not act on other organisms. In an infectious disease, such as measles, the adaptive immune system is activated during the first infection, so that upon subsequent contact with the same infectious agent no disease will occur. The immune system has learned to recognize the agent previously contacted and react specifically to it with an accelerated response. This is termed *immune memory*.

Innate Resistance

Innate defense mechanisms against foreign invaders include mechanical barriers, secreted products, and inflammatory cells (Fig. 1-1). Innate resistance is present at all times in normal individuals, modulated by physiological conditions (nutrition, age, hormones, etc.); does not distinguish among microorganisms of different species; and does not alter in intensity upon reexposure. One of the major nonspecific defense systems is the epithelial surface of the body. Externally the skin, and internally the mucous membrane linings of the gastrointestinal tract and the epithelium of the airways of the lung, provide mechanical barriers to invasion. Secreted products such as acid in the stomach, lysozyme in tears, sebaceous gland secretions, and certain proteins in the blood are toxic to potential invaders. White cells of the blood (macrophages and polymorphonuclear leukocytes) are attracted to sites of infection by products of infecting organisms or necrotic tissue and attack the invaders.

The protective epithelial barriers are frequently breached (as by a cut or abrasion of the skin or by penetration of invading organisms past the protective lining of the airways in the lung). Once organisms get through the innate defensive mechanisms and begin to grow in the tissues of the body, a more specific and more powerful backup defense system is needed. Since most infectious organisms can multiply rapidly and the defensive mechanisms in tissues must be directed specifically to the infection and not host tissue, this system must be activated quickly, be effective against relatively large numbers of organisms, and be able to react specifically with the infectious agent. This backup is provided by the adaptive immune system.

Adaptive Resistance

The adaptive immune system is quiescent until stimulated by a specific infection (*immunizing event*); it is capable of exquisitely distinguishing among microorganisms and significantly alters in its intensity and response time upon reexposure. Thus, in normal individuals, the adaptive immune system contains the potential to be activated. This potential is converted to actuality by one of two major arms of the immune response: specific antibodies (*humoral immunity*) or specifically sensitized white blood cells (*cellular immunity*). The cells responsible for antibody production are in the B lymphocyte series, those for cellular immunity in the T lymphocyte series (Table 1-2). Antibodies

Table 1-2. Two Major Arms of Immunity

	Humoral	Cellular
Cell line	B cells, plasma cells	T cells
Product	Antibody	Sensitized cells
Protection against	Bacteria	Viruses, mycobacteria, fungi

are protein molecules that react specifically with structures (*antigens*) on infecting organisms through specialized receptors (*binding sites*) on the antibody molecule. Specifically sensitized T cells also have an antibody-like receptor that recognizes antigens. Antibodies belong to a family of molecules found in the blood or external secretions, termed *immunoglobulins.* Antibodies and sensitized cells are made in response to specific stimulation after contact with an immunizing agent (*immunogen*). They are manufactured by specialized organs in the body (the *lymphoid system*) and released into the blood, which allows rapid delivery to other parts of the body.

Immunization (or vaccination) is the process of stimulating adaptive resistance; once induced, a discrete *state of immunity* exists. The response of the immune system to immunization has been compared to a motor neuron reflex arc, in that it has an afferent, an efferent, and a central limb (Fig. 1-2). *Afferent* refers to delivery of the immunogen to cells of the

Figure 1-2. Afferent, central, and efferent limbs of the immune response. Afferent: delivery of immunogen to lymphoid organ (lymph node). Central: recognition of antigen by cells of the immune system and production of specifically sensitized cells and humoral antibody. Efferent: delivery of immune products to site of antigen localization and activation of immune effector mechanisms.

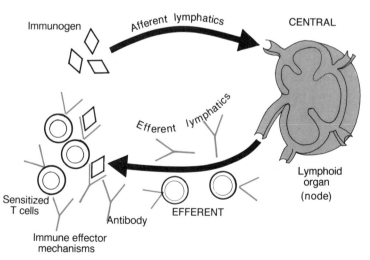

immune system; *central* to the response of the reacting organs, resulting in production of antibody and sensitized cells; *efferent* to the delivery of these products to the site of antigen deposition and activation of immune defense mechanisms. Once immunization has occurred, the immunized individual will respond with a more rapid and more intense response upon second exposure to the same immunogen.

The infectious invaders of our bodies have many ways of evading both the innate and the adaptive resistance. These include such properties as the release of *toxins*, the formation of protective coatings, the ability to localize in inaccessible sites, and the ability to exist within our own cells or even be incorporated into our DNA and thus evade recognition or destruction (see Chapter 24). Important properties for the effectiveness of the adaptive immune system are listed in Table 1-3.

Table 1-3. Functional Abilities of the Adaptive Immune System

1. *Recognition* of many different foreign invaders specifically
2. *Rapid synthesis* of immune products upon contact with invaders
3. *Delivery* of the immune products quickly to the site of infection
4. *Diversity* of effector defensive mechanisms to combat infectious agents with different properties
5. *Direction* of the defensive mechanisms specifically to foreign invaders rather than one's own tissue
6. *Deactivation* mechanisms to turn off the system when the invader has been cleared

Inflammatory Response

The response of our bodies to an infection occurs in the form of *inflammation*. The hallmark of an inflammatory response is the passage of proteins, fluid, and cells from the blood into focal areas in tissues. The result is the local delivery of agents that can effectively combat infections. During an inflammatory response, components of the innate and adaptive resistance mechanisms are shared. These include *inflammatory cells*, products of inflammatory cells, certain blood proteins *(inflammatory mediators)*, and common pathways of response (see Chapter 12).

Initiation of an inflammatory response begins with increasing blood flow to infected tissues and with the opening of the cells lining the blood vessels or capillaries (Fig. 1-3). This allows fluid and/or cells to enter into the tissues. The manifestations of acute inflammation were first clearly described by Celsus about 25 BC. The cardinal signs of inflammation (Table 1-4) are manifestations of the increased blood flow and infiltration of tissues by inflammatory proteins and cells. Increased blood flow causes redness and increased temperature. The presence of fluid and red blood cells in tissues is grossly recognized by swelling (edema) and redness. White blood cell (inflammatory cell) infiltrations cause a white color. If the site of

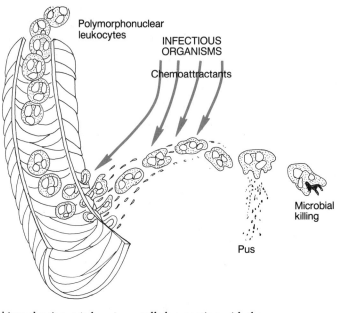

Figure 1-3. Acute inflammatory response to infection. Infectious organisms release chemicals or initiate tissue damage, which produces substances that are chemotactic toward (attract) inflammatory cells (polymorphonuclear leukocytes) and cause constriction of vascular endothelial cells. This results in release of fluid into the tissue (edema) and/or infiltration of tissue with inflammatory cells. Polymorphonuclear leukocytes may ingest and kill the infecting organisms or may release proteolytic enzymes into tissue, causing necrosis and formation of pus. Antibody serves to enhance this response and direct the inflammatory cells by reacting with the infecting organisms and activating bloodborne inflammatory mediators brought into the tissue during edema formation. These mediators react with cell surface receptors on the inflammatory cells and enhance the ability of the cells to ingest (phagocytose) the organisms.

inflammation is necrotic and filled with white cells, the inflammatory site will be seen as pus. If red blood cells are present, the pus may be yellow or bloody red depending on the proportion of red cells. The cellular evolution of an inflammatory response eventually results in the healing or scarring of the lesion. The inflammatory process is presented in detail in Chapter 12.

Table 1-4. The Four Cardinal Signs of Acute Inflammation: Celsus (25 BC)[a]

Rubor	Redness
Tumor	Swelling
Calor	Heat
Dolor	Pain

[a] The fifth classic sign of acute inflammation, *functio laesa* (loss of function), was added by Virchow (1821–1902).

Evolution of Immunity (Phylogeny)

Adaptation to the environment is the driving force in the evolution and survival of a species. Organisms must not only accommodate to changes in temperature, pH, nutrients, oxygen, and water, but also be able to defend against potentially fatal effects of other organisms. The most primitive defense system is the ability to recognize that something is foreign (nonself). This capacity may have evolved from the primitive alimentation function of phagocytosis, the ingestion of material by a cell. That is, protozoa are able to recognize other protozoa as different because of different enzymes in different species and can defend themselves by phagocytosis. In this process they are able to differentiate foreign from self (same species).

Invertebrate

A simplified phylogenetic tree as related to evolution of immune functions in invertebrates is presented in Figure 1-4. The ability to identify foreign species and strains is present in each species. Specific immunoglobulin antibody and T and B cell lymphocyte differentiation are not seen in invertebrates. The ability to recognize tissue of different species (histocompatibility differences) clearly exists in sponges. Identical pairs will fuse when mixed, whereas foreign pairs show a cytotoxic (necrotic) rejection response at their interface. The strength of rejection depends on the degree of genetic difference. A more rapid and extensive rejection occurs when two allogenic (different) species are put together a second time (secondary response or immune memory). In higher organisms this phenomenon is tested by whether or not an individual will accept a graft of tissue from another individual (graft rejection implies recognition of foreign tissue). In coral the extent of parabiotic incompatibility suggests that each clone of coral is different. This principle of the uniqueness of the individual also applies to humans (see Chapter 9).

White blood cell differentiation appears first in echinoderms and protochordates (for a description of white blood cells, see Chapter 2). In the coelomic cavity of earthworms are primitive white blood cell types that combine features of polymorphonuclear cells and lymphocytes. These cells appear to be responsible for graft rejection in these species, and some appear to respond to mitogen stimulation. Protochordates contain nodules of lymphatic cells and circulating lymphocytes that respond to stimulation. Lymphocyte-like cells also infiltrate grafts of sea urchins. Humoral factors also appear in earthworms, and hemolysins (which cause lysis of red blood cells) and hemagglutinins (which cause agglutination of red blood cells) are found in starfish and shellfish. However, these are not immunoglobulins and are not antigen specific. Tunicates express both cellular and humoral immune factors, including some differentiation of lymphocytes. Immune

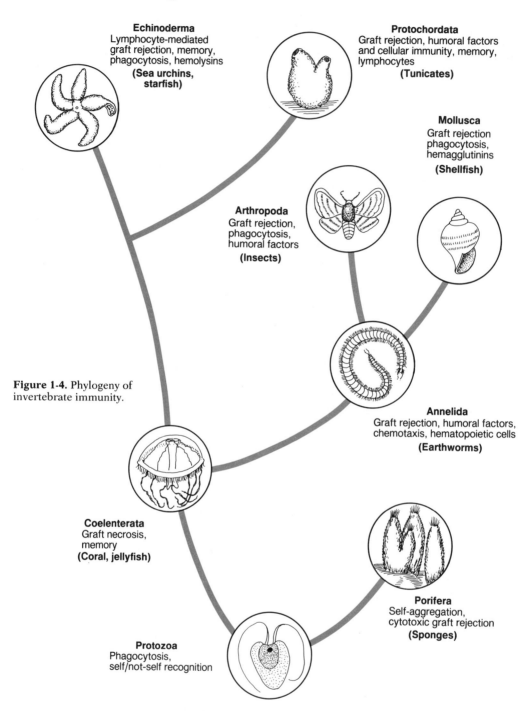

Echinoderma
Lymphocyte-mediated
graft rejection, memory,
phagocytosis, hemolysins
**(Sea urchins,
starfish)**

Protochordata
Graft rejection, humoral factors
and cellular immunity, memory,
lymphocytes
(Tunicates)

Mollusca
Graft rejection
phagocytosis,
hemagglutinins
(Shellfish)

Arthropoda
Graft rejection,
phagocytosis,
humoral factors
(Insects)

Annelida
Graft rejection, humoral factors,
chemotaxis, hematopoietic cells
(Earthworms)

Figure 1-4. Phylogeny of
invertebrate immunity.

Coelenterata
Graft necrosis,
memory
(Coral, jellyfish)

Porifera
Self-aggregation,
cytotoxic graft rejection
(Sponges)

Protozoa
Phagocytosis,
self/not-self recognition

memory, expressed as a shorter time to induce necrosis in
grafts of different strains upon second exposure, is seen in
coral. Cellular immune responses appear to precede the development of humoral responses during evolution.

Vertebrate

The phylogeny of immunity in vertebrates is illustrated in Figure 1-5. The immune system in vertebrates is characterized by a true two-component (T and B cell) system, specific immuno-

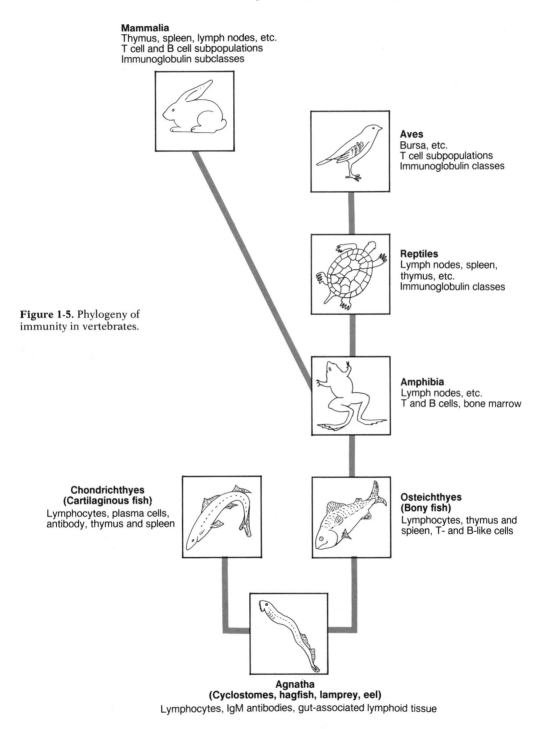

Mammalia
Thymus, spleen, lymph nodes, etc.
T cell and B cell subpopulations
Immunoglobulin subclasses

Aves
Bursa, etc.
T cell subpopulations
Immunoglobulin classes

Reptiles
Lymph nodes, spleen,
thymus, etc.
Immunoglobulin classes

Figure 1-5. Phylogeny of
immunity in vertebrates.

Amphibia
Lymph nodes, etc.
T and B cells, bone marrow

**Chondrichthyes
(Cartilaginous fish)**
Lymphocytes, plasma cells,
antibody, thymus and spleen

**Osteichthyes
(Bony fish)**
Lymphocytes, thymus and
spleen, T- and B-like cells

**Agnatha
(Cyclostomes, hagfish, lamprey, eel)**
Lymphocytes, IgM antibodies, gut-associated lymphoid tissue

globulin antibody production, highly developed specific cellular immunity, and specific immune memory. T- and B-like cells exist in teleost fishes but are not clearly defined in agnatha, although a primitive T cell response can be demonstrated. Table 1-5 outlines the evolution of lymphoid organs in vertebrates (for a description of lymphoid organs see Chapter 3).

Table 1-5. Phylogeny of the Immune System from Primitive Fishes to Mammals

Class or Group	Thymus	Bone Marrow	Lymph Glands or Nodes	Blood Granulocytes and Lymphocytes	Reactions to Primary Tissue Allografts (Cell-Mediated Immunity[a])	
					Moderate	Strong
Hagfish and lampreys	0	0	0	+	+	0
Sharks and rays	+	0	0	+	+	0
Bony fishes	+	+	0	+	+	+
Amphibians	+	+	+	+	+	+
Reptiles	+	+	+	+	+	0
Birds	+	+	+	+	+	+
Mammals	+	+	+	+	+	+

+ indicates presence of corresponding types of cells or reactivity.

[a] Moderate histocompatibility barriers are found in animals representing all vertebrate classes, but strong barriers are the rule in advanced bony fishes, anuran amphibians, and most birds and mammals.

From Hildemann WH: "Immunophylogeny," in Hildemann WH (ed): *Frontiers in Immunogenetics*, Elsevier, 1981.

Agnatha demonstrate diffuse lymphoid tissue in the gut but do not have other lymphoid organs. Thymus and spleen appear in fishes, and lymph nodes in amphibians.

Clearly defined T and B cells are first seen in amphibians, where thymectomy results in loss of cellular responses such as graft rejection, and T and B cell responses can be demonstrated. Reptiles have demonstrable T regulatory cells, cells with surface immunoglobulin, and lymphoid organs that resemble those of mammals. Most amphibians do not have graft rejection, but some have graft rejection reactions that are slow and chronic compared with those of reptiles, birds, and mammals. The evolutionary trend from slow to fast graft rejection may reflect expression of histocompatibility antigens rather than a weakness in the immune reaction.

Epithelium and Lymphoid Organ Evolution

Associations of epithelial tissue and lymphoid tissue in some lymphoid organs appear to be of critical importance in the development of the mammalian immune system. In order to make survival on land possible, changes in the gill pouches and cloacal bursa of amphibians had to evolve in birds and mammals. In primitive coelenterates the coelomic cavity serves not only to absorb nutrients, but also to absorb oxygen. To perform this function, gills evolved in the neck (foregut) of fishes and the hindgut of mollusks and arthropods. During embryogenesis of higher vertebrates the five paired gill pouches cease absorbing oxygen and develop to supply epithelium for cervical organs. The five gill pouches in fish become vestigial in amphibia, but the epithelial tissue of the third pharyngeal pouch provides the stroma of the medulla of the thymus. This epithelial stroma produces thymic hormones essential for the maturation of thymocytes (see Chapter 3). The hindgut gills evolve into the cloaca in turtles and further into the cloacal bursa of Fabricius in birds. The bursa of Fabricius is essential for the development of the B cell system in birds. In mammalia, there is evidence that the gastrointestinal associated lymphoid tissue (GALT) plays an important role in the development of the B cell system.

In Summary

1. Some form of recognition of self and nonself is present in the simplest animal species.
2. Cellular immunity precedes humoral immunity in evolution.
3. A bifunctional (T and B cell) system with developed lymphoid organs is the most recent immunological development.
4. Epithelium that evolves from the gills of fishes (i.e., pharyngeal pouches) plays a major role in the development of the lymphoid organs of mammals (thymus and GALT).

Selective pressures during evolution are believed to have resulted in the development of protective immune mechanisms. Primitive immune mechanisms may have had a number of other functions in lower organisms, such as recognition of cell surface markers required for aggregation of cell types in the early stages of development of multicellular structures (recognition of self and nonself). Immune recognition mechanisms may be variants of the cell–cell interactions that occur during embryologic development. It is likely that the immune system, as we now see it, is expanding and being modified to perform even other new functions such as regulation of neuroendocrine or hormonally expressive cells.

Immunopathology, the Double-Edged Sword

The evolution of the immune system did not occur without flaws. This same system that functions so well to protect against foreign invaders may also be turned against us. The term *immunopathology* incorporates a double meaning: *immune* means protected or exempt; *pathology* is the study of disease. Thus immunopathology literally means the study of the protection from disease, but in usage it actually means the study of how immune mechanisms cause diseases. Immunity is a double-edged sword: on the one hand immune responses protect us from infections; on the other hand, immune mechanisms may cause disease. The most compelling evidence that immune reactions are protective is provided by the naturally occurring immune deficiency diseases of man. Individuals with an inability to mount an effective immune response to infectious agents invariably succumb to infections unless vigorously treated. However, immune reactions may also cause disease. The terms *allergy* and *hypersensitivity* are used to denote deleterious immune reactions. *Allergy* is frequently used for a particular type of reaction *(anaphylactic)*, and *hypersensitivity* for delayed or cell-mediated immune reactivity. The term *immunity* was once restricted to the protective effects of immune reactions but, by common usage, this is no longer the case. In some diseases immune mechanisms may actually be directed against our own tissues. This is termed *autoimmunity*.

History of Immunology and Immunopathology

A short history of immunopathology is given in Table 1-6. Recognition of adaptive immunity occurred in the ancient societies of China and Egypt. Application of this phenomenon by introduction of smallpox organisms into lesions scratched on the skin — "variolation" — or by their inhalation into the nasal cavity was practiced by the Chinese about AD 1000, and artificial vaccination was introduced in England in 1798. In the late 1800s and early 1900s many immune-mediated phenomena were described. The cellular immune system was emphasized by Metchnikoff and the humoral system by von Behring. Modern immunology can be said to have begun in the late 1950s with the recognition of histocompatibility antigens, identification of the structure of antibodies, and study of immune mechanisms that cause disease. Today studies in immunology are revealing the nature of the different cell types involved in immune responses, how cellular receptors are made, how immune cells are activated, and the nature and expression of the genetic information required for specific immune recognition.

Summary

Higher organisms have evolved effective defense systems to protect themselves against foreign invaders. One system is constitutive and consists of mechanical barriers, pH, temperature, phagocytosis, and nonspecific inflammation (innate resistance). The other is induced and consists of specific products that recognize invaders as foreign (adaptive immunity). After induction (immunization) the adaptive system responds more rapidly and with greater intensity than after first exposure (immune memory). The two major arms of the adaptive immune response are humoral (antibody) and cellular (specifically sensitized cells). Cells of the body known as lymphocytes are responsible for the adaptive immune response (T lymphocytes for cellular immunity and B lymphocytes for humoral immunity). In response to infection both adaptive and innate inflammatory mechanisms may be activated.

During evolution the adaptive immune response has become increasingly complex. Humans have different classes of antibody and different subsets of T cells that have different functions as immune effectors.

Table 1-6. A Short History of Immunopathology

Fever	Mesopotamia	3000 BC
Recognition of adaptive immunity	Egypt, China	2000 BC
Anatomic identification of organs	Hippocrates	400 BC
Acquired resistance to poisons	Mithridates Eupator, King of Pontus	80 BC
Four cardinal signs of inflammation	Celsus	AD 25
"Snuff" variolation for smallpox	Sung Dynasty, China	1000
Renaissance of anatomy	Vesalius	1540
Bursa of birds described	Fabricius	1590
Peyer's patch	Peyer	1690
Cowpox vaccination	Jenner	1798
Tuberculous granulomas	Rokitansky	1855
Langhans' giant cell	Langhans	1868
Waldeyer's ring	Waldeyer	1870
Cellular pathology	Virchow	1880
Attenuated vaccines	Pasteur	1880
Phagocytosis	Metchnikoff	1882
Neutralization (antitoxin)	von Behring	1890
Delayed hypersensitivity skin test	Koch	1890
Bacteriolysis (antibody and complement)	Bordet	1894
Blood groups	Landsteiner	1900
Side-chain theory, tumor immunity, horror autotoxicus	Ehrlich	1900
Anaphylaxis	Richet and Portier	1902
Arthus' phenomenon	Arthus	1903
Serum sickness	von Pirquet and Schick	1905
Organ transplantation	Carrel and Guthrie	1905
Delayed hypersensitivity to viruses	von Pirquet	1906
Immune surveillance of cancer	Ehrlich	1909
Viral cancer immunity	Peyton Rous	1910
Passive cutaneous anaphylaxis	Prausnitz and Kustner	1921
Chemical mediators of inflammation	Lewis	1925
Quantitative precipitin reaction	Heidelberger	1935
Gamma globulin	Tiselius and Kabat	1938
Hemolytic disease of newborn (Rh)	Levine	1941
Immunofluorescence	Coons	1942
Concept of collagen disease	Klemperer	1942
Immune tolerance	Medawar and Burnet	1944
Mechanism of glomerulonephritis	Dixon	1956
Histocompatibility antigens	Snell, Dausset	1958
Structure of antibodies	Porter, Edelman	1959
Lymphocyte recirculation	Gowans	1959
Mitogenic activation of lymphocytes	Nowell	1961
Function of the thymus	Miller and Good	1961
Classification of immune mechanisms	Gell and Coombs	1962
Lymphocyte surface immunoglobulin and lymphocyte activation	Sell and Gell	1964
Immunoglobulin gene rearrangements	Dreyer and Bennet	1965
Identification of T and B cells	Claman	1966
In vitro primary immune response	Mischell and Dutton	1967
Accessory cell role in immune response	Mosier	1968
Immune response genes	Benacerraf and McDevitt	1969
Idiotype network	Jerne	1974
Hybridoma (monoclonal antibodies)	Kohler and Milstein	1975
T cell receptor	Allison, Kappler, et al	1982
T cell receptor gene	Hedrick, Davis	1984

The immune response is not always protective; in many instances the same immune effector mechanisms that defend against foreign invaders may be turned against us and produce disease (the double-edged sword of immunopathology). In the following chapters the immune response is described (Part 1, Immunology), the destructive effects of immune mechanisms are presented (Part 2, Immunopathology), and the role of immune mechanisms in defense is analyzed (Part 3, Immunity).

General References

Periodicals

Advances in Immunology, Academic Press, New York.

Annual Review of Immunology, Annual Reviews Inc., Palo Alto, Calif.

Comprehensive Immunology, Plenum, New York.

Progress in Allergy, Karger, Basel, Switzerland.

Immunological Reviews, Munksgard, Copenhagen.

Immunology Today, Elsevier, Amsterdam.

Basic Immunology Texts

Barrett JT: Textbook of Immunology, 4th ed. St. Louis, Mosby, 1983.

Dale MM, Foreman JC: Textbook of Immunopharmacology. London, Blackwell, 1984.

Eisen H: Immunology, 2nd ed. Hagerstown, Md., Harper & Row, 1980.

Golub ES: The Cellular Basis of the Immune Response, 2nd ed. Sunderland, Mass., Sinauer Assocs., 1981.

Hildemann WH: Fundamentals of Immunology. New York, Elsevier, 1984.

Hood L, Weissman IL, Wood WB, Wilson JH: Immunology, 2nd ed. Menlo Park, Calif., Benjamin Cummings, 1984.

Humphrey SH, White RG: Immunology for Students of Medicine, 3rd ed. Oxford, Blackwell, 1970.

McConnel I, Munro A, Waldemann H: The Immune System, 2nd ed. Oxford, Blackwell, 1981.

Roitt I: Essential Immunology, 5th ed. Oxford, Blackwell, 1984.

Stites DP, Stobo JD, Fudenberg HH, Wells JV: Basic and Clinical Immunology, 5th ed. Los Altos, Calif., Lange, 1985.

Clinical Immunology Texts

Holborow EJ, Reeves WG: Immunology in Medicine. London, Academic Press, 1977.

Lachmann PJ, Peters DK: Clinical Aspects of Immunology, 4th ed. Oxford, Blackwell, 1982.

Miescher PA, Muller-Eberhard HJ: Textbook of Immunopathology, 2nd ed. New York, Grune & Stratton, 1976.

Sampter M: Immunological Diseases, 2nd ed. Boston, Little, Brown, 1965.

Historical

Haggard HW: Mystery, Magic and Medicine. Garden City, N.Y., Doubleday, Doran and Co., 1933.

Kabat EA: Structural Concepts in Immunology and Immunochemistry. New York, Holt, Rinehart & Winston, 1968.

Landsteiner K: The Specificity of Serological Reactions. New York, Dover, 1962.

Long ER: A History of Pathology. New York, Dover, 1965.

Majno G: The Healing Hand. Cambridge, Mass., Harvard University Press, 1975.

Silverstein AM: History of immunology: a history of theories of antibody formation. Cell Immunol 91:263–283, 1985.

Phylogeny of Immunity

Cohen N: Phylogeny of lymphocyte structure and function. Am Zool 15:119–133, 1975.

Goetz D (ed): Evolution and function of the major histocompatibility system. Berlin, Springer-Verlag, 1977.

Hildemann WH (ed): Frontiers in Immunogenetics. New York, Elsevier, 1981.

Hildemann WH, Clark EA, Raison RL: Comprehensive Immunogenetics. New York, Elsevier, 1981.

2 | The Immune System I: Cells and Vessels

The organs of our bodies that provide the products (proteins and cells) of immunity make up the *lymphoid system*. The lymphoid system is a complex network of lymphatic vessels, lymphoid nodules, lymph nodes, tonsils, spleen, and other organs (Fig. 2-1). The cells and vessels of the lymphoid system are described in this chapter; the lymphoid organs and their development are the subjects of Chapters 3 and 4.

Cells of the Immune System

The major constituents of the immune system are lymphocytes. However, other cells (macrophages) are also involved in induction of immune responses, and other white blood cell types such as macrophages and polymorphonuclear leukocytes take an active part in various parts of inflammatory responses associated with immune reactions (Fig. 2-1). The term *white blood cell (leukocyte)* is applied because when unclotted blood is allowed to stand, these cells sediment in a thin, white layer between the denser erythrocytes (red blood cells) and the plasma. This layer of white cells is called the *buffy coat*. The mature forms of these cells are most easily recognized in peripheral blood smears. The basic structure and function of white blood cells are now described; their role in immune responses and inflammation is presented in more detail in the following chapters.

Blood Cells

In smears of peripheral blood stained with Wright's stain, *erythrocytes* are small and light pink and have no nuclei. Because erythrocytes are by far the most numerous cells in blood smears, it is the percentage of nonerythroid cells (white blood cells) that is normally counted.

White Blood Cells (Leukocytes)

The terms used by pathologists, immunologists, and hematologists for the different white blood cells reflect different ways of looking at complex cell populations. A simple classification is presented in Figure 2-2.

19

Cell Type	% of White Blood Cells in Blood	Diameter (μm)	Nucleus	Cytoplasm and Granules	Drawings
Erythrocytes	—	7.5	None	Pink, homogeneous cytoplasm	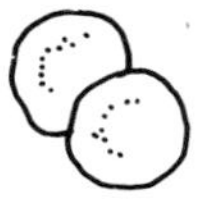
LEUKOCYTES Polymorphonuclear Neutrophils	50–70	10–12	2–5 lobules connected by thin bridges, coarse chromatin	Abundant cytoplasm/ fine pinkish granules	
Eosinophils	1–3	10–12	Usually two oval lobes connected by bridge	Abundant cytoplasm/ coarse reflective granules stained red	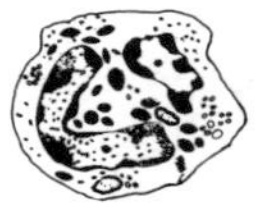
Basophils	<1	8–10	Bent in S with two or more constrictions; obscured by cytoplasmic granules	Large and irregular granules stained deep blue	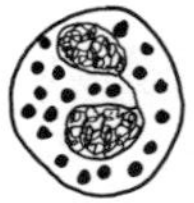
Mononuclear Lymphocytes	25–35	6–15	Round to oval; coarse chromatin	Bluish cytoplasm/ about 10% of cells fine azurophilic granules	
Monocytes	3–7	12–18	Kidney shaped, indented; fine chromatin	Bluish cytoplasm/ fine azurophilic granules	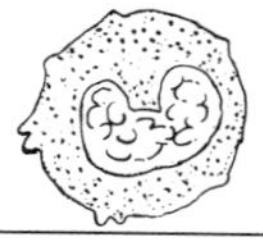

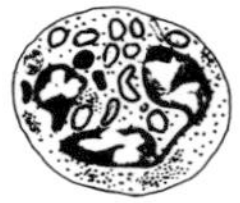

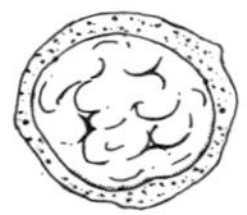

Figure 2-1. Leukocytes. Composite drawing indicating relative size (micrometers) and morphology of cells involved in immune reactions and in nonimmune inflammatory reactions. The erythrocyte is included for size reference, since it is the most easily identifed cell in blood smears and in many tissue sections. The drawings illustrate the characteristic appearance of cells in a peripheral blood smear stained with Wright's stain.

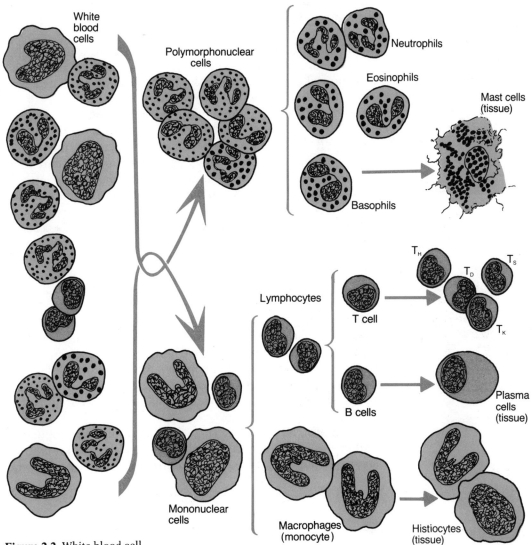

Figure 2-2. White blood cell nomenclature.

White blood cells (WBC) may be divided into two major populations on the basis of the form of their nuclei: single nuclei (*mononuclear* or *"round" cells*) or segmented nuclei (*polymorphonuclear*). Mononuclear cells are further divided into large (*macrophage* or *monocyte*) and small (*lymphocyte*). Lymphocytes may be further subdivided into two major populations, *T cells* and *B cells*, on the basis of function and cell surface phenotype (to be described later). B cells are the precursors of the cells that synthesize and secrete humoral antibodies. Subpopulations of T cells are responsible for a number of *cell-mediated* immune activities (see below). T cells and B cells cannot be differentiated on the basis of morphologic appearance, but do have different phenotypic markers. In addition, lymphocytes without distinguishing markers *(null cells)* are present in smaller numbers than T cells or B cells. Some null cells may *kill* certain other cell types in vitro (natural killer (NK) cells), and others may become "armed" by passive absorption of antibody (antibody-dependent cell-mediated cytotoxicity; killer (K) cells). The characteristics of these cells are presented in much more detail in a later chapter.

The large mononuclear cells (macrophages) are phagocytic cells. Macrophages in peripheral blood are termed *monocytes;* in tissues they are called *histiocytes*. Particular care must be taken in understanding *monocytes* and *mononuclear cells*. Hematologists use the term *monocytes* for the larger circulating mononuclear white blood cells found in the peripheral blood that are in the macrophage lineage. Pathologists use the term *mononuclear* or *"round" cells* for lymphocytes and macrophages seen in tissue, to differentiate them from polymorphonuclear cells. These similar terms must be carefully distinguished to avoid confusion.

Polymorphonuclear Leukocytes

Polymorphonuclear white blood cells are subdivided into three major populations on the basis of the staining properties of their cytoplasmic granules in standard hematologic blood smears or tissue preparations: neutrophil—pink, eosinophil—red, basophil—blue. Polymorphonuclear cells take part in both immune specific and nonspecific inflammatory reactions.

Neutrophils. Neutrophils (Fig. 2-3) are polymorphonuclear leukocytes (PMN) whose cytoplasmic granules do not take on strong acidophilic (red) or basophilic (blue) staining with the

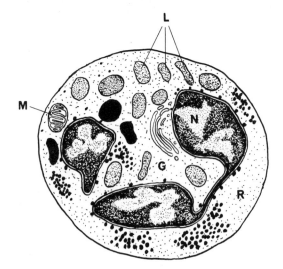

Figure 2-3. Neutrophil. The cytoplasm contains large numbers of membrane-limited bodies (lysosomes) that stain pale pink with the usual staining agents. The nucleus is divided into round or oval lobes connected to one another by thin strands of nuclear material. G, Golgi apparatus; L, lysosomes; M, mitochondrion; N, nucleus; R, ribosomes.

usual dyes used for blood smears, but show only a pale pink coloration. Such cells make up from 50 to 90% of the WBC of the peripheral blood and may be found scattered diffusely in many tissues. Like its relative, the macrophage ("large eater"), the neutrophil is active in phagocytosis and has been named by some a microphage ("small eater"). Neutrophils are rapidly migrating, phagocytic cells that appear in areas of infection or tissue damage. The nucleus of the neutrophil, characteristic of the polymorphonuclear leukocytes, is divided into round or oval lobes connected to one another by thin strands of nuclear material. The other outstanding feature of this type of WBC is the large number of uniform, membrane-limited granules. The granules of the neutrophil contain a wide variety of hydrolytic enzymes and are called primary lysosomes. These enzymes digest phagocytosed organisms. Neutrophils are the first wave of a cellular attack on invading organisms and are the characteristic cells of acute inflammation. The appearance of neutrophils in areas of inflammation may be caused by chemicals released from bacteria or factors produced nonspecifically from necrotic tissue, or may be directed by antibody reacting with antigen. The role of the neutrophil in acute inflammation is taken over by the macrophage in the chronic stage of inflammation (Chapter 12).

Eosinophils. Eosinophils (Fig. 2-4) are similar in appearance to neutrophils, except that they have prominent eosinophilic (red) granules that may contain rodlike crystalloid inclusions as viewed by electron microscopy. These eosinophilic granules are membrane limited and contain large amounts of hydrolytic enzymes, and thus are lysosomes. The granules differ from those of neutrophils in a high content of peroxidase, which is perhaps related to the crystalloid structure. The chemotactic

Figure 2-4. Eosinophil. Morphologically the cell resembles the neutrophil, but prominent cytoplasmic membrane-limited bodies (lysosomes) stain red with the usual staining agents and contain rodlike crystalloid structures as observed by electron microscopy. L, lysosomes; M, mitochondria; N, nucleus; R, ribosomes.

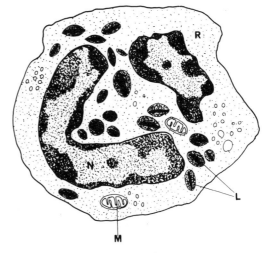

responses of the eosinophil are basically identical to those of neutrophils, but eosinophils are found in unusually high numbers around antigen–antibody complexes and parasites in tissues. Eosinophils appear to limit or modulate inflammation. Eosinophils make up from 1% to 3% of the circulating WBC.

Basophils. Basophils have prominent blue-staining cytoplasmic granules. Basophils located in solid tissue are called *mast cells,* and are found in loose (areolar) connective tissue. Blood basophils are rounded in appearance, whereas tissue mast cells may be elongated or irregular in cell outline. Blood basophils make up less than 1% of the peripheral WBC. Mast cell nuclei are round or oval, but circulating basophils have a lobulated form (polymorphonuclear). However, they, like the eosinophil, tend to have bilobed rather than multilobed nuclei. An outstanding feature of basophils is the abundance of oval basophilic (blue) granules with a finely granular or reticular ultrastructure. The predominance of granules overshadows other cytoplasmic structures: mitochondria, endoplasmic reticulum, ribosomes, and a Golgi apparatus. Basophil granules contain heparin, histamine, serotonin (5-hydroxytryptamine), membrane-like material that is metabolized to prostaglandins and leukotrienes, and a battery of hydrolytic enzymes. The presence of these pharmacologically active agents in mast cell granules and the prominence of mast cells in perivascular tissues suggest that the release of such agents would have a marked effect on the smooth muscles of arterioles and the permeability of capillaries. Release of these pharmacologically active agents by mast cells is the mechanism responsible for early inflammatory changes and for the unleashing of anaphylactic or atopic allergic reactions (see Chapter 18). Mast cell–generated factors also attract neutrophils and eosinophils to inflammatory sites.

Lymphocytes

Lymphocyte is a morphological term that includes a population of cells of similar appearance but with different immune functions. The lymphocyte is a small, round cell found in the peripheral blood, lymph nodes, spleen, thymus, tonsils, and appendix and scattered throughout many other tissues. In smears of peripheral blood, lymphocytes appear slightly larger (7–8 μm) in diameter than red blood cells (erythrocytes) and make up about 30% of the total white blood cell count. A typical lymphocyte has very little cytoplasm and is composed mostly of a circular nucleus with prominent nuclear chromatin (Fig. 2-5). The narrow rim of cytoplasm contains scattered ribosomes as well as a few ribosomal aggregates but, in unstimulated states, is virtually devoid of endoplasmic reticulum or other organelles. Although it was once believed that the lymphocyte was a short-

Figure 2-5. Lymphocyte. (a) Blood smear; (b) transmission electron micrograph; (c, d) scanning electron micrographs of two functional states of the lymphocyte surface: smooth (c) and hairy (d). Cell is composed mainly of a nucleus, with a paucity of cytoplasmic elements. A narrow rim of cytoplasm contains scattered ribosomes, a few membrane-limited bodies (lysosomes), and a few mitochondria. L, lysosome; M, mitochondria; N, nucleus; R, ribosomes.

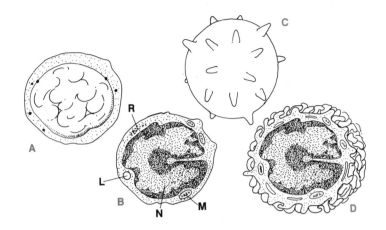

lived "end" cell, it is now known that some populations of lymphocytes may survive for months or even years and recirculate from lymph nodes to lymph and blood.

The lymphocyte is responsible for the primary recognition of antigen and is an immunologically specific effector cell. Lymphocytes produce cell surface molecules that serve as receptor sites for reaction with antigen. The lymphocyte is the carrier of immunologically specific information. *Immunologically competent cell* and *memory cell* are functional terms for specialized cells that are found in immunized individuals and that are not morphologically distinguishable from other lymphocytes. The lymphocytes that interact during the production of circulating antibody have different functional and antigenic properties, but are structurally similar.

T cells. The term T cell is applied to the thymus-derived lymphocyte. T cell precursors (prothymocytes) are produced in the bone marrow and circulate to the thymus. Thymus-derived cells originate in the thymus from these precursor cells, are rereleased into the circulation, and subsequently localize in thymus-dependent areas of the other lymphoid organs. Thymus-derived cells may be identified by specific cell surface markers (see Chapter 4). Approximately 65% to 85% of lymph node cells and 30% to 50% of spleen cells are T cells.

In the human, T cells form *rosettes* with normal sheep erythrocytes (E rosettes). A rosette is composed of a central lymphocyte surrounded by a layer of four or more erythrocytes. B cells do not form rosettes with normal sheep erythrocytes but will form rosettes with sheep cells coated with antibody and complement (EAC) because of receptor sites for the third component of complement. In addition, as stated above, human B lymphocytes contain surface immunoglobulin that is detected by immunofluorescence. These techniques have been used to characterize human lymphoid cell populations. Ninety to one

Table 2-1. Some Properties of T and B Lymphocytes

Properties	T Cells	B Cells
Site of precursor	Thymus	Fetal liver, GI tract, bone marrow
Surface markers	T antigens	Surface Ig
Rosettes	E	EAC
Tissue distribution	Interfollicular (paracortical)	Follicles (cortical)
Percentage of lymphocytes in blood	80	20
Radiation inactivation	+	++++
Mitogen response	Con A, PHA	PPD, LPS
Function	Helper, suppressor, killer	Plasma cell precursor
Mixed lymphocyte reaction	Reactive cell	Stimulator cell

E, sheep erythrocytes; EAC, sheep erythrocytes coated with antibody and complement; GI, gastrointestinal; PHA, phytohemagglutinin; PPD, purified protein derivative; LPS, lipopolysaccharide.

hundred percent of human thymus cells form rosettes with unsensitized sheep red blood cells and no rosettes with EAC. Spleen, peripheral blood, and lymph nodes contain approximately 20% to 30% B cells and 60% to 75% T cells by rosetting analysis (Table 2-1).

T cells may be further divided into subpopulations on the basis of function and other phenotypic markers. Different T cell subpopulations function to help in antibody formation (T helper cells), to kill target cells (T cytotoxic cells), to induce inflammation (T delayed hypersensitivity cells), to inhibit immune responses (T suppressor cells), etc. (see Chapter 10). T lymphocytes activated by antigens produce effector molecules that activate or deactivate other lymphocytes (interleukins), contribute to immune-mediated inflammation (lymphokines), or interact with other cell types (Table 2-2). Not only does the T cell population contain a variety of effector cells, but T cells are also the master regulators of the immune system. As Richard Gershon said, "The T cell is the director of the immunological orchestra." T cells function to turn other cells in the immune system (T suppressors, T helpers, T contrasuppressors, and B cells) off or on.

B cells. B cells arise from precursors in the bone marrow and are the precursors of the cells that synthesize immunoglobulins (plasma cells). B cells contain readily detectable surface immunoglobulin (sIg), whereas T cells do not have surface immunoglobulin. When tissues are tested by fluorescent antiimmunoglobulin sera, 10% to 20% of lymph node cells, 20% to

Table 2-2. Some Factors Produced by
Activated Lymphocytes[a]

PRODUCTS AFFECTING OTHER LYMPHOCYTES (INTERLEUKINS)

Helper factors
Growth promoting factors
Differentiating factors
Suppressor factor
Transfer factor

PRODUCTS AFFECTING MACROPHAGES (LYMPHOKINES)

Migration inhibitory factor
Activation factor
Chemotactic factor

PRODUCTS AFFECTING POLYMORPHONUCLEAR LEUKOCYTES
(LYMPHOKINES)

Chemotactic factors
Histamine releasing factor
Leukocyte inhibitory factor

PRODUCTS AFFECTING OTHER CELL TYPES (LYMPHOKINES)

Cytotoxic factor
Growth inhibitory factors
Osteoclast activating factor
Interferon
Colony stimulating factor

[a] For more details see Chapters 10 and 13.

35% of spleen cells, and 0% of thymus cells contain surface immunoglobulin. The lymphoid cells in these organs that contain T cell antigen do not have surface immunoglobulin.

B cells develop from stem cells that originate in the fetal bone marrow or liver. The site of B cell differentiation may be in the fetal liver, the gastrointestinal lymphoid tissue, or the peripheral lymph nodes. After antigenic stimulation, B cells differentiate into antibody-secreting plasma cells (see below).

Null Cells. Some lymphocytes do not have detectable surface immunoglobulin or T cell markers. Such cells are termed *null cells* and are active in certain types of lymphocyte-mediated target cell killing (see Chapter 4).

Macrophages

The macrophage ("large eater"), the primary phagocytic cell, is the largest cell in the lymphoid system, ranging from 12 to 15 μm in diameter. Macrophages in the blood are called monocytes; those in tissue are called histiocytes. The macrophage nucleus usually has a bilobed kidney shape with considerable peripheral condensation of nuclear chromatin. The cytoplasm of the macrophage contains a great variety of organelles, including endoplasmic reticulum, a Golgi complex, mitochondria, free and aggregated ribosomes, and various membrane-limited phagocytic vacuoles (lysosomes, dense bodies, myelin figures, microbodies) (Fig. 2-6). The tissue macrophage

Figure 2-6. Macrophage. (a) Blood smear (monocyte); (b) transmission electron micrograph; (c) scanning electron micrograph. Large nucleus is centrally located and bilobed or kidney shaped. Cytoplasm is extensive and contains a wide variety of organelles. ER, endoplasmic reticulum; G, Golgi apparatus; L, lysosomes; M, mitochondrion; N, nucleus; R, ribosomes.

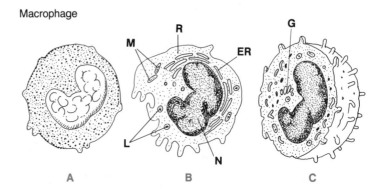

Macrophage

A   B   C

or histiocyte is larger (15–18 μm) and may contain many more cytoplasmic vacuoles than do blood monocytes. Macrophages invade sites of inflammation after polymorphonuclear cells and serve to clear the site of necrotic debris. The digestive capacity of the macrophage is more effective than that of the polymorphonuclear cell. It appears that PMN get in quickly ("attack troops") to act on infecting organisms, but macrophages are needed to finish the job ("mop-up troops").

Role of Macrophages in the Immune Response. The uptake of antigens by macrophages is the first step in the processing of antigen leading to the production of circulating antibody. In such cases, antigen is not completely degraded by the macrophage but becomes bound to macrophage RNA or membrane. The macrophage is not the cell that recognizes antigen as foreign, but the macrophage nonspecifically processes the antigen so that it may be recognized by specific antigen reactive cells. Processed antigens are expressed on the surface of antigen-presenting macrophages in conjunction with self surface markers (class II major histocompatibility markers) that are recognized by T cell receptors for antigen and for self class II MHC. Further definitions of the role of the macrophage in the induction of immunity are discussed in Chapter 10.

The macrophage also plays a prominent role in the later stages of the inflammatory response and may accumulate in large numbers in sites of inflammation. The migration of macrophages (both blood and tissue) into inflammatory sites is generally believed to be non–antigen specific. Specifically sensitized lymphocytes may, upon reaction with antigen, release substances that attract and affect the migration of macrophages or products that increase the phagocytic or digestive capacity of macrophages (see Table 2-2).

Subpopulations of cells in the macrophage family may be recognized by a combination of cell surface markers, morphological appearance, and location in tissue (Table 2-3). Fixed histiocytes lining the sinusoids of the liver are given the special

Table 2-3. Macrophage Subpopulations

Macrophage Subpopulation	Organ	Presumed Function
Stem cell	Bone marrow	Precursor
Monocyte	Blood	Circulating macrophage
Fixed histiocyte	Reticuloendothelial cells	Phagocytic cells in tissue
Dendritic histiocytes	Lymphoid organs	Process antigen for B cells
Interdigitating reticulum cells	Lymphoid organs	Process antigen for T cells
Langerhans' cells	Skin, lymph nodes	Process antigen for T cells

name *Kupffer cells.* Factors are also produced by macrophages that contribute to induction and expression of immune responses as well as inflammation (see Chapter 12). One macrophage-derived factor, interleukin 1, plays a key role in induction of immune responses.

Langerhans' Cells. Langerhans' cells (Fig. 2-7) are a population of the macrophage series found within the mammalian epidermis and certain lymph nodes. They are derived from bone marrow macrophage precursors. They are able to present antigen to T cells in vitro and are believed to be important in

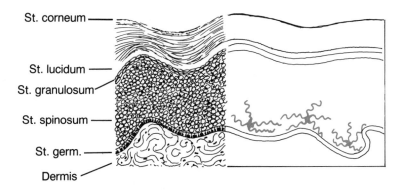

Figure 2-7. On the left is a drawing of the layers of the epithelium of the skin. On the right is depicted the location of Langerhans' cells as detected by special markers. Langerhans' cells are not distinguishable from epithelial cells by the usual methods used for staining tissue.

St. corneum

St. lucidum

St. granulosum

St. spinosum

St. germ.

Dermis

promoting certain immune-mediated lesions, such as contact dermatitis. These cells are not usually visualized in hematoxylin and eosin (H&E)–stained sections but can be distinguished by the presence of class II markers of the major histocompatibility locus, by certain antigenic markers, and by the presence of Birbeck granules seen by electron microscopy.

Figure 2-8. Plasma cell. Cell is composed of abundant cytoplasm containing mostly lamellar endoplasmic reticulum and a few other cytoplasmic organelles. Tissue sections show the polar location and the "cartwheel" appearance of the nucleus produced by the condensation of chromatin along the nuclear membrane. ER, endoplasmic reticulum; G, Golgi apparatus; M, mitochondria; N, nucleus.

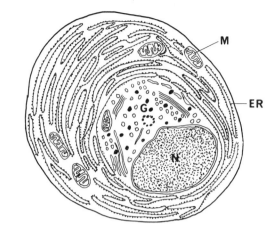

Plasma Cells

The production of immunoglobulins (antibody) is the primary function of the plasma cell. Plasma cells differentiate from activated B cells (see Chapter 6). The plasma cell is a small, round or oval cell ($9-12\ \mu$m in diameter) with a small, compact, dense nucleus located at one pole of the cell. Aggregation of the chromatin along the nuclear envelope gives rise to the characteristic "cartwheel" appearance of the plasma cell nucleus under the light microscope. The cytoplasm is dominated by rough endoplasmic reticulum organized in stacked laminae and a prominent Golgi apparatus (Fig. 2-8). The characteristic lamellar endoplasmic reticulum and the Golgi apparatus reflect immunoglobulin synthesis and rapid secretion. They are found in some other cells in which protein secretion is a major function (e.g., pancreatic acinar cells). Plasma cells are prominent in the lymph nodes, spleen, and sites of chronic inflammation. Plasma cells increase in number in lymphoid organs draining the site of antigen injection during the induction of antibody formation. Membrane-bound amorphous densities believed to contain stored immunoglobulins may be observed in more mature plasma cells (Russell bodies).

Blast Cells

A well-recognized feature of active immune responses is the presence of large *blast* cells. Blast cells are cells that are activated and are in the process of dividing. These cells have large nuclei containing finely divided chromatin and prominent nucleoli. The cytoplasm of blast cells is strongly basophilic and contains dense collections of free and aggregated ribosomes (Fig. 2-9). A variety of other subcellular organelles may be found in the cytoplasm, including a Golgi apparatus, varying amounts of endoplasmic reticulum, and mitochondria. Blast cells are found in lymphoid organs draining sites of antigen injection and in active inflammatory lesions (particularly those of delayed hypersensitivity reactions), and may be induced in vitro in pure cultures of lymphocytes by certain mitogenic

Figure 2-9. Blast cell. The blast cell has a large nucleus containing finely divided chromatin and prominent nucleoli. The cytoplasm stains blue with the usual staining agents and contains dense collections of ribosomes as well as other organelles. ER, endoplasmic reticulum; G, Golgi apparatus; M, mitochondria; N, nucleus; NU, nucleolus; R, ribosomes.

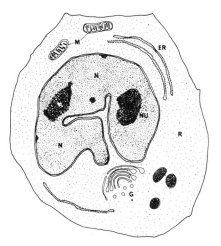

agents. Antigen-recognizing lymphocytes are stimulated by antigen to undergo transformation into blast cells that proliferate and differentiate into plasma cells or sensitized T cells.

Cellular Interactions in Immune Responses

At least three cell types are required for maximal antibody production to most antigens: T cells, B cells, and macrophages (Fig. 2-10). The characteristics and mechanisms of interactions of T and B cells in induction and expression of immune re-

Figure 2-10. Cellular interactions in induction of antibody formation. Antigen is localized by dendritic macrophage. Specific recognition of antigen requires a second cell type, thymus-derived lymphocyte (T cell), which is processed in thymus and migrates to peripheral lymphoid tissue where it comes in contact with antigen. Thymus-derived lymphocyte or macrophage presents antigen to precursor of plasma cell (B cell), which is then stimulated to divide and differentiate into antibody-producing plasma cell (see Chapter 10).

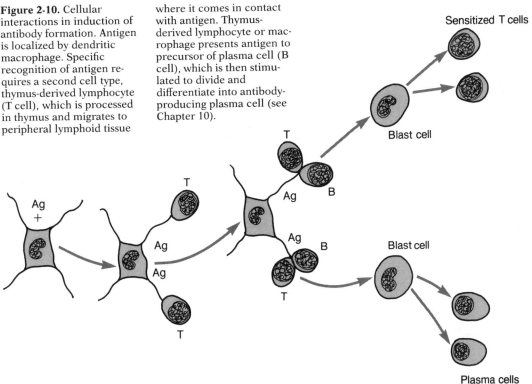

sponse are discussed in more detail in Chapter 10. Specific recognition of most antigens requires the T cell. Macrophages process the antigen. T cells recognize self markers and antigen on macrophages and provide proliferation and differentiation signals to the precursors of plasma cells (B cells). The B cell is stimulated to divide and differentiate so that large numbers of specific antibody–producing plasma cells are produced. In some instances B cells can present antigen to T cells and bypass the macrophage requirement, or B cells may be stimulated directly.

Lymphatic Vessels

The lymphatic vessels retrieve fluid (lymph) and blood proteins that escape from blood capillaries and venules, and return them to the venous system. If this function of the lymphatic circulation is impaired, fluid will collect in the involved tissues (edema). The lymphatic vessels also permit wandering white blood cells in the tissues to return to the lymphoid organs. Lymphatic vessels drain every organ of the body except parts of the central nervous system, the eye, the internal ear, cartilage, spleen, and bone marrow (Fig. 2-11). The spleen and bone marrow have specialized capillary vessels that drain into the systemic vascular system directly and do not have lymphatics.

The fluid of the lymphatic circulation is made up of interstitial fluid drained from tissues or, in the gastrointestinal tract, fluid absorbed from the gastrointestinal contents. There is no pump for the lymphatic circulation corresponding to the heart for the systemic circulation. Lymphatic fluid is propelled by contraction of skeletal muscles or, in larger vessels, by smooth muscle cells that force the fluid from one level to another past valves that permit passage of fluid and cells only in one direction.

Lymphatic vessels drain from tissues through lymph nodes to larger *efferent* lymphatics that collect into larger lymph vessels, which drain into the thoracic duct or the right lymphatic duct. The thoracic duct is the largest lymph vessel in the body and joins the left subclavian vein. The right lymphatic duct joins the right subclavian vein. Seventy-five percent of body tissues are drained by the thoracic duct, and 25% are drained by the right lymphatic duct.

Lymphoid Organs

The cells of the lymphoid system are derived from blood cell precursors in the bone marrow and become organized in specialized organs of the body known as lymphoid organs. Lymphoid organs act as sites of immune responses, producing the products that provide specific adaptive immunity against a variety of infectious agents. Mature lymphoid organs are situated in the body in places where foreign material entering the body from the external environment will be brought into contact

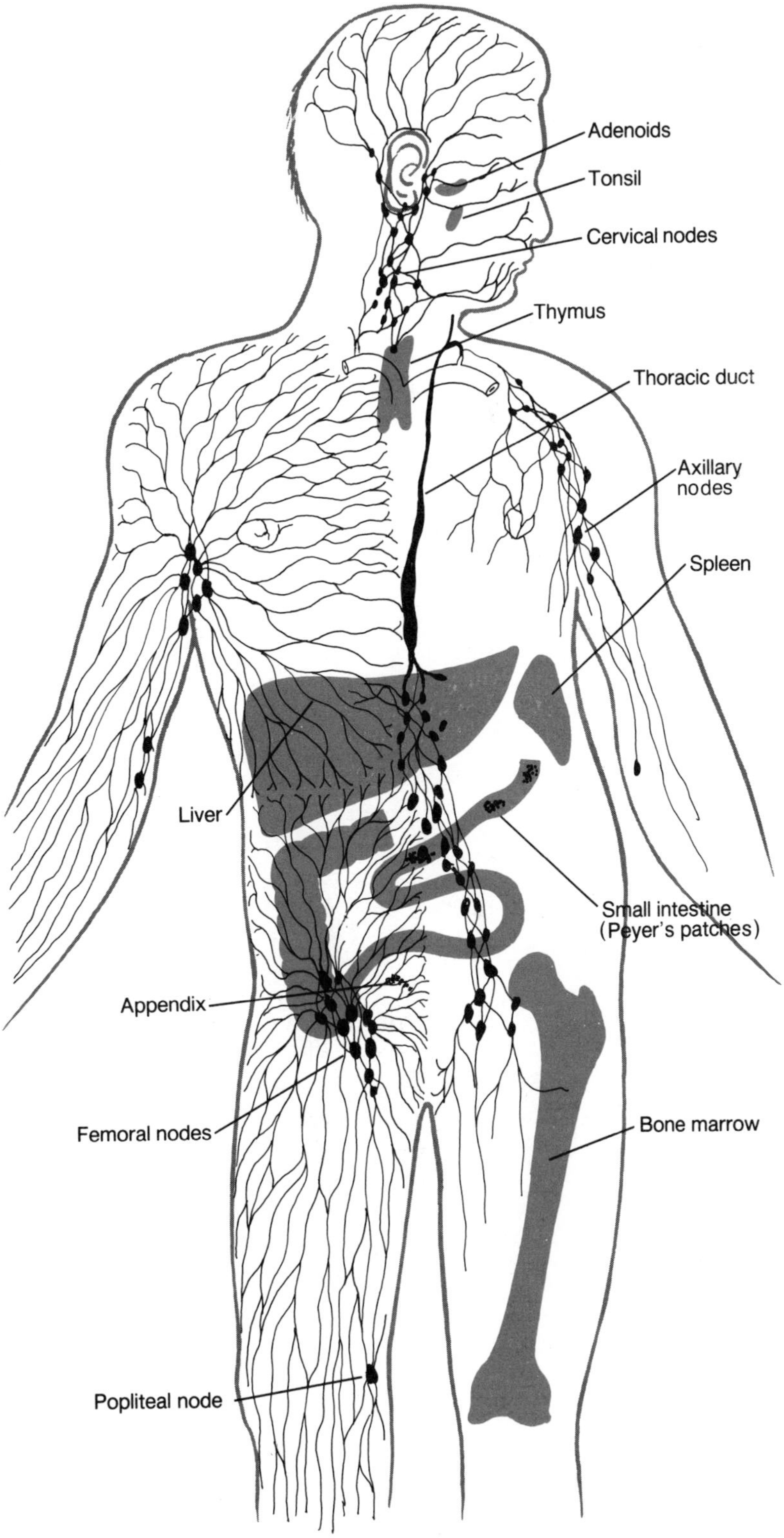

Adenoids
Tonsil
Cervical nodes
Thymus
Thoracic duct
Axillary nodes
Spleen
Small intestine (Peyer's patches)
Bone marrow
Liver
Appendix
Femoral nodes
Popliteal node

Figure 2-11. A diagram of the human lymphoid system. The system consists of circulating lymphocytes and the lymphoid organs, which include the tree of lymphatic vessels and the lymph nodes stationed along them, the bone marrow (in the long bones, only one of which is illustrated), the thymus, the spleen, the adenoids, the tonsils, the Peyer's patches of the small intestine, and the appendix. The lymphatic vessels collect the lymphocytes and antibody molecules from the tissues and lymph nodes and return them to the bloodstream at the subclavian veins.

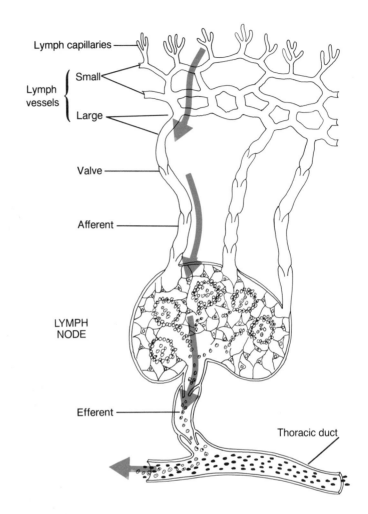

Figure 2-12. Lymphatic collecting vessels are similar to veins.

Labels on figure: Lymph capillaries; Lymph vessels — Small, Large; Valve; Afferent; LYMPH NODE; Efferent; Thoracic duct

with lymphoid organs. Thus, lymph nodes are located along the course of lymphatic vessels that drain from the skin; gastrointestinal lymphoid organs are located along the absorptive areas of the gastrointestinal tract, where they act as filters of lymphatic fluids (Fig. 2-12). Lymphatic capillaries of the gastrointestinal tract are called *lacteals*. These capillaries absorb fats in the form of chylomicra. The spleen does not have lymphatics and serves as a filter for the circulating blood. The structure and function of the lymphoid organs are described in detail in the next chapter.

Summary

The lymphoid or immune system is made up of a number of organs connected by a network of vessels. The cells of the lymphoid system are the white blood cells. This chapter compares the structure and function of leukocytes (white blood cells). Mononuclear cells (lymphoid cells) include macrophages, lymphocytes (T cells, B cells, and null cells), and plasma cells. These cells are active in inflammation and in both induction and expression of immune responses. T cells, B cells, and macrophages cooperate in the induction of antibody responses to most antigens. Upon immune induction, T cells differentiate into specifically sensitized lymphocytes responsible for cellular immune reactivity, whereas B cells differentiate into antibody-secreting plasma cells. Polymorphonuclear cells and macrophages are active in the effector states of tissue inflammation in both a specific and a nonspecific manner.

References

More recent references on differentiation, identification of phenotypic markers, and genetics of the cells of the immune system are given in later pertinent chapters.

Polymorphonuclear Cells

Benditt BP, Lagunoff D: The mast cell: its structure and function. Prog Allergy 8:195, 1964.

Braunsteiner R, Zuker-Franklin D (eds): The Physiology and Pathology of Leukocytes. New York, Grune & Stratton, 1962.

de Duve C, Wattiaux R: Function of lysosomes. Annu Rev Physiol 23:435, 1966.

Oppenheim JJ, Rosenstreich DL, Potter M: Cellular Functions in Immunity and Inflammation. New York, Elsevier/North-Holland, 1981.

Spicer SS, Hardin JH: Ultrastructure, cytochemistry, and function of neutrophil leukocyte granules. Lab Invest 20:488, 1969.

Lymphocytes

Bianco C, Patrick R, Nuzzenzweig V: A population of lymphocytes bearing a membrane receptor for antigen–antibody complement complexes. J Exp Med 132:702–718, 1970.

Cooper HL: Studies on RNA metabolism during lymphocyte activation. Transplant Rev 11:3–38, 1972.

Gowans JL, McGregor DD: The immunological activities of lymphocytes. Prog Allergy 9:1, 1965.

Jondal M, Holm G, Wigzell H: Surface markers on human T and B lymphocytes. I. A large population of lymphocytes forming non-immune rosettes with sheep red blood cells. J Exp Med 136:207, 1972.

Katz DH: Lymphocyte Differentiation, Recognition and Regulation. New York, Academic Press, 1978.

Miller JRAP, Osoba D: Current concepts of the immunological function of the thymus. Physiol Rev 47:437, 1967.

Moller G (ed): Lymphocyte immunoglobulin. Transplant Rev 14:1, 1973.

Moller G (ed): T and B lymphocytes in humans. Transplant Rev 16:1, 1973.

Raff MC: Surface antigenic markers for distinguishing T and B lymphocytes in mice. Transplant Rev 6:52, 1971.

Ross GD, Rabellino EM, Polley MJ, Grey HM: Combined studies of complement receptor and surface immunoglobulin-bearing cells and sheep erythrocyte rosette–forming cells in normal and leukemic lymphocytes. J Nat Cancer Inst 52:377–385, 1973.

Sell S, Asofsky R: Lymphocytes and immunoglobulins. Prog Allergy 12:86, 1968.

Macrophages

Anderson J, Sjoberg O, Moller G: Mitogens as probes for immunocyte activation and cellular cooperation. Transplant Rev 11:131–177, 1972.

Axline SG: Functional biochemistry of the macrophage. Semin Hematol 7:142, 1970.

Claman HN, Mosier DE: Cell–cell interactions in antibody production. Prog Allergy 16:40, 1972.

Cohn ZA: The structure and functions of monocytes and macrophages. Adv Immunol 9:163, 1968.

Fedorko ME, Hirsch JG: Structure of monocytes and macrophages. Semin Hematol 7:109, 1970.

Streilein JW, Bergstresser PR: Ia antigen and epidermal Langerhans cells. Transplantation 30:319, 1980.

Mitchison NA: The carrier effect in the secondary response to hapten–protein conjugates. II. Cellular cooperation. Eur J Immunol 1:18, 1971.

Miller JFAP, Basten A, Sprent J, Cheers C: Review: interactions between lymphocytes in immune responses. Cell Immunol 2:249, 1971.

Moller G (ed): Role of macrophages in the immune response. Immunol Rev 40:1, 1978.

Moller G (ed): Accessory cells in the immune response. Immunol Rev 53, 1980.

Lymphatics

Grey H: The lymphatic system. *In* Goss CM (ed): Anatomy of the Human Body, 29th ed. Philadelphia, Lea & Febiger, 1973, Ch 10.

Yoffey JM, Courtice FC: Lymphatics, Lymph and the Lymphomyeloid Complex. New York, Academic Press, 1970.

The Immune System II: Organs

A lymphoid organ is essentially a compartmentalized collection of lymphocytes and macrophages. Lymphoid organs have similarities as well as differences in structure. The prototype organ is encapsulated by collagenous connective tissue and divided into lobules by strands of connective tissue *(trabeculae)*. The "skeleton" of the organ is a network of interlocking reticular cells and fibers. By far the major cell type is the lymphocyte. Different populations of lymphocytes are found in different domains of a given lymphoid organ, forming functional microenvironments with macrophages of special types. The organ is supplied with blood by a single artery and, except for the spleen, is drained by both veins and lymphatics. The artery enters through an indentation in the capsule, called the *hilum*, and extends into the organ in the trabeculae. Smaller arteries and arterioles extend from the trabeculae into the parenchyma of the organ. Venous drainage begins in the parenchyma and flows out through veins in the trabeculae to the major draining veins, which exit at the hilum. The lymphatic drainage is different for each set of organs. Lymph nodes have both afferent and efferent lymphatics. The thymus has only efferent lymphatics and the spleen has no lymphatics.

Central Lymphoid Organs

The lymphoid cells in the bone marrow, liver, and thymus primarily serve as precursors for cells that develop further in other lymphoid organs; they are referred to as central lymphoid organs. The lymph nodes and spleen are classified as peripheral lymphoid organs. Gastrointestinal associated lymphoid tissue (GALT) and bronchus associated lymphoid tissue (BALT) have both central and peripheral compartments and functions.

Bone Marrow

The bone marrow is soft tissue found within the skeleton of the body in many bones. It contains fat cells and blood forming cells (hematopoietic tissue). The stem cells of all the blood elements, including the precursors of lymphoid cells, are lo-

37

cated in the bone marrow. These stem cells and their progeny are organized into islands of cells within fatty tissue. In the bone marrow the cell types are admixed so that precursors of red blood cells (erythroblasts), macrophages, platelets (megakaryocytes), polymorphonuclear leukocytes (myeloblasts), and lymphocytes (lymphoblasts) may be seen in one microscopic field. It is impossible to differentiate stem cells for one cell line from those of another cell line by morphologic appearance alone. However, stem cells are usually surrounded by more mature cells of the same cell line, so that a given cell may be identified by the company it keeps. In normal bone marrow, the myelocytic series (polymorphonuclear cells) makes up approximately 60% of the cellular elements, and the erythrocytic series 20% to 30%. Lymphocytes, monocytes, reticular cells, plasma cells, and megakaryocytes constitute only 10% to 20%. Lymphocytes make up 5% to 15% of the cells of the normal adult marrow and 20% to 30% of a child's marrow. Normally, lymphocytes are mixed diffusely with the other cellular elements, but focal collections of lymphocytes may be seen in the marrow of elderly individuals. Plasma cells normally constitute fewer than 1% of the marrow cells but increase in percentage with age. Circulating blood enters via arteries that enter through the periosteum and pass through the compact bone in small canals. The marrow is drained by venous sinuses that collect mature blood elements for distribution into the peripheral blood. The mechanism whereby mature cells escape into the bloodstream while immature ones are held back is not known.

The bone marrow is not usually a site of reaction with, or response to, antigen. Marrow lymphocytes circulate from the marrow to other lymphoid organs and differentiate into lymphocytes capable of immune function. Cells originating in the marrow populate the thymus, where they may differentiate into T cells, whereas other marrow cells differentiate into B cells. An intriguing observation is that in the human, naturally occurring tumors of plasma cells that produce immunoglobulin (multiple myeloma) are often found in the bone marrow; an extramedullary location for multiple myeloma is much less frequent. This suggests that the precursors of plasma cells with malignant potential may be located in the marrow. In vitro studies of bone marrow after fractionation of the cells suggest that some immunologically reactive cells may be present in the bone marrow and are able to respond to antigenic stimulation. The contribution of bone marrow cells to the immune response of the whole animal remains unclear. However, the bone marrow may serve as a source of memory cells.

Liver

Early in ontogeny, the liver and yolk sac of mammals constitute the primary site of blood cell formation and, along with the bone marrow, may be the original site of maturation or production of B cells. The yolk sac and liver are closely related embryologically. The fetal liver is made up of immature liver cells (hepatocytes) surrounded by many islands of blood-forming cells containing essentially the same populations of hematopoietic cells as the bone marrow. Attempts to identify a tissue site for maturation of B cell populations have largely been influenced by the finding that the bursa of Fabricius, a gastrointestinal lymphoid organ of birds, is required for normal avian B cell maturation. A mammalian equivalent to the avian bursa in this regard has not been convincingly demonstrated. The mammalian gastrointestinal lymphoid tissue may also be a site for B cell development, but studies are inconclusive. Lymphocytes derived from mouse embryo liver develop surface Ig (B cells) when cultured in vitro. On the basis of this finding it has been suggested that the fetal liver of mammals is a major tissue site of B cell maturation. The yolk sac may also serve as a site for production of immature immune cells for the embryo.

Thymus

The thymus contains a cortical area of packed lymphoid cells, a medulla, a fibrous capsule, prominent trabeculae that divide the organ into lobules, and a hilum with entering arteries and draining veins and lymphatics (Fig. 3-1). The thymus differs

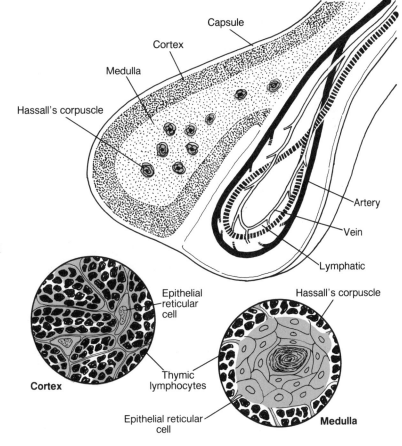

Figure 3-1. Thymus. The thymus is divided into an outer layer (cortex) and an inner layer (medulla). The stroma of both layers is made up of a reticular network formed by epithelial stromal cells. The cortex contains densely packed small thymocytes. The medulla contains less densely packed thymocytes and characteristic epithelial structures known as Hassall's corpuscles.

from the lymph nodes and the spleen in three important features: (1) Normally, there are no lymphoid follicles. The cortex consists of packed small lymphocytes and many proliferating cells in the T lymphocyte series. (2) The medulla contains remnants of epithelial islands that appear as concentric rings of eosinophilic tissue known as *Hassall's corpuscles*. (3) The medulla does not contain sinusoids but is a mesenchymal reticular network in which are found large numbers of lymphocytes. The cortex can be differentiated from the medulla because the lymphocytes are much more closely packed in the cortex. There are no afferent lymphatics in the thymus. The drainage of the thymus has not been well characterized; most drainage occurs through the vein, although significant lymphatic drainage has been claimed by some observers. The cortex is an area of active cell proliferation, with complete turnover of cells believed to occur every 3 or 4 days. The primary function of the normal adult thymus is the production of thymic lymphocytes (thymocytes). However, only about 1% of the lymphocytes produced ever leaves the thymus; the other 99% are destroyed locally. Cellular debris derived from this process is seen in the thymic cortex. The thymus is important for the development of immunity of the cellular type and for normal maturation of the paracortical areas of the lymph node and of the periarteriolar collection of lymphocytes in the white pulp of the spleen (see Lymph Node and Spleen, below). Essentially no B cells can be identified in the normal thymus.

Phenotypic characterization of both the thymocytes and stromal cells of the thymus reveals a complexity of cell types not apparent by morphology alone. The cortical epithelium is derived from an ectodermal branchial cleft, whereas the medullary epithelium is derived from the third pharyngeal pouch. The capsule is derived from mesodermal connective tissue (Table 3-1).

Table 3-1. Characterization of Thymic Stroma

Location	Tissue
Capsule	Mesodermal
Subcapsule	Endocrine epithelium
Cortex	Nonendocrine epithelium
Medulla	Endocrine epithelium

The medullary epithelial cells, including Hassall's corpuscles, represent stages of differentiation and express different phenotypes as differentiation from medullary endocrine epithelium to mature Hassall's corpuscles occurs. The differentiation parallels that seen in skin keratinocytes (Table 3-2).

Thymocytes also show differentiation-related phenotypic changes from cortex to medulla as defined by phenotypic

Table 3-2. Comparison of Differentiation Stages of Skin and Thymic Medullary Epithelium

SKIN

Basal	→	Spinosum	→	Granulosum	→	Corneum

THYMUS

Medullary endocrine epithelium	→	Epithelium around Hassall's bodies	→	Outer layer of Hassall's bodies	→	Inner layer of Hassall's bodies

markers identified by monoclonal antibodies. Most cortical thymocytes are surrounded by epithelial cell membrane extensions. These cortical epithelial cells, termed *thymic nurse cells,* may be responsible for early thymocyte differentiation. Further differentiation occurs after the cells leave the thymus (postthymic compartment). More details of the differentiation of thymocytes are presented in Chapter 4.

The term *T cell* refers to thymus-derived lymphocyte. Cells in the thymus are technically not T cells; T cells are cells that have matured in the thymus and are now present in other tissues (blood, lymph node, etc.). The role of the thymus in the development of other endocrine organs is not well known. Thymectomy leads to a reduction of pituitary hormone levels and atrophy of the gonads. Neonatal hypophysectomy results in thymic atrophy and wasting disease. Other evidence suggests that growth hormone may have an important effect on T cell maturation. Much remains to be learned about thymus–hypophysis interrelationships controlling T cell development.

Peripheral Lymphoid Organs

Lymph Node

Lymph nodes are located in areas of lymphatic drainage in the body and serve as filters for tissue fluid in lymphatic vessels (Fig. 3-2). The lymph node cortex contains nodules of lymphocytes (primary follicles), more loosely arranged nodules surrounded by a rim of tightly packed lymphoid cells (secondary follicles), and lymphocytes lying between germinal centers (paracortical areas) that extend irregularly as bulges into the medulla (deep cortex). Thymectomy of neonatal animals leads to a depletion of lymphoid cells in the paracortical and deep cortical zones; therefore, these zones have become known as the *thymus-dependent area.* On the other hand, depletion of the primary follicles and germinal centers occurs in birds upon removal of the bursa of Fabricius. The follicular areas are therefore termed *bursa dependent.* The medulla consists of a network of draining sinusoids formed by a meshwork of phagocytic reticular cells. The follicles are composed mainly of B cells *(B cell domain),* and the paracortical zone mainly of T cells *(T cell domain).* Specialized macrophages are also present in each of these domains (see Chapter 2). Afferent lymphatic vessels drain into a subcortical sinus; lymphatic sinusoids drain through the cortex around follicles and paracortical areas into the extensive sinusoidal network of the medulla. Some efferent

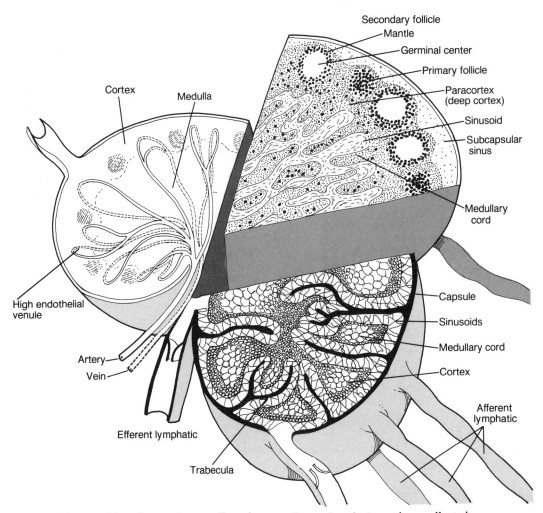

Figure 3-2. Normal lymph node. Nodes are made up of lymphoid cells contained in a meshwork of reticular fibers surrounded by connective tissue capsule. Most lymph nodes are bean-shaped, with an indented area known as the hilus. Cortex (outer layer) contains densely packed lymphoid cells and includes germinal centers responsible for production of antibody-synthesizing plasma cells and paracortical areas where lymphocytes are produced. Medulla (central area) consists of sinusoidal channels maintained by reticular cells. Columns of lymphoid cells are found between sinusoids in areas containing reticular macrophages. Afferent lymphatics drain through cortex around germinal centers into medullary sinusoids. Medullary sinusoids drain into efferent lymphatics and are collected by main efferent lymphatic that drains from the hilus. The main artery divides into capillaries supplying cortex. These capillaries drain into veins that follow trabeculae and exit at the hilus. (Modified from Bloom W, Fawcett DW: A Textbook of Histology, 9th ed. Philadelphia, Saunders, 1969.)

lymphatics arise at the junction of the paracortex and the medulla. It is here that T lymphocytes produced in the deep cortex enter the medullary sinusoids. The medullary sinuses drain into efferent lymphatics, which empty into the main efferent lymphatic vessel and exit through the hilum. The arteries divide into capillaries in the cortex. These capillaries drain into veins in the cortex, so that the cortex is supplied with circulating blood in a conventional manner, whereas the medulla is mainly supplied with lymph fluid by afferent and efferent lymphatics. Recirculating lymphocytes enter the lymph node via high endothelial postcapillary venules in the paracortex. B cells must pass through the T cell domain to home to the B cell domain (follicle).

Spleen

The lymphoid tissue of the spleen is analogous to that of the lymph node, but it is arranged differently (Fig. 3-3). Splenic lymphoid follicles are not demarcated into a cortical area as they are in the lymph node, but are scattered through the sinusoids. Lymphoid follicles and surrounding lymphoid tissue are called *white pulp*, and the sinusoidal area, which usually contains large numbers of red blood cells, is called *red pulp* because of the color seen on gross examination of the freshly cut organ. The white pulp is organized as a lumpy cylindrical sheath surrounding central arterioles. The arterioles curve back upon the white pulp to envelop it as the marginal sinus. The marginal sinus separates the white pulp from the red pulp. Circulating T and B cells enter the splenic white pulp by traversing the marginal sinus. T and B cells may be found mixed in the marginal zone, although B cells predominate. The B cells of the marginal zone appear to be in an activated state. It has been claimed that T-independent antibody responses may take place in the marginal zone. T cells are located in a tight sheath around the central arteriole called the periarteriolar lymphoid sheath; the B cell domain is the lumpy eccentric follicle of white pulp. These follicles may be primary or secondary (germinal center). There is a tightly packed zone of B cells surrounding splenic germinal centers, which is called the *mantle*. The mantle represents cells of the primary follicle pushed aside by formation of the germinal center. The spleen contains no lymphatic vessels. Blood enters through arteries running in trabeculae. The arteries branch and extend into the red pulp. The white pulp is positioned as a sleeve around the smaller arterioles. The arterioles continue out of the white pulp and supply the red pulp either by direct connection with the medullary sinusoids, by drainage into the intersinusoid reticular tissue known as the cords of Billroth, or by branching into specialized vessels of the marginal sinus before entering the sinusoids. Sinusoids have a basic structure similar to that of the lymph node, but drain into branches of the splenic vein and not into efferent lymphatics. There are three types of phagocytic–macrophage cells in the spleen: (1) cells lying free in sinusoids, (2) reticular cells lying between sinusoids that form a meshwork of reticular fibers, and (3) cells found in areas surrounding the white pulp (sometimes within the white pulp). The sinusoidal lining cells are of endothelial origin.

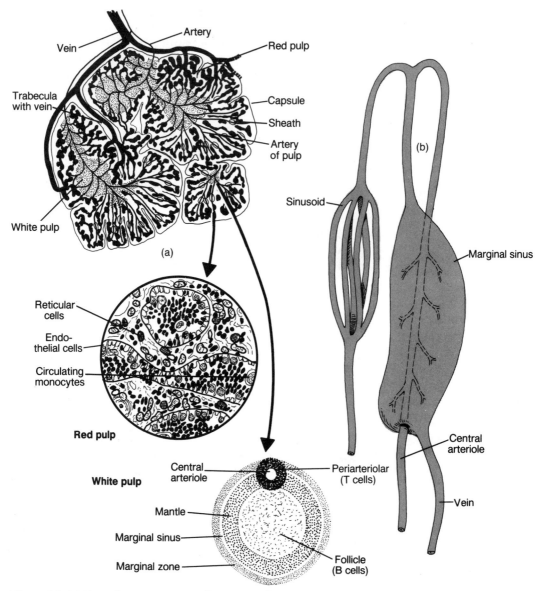

Figure 3-3. (a) Normal splenic lobule. Spleen is composed of a network of sinusoidal channels filled mainly with red blood cells (red pulp). There are no lymphatic vessels. Blood enters through arteries that may empty directly into splenic sinusoids or into reticular area between sinusoids. Sinusoids are drained by veins that exit via trabecular veins to large vein that leaves spleen at the hilus. A zone of densely packed lymphocytes surrounding a central arteriole contains T cells (thymus-dependent area), whereas B cells are found surrounding the germinal center. The mantle surrounding germinal centers is composed mainly of B cells but also of T cells, believed to be pushed aside from the B cell zone by formation of the germinal center. Overlying the mantle is the marginal zone, containing venous capillaries that permit circulating cells to enter the white pulp.

(b) The splenic microcirculation. Blood entering the spleen through central arterioles appears to circulate through either the white pulp or the red pulp. The central arteriole divides into two. One branch drains into capillaries that supply the white pulp, collects into the marginal sinuses, which surround the white pulp, and drains into the splenic vein. The other branch supplies the sinusoids of the red pulp and separately drains into the splenic vein.

It was once believed that the spleen was not an important organ for adaptive immunity; however, children who have their spleens removed surgically because of trauma, neoplastic disease, or hematologic disorders are subject to what is termed the *postsplenectomy syndrome.* Postsplenectomy syndrome is caused by bacterial sepsis, usually with large numbers of encapsulated bacteria (approximately 100 per milliliter). Thus the spleen does serve an important function in clearing the blood of infectious organisms.

Gastrointestinal and Bronchus Associated Lymphoid Tissue

Local collections of lymphoid tissue underlie the submucosa of many areas of the gastrointestinal tract and airways of the lung. In some areas, the collections become large enough to be identified individually. These areas are the tonsils (lingual, palatine, pharyngeal, and tubal) (Fig. 3-4), the appendix (Fig. 3-5), and Peyer's patches (Fig. 3-6). Different domains of lymphoid tissues may be identified in *gastrointestinal associated lymphoid tissue (GALT):* the dome, the follicle, the thymus-dependent area, and submucosal IgA-containing areas. Similar collections

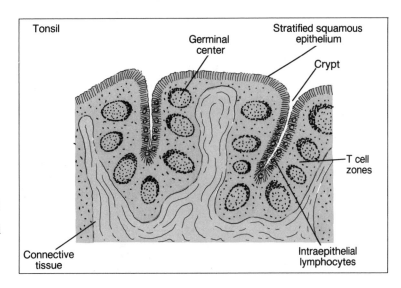

Figure 3-4. Tonsil. Tonsils are composed of a closely packed layer of germinal centers underlying epithelium. There are no afferent lymphatics, and efferent lymphatics are poorly defined. Overlying epithelium is characteristic of areas where tonsils are located (see Gastrointestinal and Bronchus Associated Lymphoid Tissue). Lymphoid cells produced by tonsil appear within overlying epithelium and are believed to emigrate into crypts.

Figure 3-5. Appendix. Appendicular lymphoid tissue is composed of a layer of germinal centers underlying mucosa. Mucosa consists of crypts of goblet cells characteristic of this part of intestine. Many cells produced in appendix appear to be discharged into the lumen. Afferent lymphatics drain around germinal centers from origin in crypts; efferent lymphatics drain from germinal centers.

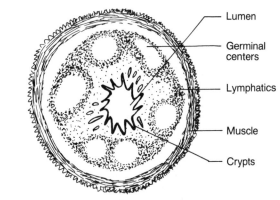

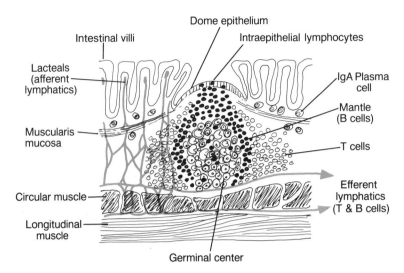

Figure 3-6. Structure of the Peyer's patch (see text).

of lymphoid tissue also occur under the epithelium of the bronchi of the lung (*bronchus associated lymphoid tissue* or *BALT*). The tonsils form a ring of lymphoid tissue at the base of the tongue and pharynx, known as *Waldeyer's ring*, which "guards" the passageway to the esophagus and trachea. The GALT is a major lymphopoietic organ in the adult and may be a source of T and B cells after thymic function declines with age. Antigen entering through the gut or lungs may stimulate cells in GALT or BALT that can then circulate to other tissues.

The overlying mucosa is characteristic of each location: lingual tonsil, stratified squamous; palatine tonsil, stratified squamous; pharyngeal tonsil, pseudostratified columnar; tubal tonsil, pseudostratified columnar; appendix, columnar goblet cells (crypts of Lieberkuhn); Peyer's patches, modified intestinal epithelium. The membranous epithelial cells overlying GALT contain less alkaline phosphatase and have shorter microvilli than adjacent mucosal cells. The GALT-associated mucosal cells are able to transport antigens and microorganisms selectively into GALT. In addition, afferent lymphatics in the form of lacteals deliver material absorbed through the intestine to the lymphatic tissue. The gastrointestinal lymphoid tissue is believed to be necessary for development of the antibody-forming organs (germinal centers, plasma cells) and to have a primary role in immunity to infectious agents entering the body through the mouth. Both immunoglobulin (antibody) and lymphoid T cells are produced by the gastrointestinal lymphoid tissue. These are delivered to the systemic circulation by draining lymphatics, but many of the proteins and cells produced are secreted into the gastrointestinal lumen.

The lactating breast is also a secretory lymphoid organ. Under the influence of prolactin, antibody-producing cells home to and proliferate in the breast, where they produce antibodies that are secreted into the milk. Upon suckling, these antibodies protect the newborn infant against diarrheal pathogens.

Comparison of Structures of Lymphoid Organs

A comparison of the characteristics of lymphoid organs is given in Table 3-3. The structure of each lymphoid organ is related to its functions, the most notable examples being:

1. The thymus, which does not normally respond to an antigenic stimulus, has no afferent lymphatics and no apparent structure associated with delivery of antigen to the organ. In addition, the thymus is the site of T cell development and does not normally contain B cell domains.
2. The lymph node, which serves as a filter for lymphatics, contains both afferent and efferent lymphatics. Both T and B cell domains are present, as well as a rapid delivery system for antibody and/or T cells into lymphatics.
3. The spleen, which is a filter for the blood and not the lymphatics, has no lymphatic vessels.
4. The bone marrow, which is the site of formation of blood cells, does not normally contain T or B cell domains.

Table 3-3. Some Characteristics of Lymphoid Organs

	Cortex	Medulla	B Cell Domain (Follicles)	Afferent Lymphatics	Efferent Lymphatics	Special Features
Thymus	+	+	0	0	+	Hassall's corpuscles, epithelial reticulum, no B cells
Spleen	0	0	+	0	0	White and red pulp, no lymphatics
Lymph node	+	+	+	+	+	Subcapsular sinus, prominent follicles, and paracortical zones
Gastrointestinal						
Tonsils	+	0	+	0	+	Zones of T and B cells, no prominent medulla or draining sinusoids, active mitoses
Appendix	+	0	+	±	+	
Peyer's patch	+	0	+	+	+	
Bone marrow	0	0	0	0	0	Hematopoietic cells in fatty tissue, few mature immune cells

+, present; 0, absent.

Lymphocyte Circulation

Histologic examination of the lymphoid organs provides a static view that belies the extensive recirculation of lymphoid cells. Lymphocytes, both T and B cells, leave their maturation sites, percolate through the lymphoid tissue, and enter other organs by circulation in the bloodstream. Entrance to the bloodstream occurs via either afferent lymphatics or draining veins. Mature lymphoid cells (memory cells?) as well as naive T and B lymphocytes may reenter lymphoid organs after circulating. Lymphocytes enter the lymph node by traversing specialized cortical capillary venules known as high endothelial venules (HEV), because of the thickness of endothelial cells. HEV have specific surface recognition sites for T and B lymphocytes, so that these cells traverse HEV located in different areas of lymphoid organs.

T cells and B cells enter at the same site but are able to go separately to their respective domains in the lymphoid organ. In the lymph node, B cells must traverse the T cell domain (paracortical zone) to reach the B cell domain (follicles). In the spleen, T cells traverse the B domain before reaching the T cell domain (periarteriolar lymphoid sheath). After traversing their respective domains, recirculating T and B cells enter the medullary or red pulp sinusoids before entering the efferent lymphatics. The lymphocyte fields of the lymph node thus contain slowly percolating masses of T and B cells, most of which are on their way from blood to lymph and back to blood. The ratio of the constitutive population of fixed cells to recirculating lymphocytes is not known. Stimulation with antigen results in a temporary increase in responding cells in lymphoid organs draining the site of antigen contact. There is some organ selectivity for lymphocyte localization, as lymph node lymphocytes preferentially localize to lymph nodes, whereas GALT lymphocytes preferentially localize to GALT (Fig. 3-7).

The GALT as well as bone marrow may be a major source of new lymphocytes in the adult animal. Both T and B lymphocytes are delivered from GALT via efferent lymphatics to the thoracic duct and to the systemic circulation. These cells may then localize in any lymphoid organ of the body (except perhaps the thymus) with preferential homing to mucosal lymphoid tissue (e.g., GI tract, lacrimal glands, mammary glands, BALT, and bladder) (Fig. 3-8).

The Effect of Antigens on Lymphoid Organs

The "normal" structure of the lymphoid organs depends upon antigenic exposure. In germ-free animals that have little antigenic contact, the lymphoid organs contain few primary or secondary follicles and sparse paracortical areas, and serum immunoglobulin levels are less than one-tenth those of ordinary animals. The medullary areas contain sinusoids relatively

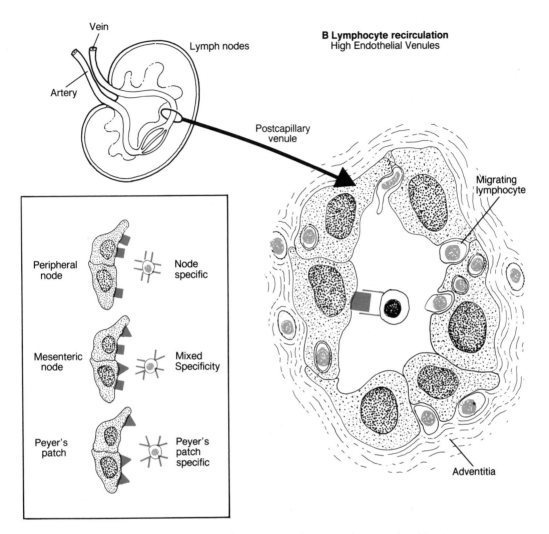

Figure 3-7. Diagram of model of B lymphocyte recognition and migration through high endothelial venules. Lymphocytes have receptors that serve to direct specific homing to lymphoid organs. Peyer's patch cells preferentially home to Peyer's patches; lymph node cells preferentially home to lymph nodes; T cells and B cells both home to the same venules, but with different preferences. In addition, T helper (H) and T suppressor cells also have slightly different homing preferences.

depleted of mononuclear cells or lymph fluid. If antigen is introduced, there is a marked increase in cortical follicles and paracortical tissue, and the serum immunoglobulin levels may increase to almost normal levels.

Antibody Production

Radiolabeled antigens that stimulate the production of both circulating antibody and nonantigens are taken up by the phagocytic cells (macrophages) of the medullary areas of lymph nodes and spleen (Fig. 3-9). However, they can also be

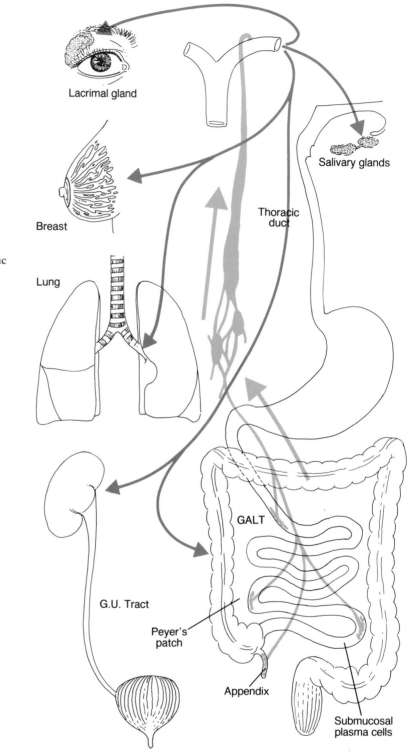

Lacrimal gland

Salivary glands

Breast

Thoracic duct

Figure 3-8. Cellular traffic in the secretory system.

Lung

GALT

G.U. Tract

Peyer's patch

Appendix

Submucosal plasma cells

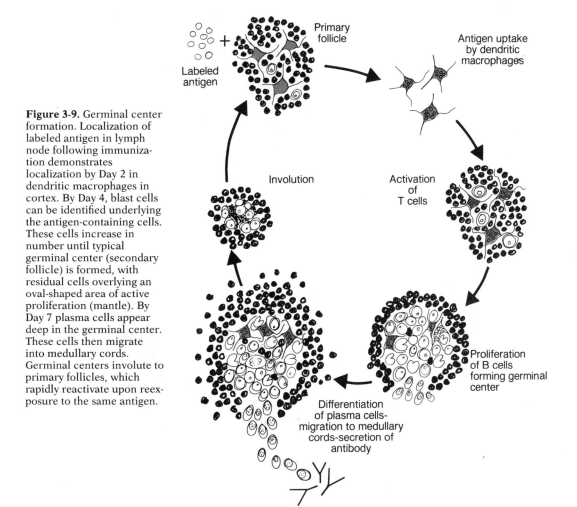

Figure 3-9. Germinal center formation. Localization of labeled antigen in lymph node following immunization demonstrates localization by Day 2 in dendritic macrophages in cortex. By Day 4, blast cells can be identified underlying the antigen-containing cells. These cells increase in number until typical germinal center (secondary follicle) is formed, with residual cells overlying an oval-shaped area of active proliferation (mantle). By Day 7 plasma cells appear deep in the germinal center. These cells then migrate into medullary cords. Germinal centers involute to primary follicles, which rapidly reactivate upon reexposure to the same antigen.

found in *dendritic* macrophages in the cortex or white pulp. Dendritic macrophages are elongated spindle-shaped cells with cytoplasmic extensions that are close to lymphocytes of the cortex or white pulp. Lymphoid follicles form around the dendritic macrophages containing the antigen. Cell proliferation leads to development of a nodule of cells *(follicle)*. The nonproliferating lymphocytes and antigen-containing macrophages are pushed aside to the periphery of the nodule to form a mantle around the follicle. Within 5 to 7 days after immunization, plasma cells appear below the germinal center and migrate into the medullary cords, where they produce and secrete immunoglobulin antibody that is released into the medullary sinusoids. Plasma cells may be observed in large numbers in the adjacent medullary cords or red pulp for periods of at least 10 weeks after immunization. The dendritic macrophages do not make antibody but interact with cells in the lymphoid series that are capable of responding (immunologically competent cells). Within 1 to 2 weeks after primary immunization, memory B cells can be identified in the lymph nodes draining the site of immunization; later, memory B cells are present in distal lymph nodes. After the active phase of antibody production the germinal center forms into a collection of lymphocytes in the cortex that is a primary follicle. Thus the primary follicles may be the location of memory cells. If this is the case, then the terms *primary* and *secondary* are inappropriate because a "primary" follicle may derive from a "secondary" follicle.

Germinal Center Cells

The morphology of cells in a germinal center is depicted in Figure 3-10. These cell types have been used to classify tumors arising from B cells (see Chapter 28).

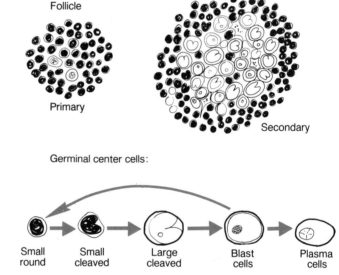

Figure 3-10. Germinal center cells. The cells seen in a germinal center range in size and shape from small round cells to large irregular "cleaved" cells on the basis of nuclear morphology. Primary follicles consist primarily of small round cells. Germinal centers contain a mixture of cells: small round, intermediate round, large round, small cleaved, medium cleaved, and large cleaved. Cleaved cells may represent "activated" B cells, with large round cells being "blast" cells that divide to form two daughter B cells that are small and round. These morphologic cell types have been used to classify tumors arising from B cells (B cell lymphomas). Small round B cell tumors have a good prognosis; large cleaved B cell tumors have a poor prognosis; cell types in between have an intermediate prognosis.

Delayed Hypersensitivity

The morphologic changes occurring in a lymph node during the development of specifically sensitized cells (delayed hypersensitivity) are different from those occurring during the production of circulating antibody (Fig. 3-11).

Figure 3-11. Morphologic response of lymph node to antigenic stimulus. Induction of essentially pure delayed hypersensitivity reaction leads to proliferation of lymphocytes in paracortical zone. Induction of pure humoral antibody formation results in germinal center formation and appearance of plasma cells in medullary cords. Immunization with most antigens produces both changes with enlargement of paracortical zones and production of germinal centers.

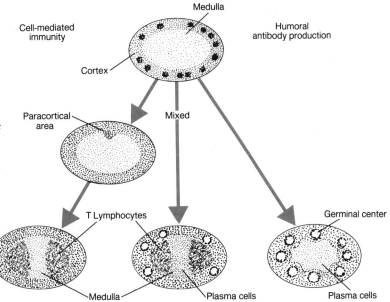

During the induction of delayed hypersensitivity, the proliferative changes in the lymph node do not occur in the follicles or germinal centers but in the other areas of the lymph node cortex that contain tightly packed T lymphocytes (the paracortical areas). Here, there is a population of macrophages known as interdigitating reticulocytes that are believed to process antigens in a manner similar to that of follicular dendritic macrophages, but to present the antigens to T cells. A few days after contact with an antigen, large "immature" blast cells and mitotic figures (dividing cells) may be recognized. A temporary increase in the number of small lymphocytes occurs in this area 2 to 5 days after immunization. It is likely that these are the specifically sensitized cells that are rapidly released into the draining lymph and disseminated throughout the body. It is not precisely clear how antigen is recognized during the development of delayed hypersensitivity. Lymphocytes may be able to recognize antigen at a site distant from the lymph node, where the sensitizing antigen is located, such as the skin. The reacting lymphocyte may return to the lymph node, lodge in the paracortical area, and undergo rapid replication, resulting in the formation of large numbers of sensitized cells that now may recognize and react with the sensitizing antigen.

In summary, different immune responses take place in different lymphoid tissue microenvironments (Table 3-4): specific T-dependent B cell proliferation in germinal centers; T cell proliferation in the paracortex or periarteriolar sheath; T-independent B cell proliferation in marginal zones; and antibody secretion in medullary cords. Memory B cells may differentiate in the mantle of germinal centers and be stored in primary follicles.

Table 3-4. Functional Lymphoid Organ Microenvironments

Microenvironment	Cells Present	Function
Germinal center	B cells, blasts, dendritic macrophages, T cells	T cell–dependent B cell proliferation and differentiation
Paracortex (lymph node), periarteriolar sheath (spleen)	T cells, interdigitating macrophages	T cell proliferation and differentiation
Marginal zones	Dendritic macrophages, B cells	T cell–independent B cell responses
Medulla (lymph node), red pulp (spleen)	Plasma cells, T cells, reticular cells	Rapid antibody production and release of sensitive T cells
Primary follicles	B cells, T cells, dendritic macrophages	Storage of memory cells
Mantle of germinal center	B cells	Memory B cell differentiation

Summary

The lymphoid cells responsible for specific immune responses are distributed in blood, lymphatics, and a number of tissues known as *lymphoid organs*. The morphologic characteristics and functional properties of lymphoid organs are different. Bone marrow serves as the major source of lymphoid stem cells. T cells develop from stem cells that migrate to the thymus and subsequently recirculate to home in thymus-dependent areas of other lymphoid organs: spleen, lymph node, and gastrointestinal tract. B cells mature in the bone marrow, liver, or gastrointestinal lymphoid tissue and migrate to B cell areas (follicles) of other lymphoid organs. Induction of antibody formation is associated with hyperplasia of follicles and plasma cell production, whereas cellular sensitivity is associated with hyperplasia of thymus-dependent areas.

References

Central Lymphoid Organs

Becker RP, DeBruyn PPH: The transmural passage of blood cells into myeloid sinusoids and the entry of platelets into the sinusoidal circulation: a scanning electron microscopic investigation. Am J Anat 145:183, 1976.

Cooper MD, Lawton AR III: The development of the immune system. Sci Am 231:58, 1974.

Cooper MD, Peterson RDA, South MA, Good RA: The functions of the thymus system and the bursa system in the chicken. J Exp Med 133:75, 1966.

Good RA, Gabrielsen AE (eds): The Thymus in Immunobiology. New York, Harper & Row, 1965.

McGregor DD: Bone marrow origin of immunologically competent lymphocytes in the rat. J Exp Med 127:953, 1968.

Melchers F: B lymphocyte development in the liver. II. Frequencies of precursor B cells during gestation. Eur J Immunol 7:482, 1977.

Metcalf D: The thymus: its role in immune responses, leukemia development, and carcinogenesis. *In* Rentchnick P (ed): Recent Results in Cancer Research, Vol 5. New York, Springer, 1966.

Miller JFAP, Marshall AHE, White RG: The immunological significance of the thymus. Adv Immunol 2:111, 1965.

Miller JFAP, Osoba D: Current concepts of the immunological function of the thymus. Physiol Rev 47:437, 1967.

Owen JJT, Cooper MD, Raff MC: In vitro generation of B lymphocytes in mouse fetal liver, a mammalian "bursa equivalent." Nature 249:361–363, 1974.

Waksman BH, Arnason BG, Jankovic BD: Role of the thymus in immune reactions in rats. III. Changes in the lymphoid organs of thymectomized rats. J Exp Med 116:187, 1962.

Peripheral Lymphoid Organs

Cantor H, Boyse EA: Lymphocytes as models for the study of mammalian cellular differentiation. Immunol Rev 33:105, 1977.

Fossum S, Ford WL: The origin of cell population within lymph nodes. Their origin, life history and functional relationship. Histopathology 9:469, 1985.

Goldschneider I, McGregor DD: Anatomical distribution of T and B lymphocytes in the rat. Development of lymphocyte specific antisera. J Exp Med 138:1433, 1973.

Makinodan T, Albright JF: Proliferative and differentiative manifestations of cellular immune potential. Prog Allergy 10:1, 1967.

Rocha B, Freitas AA, Coutinho AA: Population dynamics of T lymphocytes. Renewal rate and expansion in the peripheral lymphoid organs. J Immunol 131:2158, 1983.

Weiss L: The cells and tissues of the immune system. Structure, functions and interactions. *In* Foundations of Immunology Series. Englewood Cliffs, N.J., Prentice–Hall, 1972.

GALT–BALT

Archer OK, Sutherland DER, Good RA: Appendix of the rabbit: a homologue of the bursa in the chicken. Nature 200:337, 1963.

Brand A, Gilmour D, Goldstein G: Lymphocyte-differentiating hormone of bursa of Fabricius. Science 193:319, 1976.

Cooper MD, Lawton AR: The mammalian "bursa equivalent." Does lymphoid differentiation along plasma cell lines begin in gut-associated lymphoepithelial tissues (GALT) of mammals? Contemp Top Immunobiol 1:49, 1972.

Gallin JI, Fauci AS (eds): Advances in Host Defense Mechanisms, Vol 4, Mucosal Immunity. New York, Raven Press, 1985.

Glick B, Chang TS, Jaap RG: The bursa of Fabricius and antibody production. Poult Sci 35:224, 1956.

Nair PNR, Schroeder HE: Duct associated lymphoid tissue (DALT) of minor salivary glands and mucosal immunity. Immunology 57:171, 1986.

Waksman BH: The homing pattern of thymus-derived lymphocytes in calf and neonatal mouse Peyer's patches. J Immunol 111:878, 1973.

Waksman BH, Ozer H: Specialized amplification elements in the immune system: the role of nodular lymphoid organs in the mucous membranes. Prog Allergy 21:1, 1976.

Warner NL, Szenberg A: The immunological function of the bursa of Fabricius in the chicken. Annu Rev Microbiol 18:253, 1964.

Lymphocyte Circulation

Brahim F, Osmond DG: Migration of bone marrow lymphocytes demonstrated by selective bone marrow labeling with thymidine-H³. Anat Rec 168:139, 1970.

Ford WL: Lymphocyte migration and immune responses. Prog Allergy 19:1, 1975.

Goldschneider I, McGregor DD: Migration of lymphocytes and thymocytes in the rat. I. The route of migration from blood to spleen and lymph nodes. J Exp Med 127:155, 1968.

Gowans JL, McGregor DD: The immunological activities of lymphocytes. Prog Allergy 9:1, 1965.

Marchesi VT, Gowans JL: The migration of lymphocytes through the endothelium of venules in lymph-nodes: an electron microscopic study. Proc R Soc Lond [Biol] 159:283, 1964.

Stamper HB, Woodruff JJ: An in vitro model of lymphocyte homing. I. Characterization of the interaction between thoracic duct lymphocytes and specialized high-endothelial venules of lymph nodes. J Immunol 119:772, 1977.

Stevens SK, Weissman IL, Butcher EC: Differences in the migration of B and T lymphocytes: organ selective localization in vivo and the role of lymphocyte–endothelial cell recognition. J Immunol 128:844, 1982.

Effect of Antigen

Movat HZ, Fernando MVP: The fine structure of lymphoid tissue during antibody formation. Exp Mol Pathol 4:155, 1965.

Nossal GJV, Ada GL: Antigens, Lymphoid Cells, and the Immune Response. New York, Academic Press, 1971.

Nossal GJV, Ada GL, Austin CM: Antigens in immunity. IV. Cellular localization of 125-I and 131-I labelled flagella in lymph nodes. Aust J Exp Biol Med Sci 42:311, 1964.

Schwartz RS, Ryder RJW, Gottlieb BAA: Macrophages and antibody synthesis. Prog Allergy 14:81, 1970.

Turk JL, Oort J: Germinal center activity in relation to delayed hypersensitivity. *In* Cottier H, Odortchenko N, Schindler R, Congdon CC (eds): Germinal Centers in Immune Responses. New York, Springer, 1967.

Unanue EA: The regulatory role of macrophages in antigenic stimulation. Adv Immunol 15:95, 1972.

Wortis HH: Immunological responses of "nude" mice. Clin Exp Immunol 8:305, 1971.

4 | The Immune System III: Development of Lymphoid Organs (Ontogeny)

The most accepted model for the development of lymphoid organs is that proposed by Robert Good in the 1960s. According to this model, the precursor stem cells for all lymphoid cells are present in the bone marrow. During fetal development, the stroma for the peripheral lymphoid organs first develops in the absence of lymphoid cells and consists of epithelial or mesenchymal supportive tissue. T and B cells are derived from bone marrow precursors and acquire immune competence by maturation in inductive sites (Fig. 4-1).

T Cell Differentiation

T cell maturation involves stem cells produced in the bone marrow that circulate to and mature in the thymus (Fig. 4-2). The term *prothymocyte* is used for these cells, because they are characterized by homing to the fetal thymus. *Prothymocyte* is a functional term, as there are no phenotypic markers or other ways to identify this cell population. In the thymus these cells acquire T cell antigens such as the Thy and TL antigens found in the mouse. After proliferation in the thymus, some of the thymocytes migrate from the thymus and lodge in the thymus-dependent areas of spleen, lymph node, and other lymphoid organs. Developing thymocytes are also "educated" in the thymus to recognize self by developing receptors for self markers on the thymic epithelium (see Chapter 9). From this period on, thymocytes require recognition of self as well as foreign antigens in order to respond to an antigen. The large amount of proliferation and cell death in the thymus may be related to maintenance of tolerance to self (lack of an immune response to self antigens) through clonal elimination of self-reactive thymocytes. However, some lymphocytes must be able to recognize some self markers of the major histocompatibility system in order to function in helping B cells to respond to antigen (see Chapter 10). This type of self recognition is maintained and not eliminated during the maturation of thymocytes.

57

58

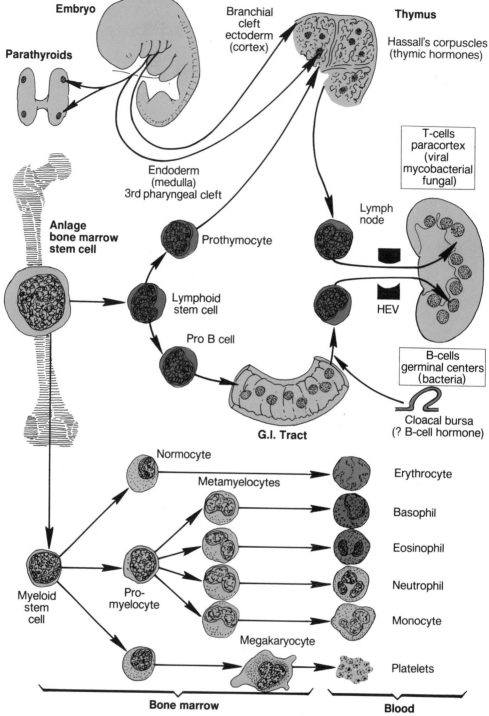

Figure 4-1. Maturation phases in the hematopoietic system. A common bone marrow hematopoietic stem cell gives rise to all elements in the blood and in the lymphoid system. In the stromal microenvironment of the lymphoid organs, specific differentiation of T and B cells occurs.

Figure 4-2. T cell differentiation (ontogeny). The model for T cell differentiation is as follows: Precursors of T cells (prothymocytes) arise from multipotent bone marrow stem cells and migrate to the thymus. In the thymic inductive microenvironment, these cells develop T cell characteristics, including the acquisition of T cell surface markers such as the Thy antigen. T cells that leave the thymus move to thymus-dependent areas, such as the lymph node paracortex, the periarteriolar sheath of the spleen, and thymus-dependent areas (TDA) of other lymphoid organs.

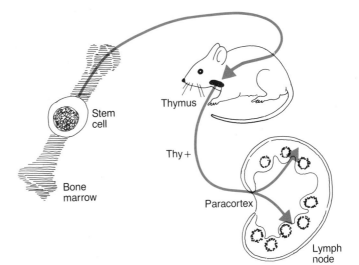

Thymectomy of newborn animals leads to an absence of T cells in the thymus-dependent areas of other lymphoid organs. The antigen receptor of T cells is fixed permanently in the thymus by rearrangement of genes coding for the T cell receptor. The expression of T cell receptor genes during development is presented further in Chapter 6.

Subpopulations of T Cells

In addition to providing help for T-dependent antibody production, T cells, as a class, have several other important functions. These include suppressor cells (T_S), which serve to limit or control immune responses; T cytotoxic or killer cells (T CTL or T_K), which are capable in vitro of lysing target cells to which they are sensitized; and T_D cells, which mediate delayed hypersensitivity in vivo through reaction with specific antigen and release of lymphokines (see Chapter 10). These functional subpopulations of T cells bear different cell surface markers. T cell surface markers are differentiation antigens that, for the most part, are found only on thymocytes or on cells derived from the maturation of thymocytes (T cells). As T cells differentiate into helper, suppressor, or killer cells, the expression of these markers changes (Fig. 4-3). There is also evidence for subpopulations of cells within these functional populations; that is, there may be at least two populations of T helper cells. In addition there is evidence for a population of T cells that counteracts the effect of T suppressor cells, called *T contrasuppressor cells* (see Chapter 10). The major phenotypes of mouse and human lymphocyte populations are given in Table 4-1. These phenotypes are based primarily on reactivity of monoclonal antibodies to different functional subpopulations of T cells. (For a discussion of monoclonal antibodies see Chapter 6.)

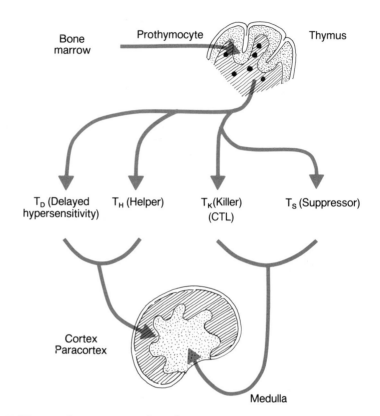

Figure 4-3. Functional differentiation of T cell subpopulations. T cells arise from prothymocyte precursors that pass through a developmental stage in the thymus. The T cell population may be identified by cell surface markers (see Table 4-1). Helper cells (T_H) are generally found in the paracortex of the lymph node, whereas T_K and T_S cells are found in the medulla.

Table 4-1. Phenotypic Markers for Major Lymphocyte Subpopulations

Human Marker[a]	Mouse Equivalent	Function
T_{11} (CD2)	Thy	Precursor
T_4 (CD4)	L3T4	Helper–inducer–DTH
T_8 (CD8)	Ly2	Suppressor, cytotoxic
9.3	—	(?) Killer

[a] See Appendix B: Cluster Designations.

Phenotypic Markers of Human T Cell Subpopulations

Human T cell differentiation markers are recognized by monoclonal antibodies (see Chapter 6) and are present on lymphocytes in different organs (Table 4-2, Fig. 4-4). The phenotypic specificities recognized by different monoclonal antibodies are now termed *cluster designations* (see Appendix B). The CD4 and CD8 subpopulations in peripheral lymphoid organs generally correlate with the major functional populations of T cells, although the major difference between these two subsets is probably their ability to recognize self markers.

Two of the monoclonal antibodies listed (anti-TAC and anti-T_9) react with activated T cells. Anti-TAC recognizes the interleukin 2 (IL2) receptor (see Chapter 10), and anti-T_9 the transferrin receptor. The fact that anti-TAC does not react with activated B cells suggests that B cell activation requires binding of IL2 by a different receptor (see Chapter 10).

Table 4-2. Monoclonal Antibodies to Human T Lymphocyte Surface Antigens

Monoclonal Antibodies	Molecular Weight of Molecules (nonreduced)	Population Defined	Comments	Commercial Names	Cluster Designation[a]
PAN-T CELL					
Anti-T$_1$	69K	All mature T cells, medullary thymocytes, and at low density on cortical thymocytes	Homologue of murine Lyt1	Anti-T$_{1A}$, Leu1, OKT1	CD5
Anti-T$_3$	20K	All mature T cells and medullary thymocytes	Modulates antigen-specific T cell responses; is mitogenic for resting T cells; is part of the T cell receptor complex	Anti-T$_{3A}$, Leu4, OKT$_3$	CD3
Anti-T$_{11}$	55K	All thymocytes and T cells	E rosette associated protein; greatest density on thymocytes and suppressor T cells	Anti-T$_{11}$, 9.6, Leu5, OKT$_{11}$	CD2
T CELL SUBSET					
Anti-T$_4$	62K	Majority of thymocytes and 50–65% of peripheral T cells	T4$^+$ T cells contain most inducer helper functions; functions are class II MHC restricted	Anti-T$_{4A}$, Leu3a,b, OKT$_4$	CD4
Anti-T$_8$(T$_5$)	76K	Majority of thymocytes and 25–35% of peripheral T cells	T8$^+$ peripheral T cells contain most suppressor functions; functions are class I MHC restricted	Anti-T$_{8A}$, Leu2a,b, OKT$_8$	CD8
Anti-T$_6$	49K	70–80% of thymocytes	Specific for cortical thymocytes, β_2 M associated, homologous to murine TL	Anti-T$_6$, Leu6, OKT$_6$, Na1/34	CD1
INDUCIBLE ACTIVATION MARKER					
Anti-TAC	55K	5% of peripheral T cells, majority of activated T cells	Recognizes IL2 receptor; blocks proliferation and IL2 binding; inducible by antigen or mitogen		CD25
Anti-T$_9$	44K	10% thymocytes, majority of activated T cells	Transferrin receptor		None
CLONOTYPE MARKER					
Anti-Ti	92K dimer	Individual T cell clones in culture, 2–5% of T cells in vivo	Anti-variable region of T cell receptor		None

Anti-T designations are available through Coulter Electronics, Hialeah, Fla.; Leu designations through Becton–Dickinson, Mountain View, Calif.; OK designations through Ortho Pharmaceutical, Raritan, N.J.; Na1/34 through Accurate Chemicals, New Jersey.

[a] See Appendix B: Cluster Designations.

Modified from Immunology Today, Sept 1982 (Reinherz E, Schlossman S, advisors).

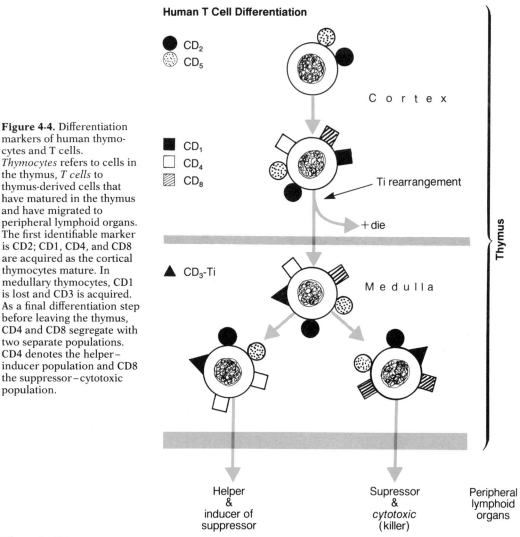

Human T Cell Differentiation

Figure 4-4. Differentiation markers of human thymocytes and T cells. *Thymocytes* refers to cells in the thymus, *T cells* to thymus-derived cells that have matured in the thymus and have migrated to peripheral lymphoid organs. The first identifiable marker is CD2; CD1, CD4, and CD8 are acquired as the cortical thymocytes mature. In medullary thymocytes, CD1 is lost and CD3 is acquired. As a final differentiation step before leaving the thymus, CD4 and CD8 segregate with two separate populations. CD4 denotes the helper–inducer population and CD8 the suppressor–cytotoxic population.

Thymic Hormones

Thymic endocrine epithelial cells produce factors known as *thymic hormones* that induce phenotypic maturation of thymocytes. Over 20 factors have been described; the four most extensively studied are listed in Table 4-3. Each of these factors added

Table 4-3. A Summary of Thymic Humoral Factor Effects

	T Cell Induction	B Cell Induction	Mitogenic	cGMP or cAMP	MLR[a]	Helper[b]	Suppressor[b]
Thymosin	+	0	+	cGMP	+	+	+
Thymopoietin	+	+	+	cGMP	+	+	+
Thymic humoral factor	+	+	+	cAMP	+	+	
Facteur thymique serique (thymulin)	+	+	0	cAMP	0	+	+

[a] MLR—induce ability to respond to mixed lymphocyte reaction.
[b] Helper, suppressor—induce these functions in thymocytes.

in vitro to thymus cells has the property of inducing the appearance of T cell differentiation markers, activating cyclic guanosine monophosphate (cGMP) or cyclic adenosine monophosphate (cAMP) and inducing mature T cell functions.

Natural Killer and Killer Cells

Natural cell-mediated cytotoxic activity is measured by lysis of selected tumor target cells (see Chapter 8). *Natural killer (NK) cells* share some properties of T cells and macrophages (Table 4-4). NK cells are nonadherent lymphocytes that reside in the

Table 4-4. Comparison of NK/K Cells with T Cells and Macrophages

Characteristic	LGL Property	Similar to T Cell	Similar to Macrophage
Size	16–20 nm		+
Cytoplasmic/ nuclear ratio	High ratio		+
Nuclear shape	Lobed or indented		+
Adherence	Nonadherent	+	
Phagocytosis	Nonphagocytic	+	
Nonspecific esterase	Absent	+	
Acid phosphatase	Present	+	+
α-Glucuronidase	In granules		+
Surface antigens	Several shared with other cell types		
Fc receptors for IgG	Shared with PMN		
Spontaneous reactivity	Present in vivo		+
Period to develop augmented effector activity	Short (minutes– hours)		+
Memory response	None		+
ADCC	Very effective		+
Activating factors	Interferon (α, β, γ)	+	+
	Interleukin 2	+	+
	Bacterial products		+
Inhibiting factors	Prostaglandin E	+	+
	Phorbol esters		+

PMN, polymorphonuclear leukocytes; ADCC, antibody-dependent cell-mediated cytotoxicity.
Modified from Ortaldo JR, Herberman RB: Annu Rev Immunol 21:359, 1984.

spleen, peripheral blood, and lungs of most mammals. Much controversy has developed as to the lineage of these cells. Although NK cells are hemopoietically derived from the bone marrow, it is not known whether these cells differentiate from classic B or T cell precursors. Even though NK cells have been found to share several surface antigens with B cells, NK lymphocytes are not involved in antibody production. NK cells also share some similar functional activities, such as their cytolytic mechanisms, with cytolytic T lymphocytes (CTL). What functionally distinguishes NK cells from CTLs is their capacity to lyse a variety of tumor cells without prior sensitization.

NK cells appear to have receptors that recognize target cells and have specificity for a given target cell, but the nature of the receptor is not known. By means of cross competition assays (cold target cell inhibition), it has been shown that suspensions of normal lymphocytes contain different subpopulations of NK cells specific for different target cells, and not all target cell lines are susceptible to NK cells.

Because of the presence of large cytoplasmic granules within NK cells these lymphocytes are referred to as LGL (large-granule lymphocytes). These cytoplasmic granules (lysosomes) of LGL contain enzymes and factors that cause lysis of target cells. Unlike that of T cells the cytotoxicity of NK cells is not MHC restricted. NK cells lyse a large variety of targets including leukemia cells, cells from carcinomas, and several types of normal cells. NK activity is increased by infections and IL2. NK cells activated by IL2 (lymphokine-activated killer cells, LAK) are now being tested for effects on cancer in humans. NK activity is regulated by suppressor cells, both T's and macrophages. The role of NK cells in vivo is not clear, but they are believed to have an important role in immunity to cancer (see Chapter 29) as well as to certain viral infections.

NK cells were not recognized for some time because investigators considered the cytolytic activity of normal cell populations as background in their assays. For instance, comparisons of killing activity were made using lymphocytes from normal donors and lymphocytes from immunized donors. The lytic effect of the normal lymphocyte cell population, such as amount of ^{51}Cr release or inhibition of target cell growth, was considered background and subtracted from the effect of the immunized cell population. However, it was discovered that the effects of the nonimmune cells were due to a population of cells different from that of the immune cells, that is, null cells, not T cytotoxic cells.

Another population of *killer* cells (K cells) have receptors for the Fc or IgG and are able to bind IgG antibodies; they are directed to lyse target cells to which the antibody is directed (antibody-dependent cell-mediated cytotoxicity, ADCC). ADCC cells have been designated K cells, but it appears that NK and K cells may be the same, the difference being the direction of the killing activity by antibody (see Chapter 8).

B Cell Differentiation

Bone marrow stem cells are influenced by the environment of the bone marrow, liver, and gastrointestinal tract to differentiate into B cells, the precursors of plasma cells (Fig. 4-5). B cells differentiate into plasma cells after induction of specific

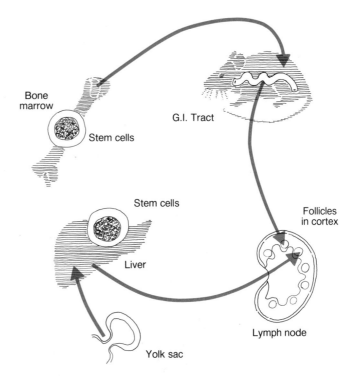

Figure 4-5. B cell differentiation. Precursors of antibody-producing plasma cells, B cells, arise from bone marrow or liver stem cells. For full development of B cells in birds, the inductive microenvironment of a gastrointestinal lymphoid organ, the bursa of Fabricius, is needed. In mammals this function may be provided by the liver or may occur in the bone marrow. B cells migrate to follicular areas of other lymphoid organs (i.e., lymph node cortex).

antibody responses by antigen. Thus, B cell differentiation is antigen independent, whereas plasma cell differentiation is antigen dependent. Differentiated plasma cells produce only one antibody of one specificity and immunoglobulin of only one class.

In mammals, the actual site of B cell differentiation remains uncertain. In birds, a special lymphoid organ, the bursa of Fabricius, located near the anus, is clearly responsible for B cell maturation. Surgical removal of the bursa at hatching leads to a lack of development of B cells and a deficiency in immunoglobulin production. In mammals, however, a clear-cut role for the gastrointestinal lymphoid tissue in B cell differentiation has not been demonstrated. There is evidence that B cells may arise in the fetal liver, or yolk sac, from stem cells that arise in the bone marrow and migrate to the liver, or from stem cells present in the fetal liver. The fetal liver and yolk sac are major blood cell–forming organs in fetal life and contain hematopoietic stem cells. Therefore B cells could arise directly in the liver in infants as well.

After B cells develop, they migrate to the B cell areas of other lymphoid organs. B cells are generally localized in lymphoid follicles of lymph node, spleen, and gastrointestinal lymphoid tissue. B cell maturation may depend on humoral factors produced by epithelial tissue in the inductive microenvironments. A factor extracted from the bursa of Fabricius of chicken, bursapoietin, apparently induces differentiation of bone marrow B cell precursors. Another factor, ubiquitin, may be extracted from thymus as well as other tissues. Ubiquitin induces differentiation of both T cells and B cells in vitro and may function as a receptor molecule for homing of circulatory lymphocytes. Again, the in vivo significance of these factors remains unclear. Attempts to restore immune competence in patients with immune deficiencies using such factors have not yet provided convincing beneficial effects. Maturation of B cells includes an antigen-independent stage and an antigen-dependent stage reflected by sequential immunoglobulin gene rearrangements and expression of cytoplasmic or cell surface immunoglobulins. Antigen-dependent B cell maturation is covered in Chapter 6.

Summary

A composite scheme of T and B cell development is shown in Figure 4-1. Both T and B cell precursors arise from a common lymphoid precursor. Lymphocytes that home to the thymus differentiate under the influence of thymic hormones produced by endocrine cells in the medulla. These cells leave the thymus as T cells (thymus-derived cells) and home via high endothelial venules to thymus-dependent pericortical zones in the lymph node. Phenotypic markers identified by monoclonal antibodies reflect T cell maturation. Functional T cells include T helper/inducer cells detected by the CD4 markers and T suppressor/cytotoxic cells detected by the CD8 markers. Functional T cells recognize antigen by a specific cell surface receptor. Cytotoxic cells without T cell or B cell markers are NK and K cells. NK cells kill certain target cells in vitro due to unstimulated recognition; K cells recognize target cells by passively absorbed antibodies (ADCC).

The site of B cell differentiation in mammals is not clearly defined. In birds, B cell maturation occurs in association with cloacal epithelium in the bursa of Fabricius. B cell maturation in mammals may occur in the gastrointestinal tract, fetal liver, yolk sac, or bone marrow.

In peripheral lymphoid organs T cells and B cells are located in different domains, but are able to cooperate in induction and control of immune responses (see Chapter 10).

References

T Cell Development

Auerbach R: Experimental analysis of the origin of cell types in the developing thymus. Dev Biol 3:336, 1961.

Cordier AC, Haumont SM: Development of thymus, parathyroids, and ultimo-branchial bodies in NMRI and nude mice. Am J Anat 15:227, 1980.

Goldstein G. Lymphocyte differentiations induced by thymopoietin, bursapoietin and ubiquitin. *In* Rutter WJ, Papaconstantinou J (eds): Molecular Control of Proliferation and Differentiation. New York, Academic Press, 1977.

Good RA, Gabrielsen AE (eds): The Thymus in Immunobiology. New York, Harper & Row, 1985.

Haynes BF: Phenotypic characterization and ontogeny of components of the human thymic microenvironment. Clin Res 32:500, 1984.

Komuro K, Boyse EA: Induction of T lymphocytes from precursor cells in vitro by a product of the thymus. J Exp Med 138:479, 1973.

Miller JFAP, Osoba D: Current concepts of the immunological function of the thymus. Physiol Rev 47:437, 1967.

Moller G (ed): Functional T cell subsets defined by monoclonal antibodies. Immunol Rev 74, 1983.

Moller G (ed): T cell antigens. Immunol Rev 82, 1984.

Owen JJT, Jenkenson EJ: Early events in T lymphocyte genesis in the fetal thymus. Am J Anat 170:301, 1984.

Romain PL, Schlossman SF: Human T lymphocyte subsets. J Clin Invest 74:1559, 1984.

Stutman O, Good RA: Thymus hormones. Contemp Top Immunol 2:299, 1973.

Tamaki K, Stingl G, Katz SI: The origin of Langerhans cells. J Invest Dermatol 74:309, 1980.

Tranin N, Small M: Thymic humoral factors. Contemp Top Immunol 2:321, 1973.

Turpen JB, Cohen N: Localization of thymocyte stem cell precursors in the pharyngeal endoderm of early amphibian embryos. Cell Immunol 24:109, 1976.

Turpen JB, Volpe EP, Cohen N: On the origin of thymic lymphocytes. Am Zool 15:51, 1975.

Van Ewjk W: Immunohistology of lymphoid and non-lymphoid cells in the thymus in relation to T cell differentiation. Am J Anat 170:311, 1984.

Natural Killer and Killer Cells

Herberman RB: Natural killer cells. Annu Rev Med 37:347, 1986.

Herberman RB, Callewert D (eds): Mechanisms of Cytotoxicity by NK cells. Orlando, Fla., Academic Press, 1985.

Herberman RB, Reynolds CW, Ortaldo JR: Mechanism of cytotoxicity by natural killer (NK) cells. Annu Rev Immunol 4:651, 1986.

Moller G (ed): Natural killer cells. Transplant Rev 44, 1979.

Ortaldo JR, Herberman RB: Heterogeneity of natural killer cells. Annu Rev Immunol 2:359, 1984.

Pross HF, Baines MG: Spontaneous human lymphocyte–mediated cytotoxicity against tumor target cells. Cancer Immunol Immunother 3:75, 1977.

Rosenberg EB, Herberman RB, Levin PH: Lymphocytotoxicity reactions to leukemia-associated antigens in identical tumors. Int J Cancer 9:648, 1972.

Timonen T, Ortaldo JR, Herberman RB: Characteristics of human large granular lymphocytes and relationship to natural killer and K cells. J Exp Med 153:569, 1982.

B Cell Development

Cooper MD, Peterson RDA, South MA, Good RA: The functions of the thymus system and the bursa system in the chicken. J Exp Med 133:75, 1966.

Cooper MD, Lawton AR: The development of the immune system. Sci Am 231:58, 1974.

Cooper MD, Lawton AR: The mammalian "bursa equivalent." Does lymphoid differentiation along plasma cell lines begin in gut-associated lymphoepithelial tissues (GALT) of mammals? Contemp Top Immunobiol 1:49, 1972.

Hamaoka T, Ono S: Regulation of B cell differentiation. Annu Rev Immunol 4:167, 1986.

Hanley-Hyde JM, Lynch RC: The physiology of B cells as studied with tumor models. Annu Rev Immunol 4:621, 1986.

Moller G (ed): Ontogeny of human lymphocyte function. Immunol Rev 57, 1981.

Moller G (ed): B cell differentiation antigens. Immunol Rev 69, 1983.

Moller G (ed): B cell growth and differentiation factors. Immunol Rev 78, 1984.

Sell S: Development of restrictions in the expression of immunoglobulin specificities by lymphoid cells. Transplant Rev 5:19, 1970.

Shields JW: Bursal dissections and gill pouch hormones. Nature 259:373, 1976.

5 | Antigenicity and Immunogenicity

The unique feature of the adaptive immune system is its ability to recognize foreign molecules and produce new products (antibodies and cells) that react specifically with the foreign molecules (antigens). This process is called immunization. The essence of an immune or allergic response is the capacity to recognize and react to an antigen.

Antigens and Immunogens

An *antigen* is a molecular species capable of inducing an immune response and of being recognized by antibody and/or sensitized cells manufactured as a consequence of the immune response (Fig. 5-1). The ability of material to induce an immune

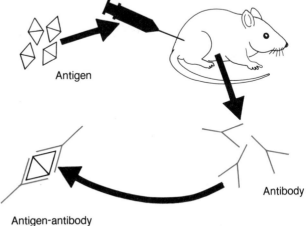

Antigen

Antibody

Antigen-antibody
reaction

Figure 5-1. Definition of *antigen* and *antibody*. A complete antigen (immunogen) is a material that is capable of inducing an immune response and of reacting with the products of the immune response. An antibody is a protein molecule formed by stimulation with antigen that reacts specifically with the antigen.

response is referred to as *immunogenicity*, and such a material is called an *immunogen*. The ability of an antigen to react with the products of an immune response is referred to as *antigenicity*. The immune products in serum (blood without fibrin and cells) that react with antigen are *antibodies*. Antibodies join to antigen by noncovalent binding of sites that can be juxtaposed

69

because of a physical "lock and key" relationship (see Chapter 7). Serum containing specific antibody activity is called *antiserum*.

Complete and Incomplete Antigens

A complete antigen is one that can both induce an immune response and react with the products of that response. An incomplete antigen (hapten) is a chemically active substance of low molecular weight that is unable to induce an immune response by itself but can, by combining with larger molecules (carriers), become immunogenic. A complete antigen is both an immunogen and an antigen, whereas an incomplete antigen is not an immunogen but is an antigen. For example, a chemically active small molecule such as dinitrophenol (an incomplete antigen) may combine with a protein of the host's such as serum albumin to form a complete antigen, so that sensitization occurs (Fig. 5-2). An individual thus sensitized reacts with the

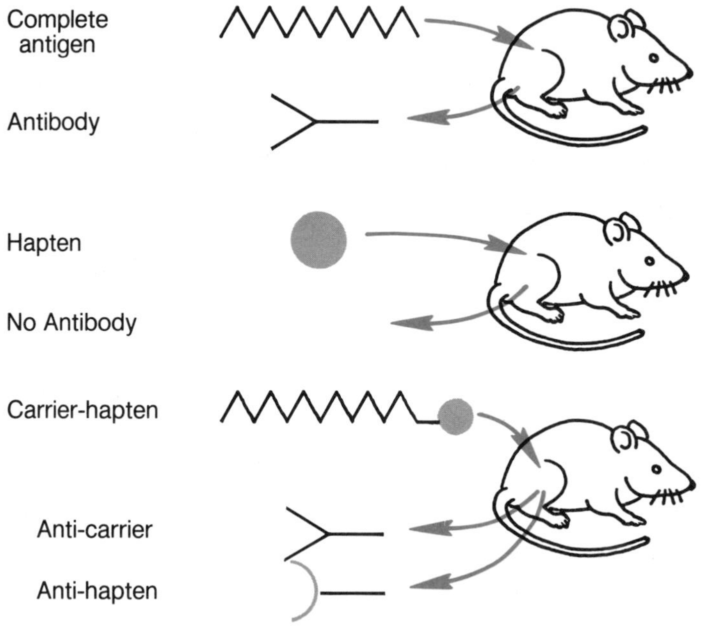

Figure 5-2. Carrier–hapten relationship in immunization. A complete antigen (immunogen) both induces an immune response and reacts with the antibody produced. Haptens are incomplete antigens. Incomplete antigens are *not* able to induce an immune response alone, but antibody can be induced if the hapten is complexed to a complete antigen.

dinitrophenol upon second contact with it because of the antibodies previously formed.

T-Dependent and T-Independent Antigens

Antibodies come from B lymphocytes, often with the help of T lymphocytes. In most hapten–carrier systems, B cells produce antibody specific for the hapten as well as the carrier, whereas T helper cells are specific for the carrier and do not recognize the hapten. Together T and B cells cooperate to induce a hapten-specific antibody response. Most protein antigens are thymus dependent.

Thymus-independent antigens, often polysaccharides, can elicit antibody production by B cells without T cell help.

Interaction of T-independent antigens directly with B cell surface receptors is sufficient to activate B cells directly.

The antibody molecules formed after immunization may express a variety of antigen-binding specificities, that is, recognize different structures on a complex multideterminant antigen. If the inducing antigenic specificity is limited to a small chemical group, the specificity of antibody binding may be exquisitely specific; if the immunogen is a large molecule, a large number of overlapping antigen-binding specificities may be represented in the antibody formed (see Chapter 7).

Epitopes and Paratopes

The parts of antigens bound by antigen-binding sites of antibody molecules (the antigenic determinants) are called *epitopes*.

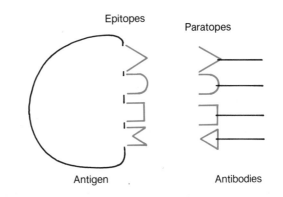

Figure 5-3. An antigen with four epitopes and antibodies with four different paratopes are represented schematically. The complexity of the antibodies is greatly increased by the fact that each epitope may be recognized from different structural aspects. Thus different antibodies with different paratopes could bind to the same epitope.

That portion of the antibody molecule that binds to the epitope is called the *paratope* (Fig. 5-3). Each antigen usually contains more than one epitope. Usually these are present on the surface of the antigen, but denaturation or unfolding of the antigen may reveal or create other epitopes. Most antigenic determinants (epitopes) are created by folding of the polypeptide chain to form overlapping antigenic surface domains (Fig. 5-4). Thus the epitopes of a protein may be sequential or assembled. Se-

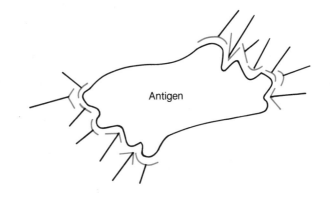

Figure 5-4. Schematic representation of antigenic determinants (epitopes) on a large antigenic macromolecule. Epitopes with which antibodies react are clustered at two "poles" of the molecule. Epitopes are determined by folding of the polypeptide chain to provide surface determinants. Amino acids distant in the linear sequence of the polypeptide chain are found together in the epitope.

quential epitopes are determined only by the amino acid sequence of the peptide sequence involved; assembled determinants are formed by bringing amino acids together by folding of the peptide chain of the molecule. Conformational folding brings together residues that are far apart in the primary sequence but end up close together on the folded protein. Most epitopes are conformational. Short polypeptides may inhibit binding of antibody to the complete native antigen but require a large molar excess to do so. Thus, these polypeptide fragments most likely contain only part of the epitope defined by the assembled determinant.

Chemical Nature of Antigens

Many different kinds of molecules may serve as antigens (Table 5-1). Heavy metals and small organic compounds may function as haptens, whereas most complete antigens are large molecules (macromolecules).

Table 5-1. Chemical Classes of Antigens

Type	Example
Metals	Nickel
Organic chemicals	Dinitrophenol, phenylarsonate
Proteins	Serum proteins, enzymes, microbial toxins
Lipoproteins	Cell membranes
Polysaccharides	Capsules of bacteria
Glycoproteins	Blood group substances (branched polysaccharides)
Polypeptides	Hormones (insulin), synthetic compounds (poly-L-lysine)
Nucleoprotein	Lupus erythematosus factor
RNA	Lupus erythematosus factor
DNA	Lupus erythematosus factor

Physical Properties of Antigens

Size, shape, rigidity, location of determinants, and tertiary structure affect antigenicity.

Size

Complete antigens (immunogens) usually have a high molecular weight (MW). Some naturally occurring immunogens may have a fairly low molecular weight, such as ribonuclease (MW 14,000), insulin (MW 6000), and angiotensin (MW 1031).

The size of an antigenic determinant or epitope may be estimated by determining the ability of a series of antigens of increasing molecular size to inhibit the reaction of antibody with the complete antigen of which the smaller compound is only a part. The smallest molecule that inhibits is considered to contain the complete epitope. Antibodies to dextran polysaccharide are optimally inhibited by six-unit saccharides (MW 990), and antibodies to polypeptides are optimally inhibited by four- to five-amino-acid oligopeptides (MW 650). Short polymers of amino acids are not usually immunogenic, but will function as haptens if added to carrier molecules such as a serum protein or if altered chemically to form a new antigenic site. Poly-L-lysine is not immunogenic, but the attachment of a dinitrophenyl (DNP) group to poly-L-lysine may establish immunogenicity of either the DNP or the poly-L-lysine. DNP-L-lysine$_7$ is immunogenic, but DNP-L-lysine$_6$ is not. In addition, L-lysine$_5$ inhibits the reaction of anti-L-lysine antibody with poly-L-lysine$_7$. Therefore a larger molecule is usually required to induce an immune response than is necessary to react with antibody. The more epitopes, the more likely that an antigen will be "complete," that is, immunogenic.

Shape

The shape of a determinant is important. Certain components, such as the DNP in DNP-L-lysine$_7$, give form to a molecule that is evidently not found in the homologous polymer. Copolymers of two amino acids may be immunogenic for some species, whereas polymers of one amino acid are not. The presence of more than one amino acid in a polymer results in a configuration not available in the polymer of a single amino acid. The location of a structure within a determinant may also be important.

The nature of antigenic determinants has been analyzed by study of the reaction of antibody with incomplete antigens (haptens). A hapten of known structure, such as *p*-azobenzoate, may be joined to an immunogen, such as bovine serum albumin. Immunization with bovine serum albumin chemically complexed with *p*-azobenzoate will stimulate antibodies to *p*-

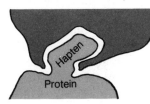

Figure 5-5. Heterogeneity of antigen-binding specificities of antibodies is demonstrated. In the serum of an animal immunized to a hapten, a mixture of antibodies with different specificities and avidities may be detected. The outline of the hapten represents van der Waal's outline of the haptenic group *p*-azobenzoate coupled to a protein carrier. The drawing on the left represents an idealized antibody for the hapten that would have a perfect fit for the haptenic determinant. Antibodies actually produced to such a hapten (right) consist of separate molecules that bind specifically to different parts of the hapten. Some antibodies bind to certain parts of the determinant and other antibodies to other parts, with varying degree of overlapping specificity. (Adapted from Kitagawa M, Yagi Y, Pressman D: J Immunol 95:455, 1965.)

azobenzoate as well as antibodies to the albumin. The heterogeneity of antibodies formed to *p*-azobenzoate is illustrated in Figure 5-5. As can be seen from this illustration, a large variety of antibodies with different binding specificities are produced. It is clear from the heterogeneity of antibodies to this relatively simple antigen that the antibodies formed to larger antigens such as the carrier albumin molecule may be extremely complex.

In many cases, immunizing with a complex antigen containing multiple epitopes leads primarily to production of antibody to one epitope, which is termed the immunodominant epitope of the antigen.

Rigidity

The role of rigidity and location of determinants in antigenicity is exemplified by the alteration in immunogenicity and antigenicity of gelatin by the addition of poly-L-tyrosine to the gelatin backbone. Gelatin, which may have a very high molecular weight, is almost completely nonimmunogenic. Addition of 1% tyrosine increases the immunogenicity and antigenicity of gelatin, and the specificity of antibody produced is directed toward the gelatin. Addition of tyrosine evidently makes the gelatin structure more stable or rigid. Addition of 3% to 10% tyrosine to gelatin changes the immunogenic capacity and results in the production of antibody with specificity directed toward the tyrosine; that is, all the antibody activity can be removed by absorption with poly-L-tyrosine and none by gelatin.

Determinant Location

Important antigenic determinants may be secluded inside large molecules and may be exposed by unfolding of the molecule. If the tyrosine is buried inside a tyrosine–gelatin molecule, it does not function as an antigen, but if the tyrosine is placed on the surface of the molecule, it is recognized. In addition, new determinants may be exposed by partial denaturation of proteins. Denaturation of a protein generally destroys its immunogenicity and antigenicity. However, partial denaturation may result in exposure of different configurations by altering the tertiary structure. This creates new antigenic determinants.

Tertiary Structure

Tertiary structure of proteins (spatial folding) is important in determining the specificity of an antibody response. Antibodies produced to the isolated alpha chains of insulin do not react with the intact molecule, which is an alpha–beta chain dimer. Reduction and reoxidation of ribonuclease under controlled conditions produce a mixture of refolded protein molecules differing only in tertiary structure. Some antisera to native ribonuclease are unreactive with these refolded, denatured molecules; other antisera to the native molecule do react with the refolded forms. Thus, the tertiary structure of antigens is recognized by antibodies and is important for affinity and specificity of binding.

Catabolism

The ability to catabolize or break down the antigen is important for the induction of an immune response. Catabolism of immunogens occurs in macrophages where they are complexed to self molecules. It is critical that the immunogen not be completely catabolized, or the antigenic determinants would be destroyed. L-Amino acid heteropolymers are catabolizable and are immunogenic, whereas D-amino acid heteropolymers are not catabolizable and are poorly immunogenic. The immunogenicity of D-amino acid polymers is dependent upon dose in mice and rabbits. The response to D-isomers exhibits a strong maximum at about 1 μg per mouse, but that to L-isomers is largely independent of dose. Therefore, the failure to detect responses to the poorly catabolized D-isomers may be due to selection of a nonimmunizing dose. Antibody formed to poorly catabolized immunogens may be difficult to demonstrate because of blocking or binding of the antibody formed with the noncatabolized antigen still present in the serum.

Partial antigen degradation or processing is a critical step in the cell–cell interactions between macrophages and T cells. Without antigen processing, T cells will not respond to the "carrier" determinants, leaving the B cells without T cell help.

Immunization

Immunogenicity is determined not only by the nature of the antigen, but also by the characteristics of the responding individual and the manner in which the antigen is presented. Contact between immunogens and responding individuals may occur by natural exposure to organisms, chemicals, or other immunogens in the environment, or may be artificially induced by controlled immunization. The following factors are involved in any controlled immunization and the detection of a subsequent immune response: (1) the source of the antigen, (2) the preparation of the antigen, (3) the form in which the antigen is given, (4) the route of immunization or anatomic location of initial contact, (5) the dose of antigen, (6) the time between the immunizing event and the testing for antibody or sensitized cells, (7) the number of immunizations given (primary or secondary response), (8) the type of test procedure employed, (9) the genetic makeup of the responding animal, and (10) the physiological condition of the responding animal (see Table 5-2). Given such a number of variables, some generalizations may be made, but in practice each immunizing situation must be evaluated individually.

Immunization is performed clinically to induce a protective response, as in vaccination with attenuated or avirulent polioviruses or diphtheria toxoid (see Chapter 25). Experimental immunization may be performed to explore immune reactions or to produce an antiserum that might be used as an immunochemical reagent. The reasons for performing a certain immunization determine, to a large extent, how it is given.

Table 5-2. Some Factors Determining Immunogenicity

Factor	Nature of Effect
ANTIGEN PROPERTY	
1. Source	Degree of foreignness; more evolutionarily distant source gives greater response
2. Preparation	Degree of purity determines extent of response and specificity
3. Form	More complex antigens are more immunogenic; particulate—DTH,[a] soluble—humoral antibody, adjuvants—enhance response
4. Route	Skin—DTH, intravascular—humoral antibody
5. Dose	Low-dose—DTH, high-dose—antibody, very low and very high doses—tolerance
6. Time	Antibody titer and type change with time after immunization
7. Number of exposures	Multiple exposures cause higher titers and sharpen specificity of response, but can also stimulate control pathways, decreasing response
8. Test procedure	Ability to detect immune products depends on sensitivity of test procedure
RESPONDER PROPERTY	
1. Genetics	High and low responders to certain antigens, genetically controlled
2. Physiological condition	Age, drugs, etc., affect response; nutrition, sex, pregnancy, hormones, stress, radiation, other infections

[a] DTH, delayed type hypersensitivity.

Source of Antigen

The source of antigen depends upon the purpose of the immunization. For protective immune responses, individuals may be immunized with living attenuated or killed infectious agents or with nontoxic extracts (see Chapter 25). In some cases, live attenuated vaccines are preferable, while in other cases, killed vaccines can immunize effectively. In experimental situations, an individual may be immunized with the serum proteins or tissues of another individual of the same or a different species, or with laboratory-synthesized material such as hapten-modified carriers or synthetic polypeptides.

As previously emphasized, one of the important features of reacting individuals is the ability to recognize foreignness. One of the ways to classify antigens is by the relationship of source of the antigen to the individual responding to the antigen. The classification given in Table 5-3 is used primarily for tissue transplantation but may be applied to all antigens.

In general the intensity of an immune response will be directly related to the degree of foreignness. Fortunately, autoimmune responses are of relatively low intensity as compared with immune responses to foreign antigens *(xenogeneic)*. An antigen that comes from the same individual or is present in that individual is an endogenous antigen; one that comes from outside the responding individual is an exogenous antigen.

Table 5-3. Source of Antigens

Source Term	Relationship to Responding Individual	Example in Humans
Xenogeneic (heterologous)[a]	Different species	Infectious organisms, animal graft
Allogeneic (homologous)	Same species, different individual	Tissue graft from another human, blood transfusion
Syngeneic (isologous)	Genetically identical individual	Tissue graft or transfusion from identical twin
Autologous	Same individual	Autoimmunity

[a] The terms in parentheses are those commonly employed in blood banks.

Preparation of Antigen

The final preparation of an antigen used for immunization depends upon the degree of specificity desired. For example, immunization of a rabbit with rat spleen produces an antiserum that reacts with various cell populations in the spleen (erythrocytes, lymphocytes, macrophages) and with as many as 30 different plasma proteins. By careful removal of the cellular elements or by immunization with rat serum (defibrinated rat plasma), a rabbit antiserum that reacts with rat serum proteins may be obtained (rabbit anti–whole rat serum). By chemical fractionation of the rat serum an antigen preparation may be obtained that contains only one serum protein. Immunization with this preparation will result in a protein-specific antiserum (rabbit anti–rat albumin). Further fractionation of an antigenic molecule may be accomplished by breaking the molecule into smaller units; an antiserum that reacts with only part of the molecule may thus be obtained.

Form in Which Antigen Is Given

The form in which an antigen is administered also may vary. A serum protein may be administered in soluble form. It may also be mixed with agents that will effectively increase the immune response (adjuvant). Precipitation with alum may result in a greater antibody response. An intense mononuclear infiltration at the site of injection is induced by injection of antigen incorporated into an oil-in-water emulsion. This greatly enhances the immune response. Many other variations may be employed to modify the nature and extent of the immune response. A partial list of adjuvants is given in Table 5-4. For more details see Chapter 27.

Table 5-4. Some Commonly Used Adjuvants

Freund's complete adjuvant (emulsion of mineral oil, water, and mycobacterial extracts)

Freund's incomplete adjuvant (emulsion of water and oil only)

Aluminum hydroxide gels (alum)

Sodium alginate

Bordatella pertussis

Synthetic polynucleotide (poly(A:U))

Muramyl dipeptide

Route of Immunization

The routes of immunization of animals include intradermal, subcutaneous, intramuscular, intraperitoneal, intravascular, and intracranial injections, as well as injection into any organ. In addition, immunization may be accomplished by ingestion, inhalation, skin application, rectal infusion, or intratracheal infusion. The type of immune response elicited depends upon the route used. Those routes that lead to distribution in vascular spaces generally lead to the formation of humoral antibodies, whereas those routes that lead to focal deposition in peripheral lymphoid tissue (intradermal injection or application on the skin surface) tend to induce cellular sensitivity. Inoculation into organs of external secretion, such as salivary glands, breast, or nasal mucosa, may result in the production of antibodies of a different class of immunoglobulin (IgA) than would be found following intramuscular injection (IgG). IgA is the major class of immunoglobulin found in secretions. (For a discussion of immunoglobulin classes of antibody, see Chapter 6.)

Dose of Antigen

The amount of antigen given is extremely important, because too little or too much may result in a loss of immune responsiveness. One microgram of any antigen is usually enough to induce an immune response. Smaller amounts (as little as 1 ng) may actually induce tolerance (see Chapter 11), depending on the purity of the antigen. If a specific antiserum is desired, the purest possible antigen preparation should be used. Otherwise, trace contamination with undesirable antigens may result in the production of an antiserum with multiple specificities.

Interval between Immunization and Testing

In most controlled immunizations circulating antibody does not appear in significant amounts until 7 to 10 days after immunization. The immunoglobulin class of antibody produced also changes with time. Early antibodies are usually of the IgM class, whereas later antibodies are of the IgG class. Also, late antibodies may bind more strongly to antigens than do early antibodies (see Chapter 7). Usually after 3 to 5 weeks the amount of antibody produced starts to decline, so that later blood analyses give lower titers of antibody.

Immunization Schedule

The amount of antibody formed after the second injection of a given antigen (secondary or memory response) usually is much greater than that formed after one injection (primary response) (Fig. 5-6). If high-titered antiserum is desired, a series of injec-

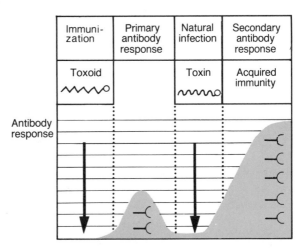

Figure 5-6. The principle of toxin immunization illustrated by the naturally induced secondary immune response to diphtheria infection following immunization with diphtheria toxoid. Diphtheria toxoid retains some of the epitopes of the diphtheria bacillus toxin, so that a primary antibody response to these epitopes is produced following vaccination with toxoid. In a natural infection the toxin restimulates B memory cells, which produce the faster and more intense secondary antibody response that neutralizes the toxin. In most individuals the circulating levels of antibodies to diphtheria and tetanus persist at high levels between exposures. (Modified from Roitt I, Brostoff J, Male D, Immunology. St. Louis, Mosby, 1985, p1.9.)

tions is commonly given. However, after three or more injections, the titer of antibody may be smaller than that after only two injections. The antibody formed after a second injection of antigen (booster) tends to be of the IgG class and more avid (binding more strongly to antigen) than the antibody formed after one injection, which may be of the IgM class. Each bleeding of an immunized animal may yield antibody of different titer, of different avidity, and perhaps of different specificity. Each blood sample must be separately tested to ensure that results obtained with different bleedings can be compared. The remarkable adaptive response to produce higher-affinity antibodies is called *maturation* of the immune response and is due to the selective expansion of clones of B cells that produce antibody of the highest affinity.

Tests for Antibody

The tests used for detection of antibody differ markedly in their ability to measure antibody activity (see Chapter 6). If a bactericidal or viral neutralization test is used, extremely small amounts of antibody may be detected within a few hours of immunization. If the double diffusion-in-agar technique utilizing a soluble protein antigen is used, a million times as much antibody may be needed for detection. In some situations antibody may be detected in vivo (by skin test or systemic anaphylaxis), while the in vitro test is negative. The procedures used for detection of antibody are discussed in more detail in Chapter 6. Whether or not antibody is found following immunization may well depend upon the test for detection.

Genetics of the Immune Response

The ability to produce an immune response and the type of response produced to some antigens are under genetic control. This subject is discussed in Chapter 9.

Condition of the Responding Animal

A wide variety of physiological factors may affect immune responses. For best results, young, healthy adult animals should be used. Very young or very old animals may not respond well to a given antigen. Diseases, immunosuppressive agents, and diet may alter immune responsiveness. Further discussion of the factors influencing the immune response may be found in Chapter 27.

Antigenic Specificity

Chemical Specificity

The specificity of an antibody may be so exact that it can be directly related to a chemically definable structure. The specificity of the antibody may be used to determine, in part, the chemical structure of unknown antigenic molecules. Antibody to pneumococcal polysaccharide Type SII is specific for a D-glucose polymer joined in 1,4,6-linkages. Anti-SII antisera react to glycogens, glycogen-limit dextran, and amylopectins, all of which contain 1,4,6 glycoside linkages. The chemical structures of some unknown carbohydrates can be predicted on the basis of the finding that these unknowns react with anti-SII sera, and direct chemical analysis will demonstrate the presence of 1,4,6-linkages in the unknowns.

Type of Antigenic Specificities

Epitopes specific for different antigenic molecules may be classified on the basis of tissue of origin, species, molecular class, and subclass, and even for individual molecular species such as individual antibodies (Table 5-5).

Table 5-5. Classification of Antigenic Specificities

Type	Example
Organ	Thyroid antigens
	Serum albumin
Species (xenotype)	Human serum albumin
Individuals within a species (allotype)	ABO blood group antigens
	Immunoglobulin allotypes
Subfamily of related molecules (isotype)	Immunoglobulin classes
Individual molecular species (idiotype)	Specific antibody (monoclonal)

Organ Specificity

The same organs of different species share some common antigenic specificities. Thus, the thyroid antigens of one species are shared by the thyroid of another species; the adrenal or brain of one species shares specificity with the adrenal or brain of another species.

Serum proteins with different functional activities have different antigenic specificities, and serum proteins that perform similar functions in different species may share antigenic specificities. The albumins, α-globulins, and immunoglobulins of a given species possess different antigenic specificities. Rabbit anti-human albumin does not react with human immunoglobulins, and vice versa. However, the albumins of different species may contain common epitopes. Rabbit antiserum to human albumin will usually also react with bovine albumin, albeit more weakly.

Species Specificity
(Xenotype)

Rabbit anti-human albumin reacts more strongly with human albumin than with the albumin of any other species. Human albumin contains some antigenic specificities unique for humans, but also contains some epitopes in common with the albumins of other species.

In some cases, for unknown reasons, an identical antigenic specificity is present in the tissues of different species. The classic example is the Forssman antigen. Anti-Forssman antibody is produced by injecting sheep red blood cells into rabbits. The resulting antiserum reacts with sheep cells, goat cells, guinea pig tissue, human type A red cells, certain bacteria, plants, and other animal or fish tissues. The Forssman antigen is a carbohydrate rich in galactosyl residues (see Chapter 29). Antibody to the Forssman antigen is clinically significant in that it appears in patients with infectious mononucleosis and was classically detected by the capacity of serum from an affected patient to bind to sheep red blood cells (Paul–Bunnell test). There is no known phylogenetic or functional relation for this antigenic specificity, only a chemical similarity. A similar relation exists between certain other organisms. For instance, the Weil–Felix reaction depends upon the fact that antiserum against *Rickettsia* reacts also with *Proteus* OX-19.

Allospecificity (Allotype)

Some individuals of a given species possess antigenic specificities not shared with other individuals of the same species. These specificities depend upon small structural differences and are best exemplified by ABO blood group specificities. Within the human species, the red blood cells of individuals of the same red blood cell group (A, B, AB, or O) have the same antigenic specificity, whereas the red blood cells of other individuals of a different blood group have different antigenic specificities. The same is true of serum proteins (immunoglobulins, α-lipoproteins) and solid tissues. The older terminology of blood group specificities referred to differences between individuals as iso-specificities; the more recent terminology introduced to cover solid tissue transplantation antigens employs the term allospecificities. The attempt to identify and classify allospecific antigens in solid tissues is an important advance in human tissue transplantation (see Chapter 19), as perfectly matched donor organs have a good chance of functioning in the new host without undergoing graft rejection.

Isotypic Specificity
(Isotype)

Some families of molecules contain subpopulations with different antigens. For example, the immunoglobulin family consists of five major classes (IgM, IgG, IgA, IgD, and IgE; see Chapter 6). The antigenic determinants that distinguish these classes are termed *isotypes.*

Idiotypic Specificity
(Idiotype)

Idiotypes are antigenic specificities on antibody molecules that are limited to a unique antibody subpopulation. Each antigen-binding site of an antibody is different and may itself be recognized as a foreign epitope. Thus the paratope of an antibody is a unique antigen determinant called an *idiotope.* A cross-reacting idiotype is shared by a subset of antibodies, whereas an individual idiotype is unique for that molecule. Anti-idiotypes (antibodies to idiotopes) may react with the antigen-binding site of the antibody (antiparatope) or with conformational structures adjacent to the paratope. Idiotype-bearing antibodies also share common allotypic and isotypic antigens with other immunoglobulins, but have the unique idiotypic determinant as well. The regulatory role of anti-idiotypes will be discussed in Chapter 11.

Antigen Prevalence

Naturally, exposure to antigens is usually provided by contact with other organisms (bacteria, viruses, fungi). Experimental or therapeutic procedures provide opportunity for contact with other potential antigens, such as artificially produced macromolecules (drugs), serum proteins, blood cells, and tissues (grafts) from other individuals of the same species or of other species. A given individual does not usually make an immune response to his own tissues, although his own tissues contain many potential antigens recognized by other genetically different individuals in the same species. An individual may react against his own tissues *(autoallergic reaction)* if they are rendered antigenic by physical (heat, necrosis) or infectious processes, or if immune regulatory mechanisms break down.

Summary

The induction of an immune response is termed *immunization.* Immunization results in new products that recognize and react with substances that induce the response. A molecular species capable of inducing an immune response is termed an *immu-*

nogen. An *antigen* is a substance that can react with the products of an immune response. A complete antigen can both induce a response and react with the products; an incomplete antigen (hapten) cannot induce a response but can react with the products of the response. The site of the antigen (antigenic determinant) with which an antibody reacts is the epitope; the binding site of the antibody is the paratope. A number of variables concerning the nature of the antigen, the relationship of the antigen to the responding individual, the route and dose of the antigen, and the condition of the responding individual determine the nature and extent of the immune response.

References

Antigens and Immunogens

Atassi MZ, Young CR: Discovery and implications of the immunogenicity of free small synthetic peptides. CRC Crit Rev Immunol 5:387, 1985.

Benjamin DC, et al.: The antigenic structure of proteins: A reappraisal. Annu Rev Immunol 2:67, 1984.

Delisi C, Berzofsky JA: T cell antigenic sites tend to be amphipathic structures. Proc Nat Acad Sci USA 82:7048, 1985.

Heidelberger M: Lectures in Immunochemistry. New York, Academic Press, 1956.

Kabat EA: The nature of an antigenic determinant. J Immunol 97:1, 1966.

Kabat, EA: Structural Concepts in Immunology and Immunochemistry. New York, Holt, Rinehart & Winston, 1968.

Mauer PH: Use of synthetic polymers of amino acids to study the basis of antigenicity. Prog Allergy 8:1, 1964.

Mills JA, Haber E: The effect on antigenic specificity of changes in the molecular structure of ribonuclease. J Immunol 91:536, 1963.

Novotny J, et al: Antigenic determinants in proteins coincide with surface regions accessible to large probes (antibody domains). Proc Nat Acad Sci USA 83:226, 1986.

Sala M: Immunological studies with synthetic polypeptides. Adv Immunol 5:30, 1969.

Todd PEE, East IJ, Leach SJ: The immunogenicity and antigenicity of proteins. Trends Biochem Sci 7:212, 1982.

Yagi Y, Maier P, Pressman D: Antibodies against the component polypeptide chains of bovine insulin. Science 147:617, 1965.

Immunization

Freund J: The mode of action of immunologic adjuvants. Adv Tuberc Res 7:130, 1956.

Munoz J: Effect of bacteria and bacterial products on antibody responses. Adv Immunol 4:397, 1964.

Uhr JW: The heterogeneity of the immune response. Science 145:457, 1964.

Warren HS, Vogel FR, Chedad LA: Current status of immunological adjuvants. Annu Rev Immunol 4:369, 1968.

For additional references, see Chapter 25.

Antigenic Specificity

Jenkin CR: Heterophile antigens and their significance in the host–parasite relationship. Adv Immunol 3:351, 1963.

Landsteiner, K. The Specificity of Serological Reactions. New York, Dover, 1962.

See Chapter 7 for a more detailed discussion of specificity of antibody–antigen reactions, and Chapter 6 for a detailed presentation of idiotypes, allotypes, and isotypes.

6 | Antibodies, Immunoglobulins, and Receptors

Antibodies belong to a group of structurally related glycoprotein molecules found in the blood and extracellular fluids and known collectively as immunoglobulins. Immunoglobulins are the products of plasma cells, which secrete these proteins into serum and tissue fluids. Each plasma cell synthesizes and secretes large numbers of a single antibody that has the same antigen-binding specificity. Whereas some immunoglobulins are produced at all times in most normal animals, specific antibodies are a unique subset of immunoglobulins produced in response to antigenic stimulation. Given the enormous number of antigen specificities (epitopes) identifiable, an individual must have the ability to produce a great variety of antibody molecules. Cell surface antibodies on B cells serve as specific receptors for antigen; T cells also bear receptor molecules similar to antibodies, but having different structural components.

Gamma Globulin

The first identification of antibodies among the serum proteins was accomplished by electrophoresis in 1938 (Fig. 6-1). It was

Figure 6-1. If serum is placed under an electric gradient, the proteins will migrate in the charged field produced. The solid line depicts the serum protein electrophoresis pattern produced after absorption of serum from a hyperimmunized animal with the immunizing antigen. The dotted line depicts the protein pattern before absorption. It was thus shown that antibodies are largely found in the gamma globulins (the least negatively charged serum proteins).

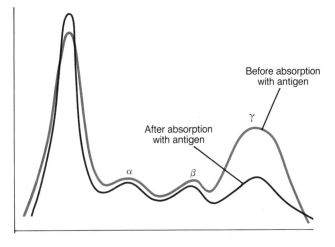

Before absorption with antigen

After absorption with antigen

α   β   γ

85

found that antibodies are part of the gamma globulin fraction of serum. With further characterization of antibody molecules, this class of proteins has been shown to be very heterogeneous and the term *immunoglobulin* has been applied to designate this group of serum proteins. Immunoglobulins possess a degree of structural heterogeneity not found in most other serum proteins, but at the same time immunoglobulins also have structural similarities.

Myeloma Proteins

The study of the structure, synthesis, and function of human immunoglobulins has been made possible by the production of homogeneous immunoglobulins by plasma cell neoplasms (multiple myeloma, macroglobulinemia). From the sera of individuals with such tumors, homogeneous proteins can be isolated. These homogeneous immunoglobulins (myeloma proteins) can then be studied and structural analysis made that is not possible using normal immunoglobulins because of the great heterogeneity of normal immunoglobulins. The clinical features of multiple myeloma are presented in Chapter 28.

Immunoglobulins

Classes (Isotypes)

Five major immunoglobulin classes have been identified in man. Some of the characteristics of these immunoglobulins are given in Table 6-1. The five classes include immunoglobulins G (IgG), A (IgA), M (IgM), D (IgD), and E (IgE). The basic structural unit of each immunoglobulin class consists of two pairs of polypeptide chains joined by disulfide bonds (Fig. 6-2). The disulfide bonds may be reduced by mercaptoethanol. In the presence of denaturing agent (e.g., acid, urea) four polypeptide chains, two L (light)- and two H (heavy)-chains, are liberated. Each antibody molecule contains two identical light chains and two identical heavy chains. The intact molecule may be digested by proteolytic enzymes to yield other fragments (Fc and Fab fragments; Fig. 6-3). The term *Fab* is used because it is this fragment that binds antigen. *Fc* was applied to a non–antibody-binding fragment of rabbit antibody that crystallized in the test tube. The Fc fragments of most antibodies do not crystallize. The L-chains are shared by immunoglobulins of the different classes and can be divided into two subclasses, kappa (κ) and lambda (λ), on the basis of their structures and amino acid sequences. A given immunoglobulin molecule is either type κ or type λ. Approximately 60% of the serum immunoglobulin molecules contain κ-type L-chains, and 40% λ-type L-chains. The H-chains are unique for each immunoglobulin class and are designated by the Greek letter corresponding to the capital letter designation of the immunoglobulin class (α-*chains* for the H-chains of IgA, γ-*chains* for the H-chains of IgG). IgM and IgA have a third chain component, the J-chain, which joins the monomeric units.

Table 6-1. Some Properties of Human Immunoglobulins

Property	Immunoglobulin Class				
	IgG	IgA	IgM	IgD	IgE
Serum concentration (g./100 ml.)	1.2	0.4	0.12	0.003	< 00005
Sedimentation coefficient (S)	7	7 (9,11,13)*	19 (24,32)*	7	8
Molecular weight	140,000	160,000△	900,000	180,000	200,000
Electrophoretic mobility	γ	Slow β	Between γ and β	Between γ and β	Slow β
H-chains	γ	α	μ	δ	ε
L-chains	λ or κ	λ or κ	λ or κ	λ or κ	λ or κ
Complement fixation	Yes	No	Yes	No	No
Placental transfer	Yes	No	No	No	No
Percent intravascular	40	40	70	—	—
Half-life (days)	23	6	5	3	2.5
Percent carbohydrate	3	10	10	13	10
Antibody activity	Most Ab to infections; major part of secondary response; Rh isoagglutinins; LE factor	Present in external secretions	First Ab formed; ABO isoagglutinins; rheumatoid factor	Antibody activity rarely demonstrated, found on lymphocyte surface	Reagin sensitizes mast cells for anaphylaxis

* Figures in parentheses indicates the existence of other molecular forms, such as polymers.
△ Serum IgA 160,000 MW; secretory IgA 350,000 MW, may activate alternate pathway (see Chap. 10) (Modified from Fahey, J.L.: J.A.M.A. 194:183, 1966).

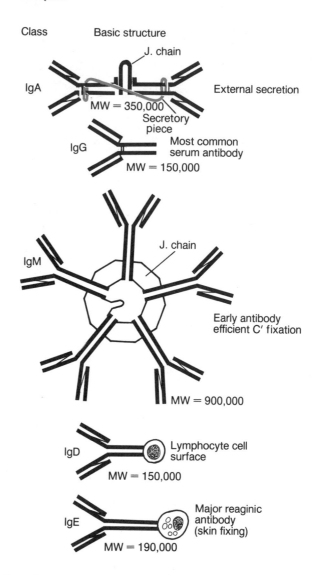

Figure 6-2. Human immunoglobulin classes. Human humoral (circulating) antibodies belong to five classes: IgA, IgG, IgM, IgD, and IgE. The basic unit of each immunoglobulin molecule consists of two pairs of polypeptide chains joined by disulfide bonds. All immunoglobulins have the same L (light)-chain components, identifiable antigenically as kappa (κ) or lambda (λ), with any given immunoglobulin molecule having two κ-chains or two λ-chains. No naturally occurring immunoglobulin molecule has one κ-chain and one λ-chain. H (heavy)-chains of each immunoglobulin class are unique for that class and determine its biologic properties. H-chains of each immunoglobulin class are designated by the Greek letter corresponding to the capital letter identifying the class.

Biological Properties of Immunoglobulins

The five classes of immunoglobulins have different biological properties and are distributed differently in the intact animal. The structure responsible for the biological properties of each immunoglobulin class is located on that part of the immunoglobulin molecule that is unique for each class (the Fc portion of the H-chain).

Each IgG molecule consists of one H_2L_2 unit with a molecular weight of about 140,000. Molecules of the IgG class are actively transported across the placenta and provide passive immunity to the newborn infant at a time when the infant's immune mechanisms are not developed. IgG is widely distributed in the tissue fluids and is about equally divided between the intravascular and extravascular spaces.

IgM is the first immunoglobulin class produced by the

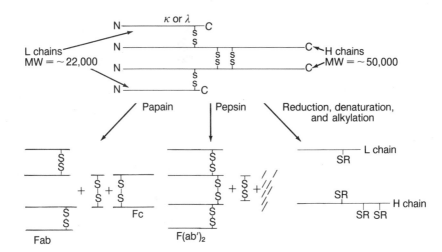

Figure 6-3. Human immunoglobulin fragments. The intact IgG molecule may be fragmented by different reagents into subunits. Digestion with papain occurs on the amino side of the interchain disulfide bond and results in three major fragments, two Fab and one Fc, and a minor fragment. Fab fragments consist of an L-chain and the amino half of an H-chain joined by a disulfide bond. The Fc fragment consists of the carboxy halves of H-chains joined by a disulfide bond. An additional small peptide from the middle of the heavy chains containing a disulfide bond is also produced. The Fab fragment contains an antigen-binding site and reacts with, but does not precipitate, antigen because it is monovalent. The Fc portion is responsible for biological properties such as complement fixation. Digestion with pepsin occurs on the carboxy side of the interchain disulfide bond and results in two F(ab') fragments joined by a disulfide bond because one of the disulfide bonds joining the H-chains is preserved. This fragment, F(ab')$_2$, reacts with and precipitates antigen because it is divalent (contains two antigen-binding sites). Additional peptide fragments, some containing disulfide bonds, are produced by the action of pepsin, presumably due to further digestion of the Fc fragment. Reduction of disulfide bonds, alkylation of free SH groups (R = CH$_2$CONH$_2$), and denaturation of ionic and hydrogen bonds result in liberation of polypeptide chains— two L-chains (MW 22,000) and two H-chains (MW 50,000). Each polypeptide chain contributes to the antigen-binding site of the intact Fab fragment. That portion of H-chain present in the Fab fragment is called the Fd piece.

maturing fetus and may be the first immunoglobulin class representing a given antibody specificity following immunization (primary response). IgM occurs as five H$_2$L$_2$ units joined to each other by disulfide bonds located on the Fc part of the molecule and to the J-chain; its molecular weight is 900,000. IgM is found mainly in the intravascular fluids (80%). It is also the most efficient class of immunoglobulin in fixing complement and therefore is highly active in cytotoxic and cytolytic reactions (see Chapter 15).

IgM does not normally cross the placenta from mother to fetus, but may be produced actively by the fetus prior to birth, especially if the fetus has been exposed to antigens by infection. Thus IgM antibodies in the cord blood of the fetus are evidence of fetal immunization by exposure to infectious agents.

IgA is found in relatively small amounts in serum and tissue fluids, but is present in high concentrations in external secretions such as colostrum, saliva, tears, and intestinal and bronchial secretions. The IgA molecules in these fluids exist as dimers (two H_2L_2 units) joined by a J-chain and bound to an extra protein (*transport piece*). This transport piece is produced by secretory mucosal or glandular cells and facilitates the secretion of the dimeric IgA into the external fluids. Because IgA antibodies are prominent in external secretions, such antibodies are part of the first line of defense against infectious agents.

IgE is present in very low concentrations in serum and tissue fluids, but binds to a specific cell surface receptor on tissue mast cells (see Chapter 18). These cells are so named because they contain cytoplasmic granules and appear to have eaten (German *Mast*, "forced fattening"). Mast cells are armed by IgE antibodies that are bound to their surface receptors. Each antigen to which an individual is allergic may interact with cell-bound IgE and trigger the release of the granules. This releases biologically active molecules, such as histamine and serotonin. Antibody with this biological property is termed *reaginic antibody* or *reagin*.

IgD is present in very low concentrations in the serum. IgD is found on the surface of a high proportion of immature human B lymphocytes, suggesting that IgD may serve as a cellular receptor for antigen. The same variable region is used for IgD on the cell surface and for the IgM, IgG, or IgA that will ultimately be secreted. Thus, when antigen binds the IgD receptor, it stimulates the cell to multiply and ultimately to differentiate and to secrete antibodies of other classes that will be specific for the antigen.

Subclasses (Isotypes)

In addition to the five major classes of immunoglobulins in humans, subclasses of IgG, IgA, and IgM have been recognized. For example, four subclasses of IgG may be identified. These subclasses are designated IgG_1, IgG_2, IgG_3, and IgG_4. The subclasses differ in the sequence of their heavy chain constant regions (Table 6-2). IgG_1 molecules predominate in normal serum (9 mg/ml). The serum content of IgG_2 is 2.5 mg/ml, and

Table 6-2. Biological Properties of IgG Subclasses

Property	IgG_1	IgG_2	IgG_3	IgG_4
Percentage of total IgG in serum	65	23	8	4
Complement fixation	++	+	+++	0
Placental transfer	+++	++	+++	+++
Passive cutaneous anaphylaxis[a]	+++	0	+++	+++
Receptor for macrophage	+++	0	+++	0
Reaction with staph protein A	+++	+++	0	+++
Prominent antibody activity	Anti-Rh	Anti-levan, anti-dextran	Anti-Rh	Anti-factor VIII

[a] Heterocytophilic antibody (see Chapter 18).

the serum content of IgG_3 and IgG_4 is 0.5 to 1.0 mg/ml. The biological significance of these immunoglobulin subclasses is not well understood. However, IgG_1 and IgG_3 are more active in fixing complement, whereas IgG_4 does not fix complement. IgG_2 predominates in the response to polysaccharide antigens and does not cross the placenta with the same efficiency as the other IgG subclasses. Therefore, the different IgG subclasses have different biological properties. In addition, the locations of the interchain disulfide bonds are different. IgA_1 and IgA_2 subclasses differ in sensitivity to bacterial proteases, and α_2 H and L chains are not joined to each other by disulfide bonds, as are α_1 chains, but are held together by electrostatic forces.

Antibodies

Primary Structure

The primary structure of a protein molecule is the sequence of amino acids that make up the light and heavy polypeptide chains (see Fig. 6-4). On the basis of antibody sequence data,

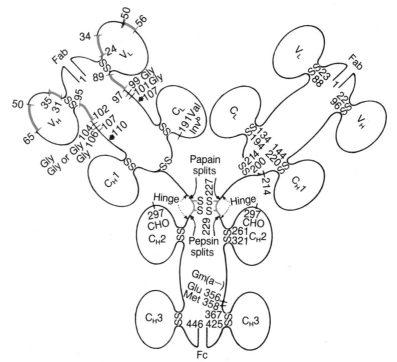

Figure 6-4. Schematic view of four-chain structure of human IgG molecule. Numbers on right side: actual residues of myeloma protein EU. Numbers of Fab fragments on left side aligned for maximum homology; light chains numbered as by E.A. Kabat (J Immunol 125:961, 1980). Hypervariable regions, complementarity-determining regions (CDR): heavier lines. V_L and V_H: light- and heavy-chain variable regions. C_H1, C_H2, and C_H3: domains of constant region of heavy chain. C_L: constant region of light chain. Hinge region in which two heavy chains are linked by disulfide bonds is indicated approximately. Attachment of carbohydrate is at residue 297. Arrows at residues 107 and 110 denote transition from variable to constant regions. Sites of action of papain before the hinge region and of pepsin after the hinge region show why papain produces Fab monomers and pepsin produces F(ab)2 dimers. Locations of a number of heritable allotypic differences (Gm, Inv) are given.

two L-chain regions have been identified. These are called *constant* (C$_L$) and *variable* (V$_L$). Of the total of 212 amino acids, those located at the carboxy terminal are virtually identical for each L-chain of κ type and each L-chain of λ type: the primary structure of the amino domain (that portion presumably containing the antigen-binding site) varies for each antibody studied. The H-chain consists of four or five structural domains, each containing about 106 amino acids in a folded β pleated sheet and a disulfide bond (Fig. 6-5). The amino-terminal struc-

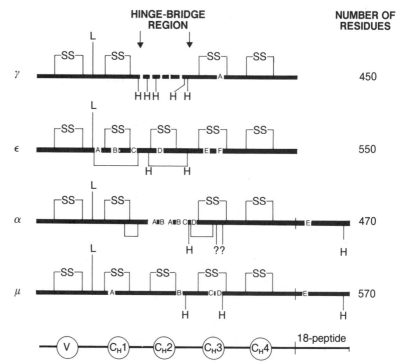

Figure 6-5. Diagrammatic comparison of the heavy chains of different immunoglobulin classes. The γ- and α-chains have three constant domains, whereas the μ- and ε-chains have four. γ- and α-chains have deletions resulting in loss of one of the domains. Other structural differences are indicated. These structural differences account for the biological properties of the different Ig classes. (Modified from Dorington KJ, Bennich HH: Immunol Rev 41:3, 1978.) The five different domains of the immunoglobulin heavy chains and the two domains of the light chains are related by homology and are believed to have evolved by gene duplication.

tural domain of the H-chain contains the H-chain variable region; the other three domains are constant for all H-chains of the same subclass. Therefore, a variable region of an immunoglobulin molecule consists of the amino terminal of the L-chain and the H-chain as they fold together to form a three-dimensional binding site for antigen.

Immunoglobulin molecules have a high degree of flexibility because of a "hinge" region between the first and second constant regions (between Fab and Fc) of the heavy chain. This section of the heavy chain is rich in proline residues, which interfere with the α-helical structure of the constant domains. The hinge region acts as a swivel allowing the Fab domain to assume angles that may vary between 0 and 180°. This permits the individual combining sites to move and assume different angles on reaction with antigenic sites. The length of the polypeptide chain between the last intra–H-chain disulfide bond and the first disulfide bond joining the L- and H-chains is not the same in each immunoglobulin class. The length of the "junction chain" determines the degree of flexibility of the antibody molecule and may influence whether or not reaction with antigen will affect the antibody structure so that functions such as fixation of complement are activated. Only IgM molecules do not have a hinge region.

The heavy chains of the different classes of immunoglobulin are not of the same length (Fig. 6-5). Deletions in the γ and α heavy chains are found in the hinge region. Thus a common ancestral heavy chain may have contained four constant domains. Deletion of some of the amino acids in one of these constant regions for IgG and IgA results in only three constant domains in γ and α heavy chains. An extra 18-amino-acid peptide is present on the carboxy-terminal end of the α and μ heavy chains. This peptide is involved in the formation of the polymeric forms of IgA and IgM molecules and of the cell membrane domain of IgM.

Antigen-Binding Sites (Paratopes)

The antigen-binding site of immunoglobulins (paratope) is located on the variable portion of the Fab of the antibody molecule (*Fab:* fragment that binds antigen). The ability to combine specifically with a given antigenic determinant (epitope) may be shared by immunoglobulins belonging to different classes. The actual site of antigen binding is small, but the complete paratope involves both the L- and the H-chains of a given antibody molecule (see Fig. 6-6). The primary structure responsible

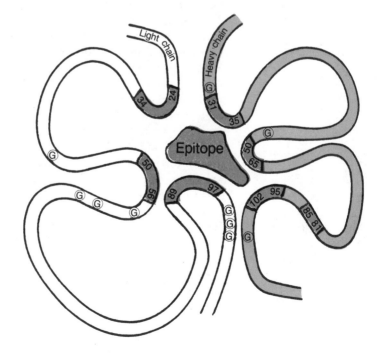

Figure 6-6. Formation of an antigen-binding site (paratope) by conformation of the hypervariable region (dark areas) on light and heavy chains. Numbers refer to amino acid residues. Glycine residues, which are always present at the positions indicated, are important in chain folding. The hypervariable amino acids occur at specific positions in the peptide chain of immunoglobulins. These "hot spots" lie relatively close together in the antigen-binding site and form a continuous surface capable of providing complementarity with a specific antigen. For a given antibody not all the hypervariable regions need be involved with binding of a given antigen.

for antigen binding is located in the variable portion of each chain. Within the variable portion are framework sequences (relatively constant segments) containing up to 30 amino acids and hypervariable sequences ("hot spots") of 4 to 7 amino acids where variability is marked (Fig. 6-4). Some amino acids not actually in the hypervariable segments may contribute indirectly to the conformational or contacting components of the site, by providing ancillary structural support. The "hot spot" segments of the variable region are folded to juxtapose in three dimensions in a manner that forms an appropriate pocket or groove for antigen to be bound (Fig. 6-6).

Biologically Active Sites

In contrast to the variable regions, found on the amino-terminal domains of the immunoglobulin chains, constant regions exist in the carboxy-terminal domains of the L-chain and the H-chain. This situation provides a structural basis for antibodies of different antigen-binding specificity (variable region) to have similar or different biologic properties due to shared constant portions. A variable region is needed to form antigen-binding sites of great diversity, whereas a constant region preserves the biological properties of each immunoglobulin class. The exact sites within the constant domains for biological properties have not been clearly identified. For instance, the site responsible for complement binding after reaction of antibody with antigen is believed to be in the C_{H2} region (see Fig. 6-5). The exact sites for placental transfer, skin fixation, or other biological functions are not known, but reside somewhere in the Fc domains of the appropriate immunoglobulin class.

The sharing of the same constant region among thousands of antibody molecules of different specificity and, hence, different variable regions presented an interesting theoretical question for molecular geneticists. The old theory of one gene – one protein required that the constant region be repeated thousands of times, contiguous with each variable region. Alternatively, immunoglobulins could be the first example of a protein that represented a composite of two genes brought together to form the V and C regions of a single portion. Then, the C region gene could be carried as a single copy on the genome but could be expressed along with any one of the thousands of V genes. This turned out to be the case, as discussed below.

Higher-Order Structure of Immunoglobulins

In addition to primary structure (amino acid sequence), immunoglobulins, like other protein molecules, have higher orders of structure: (1) *secondary*, the coiling of the individual polypeptide chains; (2) *tertiary*, the folding of the polypeptide coils; and (3) *quaternary*, the arrangement and association of the folded chains. Sedimentation, diffusion, and viscosity measurements indicate a tightly ordered structure for the polypeptide chains, with a considerable amount of helical coiling. The coiled chains of the immunoglobulin unit are folded together as well as connected by disulfide bonds. Reduction of the disulfide bonds does not separate the component chains until ionic bonds and hydrogen bonds are also broken, by denaturing agents, for example, acid, urea, or guanidine.

The folding of a constant domain of a heavy chain is illustrated in Figure 6-7. Four antiparallel chains form a β pleated

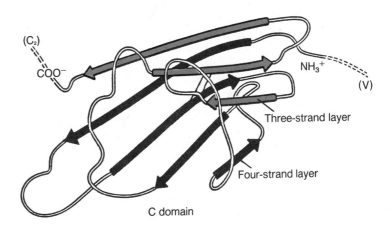

Figure 6-7. The basic folding pattern of the polypeptide chain in the constant (C) domains of an antibody molecule is cylindrical and has a sandwich-like structure: the top layer is composed of three adjacent strands of polypeptide chain (colored arrows) and the bottom layer of four (black arrows), with the two layers held together by a disulfide (sulfur–sulfur) bridge. Although the variable domain of both the light and the heavy chain has an additional loop, the overall folding pattern of the variable and constant domains is highly similar. This common domain structure is due to the presence, in the interior of both domain types, of hydrophobic amino acids that need to be protected from the aqueous environment.

sheet while three other antiparallel chain segments form another β pleated sheet. The two pleated layers enclose a hydrophobic interior and are held together by an intrachain disulfide bond as well as by hydrogen bonds. Nearly all the sharp bends in the polypeptide chains include glycine residues, which are essentially invariant. The structure of a complete light chain is depicted in Figure 6-8.

For the antigen-binding site of an antibody the hypervariable regions of the V_H and V_L domains are organized along a cylindrical surface known as "the binding site barrel." The V_L region β sheets form one side of the barrel, and the V_H β sheets the other. The hypervariable segments of the respective polypeptides are located at the free end of the barrel, forming the

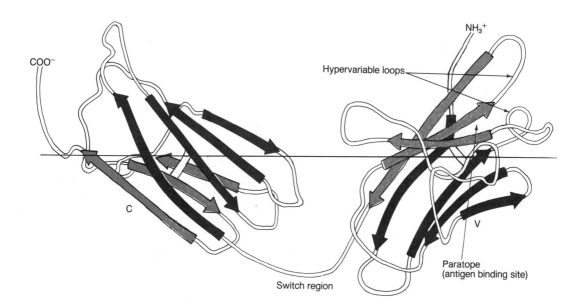

Figure 6-8. The light chain of an IgG molecule folds into a constant (C) and a variable (V) domain. The two domains are rotated 160° with respect to each other, so that their four-strand layers (colored arrows) face different directions. This rotation is accompanied by differences in the amino acid composition of the two domains that enable them to perform very different functions when they interact in pairs. For example, the association of two identical light chains in dimers forms a cavity (paratope) in which antigenic determinants (epitopes) bind. The dimers can thus be considered models for a primitive antibody. Three hypervariable regions located on three separate loops of the peptide chain lie close to one another, forming the L-chain portion of the antigen-binding site.

three-dimensional structure of the antigen-binding site. A three-dimensional model of human immunoglobulin G derived from crystallographic studies is shown in Figure 6-9.

Electron microscopic studies of IgG provide additional observations on the shape and form of the immunoglobulin molecule. IgG not bound to antigen is an irregular globular particle lacking a characteristic structure and with a maximum dimension of 120 Å. IgG antibody bound to antigen (virus particle, ferritin) appears as a Y-shaped molecule. Removal of the Fc piece of IgG causes loss of the stem of the Y. The structure identified has a thickness of 40 Å. Each arm of the Y is 65 Å long; the stem measures 50 Å. The arms and stem are inflexible, but the junction of the arms with the stem, the hinge region, is flexible. The angle between the arms may vary from 10 to 180°. The arms are the Fab pieces and contain the antibody combin-

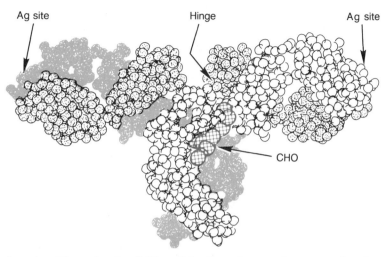

Figure 6-9. Three-dimensional structure of an immunoglobulin G molecule derived from the electron density map obtained by X-ray diffraction. One complete heavy chain is white and the other is light red. The two light chains are lightly stippled and the carbohydrate is crosshatched

ing site. Thus, the flexibility of the junction angle permits bridging of the antigen particles by binding sites that stretch between the antigen particles or looping and joining of two antigen sites on the same particle.

In fine structure, IgM consists of a central thin disk about 180 Å in diameter with five projecting arms measuring 35×125 Å; the entire molecule has a diameter of 270 Å. The structure is consistent with that postulated from chemical studies, that is, five MW 150,000 H_2L_2 units joined together. If each arm represents a Fab piece, the molecule would be expected to have 10 armlike extensions. Therefore, either each arm consists of two Fab pieces, or one of each pair of Fab pieces is incorporated into the central disk.

IgA also has a Y-shaped appearance, in which two basic units are superimposed on each other in a close-packed state. The additional fragment found in secretory IgA is located at the stem area of two Y-shaped units. This fine structure is consistent with that proposed from chemical studies.

Immunoglobulin Antigenic Specificities

The great variety of antigenic specificities that may be recognized on a given molecule is exemplified by the many specificities of antibodies that can react with immunoglobulins (anti-antibodies).

Species Cross-Reactivity

Antisera produced in distantly related species, such as rabbit anti-human immunoglobulin, not only recognize epitopes in human immunoglobulin but also react with immunoglobulin from other primate or mammalian species.

Species Specificity (Xenotypes)

The above antisera may also recognize epitopes present on essentially all human immunoglobulins but not on immunoglobulins from any other species.

Class Specificity
(Isotypes)

Antisera may also recognize epitopes limited to a given immunoglobulin class, such as anti-immunoglobulin G, which does not react with IgA, IgM, IgD, or IgE. These are located on the constant domains of the heavy chains and are H-chain specific.

Subclass Specificity
(Isotypes)

Antisera may specifically identify the IgG subclasses (IgG$_1$, IgG$_2$, IgG$_3$, IgG$_4$). Such antisera usually require absorption to remove IgG common specificities.

Fragment Specificity

Antisera may also be specific for the Fab, Fc, or Fd fragment of an immunoglobulin. This specificity may be so exact that it requires the fragment as antigen; reaction with native IgG does not occur.

Chain Specificity

Similar specificities may also be produced for L-chains only or H-chains only, because of epitopes determined by constant regions.

Allospecificity
(Allotypes)

Immunoglobulins also carry genetically controlled antigenic specificities termed *allotypes*. Allotypes are epitopes that differ among individuals of the same species. Human immunoglobulin allotypes are discussed below.

Denatured
Immunoglobulin
Specificity

Antisera produced to heat-denatured or chemically denatured immunoglobulin may react only with denatured immunoglobulins and not with native immunoglobulins. Denaturation, if not extensive, causes the unfolding or refolding of the molecule so that determinants not present on the native molecule are revealed. Many rheumatoid factors react with denatured immunoglobulin epitopes.

Antivariable Region
Specificity
(Idiotypes)

An antibody that reacts with immunoglobulin is termed anti-immunoglobulin (anti-Ig). The varieties of anti-Ig may be exemplified by the antibody produced by immunizing an animal with an antibody–antigen complex. An animal so immunized may produce (1) antibody that reacts with the antigen; (2) antibody that reacts with the antibody, but also reacts with normal immunoglobulin, for example, anti-H, anti-L, or anti-Fc; (3) antibody that reacts with the antibody–antigen complex, but not with either uncomplexed antibody or antigen (anticomplex); and (4) antibody that reacts with the antibody itself in native form, but does not react with other normal immunoglobulins. This latter specificity, which is limited to single species of proteins (antibody) within a large population of molecules (immunoglobulins), is termed an *idiotype*.

Anti-idiotypic antibodies may react with three major components of an antibody species: (1) the antigen-binding site itself (complementary determining region), (2) variable region structures away from the antigen-binding site, or (3) a combina-

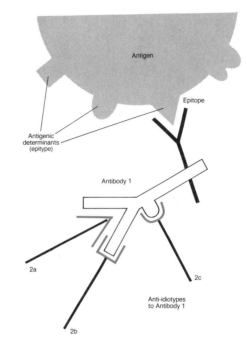

Figure 6-10. Anti-idiotypic antibodies to an antibody may react with the paratope (anti-idiotype 2a), with part of the paratope and part of the adjacent nonparatope variable region (anti-idiotype 2b), or with the nonparatope variable region (anti-idiotype 2c). The paratope of anti-idiotype 2a may mimic the antigen to which the original antibody reacts, and has been termed the *internal image* of the antigen. Anti-idiotype 2a will block the binding of the antigen to the antibody completely. Anti-idiotype 2b will block partially, and anti-idiotype 2c may not block at all unless the tertiary structure is changed by binding of anti-idiotype 2c.

tion of the two through an overlapping epitope (Fig. 6-10). The simplest explanation for the production of these anti-idiotypes is that anti-idiotypic antibodies are directed toward a site recognized as a foreign antigen because it is not present in detectable amounts in the normal immunoglobulin population. Sometimes different individuals will produce antibodies with the same idiotype when immunized with the same antigen (cross-reactive idiotype). Anti-idiotype to the antigen combining site (the paratope) will block reaction of the antibody with antigen and mimic the epitope of the antigen. Cross-reactive idiotypes often react with the antigen-binding site of the antibody. On the other hand, some anti-idiotypes do not interfere with the antigen-binding activity of the first antibody. Therefore, sites on the antibody not responsible for antigen binding but genetically codetermined with the antigen-binding site must be responsible (Fig. 6-11).

Complex Specificity

Anticomplex antibody is formed to new determinants revealed by alteration of the quaternary structure of the antibody, the antigen, or both as a result of formation of the antibody–antigen complex. This is similar to the determinants revealed by partial denaturation of immunoglobulins. Anticomplex antibody reacts with the antibody only when it is complexed with antigen. Anticomplex antibodies have been recognized that require the whole antibody molecule in complex form for reaction, whereas other anticomplex antibodies react with the Fab fragment of the complexed molecule.

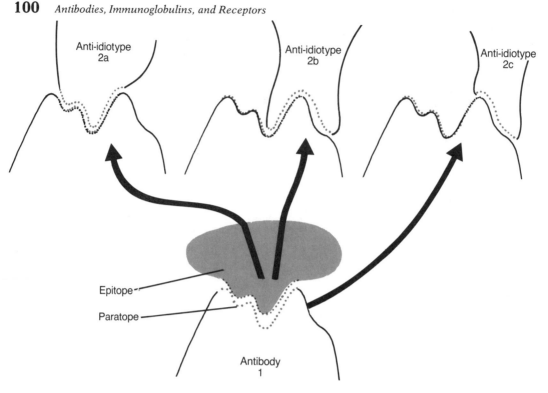

Figure 6-11. Paratopes, epitopes, and idiotopes. Depicted is an antibody combining site (paratope) and antigenic determinant (epitope) and types of anti-idiotypes. The antigen combining sites (paratopes) of anti-idiotypes are termed idiotopes. The idiotope of anti-idiotype 2a is essentially identical to the epitope of the antigen (molecular mimicry) and the mirror image of the paratope of antibody 1; the idiotope of anti-idiotype 2b shares some structures in common with the epitope, but not all; the idiotope of anti-idiotype 2c contains no structure in common with the epitope of the antigen, but contains mirror images of nonparatope regions of the antibody.

Human Immunoglobulin Allotypes

Immunoglobulin allotypes are genetic differences in the constant regions of H- or L-chains that are inherited in a codominant Mendelian pattern. Up to 30 different immunoglobulin allotypic specificities have been identified in humans. These are divided into three groups: the Gm, with up to 25 specificities; the Km, with three specificities; and allotypes restricted to IgA (Am) and IgM. The properties of these specificities are tabulated in Table 6-3. The Gm specificities are found only in IgG and are located on the γ-chain. Different specificities are found in the IgG subclasses and are inherited in fixed combinations. The Km specificities are located on the κ light chains of each immunoglobulin class and are determined by a single amino substitution at position 153 or 191 of the κ-chain.

Genetic Analysis of Human Gm Allotypes

Human immunoglobulin allotypic markers are highly specific, inbuilt, genetically determined labels that show strict adher-

Table 6-3. Some Representative Human Immunoglobulin Allotypes

Locus	Chain Location	Allotype	Amino Acid Residue
G1m	Cγ1 (CH1)	G1m (4)	Arg 214
		G1m (17)	Lys 214
	Cγ1 (CH3)	G1m (1)	Asp 356, Leu 358
		G1m (−1)	Glu 356, Met 358
G2m	Cγ2 (CH2)	G2m (23), G2m (23⁻)	N.D.
G3m	Cγ3 (CH2)	G3m (5)	N.D.
		G3m (5⁻)	N.D.
		G3m (15)	N.D.
		G3m (16)	N.D.
		G3m (21)	Tyr 296
		G3m (21⁻)	Phe 296
	Cγ3 (CH3)	G3m (6)	N.D.
		G3m (11)	Phe 436
		G3m (11⁻)	Tyr 436
		G3m (13)	
		G3m (14)	
G4m	Cγ4 (CH2)	G4m (4a)	Leu 309
		G4m (4b)	Gap at position 309
A2m	Cα2 (CH3)	A2m (1)	Phe 411, Asp 428, Val 458, Val 467
		A2m (2)	Thr 411, Glu 428, Ile 458, Ala 467
Km	Cκ	Km (1)	Val 153, Leu 191
		Km (1,2)	Ala 153, Leu 191
		Km (3)	Ala 153, Val 191

N.D., not determined.

ence to Mendelian law and are inherited as codominant alleles. The number of amino acid substitutions between two allelic allotypes is usually one, but at the most four. The known genetic markers are located on "constant" portions of the immunoglobulin chain. No human genetic marker has been found on the amino-terminal quarter of the H-chain or the amino-terminal half of the L-chain. Therefore, allotypic determinants are not involved in the antibody combining site.

The genes controlling Gm specificities are closely linked. Crossing-over between IgG genes has been directly observed in some family studies. The recombination frequencies have been estimated as follows: between IgG_1 and IgG_3, $1:1000$ to $1:10,000$; between IgG_1 and IgG_2, $1:100$ to $1:1000$. The higher frequency of recombinations suggests greater distance between the latter two loci. The IgG_4 gene may be next to that of IgG_2. This order is in agreement with linkage analysis and gene complexes in various population groups. The existence of a hybrid IgG_1–IgG_3 molecule in rare individuals is direct evidence for the existence of gene crossover or deletion.

Synthesis and Assembly of Immunoglobulins

Immunoglobulin molecules are synthesized, assembled, and secreted by plasma cells. This process is generally the same as synthesis of secretory proteins in other mammalian cells. Genetic information is encoded in DNA (deoxyribonucleic acid) of the nucleus and is transcribed into messenger RNA (ribonucleic acid). The messenger RNA molecules are released into the cytoplasm, where they become associated with a number of ribosomes to form a polyribosome. The polyribosome associated with rough endoplasmic reticulum is the basic unit of protein synthesis. The messenger RNA is translated, and the amino acids are linked into a polypeptide chain. When translation of the message is completed, the newly synthesized polypeptide is released into the lumen of rough endoplasmic reticulum, carbohydrate added, and the protein secreted.

The production of immunoglobulins by myelomas (plasma cell tumors) is the model system used to study immunoglobulin synthesis. L-chains and H-chains are produced on different-size ribosomes. H-chain polyribosomes contain 12–18 ribosomes, and L-chain polyribosomes 7 or 8. Newly synthesized L-chains enter a rapidly turning-over pool and then become associated with H-chains. Disulfide bonds usually form between free L-chains and H-chains still on the H-chain ribosome. However, assembly differs among different myelomas. In some cases, one L- and one H-chain are joined prior to formation of the inter-H-chain bond, whereas in others, the inter-H-chain bond forms first, followed by binding of the L-chains. Partially assembled molecules, such as half molecules of one L- and one H-chain joined together, may be formed, as well as L-chains alone (Bence Jones proteins) or H-chains alone (H-chain disease). However, normal lymphoid cells produce essentially equal numbers of L- and H-chains.

Immunoglobulin Gene Rearrangements

Synthesis of immunoglobulin by a given B lymphocyte is preceded by rearrangement of the immunoglobulin genes. In humans, H-chain genes are on chromosome No. 8, κ-chain genes are on chromosome No. 2, and λ-chain genes are on chromosome No. 22. The germ line DNA (Fig. 6-12) for the heavy and light chains of immunoglobulin contains multiple copies of variable region genes (V), joining region genes (J), and constant region genes (C). In addition heavy chain genes contain a diversity or "D" region. During B cell maturation, deletion of intervening sequences occurs between V and J or V and D and J, so the immunoglobulin-producing plasma cell contains DNA with juxtaposition of VJ or VDJ genomic regions required for encoding a given heavy or light chain. These rearrangements delete V region genes and J region genes that are not needed, and also bring together the V region promoter site and the J region enhancing site, which makes the new V–J–C

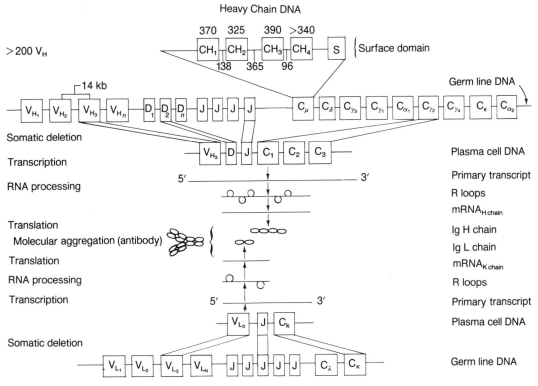

Figure 6-12. Immunoglobulin gene rearrangements associated with Ig synthesis by B cells. The example depicted has a μ_2 heavy chain and a κ light chain. The detailed genetic structure for the μ_2-chain constant regions, including four constant region domains and a sequence believed to be present on IgM molecules on the cell surface, is shown above the heavy chain germ line DNA. The numbers indicate the numbers of base pairs in each segment. The D region may also contribute to diversity by providing different sequences between V_H and J. During B cell development into an Ig synthesizing plasma cell the germ line DNA undergoes rearrangement so that one V_H region is combined with a set of constant region genes through deletion of the intervening sequences. The final mixture of mRNA is translated into the polypeptide chain including the short hydrophobic leader peptide responsible for transmembrane passage of the immunoglobulin, which is cleaved off during secretion.

transcriptionally active. Transcription of this genomic sequence results in production of a primary nuclear RNA transcript containing the base sequences necessary for translation into the protein chain (exons), separated by untranslated intervening sequences (introns). The introns are removed during RNA processing, resulting in a translationally active messenger RNA molecule. In a given plasma cell only one type of light chain and one type of heavy chain are synthesized. These then combine in the cytoplasm and are secreted as a four-chain immunoglobulin antibody molecule.

In order to attain a productive gene rearrangement DNA sequences between V and J must be removed. These sequences are flanked by a specific set of nucleic acids that match a homologous set of nucleotides (palindrome) to form a stem-and-loop:

$$-CACTGTG-$$
$$-GTGACAC-$$

A palindrome is a sequence that reads the same backward as forward (e.g., "Madam, I'm Adam"). Through this mechanism a loop of DNA is formed and chopped off (Fig. 6-13), which permits the splicing together of the DNA regions coding for V and J. All immunoglobulin-producing B cells and plasma cells

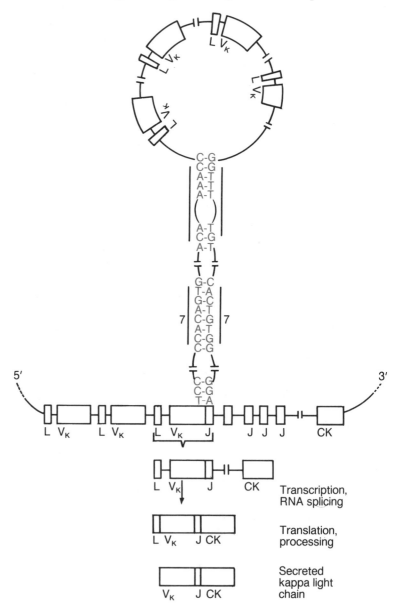

Figure 6-13. Model of V_H/J joining during immunoglobulin gene rearrangement. L = leader sequence, V_κ = kappa variable region, J = joining region, C_κ = constant region of κ light chains. Intervening L and V_κ regions are cut out as a loop formed from a stem structure of palindromic nucleotides on the 3′ end of the variable region that occur in reverse order on the 5′ end of the J region (red). DNA located between the V_κ and J region is deleted. Similar looping allows the J region to be spliced next to the C region so that the mRNA will be translated with the V_κ, J, and C_κ regions together.

must have rearranged immunoglobulin genes in order to produce immunoglobulins. To be productive the immunoglobulin genes must be rearranged correctly. In B cell differentiation, heavy chain genes appear to be rearranged before light chain genes and both κ genes appear to be rearranged before λ genes. If both κ genes are rearranged, only one will be a correct productive rearrangement (allelic exclusion). Each B cell usually produces one L-chain, which will be either κ or λ. The nonexpressed genes either will be in the germ line arrangement or will be aberrantly rearranged or deleted. The heavy chain genes are rearranged in a manner similar to the light chain genes. The heavy chains contain an additional region, the D region, which is incorporated into the V region of the heavy chain as V–D–J–C.

Cell Surface Immunoglobulin

In addition to serum antibodies, immunoglobulins also serve as cell surface antigen receptors for B cells. The mRNAs for the membrane and secreted forms of IgM are transcribed from the same gene, but the message for membrane IgM is processed differently, resulting in two additional carboxy-terminal exons coding for (1) a hydrophobic amino acid sequence that holds the molecule in the membrane lipid, and (2) a hydrophilic carboxy-terminal end on the cytoplasmic side (Fig. 6-14). The two

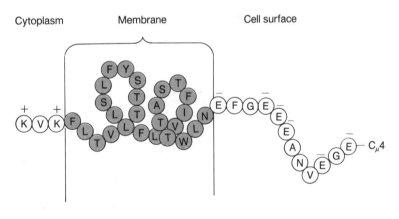

Figure 6-14. Configuration of the IgM membrane segment in the cell membrane. The μ chain is anchored in the cell membrane by the membrane (M) segment. The uncharged 26-residue sequence in the M segment is an α-helix spanning the membrane, depicted by the coiled segment in the diagram. Positive and negative charged residues that flank the transmembrane sequence are indicated.

forms of IgM are designated IgM_s (serum IgM) and IgM_m (membrane IgM) and the heavy chains μ_s and μ_m. The μ_m mRNA is assembled identically to the μ_s mRNA except that the additional coding segment containing the M polypeptide remains attached to the $C\mu4$ gene with an intervening sequence cut out during RNA processing (Fig. 6-15). This results in a mRNA for μ_m with an additional M polypeptide of 41 residues, 26 of which are uncharged and represent the hydrophobic membrane domain (Fig. 6-14).

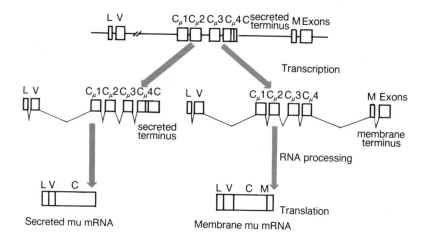

Figure 6-15. Splicing of μ_s and μ_m mRNAs. The expressed μ gene as shown has been constructed by a $V_H/D_H/J_H$ rearrangement. L = DNA coding for the signal (leader) peptide; V = V_H region; $C\mu 1$, $C\mu 2$, $C\mu 3$, and $C\mu 4$ = four constant coding segments; M = DNA for the membrane segment; Exons = 3' untranslated sequence; CT = the terminal segment of μ_s. The choice of the 3' coding segments to give μ_s or μ_m is made at the level of RNA transcription, processing, and splicing. The bent lines indicate RNA splicing between exons.

Differentiation of B Cells and Expression of Immunoglobulin

During antigen-driven maturation of B cells to plasma cells a switch in immunoglobulin class expression occurs. Most B cells express IgM and IgD on the surface. Antigen stimulation results in the appearance of B cells restricted to surface expression of one of the other immunoglobulin classes, IgG, IgA, or IgE. This is accomplished by recombination between repetitive DNA sequence elements (Fig. 6-16). Ig class switching occurs

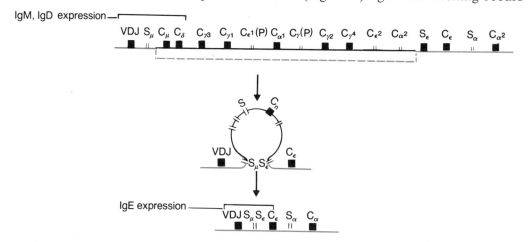

Figure 6-16. Immunoglobulin class (isotype) switching. Depicted is the sequence of constant gene regions of the immunoglobulin heavy chains of the human ($C\mu$, $C\delta$, $C\gamma$, etc). In the B cell, IgM and IgD are expressed. This expressing correlates with the juxtaposition of the VDJ region next to $C\mu$ and $C\delta$. When a cell line switches to IgE expression there is looping between the switch regions of $C\mu$ ($S\mu$) and $C\epsilon_1$ ($S\epsilon_1$) with deletion of the intervening genes. (P) refers to pseudogenes.

by genetic recombinations between switch regions that lie in front of each constant region gene. The switch regions are as long as 1600 nucleotides and contain repetitive sequences that permit "looping out" of the intervening sequences by palindromic heterodimer formation. In B cell differentiation a switch from a pre-B cell expressing μ and δ to another class is accomplished by genetic recombination between the switch region lying before $C\mu$ and that lying before the $C\gamma$ or $C\alpha$ or $C\epsilon$ region to be expressed. The arrangement of the heavy chain genes also permits switching from one upstream C_H gene to another, for example, from $C\gamma1$ to $C\gamma2$ or from a $C\gamma1$ to $C\epsilon$ with deletion of the intervening DNA. Two observations must be reconciled with this mechanism. First, occasional "back switching" may occur. In this situation a cell line expressing IgA may revert to expression of IgM. This may be explained by recombination of the other chromosome, by a mechanism that permits functional looping out without deletion and reestablishment of the original sequence, or by mRNA processing. Second, cells that express two or three isotypes at the same time are often found, usually μ and δ with another class. This may be explained by cells in transition from one class to another or by control of class switching during RNA processing.

A model for B cell maturation and generation of immunoglobulin class constant region (isotype) diversity is illustrated in Figure 6-17. There are two major phases of B cell develop-

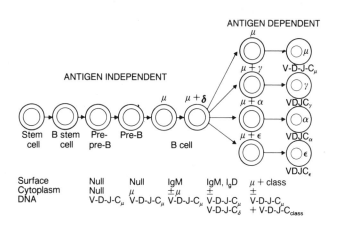

Figure 6-17. A model of B cell differentiation (for a description, see the text).

ment: antigen independent and antigen dependent. B cell maturation from a multipotent hematopoietic stem cell (see Fig. 4-1) to mature B cells expressing cell surface IgM and IgD is believed to be antigen independent. By rearranging a given V–D–J combination the antigen-recognizing specificity of the B cell may be determined at these steps before antigen enters the system. The first identifiable cell in the B cell lineage is the *pre-pre-B cell*, in which rearrangement of immunoglobulin heavy chain genes with juxtaposition of $V_H - D - J - C\mu$ has occurred but rearrangement of the light chain genes has not. The pre-pre-B cell does not express either cytoplasmic or cell surface immunoglobulin. The next cell, the *pre-B cell*, expresses cytoplasmic μ-chains but not cell surface immunoglobulin and still has not rearranged or expressed light chain genes. Immature *B cells* have rearranged heavy and light chain genes and express both. They exist in two classes, those that express cell surface IgM only and those that express cell surface IgM and IgD. Upon antigenic stimulation and given appropriate signals from helper T cells (see Chapter 10), B cells proliferate to expand the clone and differentiate into plasma cells that express the same $V - D - J$ combination as before but may now use a different constant region gene, which results in the same antigen recognition specificity but a different isotype (IgG, IgA, or IgE) or subclass of the secreted antibody molecule. Plasma cells have little surface immunoglobulin, but rapidly synthesize and secrete antibody of only one immunoglobulin class.

T Cell Receptor Expression

Similarities between T cell receptor domains and immunoglobulin domains indicate their common origin by duplication of a common ancestral gene. In contrast to antibody molecules as receptors for B cells, the receptor(s) on the T cell for antigen recognition has been difficult to characterize at the protein level. However, extensive structural studies of the T cell receptor have been possible through recombinant DNA methods. The specificity of recognition of antigen implies that the T cell receptor could be like an immunoglobulin molecule, but monoclonal antibodies to immunoglobulin epitopes do not react with T cells. In addition, T cells do not contain mRNA that hybridizes with cDNA probes for immunoglobulin. Three approaches have shed considerable light on the T cell receptor: (1) generation of T cell clones that produce homogeneous receptors, (2) production of monoclonal antibodies to T cell receptors, and (3) development of cDNA probes for the T cell receptor mRNA. Monoclonal antibodies have permitted isolation of an MW 80,000 – 90,000 heterodimer T cell receptor from T cell lines that contains an acidic (α) chain and a basic (β) chain (Fig. 6-18). Monoclonal antibodies to this receptor can activate T cells to proliferate. This receptor is quite variable among different T cell lines. It contains idiotypes and has constant and variable regions similar to those of immunoglobulin. The α and β chains are very different and are coded for by different genes. The DNA of T cells shows gene rearrangements in the genes for the T cell receptor that are characteristic of each T cell clone, similar to what occurs for immunoglobulin genes in plasma cells producing immunoglobulin. Sequence data from many clones have shown additional similarities be-

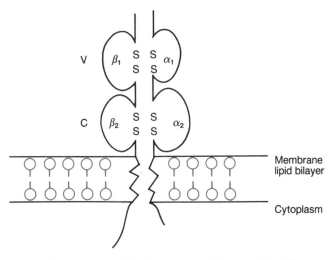

Figure 6-18. The T cell receptor contains extracellular, transmembrane, and cytoplasmic domains. It is a heterodimer of two polypeptide chains α and β. The β-chain contains variable and constant regions. The α-chain has not been well characterized.

tween B cell immunoglobulin expression and T cell receptor expression (Fig. 6-19). No clear correlation exists between T

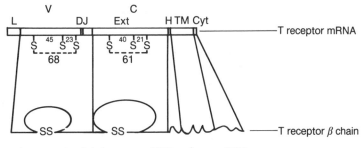

Figure 6-19. Gene rearrangements and predicted protein structure of the β-chain subunit of the T cell receptor indicate similarities to immunoglobulin gene expression. L = leader, D = diversity, J = joining, V = variable, C = constant, Ext = external, H = hinge, T$_M$ = transmembrane, and Cyt = cytoplasmic. VDJ joining of genomic DNA and processing of transcripted RNA to form mRNA are similar to those of immunoglobulin genes. (Modified from Davis M, et al: Immunol Rev 8:235, 1984.)

cell receptor gene rearrangement and major histocompatibility complex (MHC) expression.

Origin of Immunoglobulin Gene Diversity

Two major mechanisms have been hypothesized to account for the great diversity seen in immunoglobulin molecules: germ line (evolution) and somatic mutation.

Germ Line

On the basis of comparison of the immunoglobulins of different species, it is postulated that a primitive immunoglobulin gene coding for a peptide chain equal in length to one-half of an L-chain developed in the prevertebrate era. The most primitive immunoglobulins yet found in vertebrates consist of fully developed L- and H-chains. The genes responsible for fully developed chains are believed to have evolved through gene

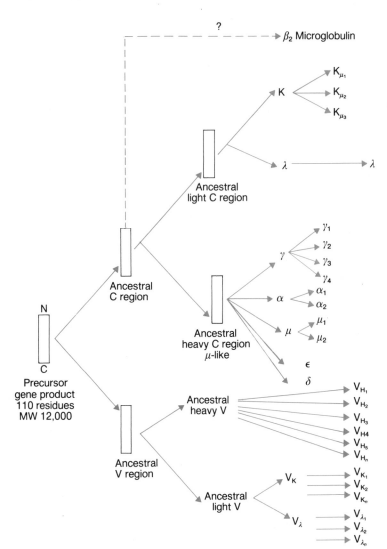

Figure 6-20. Immunoglobulin genes may have evolved from a single precursor gene by duplication and mutation. This has resulted in multiple V_H, V_κ, and V_λ genes in the different chromosomes that combine with a limited member of C_H, C_κ and C_λ genes to form the transcribed gene for the immunoglobulin mRNA.

duplication (Fig. 6-20). One duplication would result in a gene for a complete L-chain (constant and variable regions). Additional duplications would be required for production of a polypeptide chain the length of the H chain (four primitive units). A subsequent duplication of the L-chain gene would result in two L-chains, κ and λ. The most primitive H-chain identified (cyclostomes) is homologous to the μ-chain of IgM. Further gene duplication and divergence in teleosts and amphibians resulted in a gene coding for a chain homologous to the γ-chain of IgG. The α-, δ- and ϵ-chains may have resulted from further duplication of the μ-like ancestral gene chain gene. Later duplication of the γ-chain resulted in evolution of the IgG subclasses. This scheme is highly speculative and is dependent mainly on the observation that the L-chain consists of two MW 12,000 units (variable and constant regions) and the H-chain consists of four

MW 12,000 units (one variable region similar to that of the L-chain and three constant regions). Thus duplication of a gene coding for a MW 12,000 polypeptide chain could account for the evolution of human immunoglobulins.

It is not clear, however, how such duplication could lead to the genetic information required for the vast numbers of V_H and V_L regions needed for the many antigenic building sites possible. To account for these many specificities, further gene modification by somatic mutation is postulated.

Somatic Mutation

According to the somatic mutation theories, a small number of germ line genes become highly diversified during development of the individual, resulting in the formation of a large number of differentiated immunocompetent cells capable of individually recognizing a variety of antigens. This may be accomplished by point mutations occurring successively, perhaps through the influence of antigenic contact or by recombination of inherited germ line V genes during somatic cell division. The basic genetic information is probably derived from germ line diversity developed during evolution, and additional diversity arises during somatic development.

The complexity of the immunoglobulin genes permits great potential for generation of diversity. For instance in the heavy chain three segments of DNA, V_H, D, and J, must be joined together to assemble a gene coding for the entire variable region of the heavy chain. The D (diversity) region segments frequently have more than one open coding frame permitting several amino acid sequences to be produced by a single gene sequence. The D_H sequence codes for a sizable part of the third hypervariable region of the V_H domain. In this position it plays a major part in antibody specificity and is often recognized as an idiotype. The three segments, $V_H/D_H/J_H$, can use several frames for recombination, providing a molecular basis for diversity.

Summary

Antibodies are glycoprotein molecules that have the capacity to bind specifically to an antigen. Antibodies belong to a group of structurally related molecules termed *immunoglobulins*. There are five major classes of immunoglobulins with different biological properties. The basic immunoglobulin molecule consists of two pairs of polypeptide chains joined by disulfide bonds. Each chain contains regions of variable amino acid sequences and regions of constant amino acid sequences. This provides the uniqueness required for binding to different antigens and the commonality needed for the biological function of each immunoglobulin class. The genes coding for the two chains of immunoglobulin (heavy and light chains) are located on different chromosomes. The variable region genes (up to 500) and constant region genes (1 per subclass of Ig) are rearranged during development of B cells so that one V_H and one C_H region are joined in a productive sequence. During antigen-stimulated B cell development the same variable region may be joined to different constant region genes — "isotype switching." T cells also have receptors whose expression is controlled by similar mechanisms. This permits great diversity in antigen binding. One V_H region may be joined to different C_H regions in different cells and V_H regions may be altered by the process of rearrangement to permit different amino acid substitutions.

References

General

Kindt TS, Capra JD: The Antibody Enigma. New York, Plenum, 1984.

Nisonoff A: Introduction to Molecular Immunology. Sunderland, Mass., Sinauer Assoc., 1982.

Immunoglobulins

Cohen S, Milstein C: Structure and biologic properties of immunoglobulins. Adv Immunol 7:1, 1967.

Committee on Nomenclature of Human Immunoglobulins: Notation for genetic factors of human immunoglobulins. Bull WHO 30:447, 1964.

Edelman GM, Cunningham BA, Gall WE, Gottlieb PD, Rutishauser U, Waxdal MD: The covalent structure of an entire γ-immunoglobulin molecule. Biochemistry 63:78, 1969.

Fahey JL: Antibodies and immunoglobulins. JAMA 194:141, 183, 1966.

Franklin EC: Immune globulins: their structure and function and some techniques for their isolation. Prog Allergy 8:58, 1964.

Halpern MS, Koshland ME: The stoichiometry of J chain in human secretory IgA. J Immunol 111:1563–1660, 1973.

Kabat EA: General features of antibody molecules. *In* Pressman D, Tomasi TB, Jr, Grossberg AL, Rose NR (eds): Specific Receptors of Antibodies, Antigens and Cells. Basel, Karger, 1973.

Merler E, Rosen FS: The gamma globulins. I. The structure and synthesis of the immunoglobulins. N Engl J Med 275:480–536, 1964.

Metzer H: The chemistry of the immunoglobulins. JAMA 202:129, 1967.

Osserman EF, Takatsuki K: Plasma cell myeloma: gamma globulin synthesis and structure. Medicine 42:357, 1963.

Painter RH: The C1q receptor site on human immunoglobulin G. Can J Biochem Cell Biol 62:418, 1984.

Rowe DS, Hug K, Forni L, Pernis B: Immunoglobulin D as a lymphocyte receptor. J Exp Med 138:965, 1973.

Scharff MD, Laskov R: Synthesis and assembly of immunoglobulin polypeptide chains. Prog Allergy 14:37, 1970.

Silverton EW, Navia MA, Davies DR: Three dimensional structure of an intact human immunoglobulin. Proc Nat Acad Sci USA 74:5140, 1977.

Speigelberg HL: D Immunoglobulin. *In* Inman FP (ed): Contemporary Topics in Immunochemistry. New York, Plenum, 1972, pp165–180.

Spiegelberg HL: Biological activities of immunoglobulins of different classes and subclasses. Adv Immunol 19:259, 1974.

Tomasi TB, Bienenstock J: Secretory immunoglobulins. Adv Immunol 9:1, 1968.

Thorebecke GJ, Leslie GA (eds): Immunoglobulin D: Structure and Function. New York, Academy of Science, 1982.

Wilkelhake JL: Immunoglobulin structure and effector functions. Immunochemistry 15:695, 1978.

Antibody Structure

Bernier GM: Structure of human immunoglobulins: myeloma proteins as analogues of antibody. Prog Allergy 14:1, 1970.

Capra JD, Edmundson AB: The antibody combining site. Sci Am 236:50, 1977.

Givol D: Structural analysis of the antibody containing site. *In* Reisfeld R, Mandy W (eds): Contemporary Topics in Molecular Immunology. New York, Plenum, 1973, p27.

Gottlieb PD: Immunoglobulin genes. Mol Immunol 17:1423, 1980.

Green NM: Electron microscopy of the immunoglobulins. Adv Immunol 11:1, 1969.

Kabat EA: Origins of antibody complementarity and specificity— hypervariable regions and the minigene hypothesis. J Immunol 125:96, 1980.

Marquart M, Deisenhofer J, Huber R, Palm W: Crystallographic refinement and atomic models of the intact immunoglobulin molecule Ko1 and its antigen binding fragment at 3.0 Å and 1.9 Å resolution. J Mol Biol 141:369, 1980.

Novotony J, et al: Molecular anatomy of the antibody binding site. J Biol Chem 258:14433, 1983.

Ohno S, Mori N, Matsunaga T: Antigen binding specificities of antibodies are primarily determined by seven residues of V_H. Proc Nat Acad Sci USA 82:2945, 1985.

Padlan EA: Structural basis for the specificity of antibody–antigen reactions and structural mechanisms for the diversification of antigen-binding specificities. Rev Biophys 10:35, 1977.

Svehag SE, Bloth B: Ultrastructure of secretory and high-polymer serum immunoglobulin A of human and rabbit origin. Science 168:847, 1970.

Talmadge DW, Cann JR: The Chemistry of Immunity in Health and Disease. Springfield, Ill., Thomas, 1961.

Allotypes and Idiotypes

Bankert RB, Bloor AG, Jou Y-H: Idiotypes, their presence on B- and T-lymphocytes and their role in the regulation of the immune response. Vet Immunol Immunopathol 3:147, 1982.

Brient BW, Nisonoff A: Quantitative investigations of idiotypic antibodies. IV. Inhibition of specific haptens of the reaction of anti-hapten antibody with its anti-idiotypic antibody. J Exp Med 132:951, 1970.

Davis J, et al: Structural correlates of idiotypes 4:147, 1986.

Fudenberg HH, Pink JRL, Stites DP, Wang A-C: Basic Immunogenetics. New York, Oxford University Press, 1972.

Kelus AS, Cell PGH: Immunoglobulin allotypes of experimental animals. Prog Allergy 11:141, 1967.

Kohler H, Urbain J, Cazenave P (eds): Idiotypes in Biology and Medicine. Orlando, Fla., Academic Press, 1984.

Grubb R: The genetic markers of human immunoglobulins. *In* Kleinzeller A, Springer GF, Whittmann HC (eds): Molecular Biology, Biochemistry, and Biophysics, Vol 9. Berlin, Springer, 1970.

Moller G (ed): Anti-idiotypic antibodies as immunogens. Immunol Rev 90, 1986.

Moller G (ed): Idiotype networks. Immunol Rev 79, 1984.

Natvig JB, Kunkel HG: Genetic markers of human immunoglobulins: the Gm and InV systems. Semin Hematol 1:66, 1968.

Natvig JB, Kunkel HG: Human immunoglobulins: classes, subclasses, genetic variants and idiotypes. Adv Immunol 16:1, 1973.

Rajewsky K, Takemori T: Genetics, expression and function of idiotypes. Annu Rev Immunol 1:569, 1983.

Rodkey LS: Autoregulation of the immune response via idiotype network interaction. Microbiol Rev 44:631, 1980.

Immunoglobulin Genes

Calame KL: Mechanisms that regulate immunoglobulin gene expression. Annu Rev Immunol 3:159, 1985.

Cushley W, Williamson AR: Expression of immunoglobulin genes. Essays Biochem 18:1, 1982.

Honjo T: Immunoglobulin genes. 1:499, 1983.

Hood L, Campbell JH, Elgin SCR: The organization, expression, and evolution of antibody genes and other multigene families. Annu Rev Genet 9:305, 1975.

Moller G (ed): Molecular aspects of V genes. Immunol Rev 36, 1977.

Moller G (ed): Control of immunoglobulin gene expression. Immunol Rev 89, 1986.

Seidman JG, Leder A, Nau M, Norman B, Leder P: Antibody diversity. The structure of cloned immunoglobulin genes suggests a mechanism for generating new sequences. Science 202:11, 1978.

Wall R, Kuehl M: Biosynthesis and regulation of immunoglobulins. Annu Rev Immunol 1:393, 1983.

Yancopoulos CD, Alt F: Regulation and expression of variable region genes. Annu Rev Immunol 4:339, 1986.

B Cell Differentiation and Ig Expression

Brandtzaeg P: Role of J chain and secretory component in receptor mediated glandular and hepatic transport of immunoglobulins in man. Scand J Immunol 22:111, 1985.

Cebra JJ, Komisar JL, Schweitzer PA: C_H isotype switching during normal B cell development. Annu Rev Immunol 2:493, 1984.

Moller G (ed): B cell differentiation antigens. Immunol Rev 69, 1983.

Nossal CJV, Szenberg A, Ada CL, Austin G: Single cell studies in antibody production. J Exp Med 119:485, 1964.

Parkhouse RME, Cooper MD: A model for the differentiation of B lymphocytes with implications for the biological role of IgD. Immunol Rev 37:105, 1977.

Sell S: Development of restrictions in the expression of immunoglobulin specificities by lymphoid cells. Transplant Rev 5:19, 1970.

Whitlock C, Denis K, Robertson D, Witte O: In vitro analysis of B cell development. Annu Rev Immunol 3:213, 1985.

T Cell Receptor

Binz H, Lindeman J, Wigzell H: Cell-bound receptors for alloantigens on normal lymphocytes. II. Antialloantibody serum contains specific factors reacting with relevant immunocompetent T lymphocytes. J Exp Med 140:731, 1974.

Cosenza H, Kohler H: Specific suppression of the antibody response by antibodies to receptors. Proc Nat Acad Sci USA 69:2710, 1972.

Delisi C, Berzofsky JA: T-cell antigenic sites tend to be amphipathic structures. Proc Nat Acad Sci USA 82:7048, 1985.

Kronenberg M, Siu G, Hood L, Shastri N: The molecular genetics of the T cell antigen receptor and T cell antigen recognition. Annu Rev Immunol 4:529, 1986.

Meuer SC, et al: The human T cell receptor. Annu Rev Immunol 2:23, 1984.

Moller G (ed): Idiotypes on T and B cells. Immunol Rev 34, 1977.

Moller G (ed): T cell receptors and genes. Immunol Rev 81, 1984.

Watts TH, Gariepy J, Schoolnik GK, McConnel HM: T cell activation by peptide antigen: effect of peptide sequence and method of antigen presentation. Proc Nat Acad Sci USA 82:5480, 1985.

Weiss A, et al: The role of the T3/Ti antigen receptor complex in T cell activation. Annu Rev Immunol 4:593, 1986.

Generation of Diversity

Burnet FM: The Clonal Selection Theory of Acquired Immunity. Nashville, Tenn., Vanderbilt University Press, 1959.

Cohen EP: On the mechanism of immunity: in defense of evolution. Annu Rev Microbiol (Stanford) 22:283, 1968.

Gally JA, Edelman GM: Genetic control of immunoglobulin synthesis. Annu Rev Genet 6:1, 1972.

Grey HM: Phylogeny of immunoglobulins. Adv Immunol 10:51, 1969.

Hood L, Talmadge DW: Mechanism of antibody diversity: germ line basis for variability. Science 168:325, 1970.

Matsunaga T: Evolution of antibody diversity. Somatic mutation as a late event. Dev Exp Immunol 9:585, 1985.

Milstein C, Pink JRL: Structure and evolution of immunoglobulins. Prog Biophys Mol Biol 21:211, 1970.

7 | Antigen–Antibody Reactions

Antibodies are defined by their ability to react specifically with antigen. Antibody molecules are made up of constant parts, which are responsible for the biological properties of the different classes, and variable parts, which are responsible for the ability to react with and bind to antigen. The antigen-binding site or *paratope* is formed by the folding and special arrangement of hypervariable regions of the heavy and light chains of the immunoglobulin molecule. A molecular site (paratope) is formed, which permits close juxtaposition of amino acid chains and other short range reactions of the antigen-binding site of the antibody and the antigenic determinant *(epitope)* of the antigen. An antigenic determinant or epitope is defined as that part of the antigen molecule that reacts with antibody (see Chapter 5).

Polyfunctional Antibody (Cross-Reactions)

A single antibody species may be able to react with more than one antigenic determinant. This is possible if the configuration of the antigen-binding site has the flexibility or capability to fit, and bind, to small parts of structurally different antigenic determinants. The nature of polyfunctional antigen combining sites of antibody is depicted in Figure 7-1. The activity of polyfunc-

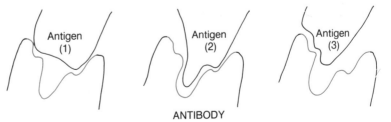

Figure 7-1. A single molecular species of antibody, termed *polyfunctional antibody,* may be able to react with seemingly different antigenic determinants that show some configurations recognizable by the antibody molecule. In this figure, antigens 1, 2, and 3 are different but each has a structure that is recognized by some part of the antigen combining site of the antibody (paratope, outlined in red).

117

tional antibodies helps explain the vast number of different antigens to which an individual can produce antibody. Antibody stimulated by one antigen may also cross-react with another antigen because of shared parts of the antigenic determinants or circumstantial fitting of the antibody-binding site to other antigens. Experimentally this is measured as the "cross-reaction" of the antibody with a seemingly unrelated second antigen.

Monoclonal Antibodies

The degree of complexity of the antigen-binding specificity of antibody is exemplified by the study of monoclonal antibodies (Fig. 7-2). Monoclonal antibodies may be produced by anti-

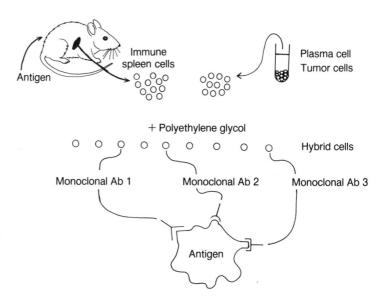

Figure 7-2. Each monoclonal antibody is the product of a single cell line produced by fusion of spleen cells from an immunized animal with cells from a plasma cell tumor. Hybrid cells with the capacity to produce and secrete a single molecular species of antibody can be produced, identified, isolated, and maintained in long-term culture. Since each individual antibody-producing hybridoma cell line produces antibody of only one specificity, more complete analysis of the possible antigenic determinant of an antigen is possible than with the mixtures of antibodies of different specificities produced by active immunization of the whole animal.

body-producing cells fused with tumors of plasma cells (myelomas). Most myeloma proteins do not react with known antigens. Monoclonal antibodies are engineered by fusion in vitro of lymphoid cells from an immunized animal with non-immunoglobulin-producing plasma cell tumor lines that have all the machinery necessary for antibody production and secretion, and also confer the ability for continuous growth in culture. Clones of hybrid cells are grown from single fused cells in vitro. Some of these cloned cell lines will retain the proliferative capacity of the tumor cell line and will also acquire the ability to produce specific antibodies coded for by the chromosomes of the cells from the immunized animal. Since each antibody-producing clone makes only one *(monoclonal)* antibody, characterization of the specificity of the reaction of a number of monoclonal antibodies to the same antigen leads to an understanding of the range of specificities produced by the immunized animal. In this way, the number and relationship of the antigenic determinants of an immunogenic molecule may be more precisely determined than was previously possible with conventional polyclonal antisera.

Primary Antigen– Antibody Reaction

The combination of antibody with antigen to form an antibody–antigen complex is termed the *primary reaction*. The strength of the antibody–antigen bond is determined by the closeness of the geometric apposition of the antigen combining site with the antigenic determinant and the number and strength of bonds formed, including charge–charge, hydrogen, and hydrophilic bonds. The strength and specificity are determined by the complementarity of antibody and antigen. A tight fit is important because each bond acts at very short distance and is relatively weak, so that multiple bonds are needed to give a high-affinity interaction. The relationship between antibody and antigen has been likened to that of a lock (antibody) and key (antigen). The primary reaction of antibody (Ab) and antigen (Ag) may be expressed as an equilibrium reaction: $Ab + Ag \rightleftharpoons AgAb$.

Affinity and Avidity

The strength of the noncovalent bond between the paratope of an antibody and the epitope of an antigen is termed *affinity;* the strength of the bond formed between a complete (divalent) antibody and antigen is termed the *avidity*. The presence of two or more antigen-binding sites on an antibody will increase the functional strength of its binding to antigen over a univalent antibody fragment; the avidity of an antibody is dependent on the affinities of its individual antigen-binding sites. Since most antigens have multiple determinants and both paratopes of an antibody may react with the antigen, it is difficult to measure affinity and avidity separately. This can be done using hapten antigens in excess (see below).

Equilibrium Dialysis

The actual affinity constant of an antibody can be measured by equilibrium dialysis (Fig. 7-3). Given the antibody–antigen binding equation

$$Ag + Ab \underset{K_2}{\overset{K_1}{\rightleftharpoons}} AgAb,$$

in which K_1 and K_2 are the rate constants for the association and dissociation of the antigen and antibody, the affinity constant K of equilibrium is

$$K_A = \frac{[AgAb]}{[Ag][Ab]} = \frac{K_1}{K_2},$$

where the brackets indicate the concentrations of the antigen [Ag], the antibody [Ab], and the complex [AgAb]. Since K is an

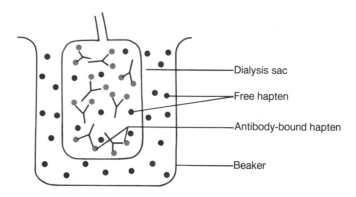

Dialysis sac

Free hapten

Antibody-bound hapten

Beaker

Figure 7-3. Equilibrium dialysis. A solution of antibody is placed inside a dialysis sac and the sac placed in a solution of free hapten. The dialysis sac is chosen to be permeable to the hapten but not to the antibody. Free hapten will dialyse into the sac where it will be bound by larger antibody. When the system reaches equilibrium the concentration of hapten in- side the sac will be equal to the concentration of free hapten outside the sac, plus the concentration of the hapten bound to the antibody inside the sac.

"association constant," it will be a large number ($>10^5$) for high affinity complexes and a small number ($<10^3$) for low affinity complexes.

The affinity of antibody for monovalent antigens (haptens) is determined by equilibrium dialysis from the relationship

$$r = Kn - Kcr$$

where r is the ratio of moles of hapten bound to moles of anti- body present, c is the concentration of unbound hapten, and n is the number of binding sides per antibody molecule. The moles of hapten bound are determined by subtracting the con-

Figure 7-4. Plot of $r/c \times 10^4$ versus r for a monovalent hapten and a divalent IgG antibody. The r intercept is 2, the number of hapten molecules bound to each an- tibody molecule at infinite concentrations of hapten. The average association constant $(K_0) = 3.5 \times 10^5$ liters/mole.

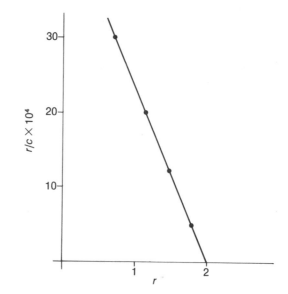

centration of hapten outside the dialysis sac from that within the sac containing the antibody. Since Kn is a constant, a plot of r/c versus r for different hapten concentrations (Fig. 7-4) will give a straight line with a slope of $-k$ and the valence of the antibody at the r intercept (infinite hapten concentration). Most antibodies have association constants from 10^5 to 10^{11} liters/mole, and most antibodies have a valence of 2.

The Farr Technique

A useful system for measuring the primary reaction of antibody and antigen was developed by Richard S. Farr. The principle of the Farr technique is the phase separation of bound antigen from free antigen. This assay forms the basis for many radioimmunoassays used for clinical and experimental quantification. The Farr procedure relies on the fact that the solubility properties of the AgAb complex may be different from those of the soluble antigen. The reaction used by Farr was that of bovine serum albumin (BSA) and rabbit antibody to BSA. The method relies on the fact that BSA is soluble in 50% saturated ammonium sulfate and that anti-BSA and BSA–anti-BSA complexes are not. The BSA is radiolabeled with ^{125}I or ^{131}I. The presence of radiolabeled BSA (*BSA) in the supernatant fluid or precipitate formed at 50% ammonium sulfate is determined by counting the radioactivity in each phase separately. Since the immunoglobulin antibody is precipitated at 50% ammonium sulfate normally, the *BSA bound to the antibody will precipitate along with the free antibody. The *BSA not attached to antibody, however, will remain soluble (Fig. 7-5). This method

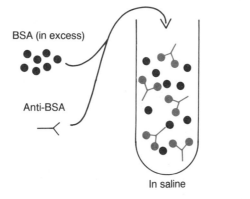
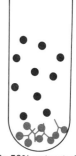

BSA (in excess)

Anti-BSA

In saline

In 50% saturated ammonium sulfate

Figure 7-5. This figure demonstrates the principle of the Farr assay. The mixture of bovine serum albumin (BSA) and anti-BSA in saline (BSA in excess) results in complexation of all the antibody molecules to antigen. The free BSA molecules and the complexes are soluble in saline. However, if ammonium sulfate is added to form a half-saturated solution, the soluble antibody–antigen complexes become insolu-ble. By determining the distribution of radiolabeled BSA (in the supernatant fluid or in the precipitate), the amount of specific antibody can be quantified.

can be used to quantitate the binding capacity of an anti-BSA antiserum or the amount of competing, unlabeled BSA present in an unknown solution.

Antigen-Binding Capacity

One way to estimate the avidity of an antibody is based on the ability of antibody at different dilutions to bind antigen. Antibody of strong avidity is able to bind antigen at high dilutions, whereas the binding of a weak antibody is quickly lost upon dilution. In general, antibodies obtained early after immunization (2–4 weeks) do not have the ability to bind antigen at high dilutions, whereas antibodies collected late after immunization continue to bind antigen at high dilutions.

The antigen-binding capacity of an antiserum is determined by diluting the antiserum with normal serum until 33% of a constant amount of *BSA is precipitated as BSA–anti-BSA complexes in 50% ammonium sulfate. The antibody-binding capacity (ABC33) is calculated from the dilution of antiserum that results in precipitation of 33% of the *BSA. It is expressed as micrograms of BSA bound per milliliter of antiserum. To make this calculation, the radioactivity of the *BSA must be converted to micrograms of BSA. (The specific activity of the *BSA must be known.)

The strength of an antibody–antigen reaction also depends on the stability of the antibody–antigen bond after a complex has been formed. This property is a measure of the dissociation of antibody–antigen complexes or, in other words, the reaction to the left of the equilibrium reaction $Ag + Ab \leftarrow AgAb$.

This reaction can be measured by adding excess unlabeled antigen (BSA) to preformed complexes of antibody and labeled antigen (anti-BSA–*BSA). If the antibody–antigen complex is strong, a long time will be required for the radiolabeled antigen to appear in the supernatant fluid, whereas radiolabeled antigen will be rapidly displaced from the AgAb complexes by unlabeled antigen if the antibody–antigen complex is weakly bound.

Secondary Antigen–Antibody Reactions

After the binding of antibody and antigen in vitro, a number of different phenomena may be observed. These are termed *secondary reactions* and depend upon the nature of the antigen, the properties of the antibody, and the presence of other factors such as complement. Secondary reactions include precipitation, agglutination, cytolysis, complement fixation, immobilization, and neutralization (Table 7-1).

In the older literature, the secondary effect of the antibody–antigen reaction was used to apply a functional name to an antiserum. Thus, an antibody in a serum that caused precipitation upon reaction with a soluble antigen was called a *precipitin*. Other terms include *hemolysin* (lysis of red blood

Table 7-1. Examples of Primary and Secondary Antigen–Antibody Reactions

Primary Reaction Ag + Ab ⇌	Secondary Reaction Ag Ab
Antigen-binding assays (Farr)	Precipitation
Equilibrium dialysis	Agglutination
Radioimmunoassays	Complement fixation
	Neutralization
	Opsonification
	Hemolysis
	Toxin neutralization
	Bacteriolysis
	Immune labeling of tissues

cells), *agglutinin* (agglutination of particulate antigens), and *opsonin* (enhancement of phagocytosis of the antigen). The terms do not imply exclusive functions of an antibody. A precipitin may also be a hemolysin, an agglutinin, or an opsonin, depending upon the secondary reaction used to measure it. The antigen used to elicit a secondary response was given the suffix *-ogen*. For example, an antigen used to elicit precipitation is called a *precipitogen*, one that is used to produce agglutination an *agglutinogen*, etc.

Precipitin Reaction

The precipitin reaction depends upon formation of an insoluble antibody–antigen complex upon reaction of soluble antibody and soluble antigen. Most naturally occurring circulating antibody molecules (except for IgM antibodies) contain two antigen-binding sites of identical specificity (are divalent), and most antigens contain more than two antigenic determinant sites (are multivalent). Thus, when multivalent antigens are mixed in the proper proportions with divalent antibodies, each antibody molecule usually combines with two antigen molecules. As antibody molecules connect molecules of soluble antigen, a lattice-like conglomeration of antigen molecules connected by antibody molecules occurs. This results in the formation of large aggregates, which become insoluble, because of a decrease in affinity for water as a result of the interaction of the solubilizing polar groups of the antigen and antibody and an increase in density of the aggregates. If the antigen is soluble, this reaction with antibody results in precipitation of the complex, and visible precipitates may be observed when the appropriate amounts of antibody and antigen are mixed. If the antigen is particulate (large enough to be visible by itself), agglutination of the particulate antigen occurs as the individual particles of antigen are joined together by the antibody. Both precipitation and agglutination can be seen with the naked eye.

Soluble Antibody–Antigen Complexes

If the antigen is soluble and contains one or two determinant sites (is monovalent or divalent as opposed to multivalent), precipitation does not occur and soluble complexes are formed. Similar soluble antibody–antigen complexes are formed if the antibody is monovalent (Fab fragment) and the antigen multivalent. In these last two situations the number of combining sites of antigen or antibody is insufficient for a lattice-like structure to be built up.

Nonprecipitating (soluble) antibody–antigen complexes are also formed if the proportions of soluble antigen and specific antibody are such that a latticelike conglomeration of antibody and antigen is not formed. This situation exists in reactions where antigen or antibody is in excess. At antigen excess, each divalent antibody reacts with two separate multivalent antigen molecules, and there are not enough antibody molecules to form larger complexes. The complexes formed consist of only two antigen molecules and one antibody molecule. A complex of this size may not be large enough to be insoluble. Similarly, at antibody excess, each binding site of a multivalent antigen molecule is occupied by a separate antibody molecule, and not enough antigen sites are available for a divalent antibody molecule to join or bridge two antigen molecules. The resulting complex consists of one antigen molecule and the number of antibody molecules sufficient to cover its antigenic sites. Such a complex may not be of a form or size to be insoluble, and a soluble antigen–antibody complex is the result.

Quantitative Precipitin Reaction

A precipitin reaction may be divided into three zones in relation to increasing amounts of antigen (Fig. 7-6): (1) zone of antibody excess—free antibody remains after all the antigen sites are covered by the antibody and soluble complexes are formed; (2) zone of equivalence—the amount of antigen is sufficient to bind all or most of the antibody so that the antigen–antibody complexes are insoluble and precipitate, with little or no unbound antibody or antigen remaining in soluble form; and (3) zone of antigen excess—the amount of antigen is sufficient to bind all the antibody to the extent that few, if any, antibody molecules can bind two antigen molecules together so that soluble complexes are formed.

Early tests for antibody activity depended upon effects such as neutralization of toxins, lysis, or agglutination of bacteria, which gave endpoints in the dilution of the antiserum that was still effective. The results of such tests were expressed as titers (dilutions). Expression of the activity of an antiserum as a titer or the highest dilution effective for a certain secondary reaction does not actually indicate the quantity of antibody present. For example, comparisons of titers of antipneumococcal sera and antityphoid sera cannot be made directly because the biological endpoints are different. Although the titer (effective dilution) of one antiserum may be higher than that of an-

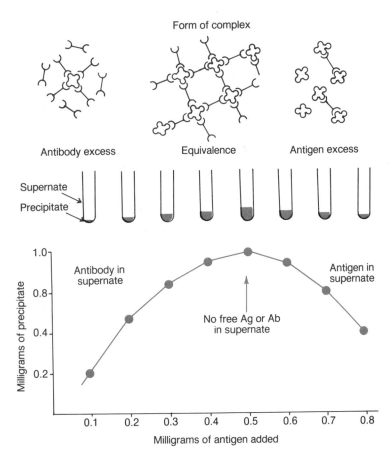

Figure 7-6. The quantitative precipitin reaction. If increasing amounts of antigen are separately added to constant amounts of antiserum, an increase in the amount of precipitate occurs to the maximum point. Further addition of antigen results in a decrease in the amount of total precipitate. This phenomenon is due to formation of antibody–antigen complexes of different compositions. At antibody excess, all the antigenic determinants are covered with antibody and no determinants are available for an antibody to form a bridge between two molecules of antigen. At equivalence, divalent antibodies bind antigenic determinants on different antigen molecules to produce a latticelike structure, which becomes insoluble. At antigen excess, each antibody molecule binds two antigen molecules together to form a lattice. At the point of maximum precipitation, all antibody and antigen should be in the precipitate (equivalence zone). If the antigen is a sugar the amount of antibody can be determined by measuring the amount of protein in the total precipitate formed.

other antiserum, much more antibody may be required to agglutinate or neutralize one kind of microorganism than another. Therefore, a direct comparison of titers in different systems is not possible.

The quantitative precipitin reaction permits measurement of antibody on a weight basis (Fig. 7-6). A series of test tubes each containing the same amount of antiserum is prepared. Increasing amounts of antigen of known quantity are added to this series of test tubes. At the equivalence zone, all of the antibody and all of the antigen added precipitate. The quantity of protein in the precipitate is determined by chemical or spectrophotometric measurement. Since the amount of antigen added is known, this quantity can be subtracted from the value of total precipitate to determine the amount of specific antibody present. The validity of this technique depends upon at least three factors:

1. The antibody–antigen rection must be specific. If a reaction of mixed specificity (more than one antigen and more than one antibody) occurs, it is virtually impossible to reach an equivalence zone as two or more separate antigen–antibody reactions are occurring at the same time.
2. The antiserum being measured must not contain monovalent (nonprecipitating) antibody, as this may not be carried down with precipitate.
3. Other proteins that may affix to antigen–antibody complexes (such as complement) must be eliminated, or an erroneously high value for specific antibody will be obtained because of nonspecific binding of the other proteins.

Nephelometry

Small aggregates of an antibody–antigen complex in a solution create turbidity. This turbidity can be measured by scattering of light passed into the turbid solution. Measurement of the degree of turbidity after addition of a constant amount of antigen to antibody solutions provides a rapid and more sensitive method than the precipitation reaction for quantitation of antigen. High levels of sensitivity are obtained using monochromatic light from a laser. Addition of polyethyleneglycol to the solution increases aggregate size and also increases sensitivity.

Precipitation in Agar

Precipitation reactions resulting from antibody–antigen combinations also occur in agar media. The agar prevents convection currents from disrupting the precipitation pattern. Precipitation-in-agar reactions are extremely valuable for analysis of multiple antigenic components in which each AgAb complex forms a distinct zone of precipitation.

Simple Gel Diffusion

The simple gel diffusion technique evolved directly from the precipitin reaction in solution. If a solution of soluble antigen is layered over antiserum in a small-caliber tube, a line appears at the interface of these solutions as a precipitation reaction occurs. If the antiserum is placed in agar in the tube and a solution of antigen is layered over the antiserum–agar base, a precipitation line appears at the interface. This is known as an *Oudin tube* (Fig. 7-7).

Since the antigen is in solution and the antiserum is distributed evenly in the agar, the location that the precipitation line assumes depends upon six factors: (1) concentration of

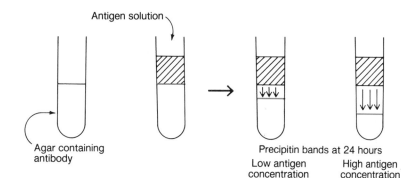

Antigen solution

Agar containing antibody

Precipitin bands at 24 hours
Low antigen concentration
High antigen concentration

Figure 7-7. Simple gel diffusion, or Oudin tube. If a solution of antigen is placed over agar containing antibody in a tube, a precipitin band will form where the antigen solution meets the antibody. The precipitin band will move into the agar as more antigen from the solution diffuses into the agar. The distance that the precipitin band moves into the agar at any time point is a function of the concentration of the antigen added (higher concentration results in further diffusion into the agar). By comparison of the distance of migration of bands formed by known concentrations of antigen with the distance of migration of bands produced by solutions containing unknown amounts of the same antigen, an accurate measure of the antigen concentration in the unknown can be made.

antigen, (2) diffusion coefficient of antigen, (3) concentration of antibody, (4) time, (5) temperature, and (6) concentration or density of agar. If the last five variables are held constant, the distance the precipitation line moves into the antiserum–agar layer depends on the concentration of antigen.

Simple gel diffusion may also be carried out on a flat surface (radial diffusion technique). Antiserum is incorporated into agar, which is allowed to gel as a layer on a glass slide. A hole is cut into the agar, and antigen solution is placed into the hole. The antigen will diffuse out into the antibody-containing agar, producing a ring of precipitation. The square of the radius of this precipitation ring depends upon the relative concentration of antigen and antibody. Using a constant dilution of antiserum, antigen concentration may be determined by comparing the diameter of the ring of precipitation produced by a solution of known antigen concentration with that of a ring produced by an unknown solution.

Double Diffusion in Agar   A better technique for analysis of mixtures of antibody–antigen systems is provided by the double diffusion-in-agar (Ouchterlony) technique. When this technique is used, antigen and antisera are separately placed in small wells cut out of a layer of agar on a plate. The antibody and antigen diffuse toward each other. A precipitation band forms where the antibody and antigen interact in the concentrations necessary to meet the requirements of the equivalence zone of the precipitin reaction. If the concentration of the antigen is relatively greater than the concentration of the antibody, the precipitation line appears nearer the antibody well. If the concentrations are equal, the line appears midway between the antibody and the antigen wells. If the antibody concentration is greater than the antigen concentration, the precipitation line appears closer to the antigen well. If multiple antibody–antigen systems are present, a separate line may be observed for each system. The patterns formed by precipitation lines when two or more antigens are compared with one antiserum, or vice versa, may be used to characterize an antigen or antibody preparation (Fig. 7-8).

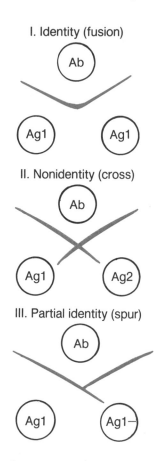

Figure 7-8. Double diffusion in agar reactions. If solution of antigen is placed in one well on the flat layer of agar and the appropriate antiserum placed in an adjacent well, antigen and antibody migrate toward each other, and a precipitation line forms when concentrations of antibody and antigen are at equivalence. If two identical antigen solutions (Ag1) are placed in wells in agar at the base of a triangle, and an appropriate antiserum (Ab) is placed in a well at the apex of the triangle, a precipitation line forms between each antigen well and antiserum well. Since both antigen solutions are the same, separate lines fuse where they meet in the center of a triangle (reaction of identity). If different antigen (Ag1 and Ag2) solutions are placed in base wells, and antiserum-containing antibodies (Ab) directed against both antigens are placed in an apex well, precipitation lines do not fuse; they cross. The reaction of antibody 1 with antigen 1 essentially does not affect the reaction of antibody 2 with antigen 2, and vice versa, so that the two precipitin lines form independently (reaction of nonidentity). If one antigen solution containing molecules with several antigenic specificities present on the same molecule (Ag1) and a second antigen solution containing molecules with only some of the antigenic specificities of the first antigen (Ag1−) are placed in adjacent wells against antiserum (Ab) which contains antibodies directed toward all specificities present in the first antigen solution, a line of partial identity, or spur formation, is observed. The precipitation line formed between antiserum and antigen with limited antigenic specificities fuses with the line formed by antiserum and antigen containing additional specificities, but this second line extends past the first line, resulting in a spur effect.

If multiple antigen–antibody systems react in agar, it may be difficult to identify and differentiate the number of precipitation bands present. An example is an antiserum prepared in one species (rabbit) by immunization with whole serum proteins of another species (rat). The rabbit antiserum to whole rat serum may produce up to 30 separate precipitation bands when reacted in agar with rat serum. However, it is not possible to differentiate the many different lines by double diffusion in agar. Such a mixture may be analyzed by combining serum protein electrophoresis and immune precipitation in agar.

Immunoelectrophoresis

Many variations combining electrophoresis and immunoprecipitation have been applied to the analysis of mixtures of antigens or antibodies. These include classic immunoelectrophoresis, rocket electrophoresis, two-dimensional electrophoresis, and immune labeling of polyacrylamide gel patterns (Western blot).

Classic Immunoelectrophoresis

The classic combination of electrophoresis in agar followed by reaction with antiserum is illustrated in Figure 7-9. The method is called immunoelectrophoresis.

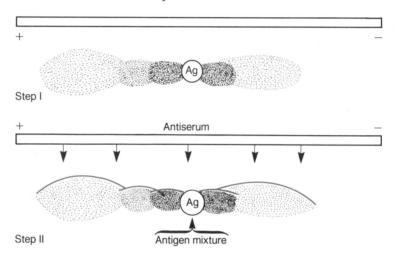

Figure 7-9. Reaction of polyvalent antiserum with a mixture of protein antigens separated by electrophoresis in agar. In step I the mixture of antigens is placed in a small well in a layer of agar on a glass plate or slide. An electric current is applied to the agar. This current acts upon the proteins and results in their migration into the agar. The distance each protein migrates is proportional to the electrostatic charge of the protein. Since proteins in the mixture of antigens differ in charge, separation of proteins due to different migration distances occurs. Location of proteins as they diffuse in agar is represented by shaded areas. In step II following electrophoretic separation, a trough is cut in the agar, a short distance from the well in which the antigen mixture was originally placed. The trough is cut so that its long axis is parallel to electrophoretic separation. Antiserum is then placed in the trough and allowed to diffuse into agar. Antibody to each antigenic protein then separately reacts with that protein in agar, forming precipitation lines where antibody and antigen are in equivalence (solid red lines). Individual antibody–antigen reactions are easier to identify and differentiate because the mixture of antigens has been separated by electrophoresis. Many variations in this basic procedure have been used to provide more exact immunochemical analysis of complex antibody–antigen systems.

Electroimmunodiffusion

A variation of single radial immunodiffusion employing electrophoresis (electroimmunodiffusion) may be used to quantify antigens in dilute fluids. Antiserum is incorporated into the agar layer and an electric current applied across the agar after an antigen solution is placed in a well cut into the agar. The electric field pulls the antigen into the antibody–agar layer. The distance that the antigen–antibody precipitate migrates into the agar layer is proportional to the amount of antigen in the solution.

Rocket Electrophoresis

In this procedure quantitation of antigen may be accomplished by determining the length of an arc of precipitation formed when antigen is electrophoresed into an agar layer containing antibody. This method is not suitable for antigens that migrate to the negative electrode, as the migration must be different from that of the antibody used (Fig. 7-10).

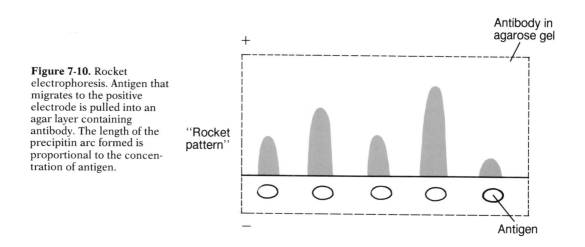

Figure 7-10. Rocket electrophoresis. Antigen that migrates to the positive electrode is pulled into an agar layer containing antibody. The length of the precipitin arc formed is proportional to the concentration of antigen.

Two-Dimensional Electrophoresis

In this variation of rocket electrophoresis an antigen mixture is electrophoresed in agar in one direction; then the antigens are pulled into agar containing antibody by electrophoresis in the perpendicular direction (Fig. 7-11). Using this method several antigens in a mixture may be quantitated.

Two Dimensional Immunoelectrophoresis

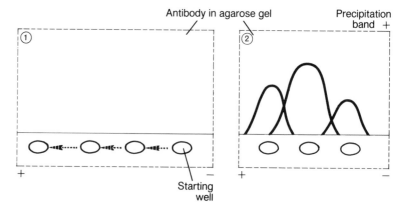

Figure 7-11. Two-dimensional electrophoresis. A mixture of antigens is separated by electrophoresis in agar in one dimension (step I). Then the separated antigens are pulled into a layer of agar containing antibody by electrophoresis in the second dimension (step II).

Immunolabeling of Polyacrylamide Gel Patterns (Western Blot or Immunoblot)

Analysis of complex mixtures of antigens may be accomplished by application of labeled antibodies to mixtures of proteins separated by one- or two-dimensional gel electrophoresis (Fig. 7-12). For one-dimensional gel electrophoresis, proteins are

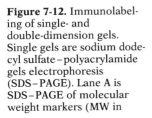

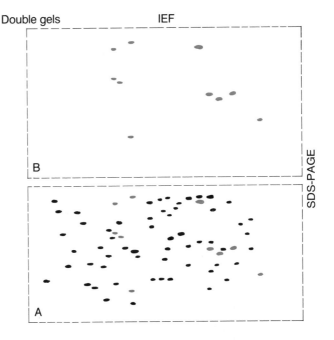

Figure 7-12. Immunolabeling of single- and double-dimension gels. Single gels are sodium dodecyl sulfate–polyacrylamide gels electrophoresis (SDS–PAGE). Lane A is SDS–PAGE of molecular weight markers (MW in thousands); lane B, the presence of all proteins as determined by a protein stain; lane C, labeled by specific antibody. Thus of the 23 proteins identified, 6 are antigens labeled by the antibody. Two-dimensional gels separate the proteins into spots on the basis of isoelectric focusing (IEF) followed by SDS–PAGE. The total proteins are stained in A and immune-labeled in B. Of the 70 proteins identified, 9 are shown to be antigenic.

placed in a charged field in a polyacrylamide gel slab. The proteins in the mixture will migrate largely on the basis of their molecular weights to form bands in the gel. For two-dimensional gels, the protein mixture is first separated on the basis of charge by isoelectric focusing, then on the basis of molecular weight by polyacrylamide electrophoresis. The gels containing the separated proteins are then electrophoretically transferred to nitrocellulose sheets. These sheets are labeled by specific antibody either directly using labeled antibody or indirectly where the first antibody is unlabeled and labeling is accomplished by a second labeled antibody, or by any of the labeling procedures described (peroxidase–antiperoxidase, biotin–avidin, labeled protein A). These procedures permit the identification of antigens in complex mixtures of proteins and are very useful in analysis of the antigens in bacteria or other infectious agents.

Agglutination

Agglutination of visible antigen particles by antibody occurs by the same mechanism as precipitation of soluble antigen (Fig. 7-13). Simple agglutination results when the antigen is an inte-

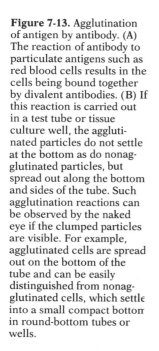

Figure 7-13. Agglutination of antigen by antibody. (A) The reaction of antibody to particulate antigens such as red blood cells results in the cells being bound together by divalent antibodies. (B) If this reaction is carried out in a test tube or tissue culture well, the agglutinated particles do not settle at the bottom as do nonagglutinated particles, but spread out along the bottom and sides of the tube. Such agglutination reactions can be observed by the naked eye if the clumped particles are visible. For example, agglutinated cells are spread out on the bottom of the tube and can be easily distinguished from nonagglutinated cells, which settle into a small compact bottom in round-bottom tubes or wells.

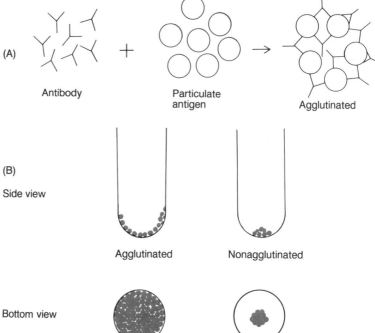

gral part of the particle, for example, when antibody to erythrocytes, or to bacteria, causes the agglutination of these particles. Passive agglutination results when a soluble antigen is chemically attached to a particle, and antibody is used to agglutinate the coated particle. Materials that have been used for this purpose include latex and bentonite particles and erythrocytes (passive hemagglutination). Addition of the soluble antigen in sufficient amounts to compete for the antibody inhibits the agglutination of the coated particles. Inhibition of passive hemagglutination reactions is an extremely sensitive method for detecting antigen.

Complement Fixation

The reaction of specific antibody with erythrocytes, bacteria, or other cells in the presence of complement results in the eventual destruction of red cells (hemolysis) or other target cells (e.g., bacteriolysis) (see Chapter 12).

The effect of antibody and antigen on the complement system may be used to measure formation of antibody–antigen complexes. The reaction of antibody and antigen in the presence of complement consumes components of the complement system (complement fixation). If a separate antibody–antigen reaction is allowed to take place in a volume of normal complement-containing serum, the complement activity is depleted by adsorption of active complement components to the antibody–antigen complexes formed. If this mixture is then added to sensitized erythrocytes, lysis does not occur, as the necessary components have been exhausted. This complement fixation reaction provides a sensitive and accurate measurement of antibody or antigen, when one of the reactants is unknown. For complement fixation to occur, a class of antibody (isotype) that can react with complement must be active (complement-fixing antibody); not all immunoglobulins have the capacity to fix complement.

Immunoabsorption

Specific antibody or antigen may be coupled to insoluble carriers, such as cellulose, bentonite, Sepharose, or glass beads, or made insoluble by crosslinking. These solid phase antibody or antigen reagents provide valuable methods for isolation of antigen (by insoluble antibody) or antibody (by insoluble antigen). For instance, a specific antiserum to a given antigen may be utilized to purify that antigen. The gamma globulin fraction of antiserum is coupled to an insoluble carrier, and a solution containing a mixture of antigen and other molecules is added. The specific antigen attaches to the insoluble specific antibody. The contaminating molecules are washed off, and the bound specific antigen is then eluted from the insoluble antibody by lowering the pH of the buffer sufficiently to disrupt the antibody–antigen electrostatic bonds, but not the covalent bond linking the antibody to the insoluble carrier.

Radioimmunoassay

The practical importance of the use of antigen–antibody reactions for the quantification of antigenic material is exemplified by the use of radioimmunoassay for measurement of peptide hormones and other biologically active molecules (Fig. 7-14). Human hormones may have species-specific differences which can elicit specific antiserum in other species. This antiserum may be used to identify and quantify the hormone, even if the hormone represents only a small fraction of the protein in serum. The basic principle is the inhibition of the reaction of a specific antibody and a known amount of antigen by the addition of unknown amounts of antigen. This principle is also used in other secondary antigen–antibody reactions, such as hemagglutination inhibition and precipitation inhibition. However, the use of radiolabeled antigen greatly increases the sensitivity of the test. Radioimmunoassay has been used to measure a large variety of antigenic molecules including hormones, enzymes, and serum proteins.

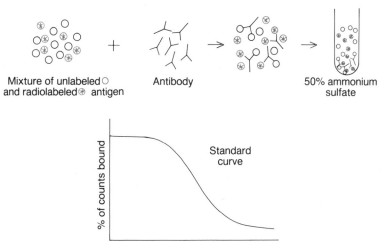

Mixture of unlabeled○   Antibody   50% ammonium
and radiolabeled⊕ antigen   sulfate

Figure 7-14. Very small amounts of antigen may be measured by the ability of the antigen to compete with radiolabeled antigen binding to antibody in this radioimmunoassay. If a mixture of unlabeled and radiolabeled antigen is added to an antibody solution in slight antigen excess, the amount of labeled antigen bound to antibody is a function of the amount of unlabeled antigen present. On the basis of this competition, a standard curve can be constructed by adding increasing amounts of unlabeled antigen to constant amounts of labeled antigen and antibody. When relatively small amounts of unlabeled antigen are present, all of the radiolabeled antigens are precipitated. As the amount of unlabeled antigen is increased, less radiolabeled antigen is bound to the antibody. When a standard curve using increasing known amounts of unlabeled antigen has been constructed, the amount of antigen in an unknown solution can be determined by comparing the degree of inhibition of binding of labeled antigen by the unknown antigen solution with that produced by known amounts of the same antigen.

Competitive Inhibition Radioimmunoassay

The principle of radioimmunoassay is given in the following reactions:

$$Ab + {}^*Ag \rightleftharpoons Ab{}^*Ag$$
$$Ab + Ag + {}^*Ag \rightleftharpoons AbAg + {}^*Ag + Ab{}^*Ag$$

In the first reaction, antibody (Ab) is reacted with a radiolabeled antigen (*Ag) under conditions that result in about 60–70% binding of the antigen. In the second reaction, unlabeled antigen (Ag) is included in the reaction mixture. Because the unlabeled antigen is present, less bound radiolabeled antigen is obtained. By varying the amount of unlabeled antigen present, a quantitative relation can be obtained between the amount of antigen present and the amount of radioactivity in the bound fractions. Once this relationship is determined, a standard curve may be constructed by plotting the percentage of bound label (or, inversely, the percentage in the supernate) against the amount of unlabeled antigen added. The amount of antigen in an unknown mixture can be found by determining the effect of the addition of dilutions of the unknown upon the antibody-labeled antigen system. The amounts of antibody and labeled antigen are kept constant in each determination.

Other properties of an antibody–antigen system may be used to quantify an antigen. Most involve the reaction of varying amounts of antigen or unknown with constant amounts of specific antiserum. As increasing amounts of antigen are added, (1) the amount of unbound antibody decreases; (2) the amount of complex increases; and (3) after equivalence is exceeded, increasing amounts of free antigen are present. The extent of any of these changes, in the presence of a fixed amount of antibody, depends upon the amount of antigen added. This permits variation in the final measurement used to quantify an antigen by immunoassay.

Immunoradiometric Assay

A variation of radioimmunoassay, *immunoradiometric assay,* uses purified radiolabeled antibody instead of labeled antigen. Radiolabeled antibody is added to a solution of antigen. Then, a solid immunoabsorbent antigen is used to separate unbound antibody, leaving the labeled antibody bound to the soluble antigen in the supernatant fluid. The sensitivity of immunoradiometric assays is comparable to that of radioimmunoassays. The choice of assay depends on the feasibility and applicability of an antibody–antigen system to the method.

Enzyme-Linked Immunosorbent Assay

The enzyme-linked immunosorbent assay (ELISA) is similar to the immunoradiometric assay except that the antibody is labeled with an enzyme instead of a radioisotope (Fig. 7-15). For example, unlabeled antibody specific for the antigen in question is allowed to adhere to the bottom of a microplate well, and unbound antibody is washed off. Solution containing an unknown amount of the antigen is added. In the appropriate sensitivity range, the absorbed antibody will be in excess and, therefore, all of the antigen will be bound by antibody. After binding of antigen, a second enzyme-labeled antibody directed against the antigen is added in excess (double-antibody technique). The amount of this second antibody that binds to the antigen depends upon the amount of antigen present. The unbound enzyme-linked antibody is then washed off, and a substrate is added that changes color when acted upon by the enzyme. The intensity of color developed over a certain amount of time depends on the amount of enzyme-linked antibody bound to the antigen in the well. By colorimetric analysis and comparison to known amounts of antigen, a quantitative standard curve is developed. Two of the enzymes commonly used are horseradish peroxidase, which turns a colorless solution of 5-aminosalicylic acid to reddish brown, and alkaline phosphatase, which turns a colorless solution of *p*-nitrophenol to yellow. In practice, the method of running ELISA assays varies. The two most commonly used are the indirect method, similar

Figure 7-15. Quantification of the enzyme-linked immunosorbent assay (ELISA) depends on the conversion of a colorless substrate to a colored compound by an enzyme coupled to antibody or to antigen. The amount of substrate converted is measured colorimetrically and is dependent upon the amount of enzyme-labeled antibody bound. The amount of antibody bound is in turn dependent upon the amount of antigen bound to unlabeled antibody absorbed to the bottom of the well. The unlabeled antibody absorbed to the well must be added in excess, and the unbound antibody washed off. Then, a standard curve similar to the one shown in Figure 7-14 can be constructed. Variation of the ELISA procedure employing mixtures of antibodies and antigens similar to those shown for immunofluorescence in Figure 7-15 may be used.

(1) Antibody absorbed to well

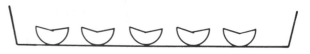

(2) Unlabeled antigen added

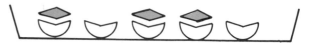

(3) Enzyme-labeled antibody added

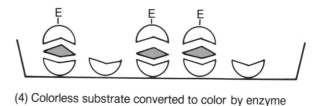

(4) Colorless substrate converted to color by enzyme

to a competitive radioimmunoassay, and the double-antibody method.

Tissue Labeling by Antibody

The location and distribution of antigens in tissues or cells can be accomplished using a variety of techniques that employ markers localized by antigen–antibody reactions.

Immunofluorescence

The most commonly employed dyes for tissue labeling by immunofluorescence are fluorescein (green fluorescence) and rhodamine (red fluorescence). Those compounds may be covalently attached to antibody molecules and emit visible light (fluoresce) when exposed to ultraviolet light of the appropriate wavelength. Fluorescein- or rhodamine-labeled antibody preparations are applied to sections of the unfixed tissue to be examined. The antibody binds to the antigen, if the latter is present in sufficient amounts in the tissue section, forming microprecipitates. If the treated tissue section is washed to remove excess unbound labeled antibody and observed under ultraviolet light, the areas of the tissue section containing the antigen give off visible light that can be observed under the microscope as a red or green fluorescence. Variations of this technique are illustrated in Figure 7-16.

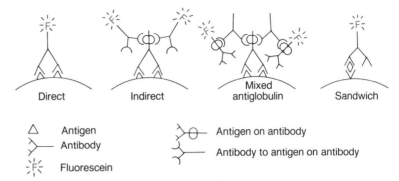

Direct	Indirect	Mixed antiglobulin	Sandwich

△ Antigen   ⊃⊖ Antigen on antibody

⊃ — Antibody   Antibody to antigen on antibody

⊃F Fluorescein

Figure 7-16. Fluorescent antibody techniques. In the direct technique, specific antibody is labeled with fluorescent compound and added to tissue sections. The reaction of specific antibody to antigenic sites in the tissue sections is detected by exposing the section to ultraviolet light and visualizing areas of fluorescence. By means of the indirect technique, unlabeled antibody is reacted with tissue antigen. Fluorescein-labeled antibody to the first antibody is added. The second antibody reacts with the first, which in turn has reacted with tissue antigen. The first antibody added provides more binding sites for second antibody than was provided by tissue antigen, in this way increasing the sensitivity of the technique. In the mixed antiglobulin technique, antigens present on the first antibody are used to react to binding sites of the second antibody. The label can be fluorescent-labeled immunoglobulin of the same species as that of the first antibody. This technique can be particularly useful in labeling surface immunoglobulin molecules. In such a system, the Ig antigens are already present on the cell to be labeled. Anti-immunoglobulin antibody is used to bind labeled Ig to the cell surface Ig. To identify antibody rather than antigen in tissue sections, a "sandwich" technique is used. Antigen is added to tissue and is bound by specific antibody present in the tissue. Specific fluorescein-labeled antibody to antigen is added, which reacts with antigen now fixed to the antibody in the tissue.

Immunofluorescence studies must be carefully controlled to prevent misinterpretation of the staining patterns. (1) Because minute amounts of contaminating antibody to an antigen other than the one of interest may give erroneous results, the specificity of the labeled antibody must be carefully checked by immunochemical controls. (2) The fluorescence produced by the labeled antibody must also be differentiated from nonspecific tissue fluorescence. This can usually be done, because natural tissue fluorescence gives a different color than fluorescein or rhodamine fluorescence. (3) The staining pattern produced by the labeled specific antibody must be clearly different from that which may occur if an adjacent tissue section is treated with labeled nonantibody (normal) immunoglobulins, since the labeled antibody may be nonimmunologically (nonspecifically) bound to the tissue section. (4) The staining pattern should not occur if the tissue section is treated with nonlabeled antibody prior to the addition of the labeled antibody. (5) Specific blocking should also occur if the labeled antiserum is absorbed with authentic nonlabeled antigen prior to the addition of antiserum to the tissue section. Even if these controls are carefully done, the investigator must be careful not to overinterpret the results of immunofluorescence.

Fluorescence Activated Flow Cytometry

Cells that are labeled by a fluoresceinated antibody may be quantitated and separated using a fluorescence-activated cell sorter (FACS) (Fig. 7-17). The FACS delivers single cells in a

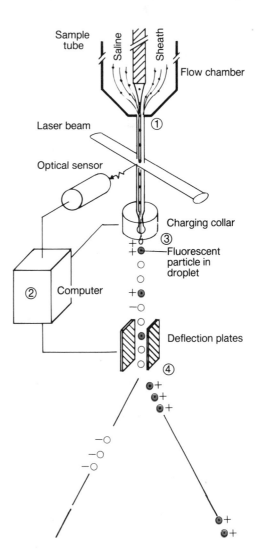

Figure 7-17. Cell separation by sorting. (1) Fluorescently stained cells are forced out of a small nozzle in a liquid jet. (2) Cellular fluorescence, measured immediately below the nozzle, is used to select the cells to be sorted. (3) The jet is broken into droplets. Droplets containing selected cells are electrically charged in a high-voltage field between deflection plates. (4) The charged droplets are electrically deflected into collection tubes.

stream that passes through a laser beam. Light from a laser beam excites the fluorescent dye, which gives a greater or lesser signal depending on the amount of antibody bound. The machine analyzes the distribution of fluorescence in large numbers of cells, giving data as shown in Figure 7-18. Alternatively, the machine can be set up as a cell sorter to separate brightly

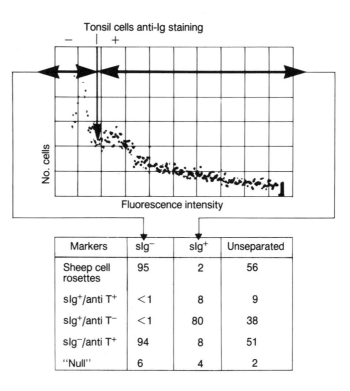

Figure 7-18. Separation of B and T cells with the fluorescence-activated cell sorter. After they are stained with fluorescein-conjugated anti-Ig, the viable cells are analyzed by flow cytofluorometry to give a histogram. The lymphocytes are separated into surface membrane Ig positive (SmIg$^+$) and negative (SmIg$^-$) populations depending on whether the fluorescence intensity is above or below the arbitrary cutoff point. The separated populations may then be reanalyzed for surface Ig and T cell surface markers as shown in the table. Null cells are negative with both anti-Ig and anti-T reagents. (Modified from Roitt I, Essential Immunology, 5th ed. Oxford, Blackwell, 1984, p. 63.)

Tonsil cells anti-Ig staining

Markers	sIg$^-$	sIg$^+$	Unseparated
Sheep cell rosettes	95	2	56
sIg$^+$/anti T$^+$	<1	8	9
sIg$^+$/anti T$^-$	<1	80	38
sIg$^-$/anti T$^+$	94	8	51
"Null"	6	4	2

fluorescent cells from dark ones. This is done by breaking up the stream of negatively charged cells into droplets. The droplets fall between charged plates that direct brightly fluorescence-labeled cells into one stream and unstained cells into another stream, and thusly into separate collection vessels. A recording apparatus measures the intensity of fluorescent staining of each cell as well as the cell size (Fig. 7-18).

Immunoperoxidase

Tissue localization of antigens or antibodies may also be accomplished using enzyme-labeled reagents, such as peroxidase-labeled antibody. Identification of bound antibody is possible through conversion of a colorless soluble substrate to a colored insoluble product by the enzyme. Since different substrates may be activated by the same enzyme, it is possible to localize more than one antigen by the serial addition of peroxidase-labeled antibodies. For instance, double staining of adrenocorticotropin (ACTH) and growth hormone (GH) in the rat anterior pituitary may be accomplished by reaction with rabbit anti-ACTH followed by peroxidase-labeled horse anti-rabbit IgG (double-antibody technique) and incubation with 3,3′-diaminobenzene as substrate. This will produce a known reaction product, which is orange and which will remain fixed on the slide. The slide can then be treated with rabbit anti-GH, peroxidase-labeled horse anti-rabbit IgG, and 4-Cl-1-naphthol. The naphthol substrate will produce a blue reaction product. In this manner, the same section may be examined for localization of ACTH (orange color) and GH (blue color).

Immunoelectron Microscopy

Ultrastructural localization of antigens may be accomplished using essentially the same type of reactions used for immunofluorescence. However, the markers used for electron microscopy are different. These include large or electron-dense molecules such as ferritin, hemocyanin, gold, or virus particles, which are large enough to be visualized by electron microscopy yet can be coupled to antibody or to antigen by chemical means. In addition, peroxidase-labeled antibodies may be used, as the products produced by reaction with the substrates can be seen under the electron microscope. The peroxidase method is more suitable for cytoplasmic localization, the larger particles for cell surface labeling. Even larger particles such as latex beads or larger viruses may be adapted for localization by scanning electron microscopy. Radiolabeled antigens may also be used to detect antigen receptors on cells or in tissues by electron microscopic autoradiography.

The Avidin–Biotin Complex

The extremely high affinity of the glycoprotein avidin for the vitamin biotin provides a system that greatly increases the sensitivity of many immune assays. Avidin has four high-affinity binding sites for biotin ($K_D = 10-15$ moles/liter). Biotin or avidin may be conjugated chemically to antibody, to antigen, or to enzymes or other labeled probes. The variations of labeling permit the use of the avidin–biotin system in immune assay and in immune absorption isolation procedures (Fig. 7-19). Techniques using avidin–biotin labeling are more sensitive and more specific than other enzyme labeling or fluorescent systems. It is estimated that avidin–biotin systems are five times more sensitive than conventional fluorescence for labeling tissue sections.

Microbiological Tests

The effect of bactericidal antibody and complement on certain organisms provides the basis for many microbiological laboratory tests.

Treponema pallidum Immobilization

A specific serologic test for syphilis, *Treponema pallidum* immobilization (TPI), depends upon the presence in an affected individual's serum of antibodies to the causative agent, *T. pallidum*. Motile organisms are mixed with the test serum and normal guinea pig serum (complement source). The mixture is incubated for 16 to 18 hours at 35°C under anaerobic conditions and then examined microscopically. Normally, the *T. pallidum* organisms are motile and are observed to move actively. The action of specific antibody and complement results in loss of this motility.

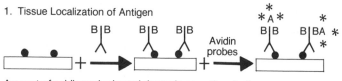

1. Tissue Localization of Antigen

Amount of avidin probe bound depends on antigen in tissue

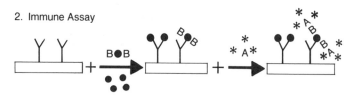

2. Immune Assay

Amount of avidin probe bound related to amount of biotin labeled antigen bounded to antibody; unlabeled antigen competes as in radioimmunoassay

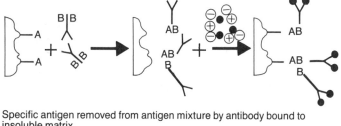

3. Ultrastructural Cell Surface Labeling

Ferritin detected on cell surface by electron microscopy

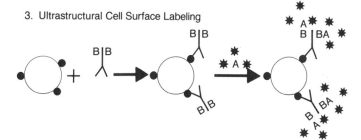

4. Immune Absorption

Specific antigen removed from antigen mixture by antibody bound to insoluble matrix

Legend

✱ Enzyme label ✹ Ferritin ● Antigen B Biotin A Avidin

Figure 7-19. Some uses of the avidin–biotin complex in immune assays. Biotin or avidin may be chemically conjugated to antigen, antibody, or a probe (enzyme, fluorescence, ferritin). The strong binding of avidin to biotin permits the use of a variety of binding complexes for immune assay and immune labeling procedures.

Opsonization

Opsonization is the reaction of specific antibody and complement with a particle or organism that facilitates or augments phagocytosis of the organism. An opsonic index can be obtained by determining the ratio of activity of a patient's serum to that of normal serum. The activity is determined by the degree of phagocytosis of the test material by microscopic examination of mixtures of serum, complement, and organisms cultured in the presence of macrophages, or by using an O_2

electrode to measure the "O_2 burst" that accompanies phagocytosis.

Neutralization Tests

The activity of antisera to bacteria or viruses may be tested by the ability of such sera to reduce the viability of suspensions of these organisms when cultured in vitro. The effect is usually measured by the activity of dilutions of the antisera or by the rate of neutralization of the target organism by the dilution of the antiserum. The ability to elicit neutralizing antibodies is particularly critical for vaccine development (see Chapter 25). For example, current efforts to produce a vaccine for AIDS may depend on the ability to demonstrate virus-neutralizing antibodies.

Neutralization of the activity of a biologically active molecule or infective organism may also be tested in vivo. A classic example is the toxin neutralization test for anti-diphtheria toxin serum.

Diphtheria Toxin Neutralization. The neutralization potency of an antiserum to diphtheria toxin (antitoxin) is measured by comparison with a standard sample of antitoxin. To test a toxin preparation, increasing amounts of toxin are added to a series of tubes containing 1 unit of a standard antitoxin, and each of the mixtures is injected into a 250-g guinea pig. The amount of toxin that must be mixed with 1 unit of antitoxin to cause death in 4 days is taken as the endpoint and is called the L_+ dose. Conversely, the potency of the unknown antiserum can be determined by mixing increasing dilutions of the antitoxin with one L_+ dose of the toxin and injecting the mixture into guinea pigs. The volume of serum that, when mixed with one L_+ dose of toxin, results in death in 4 days contains 1 unit of antitoxin.

Antigen–Antibody Reactions in Vivo

Antigen–antibody reactions in vivo initiate a number of inflammatory reactions that may be viewed as tertiary effects of antigen–antibody reactions. The manifestations of antibody–antigen reaction in vivo are the subject of Chapters 14–18 of this text.

Immune Elimination

The presence of antibody in the circulation leads to rapid clearance of antigens injected into the blood (Fig. 7-20). Reaction of antibody with antigen results in formation of aggregated Ig components and activation of complement, which *opsonizes* the complexes and results in clearance of the antigen complexes by the reticuloendothelial system. During the induction phase of antibody formation, antigen will be catabolized at a slow "nonimmune" rate. However, when antibodies are formed, catabolism occurs much more rapidly. During the early phase of immune elimination soluble antigen–antibody complexes in antigen excess are found in the circulation. Solu-

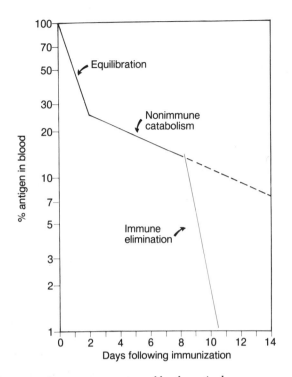

Figure 7-20. Immune elimination. If antibody is present in vivo, antigen is rapidly cleared from the bloodstream. A three-stage elimination of diffusible antigen from the bloodstream of a previously nonimmunized animal has been recognized. Upon intravascular injection of antigen, the blood level of antigen drops rapidly until only about 40% of injected antigen remains in blood. This is due to equilibrium of diffusible antigen between intravascular and extravascular fluids. Following this rapid equilibration, antigen is slowly removed by normal metabolic processes (nonimmune catabolism) until the onset of antibody production between 7 and 10 days after antigen injection. Appearance of antibody results in rapid elimination of antigen (immune elimination) due to formation of antibody–antigen complexes and their removal by the reticuloendothelial system. During the phase of immune elimination, soluble antibody-antigen complex (formed in antigen excess) may be demonstrated in blood. After antigen is completely removed, free antibody appears. If antigen is injected into an animal that already has circulating antibody, antigen is removed in one rapid immune elimination phase.

ble complexes in antigen excess do not contain Fc aggregates, are not opsonized, and may deposit in tissue and be responsible for the lesions of serum sickness (see Chapter 16).

Antibody–Mediated Inflammatory Reactions

The activity of antibodies in vivo in an actively immunized animal, or an animal that has received antibody by passive transfer of an antiserum prepared in another animal, may result in a reaction involving accessory inflammatory mechanisms. Intravenous injection of antigen into an actively or passively sensitized animal may cause an acute systemic reaction (anaphylaxis). If the antigen is injected into the skin of sensitized animals, erythema (redness) and swelling may be observed. These reactions depend upon tissue inflammatory responses initiated by reactions of antibody or sensitized cells with antigen.

Schick Test

In some cases, antibody can neutralize the inflammatory activity of bacterial toxins, resulting in the absence of a reaction in immune individuals. Historically, in vivo neutralization of diphtheria toxin by antibody was determined by skin testing. A small amount of diphtheria toxin injected intradermally produces a local inflammatory reaction that is maximal at 4 to 5 hours and then fades. In an immunized individual who has antibody to diphtheria toxin, no reaction occurs; the antibody neutralizes the effect of the toxin. This test was pioneered by Bela Schick between 1910 and 1930 and is known as the Schick test. A delayed hypersensitivity reaction to diphtheria toxin may also occur. This is known as a pseudoreaction and can usually be differentiated from the effects of the toxin, as the delayed reaction reaches a maximum at 2 to 3 days and fades by 4 to 5 days.

Dick Test

Some human sera injected into patients with a characteristic scarlet fever rash (scarlatina) can produce a blanching of the rash at the site of injection. Not all human sera can induce this blanching. The effect is due to the presence of specific antibody to the erythrogenic toxin produced by the streptococcal organism responsible. These observations led to the development of the Dick test for antibody to hemolytic streptococcal antigens. Filtrates of cultures of the scarlatinal strains (strains responsible for scarlet fever) of streptococci contain a toxic substance that produces a typical skin reaction in nonimmunized individuals. Individuals with neutralizing antibody do not react to this erythrogenic toxin. The reaction induced by erythrogenic toxin appears as a bright red flush within 6 to 12 hours, is maximum at 24 hours, and fades rapidly. This test measures only resistance to strains of streptococci causing scarlet fever and does not measure protection from or susceptibility to streptococcal throat infection.

Sensitivity of Antigen–Antibody Reactions

The sensitivity of some methods for detection of antibody–antigen reactions is given in Table 7-2. For further information on how to detect and measure both primary and secondary antibody–antigen reactions, the American Society of Microbiology's *Manual of Clinical Immunology* is recommended.

Summary

Antigens react with antibodies to produce antigen–antibody complexes that in turn are responsible for a number of in vitro and in vivo effects. The primary reaction of antigen with antibody involves close approximation of structures on the surface of the antigen (epitopes) with the antibody combining sites

Table 7-2. Sensitivity of Some Methods for Measuring Antibody–Antigen Reactions

Method	Sensitivity (μg antibody N/ml)
Quantitative precipitin	4–10
Simple agar diffusion	5–10
Bacterial agglutination	0.01
Bactericidal	0.0001–0.001
Hemagglutination	0.003–0.006
Hemolysis	0.001–0.03
Complement fixation	0.1
Toxin neutralization	0.01
Passive systemic anaphylaxis (guinea pig)	30
Uterine muscle in vitro	0.01
Passive cutaneous anaphylaxis	0.003
Radioimmunoassay	<0.001

Adapted from Humphrey JH, White RG: Immunology for Students of Medicine, 2nd ed. Oxford, Blackwell, 1963, p201.

(paratopes) so that oppositely charged groups interact and hydrogen bonds and hydrophilic bonds form to join the antigen and the antibody. The strength of these bonds is termed *affinity*. As antibodies have more than one identical paratope and most antigens have many different epitopes, a latticelike complex of antigen and antibody may be formed, which precipitates. This precipitation may be used to quantitate the amount of antibody or antigen in a solution. Other in vitro reactions include agglutination, neutralization, and opsonization. The reaction of antibody with antigen may activate accessory systems such as complement (see Chapter 11) or inactivate biologically active molecules such as bacterial toxins. These effects are the basis for a number of in vitro secondary effects that may be used to measure antibody (or antigen) or to localize antigen cells on tissues. The reaction of antibody with antigens in vivo may activate a number of effector mechanisms. The manifestations of in vivo effects will be presented in more detail in later chapters.

References

Primary Antigen–Antibody Reactions

Benjamin DC, Berzofsky JA, East IJ, et al: The antigenic structure of proteins: a reappraisal. Ann Rev Immunol 2:67, 1984.

Farr RS: A quantitative immunochemical measure of the primary interaction between I*BSA and antibody. J Infect Dis 103:239, 1958.

Kabat EA: The nature of an antigenic determinant. J Immunol 97:1, 1966.

Karush F: Immunological specificity and molecular structure. Adv Immunol 2:1, 1962.

Kitagawa M, Yagi Y, Pressman D: The heterogeneity of combining sites of antibodies as determined by specific immunoabsorbents. J Immunol 95:446, 1965.

Landsteiner K: The Specificity of Serologic Reactions. Springfield, Ill., Thomas, 1936.

Pressman D, Grossberg AL: The Structural Basis of Antibody Specificity. New York, Benjamin, 1968.

Richards FF, Konigsberg WH, Rosenstein RW, et al: On the specificity of antibodies. Biochemical and biophysical evidence indicates the existence of polyfunctional antibody combining regions. Science 187:130, 1975.

Schick AF, Singer SJ: On the formation of covalent linkages between two protein molecules. J Biol Chem 236:2477, 1961.

Monoclonal Antibodies

Cotton RGH: Monoclonal antibodies in the study of structure–functional relationships of proteins. Med Res Rev 5:77, 1985.

Godino J: Monoclonal Antibodies. Principles and Practices. Orlando, Fla., Academic Press, 1983.

Kohler G, Milstein C: Continuous cultures of fused cells secreting antibody of predefined specificity. Nature 256:495, 1976.

Mariuzza R, Strand M: Chemical basis for diversity in antibody specificity analyzed by hapten binding to monoclonal anti-4-hydroxy-3-nitrophenacetyl (NP) immunoglobulins. Mol Immunol 18:847, 1981.

Secondary Antigen–Antibody Reactions

Ackroyd JF: Immunological Methods. Oxford, Blackwell, 1964.

Avrameas S, Ternynck T: The cross-linking of proteins with glutaraldehyde and its use for the preparation of immunoadsorbents. Immunochemistry 6:53–66, 1969.

Bullock G (ed): Techniques in Immunochemistry. Orlando, Fla., Academic Press, Vol 1, 1982; Vol 2, 1983.

Campbell DH, Luescher E, Lerman LS: Immunologic absorbents. I. Isolation of antibody by means of cellulose protein antigen. Proc Nat Acad Sci USA 37:575, 1951.

Crowle AJ: Immunodiffusion. New York, Academic Press, 1961.

Hapke M, Patil K: The establishment of normal limits for serum proteins measured by the rate nephelometer. Hum Pathol 12:1011, 1981.

Heidelberger M: Lectures in Immunochemistry. New York, Academic Press, 1956.

Kabat EA, Mayer MM: Experimental Immunochemistry, 2nd ed. Springfield, Ill., Thomas, 1961.

Lefkowits I, Pernis B: Immunological Methods. Orlando, Fla., Academic Press, Vol 1, 1979; Vol 2, 1980.

Loken MR, Stall AM: Flow cytometry as an analytical and preparative tool in immunology. J Immunol Methods 50:85, 1982.

Mancini G, Carbonara AO, Heremans JF: Immunochemical quantitation of antigens by single radial immunodiffusion. Immunochemistry 2:235, 1965.

Merrill D, Hartley TF, Claman HN: Electroimmunodiffusion (EID): a simple, rapid method for quantitation of immunoglobulins in dilute biological fluids. J Lab Clin Med 69:151, 1967.

Ouchterlony O: Diffusion-in-gel methods for immunological analysis. Prog Allergy 6:30, 1962.

Oudin J: Method of immunochemical analysis by specific precipitation in gel medium. C R Acad Sci (Paris) Ser D 222:115, 1946.

Towbin H, Gordon J: Immunoblotting and dot immunoblotting—current status and outlook. J Immunol Methods 72:313, 1984.

Weetall HH: Preparation and characterization of antigen and antibody adsorbents covalently coupled to an inorganic carrier. J Biochem 117:257–261, 1970.

Weir DM: Antigen–antibody reactions. *In* Cruickshank R (ed): Modern Trends in Immunology. London, Whitefriar, 1963.

Wilchek M, Bocchini V, Becker M, Givol D: A general method for the specific isolation of peptides containing modified residues, using insoluble antibody columns. Biochemistry 10:2828–2834, 1971.

Radioimmunoassay and Enzyme-Linked Immunosorbent Assay

Engvall E, Perlmann P: Enzyme linked immunoabsorbent assay (ELISA). Quantitative assay of immunoglobulin G. Immunochemistry 8:871, 1971.

Rodbard D, Catt KJ: Mathematical theory of radioligand assays: the kinetics of separation of bound from free. J Steroid Biochem 3:255–273, 1972.

Rodbard D, Weiss GH: Mathematical theory of immunoradiometric (labeled antibody) assays. Anal Biochem 52:10–44, 1973.

Schuurs AHWM, Van Weemen BK: Enzyme-immunoassay. Clin Chim Acta 81:1, 1977.

Skelley DS, Brown LP, Besch PK: Radioimmunoassay. Clin Chem 19:146–186, 1973.

Yalow RS: Radioimmunoassay: A probe for the fine structure of biologic systems. Science 200:1236, 1978.

Cell and Tissue Labeling

Avrameas S: Indirect microenzyme techniques for intracellular detection of antigens. Immunochemistry 6:825, 1969.

Coons AH: Histochemistry with labelled antibody. Int Rev Cytol 5:1, 1956.

Hsu SM, Cossman J, Jaffe ES: A comparison of ABC, unlabeled antibody and conjugated immunochemical methods with monoclonal and polyclonal antibodies. An examination of the germinal centers of tonsils. Am J Clin Pathol 80:429, 1983.

Kraenenbuhl JP, Galardy RE, Jamieson JD: Preparation and characterization of an immunoglobulin microscope tracer consisting of a heme-octopeptide coupled to Fab. J Exp Med 139:208, 1974.

Linthicum DS, Sell S: Topography of lymphocyte surface immunoglobulin using scanning immunoelectron microscopy. J Ultrastruct Res 51:55, 1975.

Nakane PK, Pierce GB Jr: Enzyme labeled antibodies for the light and electron microscopic localization of tissue antigens. J Cell Biol 33:307, 1967.

Reisberg MA, Rossen RD, Butler WT: A method for preparing specific fluorescein-conjugated antibody reagents using bentonite immunoadsorbents. J Immunol 105:1151–1161, 1970.

Santer V, Bankhurst AD, Nossal GJV: Ultrastructural distribution of surface immunoglobulin determinants on mouse lymphoid cells. Exp Cell Res 72:377, 1972.

Shnitka TK, Seligman, AM: Ultrastructural localization of enzymes. Annu Rev Biochem 40:375, 1971.

Stein H, Gatter K, Asbahr H, Mason DY: Use of freeze-dried paraffin-embedded sections for immunohistologic staining with monoclonal antibodies. Lab Invest 51:676, 1985.

Microbiological Tests

Dick GF, Dick GH: A skin test for susceptibility to scarlet fever. JAMA 82:265, 1924.

Dick GF, Dick GH: Results with the skin test for susceptibility to scarlet fever. Preventive immunization with scarlet fever toxin. JAMA 84:1477, 1925.

Dochez AR: Etiology of scarlet fever. Medicine 4:251, 1925.

Romer PH: Über den Nachweis sehr kleiner Mengen des Diphtheriegiftes. Z Immunitaetsforsch 3:208, 1909.

Schick B: Die Diphtherietoxin-Hautreaktion des Menschen als Vorprobe der prophylaktischen Diphtherieheilserum-Injection. Munch Med Wochenschr 60:2608, 1913.

Schultz W, Charlton W: Serologische Beobachtungen am Scharlachexanthum. Z Kinderheikd 17:328, 1917.

Schwentker FF, Hodes HL, Kingland LC, Chenoweth BM, Pek JL: Streptococcal infections in a naval training station. Am J Public Health 33:1455, 1943.

Antigen–Antibody Reactions in Vivo

Dixon FJ: The metabolism of antigen and antibody. J Allergy 25:487, 1954.

Talmadge DW, Dixon FJ, Bukantz SC, Dammin GJ: Antigen elimination from the blood as an early manifestation of the immune response. J Immunol 67:243, 1951.

Weigle WO, Dixon FJ: The elimination of heterologous serum proteins and associated antibody response to guinea pigs and rats. J Immunol 79:24, 1957.

Sensitivity of Assays

Gill TJ III: Methods for detecting antibody. Immunochemistry 7:997–1000, 1970.

Minden P, Reid RT, Farr RS: A comparison of some commonly used methods for detecting antibodies to bovine albumin in human serum. J Immunol 96:180, 1966.

8 | Cell-Mediated Immunity in Vitro

In the preceding chapter in vitro immune reactions mediated by antibody were described. This chapter covers reactions of immune cells in vitro. *Cell-mediated immunity* refers to the effects of cells of the immune system. As with the reaction of antibodies with antigens in vitro, the reaction of specifically sensitized lymphocytes with antigen may also be measured in vitro. These reactions may also be divided into *primary* and *secondary* reactions. *Primary reactions* refers to direct effects of antigens on sensitized cells, such as binding of antigen or induction of proliferation of the reacting cells. *Secondary reactions* are a result of the effects of immune activated cells on other cells, such as killing of target cells by sensitized lymphocytes, or of the effects of products released from cells (i.e., *lymphokines*). The effect of cell-mediated immunity (CMI) in vivo is exemplified by delayed hypersensitivity (Chapter 19) and granulomatous reactions (Chapter 21). It is not yet possible to duplicate these reactions in vitro. However, in many instances a correlation exists between the effect of cells or cell products as measured by in vitro tests and by in vivo responses. In most instances, T cell populations mediate these effects, but lymphocytes without markers (*null cells*) may also act as effector cells. In addition, accessory cells such as macrophages or polymorphonuclear leukocytes may be recruited (see Chapter 12).

Sensitization of T Cells

The mechanism of sensitization of T cells by antigen has been characterized through in vitro studies. The basic cellular requirements are for immune T lymphocytes and antigen presenting cells to match at the major histocompatibility locus (this subject is presented in detail in Chapters 9 and 10). The antigen-presenting cells are usually macrophages, which are phagocytic, take up the antigen, and also have on their surfaces self antigens that are often used to present soluble protein antigens. The antigen is displayed on the surface of the antigen

149

presenting cell in association with self markers. Then, the T cell receptor binds the antigen and triggers the T cell response.

Primary Cellular Reaction with Antigen

Antigen Binding by Sensitized Cells

T cells that react specifically with antigen as a result of immunization are termed *sensitized cells*. The direct binding of antigen by specifically sensitized cells is measured by using labeled antigens. Radiolabeled antigen, fluorescent or enzyme-labeled antigen, or particulate forms of antigen may be used to demonstrate binding by radioisotopic counting, microscopy, or electron microscopy (Fig. 8-1). Sensitized lymphocytes have cell

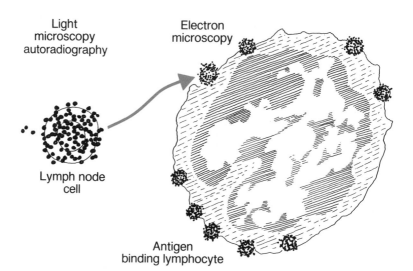

Figure 8-1. Labeling of antigen on surface of lymphocytes. Left: lymph node cell labeled with radiolabeled antigen. (From Diener and Poetkav: Proc Nat Acad Sci USA 69:2366, 1972.) Right: electron microscopic autoradiography of antigen-binding lymphocyte. (From Ada GL: Transplant Rev 5:110, 1970.) In addition, electron-dense antigenic particles, such as whelk hemocyanin, virus, or particles coated with antigen, may be used to label cell surface receptors. Labeling results in a patchy distribution of antigen on the cell surface if carried out at 4°C or in the presence of metabolic inhibitors such as azide. Under physiological conditions the cell surface labeling is lost by modulation (capping, endocytosis, or shedding) of the receptors (see Fig. 8-3). Capping and shedding are energy-dependent processes.

surface receptors that may bind antigens and activate cell proliferation (blast transformation).

Blast Transformation

Blast transformation measures the proliferation response of sensitized T cells to antigen (Fig. 8-2). The responding cells may have different T cell functions including T_K (killer or cytotoxic), T_D (delayed hypersensitivity), T_H (helper), and T_S (suppressor). The degree of response is measured by visual observation of enlarged "blast" cells or by incorporation of radiolabeled precursors into protein, RNA, or DNA. Because these assays are done in cell culture, the cell numbers can be carefully con-

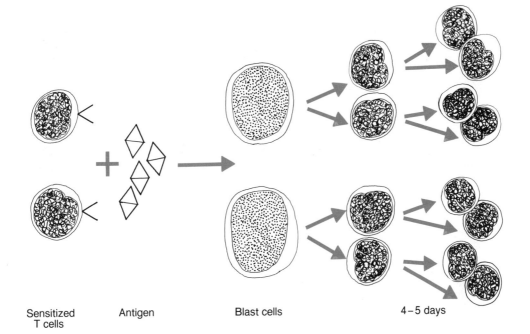

Sensitized   Antigen   Blast cells   4 – 5 days
T cells

Figure 8-2. Antigen-induced T lymphocyte blast transformation. Antigen added to sensitized T cells in the presence of self-matched antigen-presenting cells stimulates enlargement of cells to "immature blast cells." This enlargement requires RNA and protein synthesis, and is followed by DNA synthesis and mitosis. The response is usually measured by adding one of the four building blocks of DNA as radiolabeled precursors, such as tritiated thymidine, and determining the incorporation of this isotope into new DNA synthesized by the growing cells.

trolled. In such cultures it has been shown that an antigen-processing cell must present the antigen to the responding T cell. The antigen-processing cell displays the antigen on its surface in association with self markers. In addition, T_s cells may inhibit blast transformation of other T cell types, while initially being stimulated to proliferate by antigen.

The early events that occur during activation of blast transformation of T or B cells are very similar to those that are associated with degranulation of mast cells (see Fig. 12-3). Reaction of antigens or mitogens with cell membrane receptors activates phospholipase C in the membrane that cleaves phosphatidylinositol into two second messengers: diacylglycerol and inositol triphosphate. How reaction of mitogen with receptor activates phospholipase C is not known. Diacylglycerol activates protein kinase C, and inositol triphosphate mobilizes Ca^{++} from internal storage sites in the cell into the cytoplasm. Activated protein kinase C in the presence of free Ca^{++} phosphorylates receptor-associated membrane proteins. Subsequent events are not well understood, but may involve increased receptors for, or sensitivity to, activators or growth factors such as interleukins. Mor-

I. Capping

II. Endocytosis

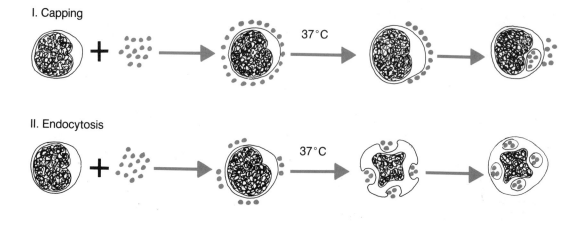

Figure 8-3. Cell surface events associated with lymphocyte activation. Two cell membrane events occur when antigens (or mitogens) react with the cell surface of lymphocytes: (I) diffuse pericellular labeling followed by capping with endocytosis and shedding, or (II) patchy labeling with endocytosis of patches. Both events result in clearing of the cell surface receptor. Activation to proliferation correlates with endocytosis, but not with capping.

phologic studies demonstrate two events at the cell surface: capping and endocytosis (Fig. 8-3). Capping refers to redistribution of the cell surface receptors from over the cell surface to one pole of the lymphocyte. This occurs with many agents that bind to the cell surface and does not necessarily lead to activation of the cell. Endocytosis refers to internalization of the cell surface receptor and bound antigen. This may occur in small patches (clusters of receptors) over the cell surface or in association with capping. Endocytosis does correlate with activation of the lymphocyte to proliferate. The membrane events described above may be required for endocytosis of antigen receptors. The events that follow endocytosis to signal the cell to begin the cell cycle remain unknown. The role of cell–cell interactions and soluble factors in lymphocyte activation and the immune response is discussed in Chapter 10.

The proliferation of immune T cells in culture allows the enrichment of antigen-specific clones: the frequency rises from less than 1 to 10,000 to about 1 in 100. Repeated stimulation in culture can result in pure populations of antigen-specific T cells. These can be diluted to one cell per well and grown in the presence of growth factors to give homogeneous populations of antigen-specific T cells (T cell clones). This form of positive selection in vitro mimics the clonal expansion that occurs in vivo. The ability to call up antigen-specific T cells when they are needed is an essential function of the immune system. T and B cells are committed to producing a single receptor with predetermined specificity prior to antigen stimulation, and a tremendous diversity of antigens must be recognized with a high specificity. Therefore the subset of cells with the desired specificity is quite rare. So antigen-specific cells must be rapidly expanded as they are needed to mount a timely and effective immune response.

Secondary Effects of Antigen Activation of Lymphocytes

Cell-Mediated Cytotoxicity

Five general cell-mediated cytotoxic effector mechanisms have been recognized in vitro (Table 8-1): (1) specifically sensitized effector cytotoxic T cells reacting directly with target cells; (2) specifically sensitized effector lymphocytes (T_D) reacting with antigen and releasing mediators that kill target cells (cytotoxins) or activate other effector cells (macrophages); (3) nonsensitized lymphocytes (null cells) activated by immunoglobulin antibody by Fc binding (antibody-dependent cell-mediated cytotoxicity or ADCC); (4) nonsensitized lymphocytes (natural killer cells, NK) reacting directly with target cells, and (5) activated macrophages. The basis of the reactivity of NK cells is not known. In addition, other cell types such as polymorphonuclear leukocytes or macrophages may function as killer cells via cytophilic antibody. Macrophages may also be activated by nonspecific stimulators such as phorbol esters or polynucleotides. Immune specific delayed hypersensitivity reactions mediated by the first two mechanisms involve T_D (delayed hypersensitivity) or T_K cells. T_K cells are also referred to as cytotoxic T lymphocytes (CTL). T_D activity correlates in vitro with antigen-induced blast transformation.

Table 8-1. Mechanisms of Lymphoid Cell-Mediated Immunity

T_K cells (CTL)	Sensitized to target cell—direct killing
T_D cells	Sensitized to target cell—lymphokine release, indirect killing (accessory cells)
Null cells + specific antibody	Antibody-dependent cell-mediated cytotoxicity (ADCC)
NK cells	Natural killing
Activated macrophages	Phagocytosis and digestion

Cytotoxic T lymphocyte activity is measured as the ability of T cell populations to kill target cells in vitro. Intracellular components of target cells may be labeled by addition of isotopes such as ^{51}Cr and cytolysis determined by the release of label from the target cell (Fig. 8-4). The cytotoxic effect of a population of T cells is expressed as the percentage of specific killing at a given effector-to-target-cell ratio (E/T ratio). This does not necessarily relate directly to the number of killer cells present. Different CTL may express different lytic capacity. In addition, one CTL may lyse more than one target cell. Thus, in measuring cytolysis by release of intracellular components, the

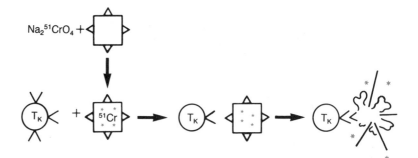

Figure 8-4. ^{51}Cr release assay for lymphocyte-mediated cytotoxicity. The release of intracellular components by the action of killer cells is determined. Target cells are labeled by incubation with $Na_2{}^{51}CrO_4$. Killer cells are then added to the labeled target cells. After incubation, the amount of intracellular and extracellular label remaining is determined by counting the radioactivity in the supernate and/or centrifuged cells. The percentage of specific lysis is calculated from the formula

$$\frac{\text{experimental } {}^{51}\text{Cr release} - \text{spontaneous release}}{\text{maximal release} - \text{spontaneous release,}} \times 100$$

where the experimental release is that from the target cells treated with killer cells, the spontaneous release is that from untreated target cells, and the maximal release is that observed by lysing the target cells by freezing and thawing or by solubilizing them in detergent.

relative degree of activity of two populations of killer cells can be estimated by the E/T ratio of each that gives the same percentage of specific release. The T cell population that has greater cytotoxic activity will give 50% release at a lower E/T ratio.

The specificity of killing can be assayed by cold target inhibition of specific ^{51}Cr release (Fig. 8-5). Cytotoxic T lympho-

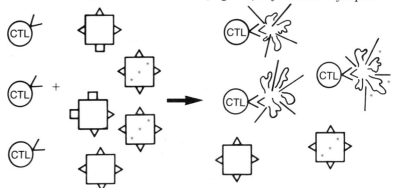

Figure 8-5. Cold target inhibition assay. Unlabeled target cells may be used to compete with labeled target cells in a lymphocyte-mediated cytotoxicity assay. The killer cells are added to a mixture of labeled and unlabeled target cells. If the unlabeled target cells contain some of the same antigenic specificities as the labeled target cells to which the CTL are reactive, the amount of ^{51}Cr released from the labeled target cells in a given period of time will be decreased. Quantitation of this inhibition of the CTL-mediated lysis may be used to determine antigenic relationships among different target cell populations and the specificity of reactivity of different CTL in a mixed population. In the example shown, only half as much radiolabel is released as would have occurred if no unlabeled target cells were present, because the CTL act on a mixture of labeled and unlabeled target cells.

cytes (T_K) are added to a mixture of unlabeled target cells and labeled target cells. The unlabeled target cells compete for the specific CTL and decrease the amount of label released from the labeled target cells. In a manner similar to a radioimmuno-assay, the degree of antigenic cross-reactivity may be estimated by the amount of cold target inhibition obtained. In this manner, shared antigens recognized by CTL cells in different tissues may be identified.

Killing of target cells by specifically sensitized lymphocytes is an immune-specific effector function of the cellular arm of the immune response. Immunization with cells expressing foreign antigens on the cell surface results in expansion of populations of T_K (or cytotoxic T) lymphocytes with specific receptors for the antigen. CTL activity is specific for antigens on the target cells, does not require antiserum or complement to be effective, and is active against foreign MHC class I antigens (graft rejections), viral antigens expressed on cell surfaces, or tumor antigens. Upon second contact with antigen in vivo this population of cells is available to kill cells expressing the antigen (memory).

Agents that inhibit direct lymphocyte-mediated cytolysis have been used to study the mechanism of direct killing of target cells by specifically sensitized T_K lymphocytes. The activity of the killer cell during killing may be divided into three phases: (1) initial recognition of target cell antigens by sensitized CTL; (2) CTL activation and lethal attack; and (3) target cell lysis (Fig. 8-6). Following killing of a target cell, a CTL may go on and kill other target cells. A direct transfer of killer cell products to target cells is thought to produce a membrane defect in the target cell similar to that produced by the membrane-attack complex of complement (see Chapter 12), which results in a lethal hole in the target cell membrane. Intimate contact between killer T cells and target cells is required for cell killing.

Monolayer Plaques

The interaction of sensitized lymphocytes and target cells may be studied morphologically by observing the effect of sensitized lymphocytes on target cells growing in monolayers. Plaques or holes occur in the monolayer when sensitized lymphocytes are added. Sensitized lymphocytes surround the target cells and eventually cause their detachment from the monolayer. Figure 8-7 depicts the destruction of monolayer target cells. As long as the target cells remain attached to the monolayer, they appear to be viable; however, upon separation from the monolayer, the target cell undergoes morphologic alterations indicative of cell death. These alterations include vacuolization and disintegration of the cytoplasm and condensation of nucleus and cytoplasm. Although close contact between the sensitized lymphocytes and target cells occurs, the exact mechanism of target cell death remains unclear.

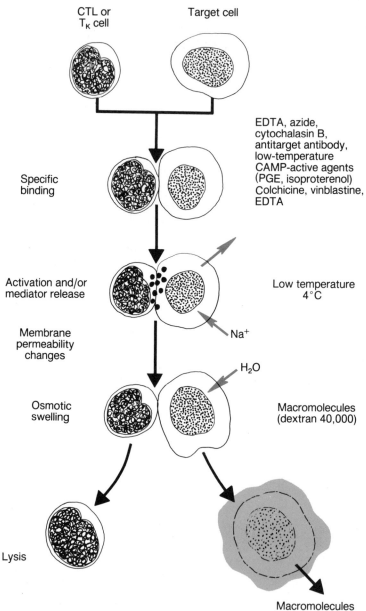

Figure 8-6. Stages of CTL (T_K)-mediated target cell lysis. Reaction of specifically sensitized T_K cell with target cell is followed by sequential changes culminating in lysis of the target cell. The T_K cell can then detach and attack another target cell. The use of inhibitors suggests that binding occurs via an antigen receptor and is an energy-requiring process involving membrane modulation. Following binding, energy-requiring activation of T_K cells may occur in some situations, as indicated by the effect of metabolic inhibitors. However, membrane permeability changes in the target cell occur within minutes of killer cell binding. Further lysis proceeds without an energy requirement. Activated T_K cells have granules containing lysosomal enzymes, which may be released after contact with the target cell. The terminal stages of lysis involve continued osmotic uptake of H_2O into the cell due to the increase in membrane permeability. (Modified from Henney CS: J Reticuloendothel Soc 17:4, 1975.)

An identical type of interaction between lymphocytes and target cells may occur in vivo in tissue reactions mediated by lymphocytes. Figure 8-8 shows the pathologic changes occurring during the development of experimental allergic thyroiditis. As in the target cell monolayer system, lymphocytes pass between the thyroid-follicle-lining cells, causing them to separate from each other and from the basement membrane, eventually destroying the thyroid cells. The basement membrane appears intact during the development of the lesion. Infiltra-

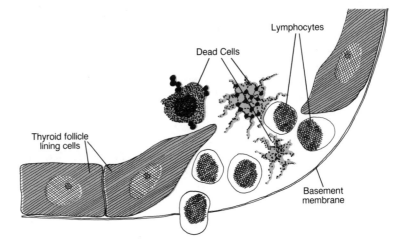

Figure 8-7. Reaction of sensitized lymphocytes with target cells in vitro. T lymphocytes from a sensitized donor infiltrate and surround monolayer target cells, seemingly without effect on viability or morphologic appearance of target cells. As a result of this infiltration, monolayer cells become separated from each other and from culture surface. Monolayer cells that retain contact with the monolayer remain viable, but when they are separated from other monolayer cells, morphologic changes consistent with cell death occur. These alterations do not occur in tissue culture cells that become separated from the monolayer in the presence of normal lymphocytes. Fluids and washings taken from monolayers treated with sensitized lymphocytes cannot be used to initiate new cultures, whereas fluids or washings of cultures treated with normal lymphocytes can. DC, dead or dying cells separated from monolayers; L, lymphocytes; MTC, monolayer target cells. (Modified from Biberfield P, Holm G, Perlmann P: Exp Cell Res 52:672, 1968. Copyright © Academic Press.)

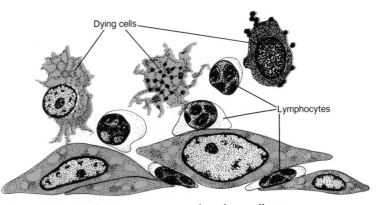

Figure 8-8. Reaction of sensitized lymphocytes with target cells in vivo (morphologic changes in experimental allergic thyroiditis). Changes similar to those illustrated in Figure 8-7 for reaction of sensitized lymphocytes with tissue culture monolayers occur with thyroid-follicle-lining cells in allergic thyroiditis. Mononuclear cells appear first in perivenular areas and then invade stroma of thyroid. Invasion of follicles follows. Lymphocytes appear to pass through the basement membrane of the thyroid follicle, separating thyroid-follicle-lining cells from basement membrane and from other follicular cells. Death of lining cells occurs when these cells are isolated from basement membrane and from other follicular cells. DC, dead or dying cells; L, lymphocytes; TFC, thyroid-follicle-lining cells. (Modified from Flax MH: Lab Invest 12:199, 1963. Copyright © 1963, International Academy of Pathology.)

tion of mononuclear cells, with separation, isolation, and destruction of target cells, may be observed in contact dermatitis, classic graft rejection, and many autoallergic diseases believed to be mediated by specifically sensitized cells (e.g., destruction of thyroid-follicle-lining cells in experimental allergic thyroiditis and destruction of germinal epithelium in experimental allergic orchitis) (see Chapter 20).

T_D Lymphocytes

T_D lymphocytes initiate delayed hypersensitivity inflammatory reactions in vivo. The activity of these cells may also be measured in vitro (Fig. 8-9). Sensitized T_D cells are activated to

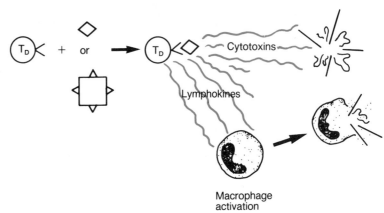

Figure 8-9. T_D cell-mediated immunity. T_D cells are activated by reaction with antigen, either soluble or cell surface, to release lymphocytic mediators (lymphokines). These mediators attract and activate accessory cells, in particular macrophages, which destroy the target cell.

proliferate in the presence of antigen and to produce and release a variety of lymphocyte mediators termed *lymphokines.* Proliferation may be directly measured as blast transformation (see above). Lymphokine production may be measured by determining a variety of effects on other cells, some of which may be measured in vitro. The role of lymphocytes and lymphokines in inflammation is presented in Chapter 12. Lymphokines may activate macrophages to produce damage to cells not bearing the specific antigen recognized by the T_D effector cell ("innocent bystander" effect). Thus reactions of T_D cells with antigen on one cell may ultimately cause damage to an antigenically unrelated cell if a severe inflammatory response is generated. Experimentally, measurement of the activity of lymphokines may often be used to detect T_D cell-mediated immunity. However, some of the techniques used are not readily applicable for widespread use. Another in vitro technique used to measure the effects of antigen on T_D cells is leukocyte (macrophage) migration inhibition.

Migration Inhibition

Migration inhibition measures the effect of mediators from sensitized lymphocytes (lymphokines) on migration of peritoneal exudate macrophages in the presence or absence of antigen. Extracts of antigen-treated lymphocytes may also be assayed for migration inhibition factor (MIF). Quantitation is achieved by measuring the area of migration of antigen- or MIF-treated cells on an agar layer, comparing the area to that of nontreated cells, and calculating the percentage of migration inhibition (Fig. 8-10). This assay has been used extensively in experimental and clinical studies.

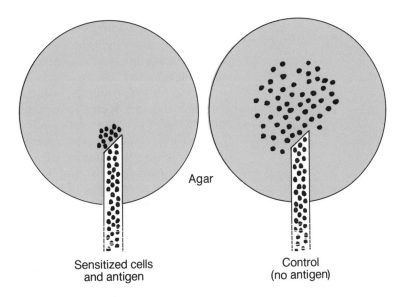

Figure 8-10. Macrophage migration inhibition. To measure the migration of macrophages a population of cells is collected in a capillary pipette. The pipette is placed on an agar layer. After incubation in vitro the cells migrate over the agar (control). However, if sensitized lymphocytes and antigen or migration inhibition factor (MIF) are present, the macrophages do not migrate out of the capillary pipette.

Agar

Sensitized cells and antigen

Control (no antigen)

Lymphokine-Activated Cells

Normal unsensitized T lymphocytes may be activated to become killers following non-antigen-specific stimulation with a variety of mitogens (Fig. 8-11). This activation may be caused by

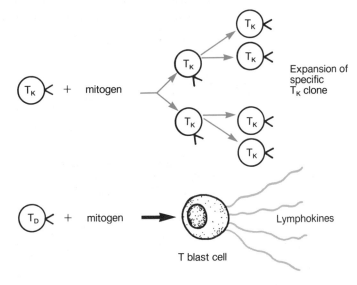

Figure 8-11. Mitogen-activated cell-mediated immunity. Mitogens activate T cell killing either by expanding the numbers of T_K cells by proliferation or by nonspecifically inducing the production of lymphokines by T_D cells.

T_K + mitogen

T_K

T_K

T_K

T_K

T_K

Expansion of specific T_K clone

T_D + mitogen

T blast cell

Lymphokines

the increased numbers of T killer cells generated by mitogen stimulation or the generation of cytotoxic or macrophage-activating lymphokines (see above). Whereas some evidence exists that mitogens may act at least in part by agglutinating activated killer cells to target cells, this is not the case with concanavalin A (ConA)-activated killer cells. ConA presumably acts by stimulating preexisting T_K cell populations to expand and thus express their genetically determined immune specificity to foreign target cells. The in vivo significance of mitogen-induced cytotoxicity remains uncertain. However, this phenomenon does indicate the inherent killing spectrum of activated T cells and suggests that nonspecific activation produces killer cells that might act on foreign cells or organisms.

In a somewhat similar fashion one lymphocyte mediator, interleukin 2, has been shown capable of expanding and activating a new class of cytolytic cells, lymphokine-activated cells (LAC). These cells can be shown to be potent killers of fresh tumor cells in vitro and in vivo. Unlike that caused by CTL, chromium release caused by LAC in vitro is not antigen specific, more than one type of tumor may be lysed, and killing is not self restricted. However, on the basis of cell surface markers, IL2 works on a precursor cell that differentiates into the activated killer, LAC. These cells, when given back to donor mice along with high doses of IL2, have been shown to proliferate in vivo and to kill tumor cells actively. They are totally dependent on exogenous IL2 and disappear when the interleukin is not given. However, LAC therapy at the present time is associated with considerable toxicity to the lungs, generalized edema apparently of nonspecific localization, and release of various lymphokines. The basis of the tumor-specific killing is unknown at this time. Recent reports of clinical efficacy in treating melanomas and certain carcinomas need to be verified (see Chapter 29).

Sensitization of Killer Cells in Vitro

CTL may be induced in vitro. Cell populations containing non-sensitized CTL are mixed with stimulator cells and incubated for 4 to 7 days (Fig. 8-12). During this time the specifically reactive cells proliferate and develop the specific capacity to kill the target cells. Cells that respond in mixed lymphocyte reactions with stimulator cells of foreign histocompatibility type develop cytotoxic activity to specific histocompatibility antigens. Fibroblast cultures have been used for this purpose. Using fibroblast monolayers, it is possible to sensitize lymphocytes to foreign histocompatibility antigens. Tumor cell monolayers may be used to sensitize to tumor specific transplantation antigen. Virus-infected target cells may be used to induce CTL specific for viral antigens. Self antigens may be

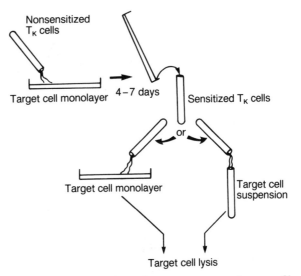

Figure 8-12. Sensitization of CTL in vitro. Nonsensitized populations of CTL may be sensitized in vitro by incubation with target cells. After 4 to 7 days, the CTL removed specifically lyse target cells containing antigens to which they were exposed in vitro. This is due to a specific expansion of CTL (proliferation).

recognized by culturing lymphocytes on autologous fibroblast cultures, thus inducing autoallergy in vitro. Macrophages are required for optimal sensitization of T cells in vitro, but macrophages do not usually take part in the killer cell effector stage of the reaction.

In vitro secondary sensitization or boosting may also be used to demonstrate antigenic cross-reactivity between different target cell populations. In vitro boosting is accomplished in the same manner as in vitro priming, except that the lymphoid cells are obtained from donor animals that have been immunized to a given target cell line. If a marked increase in killing is evidenced after in vitro exposure to a second target cell line as compared with the effect of exposure of lymphoid cells from unimmunized donors to that cell line, then an antigenic relationship between the cell line used for in vivo priming and that used for in vitro boosting has been demonstrated.

Antibody-Dependent Cell-Mediated Cytotoxicity

Target cells may be lysed by effector cells that are not themselves specifically sensitized, but bind onto the target cell by antibodies on the target cell surface (Fig. 8-13). The cells active as effectors in antibody-dependent cell-mediated cytotoxicity (ADCC) bear cell surface receptors for the Fc domains of aggregated immunoglobulin that is usually of the IgG class. ADCC effector populations include polymorphonuclear leukocytes and macrophages as well as lymphocytes. Killing requires effector target cell interaction that is accomplished by the antibody attaching to the target cell by its antigen-binding site and to the effector cell by its Fc piece. The in vivo significance of ADCC is also not clear, but such a mechanism could act to augment antibody-mediated effector mechanisms and can be shown to kill larval stage parasites in vitro.

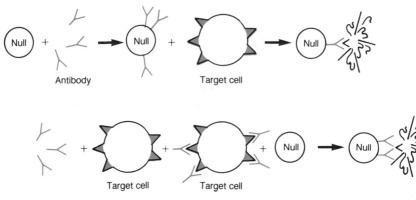

Figure 8-13. Antibody-dependent cell-mediated cytotoxicity (ADCC) is due to the attachment of effector cells to aggregated antibody on target cells. This bestows on previously nonimmune reactive cells the capacity to react specifically with antigens on cells and kill them. Other cells such as polymorphonuclear leukocytes and macrophages may also function as effector cells through passively absorbed antibody.

Natural Killer Cells

Some lymphocytes with neither T nor B cell markers are able to cause death of certain target cells without specific antibody-mediated direction. These cells are called *NK (natural killer)* cells. Natural killer cell activity is also measured by a cytotoxic assay (Fig. 8-14). It is directed against a variety of target cell

Figure 8-14. Natural killer cells. Nonimmune persons have cells that are able to kill target cells. The nature of the antigen receptor for such cells is unknown, although the effect appears to be target cell antigen specific.

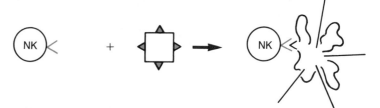

lines and may be inhibited by carbohydrates, suggesting that NK cell receptors react to carbohydrate antigens. NK activity exists without stimulation but may be enhanced by interferon (see Chapter 29).

Activated Macrophages

The macrophage has an important accessory role for CMI (Fig. 8-15). In delayed hypersensitivity reactions in vivo it is usually

Figure 8-15. Activated macrophages. Macrophages may be activated nonspecifically by endotoxin or polynucleotides or by lymphokines released by T_D cells reacting with specific antigens. Activated macrophages will kill target cells nonspecifically.

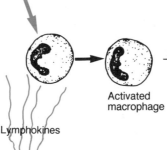

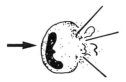

the macrophage that actually performs the lytic or destructive step. Thus, T_D cells kill indirectly by producing lymphokines that activate macrophages to become killers. Macrophages also may become *armed* by attachment of *cytophilic antibody* and function as immune specific killers. In addition, macrophages may be activated by a variety of agents (biological response modifiers) to become more efficient killers, presumably by increasing the amount of lysosomal enzymes and cellular metabolism. Increased in vitro activity of the macrophage may reflect an enhanced state of resistance to infectious agents in vivo. (See Chapters 12 and 27.)

Summary

Cell-mediated immunity refers to the measurement of reactions mediated by immune lymphocytes. Primary reactions are the direct effect of antigen on sensitized cells; secondary reactions are the result of immune-activated lymphocytes on other cells. Direct effects include antigen binding and activation of sensitized cells to proliferate. Secondary effects include T_K (killer) or T cytotoxic cell (CTL) activity, mitogen-induced killing or lymphokine production, antibody-dependent cell-mediated cytotoxicity, natural killer cell activity, and killing by activated macrophages. The mechanisms responsible for most cellular reactions in vivo are T_K (CTL) and T_D. T_K activity is measured by the effect of specifically sensitized T_K cells on target cells in vitro (cytotoxicity); T_D activity is measured by proliferation or lymphokine production after antigen stimulation.

References

General

Bloom BR, David JR: In Vitro Methods in Cell Mediated and Tumor Immunology. New York, Academic Press, 1976.

Cohen S: The role of cell-mediated immunity in the induction of inflammatory responses. Am J Pathol 88:502, 1977.

Antigen Binding

Ada GL: Antigen binding cells in tolerance and immunity. Transplant Rev 5:105, 1970.

Ada GL, Ev PL: Lymphocyte receptors and antigen receptors on B and T cells. *In* Sela M (ed): The Antigens, vol 3. Academic Press, New York, 1975, p 190.

Basten A, Miller JFAP, Warner NL, Dye J: Specific infection of thymus-derived (T) and non-thymus derived (B) lymphocytes by [135]I labeled antigen. Nature 231:104, 1971.

Cone RE, Gershon RK, Askenase PW: Nylon adherent antigen-specific rosette-forming T cells. J Exp Med 146:1390, 1977.

Greaves MF, Moller E: Studies on antigen binding cells. I. The origin of reactive cells. Cell Immunol 1:372, 1970.

Noar D, Sulitzeanu D: Binding of radiolabeled bovine serum albumin to mouse spleen cells. Nature 214:687, 1967.

Sell S, Asofsky R: Lymphocytes and immunoglobulins. Prog Allergy 86:95, 1968.

T Cell Activation and Blast Transformation

Dutton RW, Bulman RW: The significance of the protein carrier in the stimulation of DNA synthesis by hapten–protein conjugates in the secondary response. Immunology 7:54, 1964.

Hirschhorn K, Back F, Kolodny RL, Firschein IL, Hashem N: Immune response and mitoses of human peripheral blood lymphocytes in vitro. Science 142:1185, 1963.

Kirchner H, Blaese RM: Pokeweed mitogen-, concanavalin A-, and phytohemagglutinin-induced development of cytotoxic effector lymphocytes. An evaluation of the mechanisms of T cell-mediated cytotoxicity. J Exp Med 138:812, 1973.

Ling NR: Lymphocyte Stimulation. Amsterdam, North-Holland, 1968.

Marshall WH, Valentine FT, Lawrence HS: Cellular immunity in vitro: clonal proliferation of antigen stimulated lymphocytes. J Exp Med 128:327, 1969.

Moller G (ed): Interleukins and lymphocyte activation. Immunol Rev 63, 1982.

Nedrud J, Touton M, Clark WR: The requirement for DNA synthesis and gene expression in the generation of cytotoxicity in vitro. J Exp Med 142:960, 1975.

Oppenheim JJ, Rosenstreich DL: Mitogens in Immunobiology. Academic Press, New York, 1976.

Pearmain G, Lycette RR, Fitzgerald PH: Tuberculin-induced mitosis in peripheral blood leukocytes. Lancet 1:637, 1963.

Robbins AH: Tissue culture studies of the human lymphocyte. Science 146:1648, 1964.

Valentine IT: The transformation and proliferation of lymphocytes in vitro. *In* Revillard JP (ed): Cell Mediated Immunity: In Vitro Correlates. Baltimore, University Park Press, 1971, p6.

T_D Activities in Vitro

Aarden LA, et al: Letter to the Editor. Revised nomenclature for antigen nonspecific T cell proliferation and helper factors. Mol Immunol 17:641, 1980.

Bennett B, Bloom BR: Reactions in vivo and in vitro produced by a soluble substance associated with delayed-type hypersensitivity. Proc Nat Acad Sci USA 59:756, 1968.

Bloom BR, Bennett B: Mechanism of a reaction in vitro associated with delayed hypersensitivity. Science 153:80, 1966.

Bloom BR, Jimenez L: Migration inhibitor factor and the cellular basis of delayed hypersensitivity reactions. Am J Pathol 60:453, 1970.

Carpenter RR: In vitro studies of cellular hypersensitivity. I. Specific inhibition of migration of cells from adjuvant-immunized animals by purified protein derivative and other protein antigens. J Immunol 91:803, 1963.

David JR: Delayed hypersensitivity in vitro: its mediation by cell free substances formed by lymphoid cell–antigen interaction. Proc Nat Acad Sci USA 56:72, 1966.

David JR, Al-Askari S, Lawrence HS, Thomas L: Delayed hypersensitivity in vitro. I. The specificity of inhibition of cell migrations by antigen. J Immunol 93:264, 1964.

George M, Vaughan JH: In vitro cell migration as a model for delayed hypersensitivity. Proc Soc Exp Biol Med 111:514, 1962.

Green JA, Cooperband SR, Kibrick S: Immune specific induction of interferon production in cultures of human blood lymphocytes. Science 164:1415, 1969.

Heise ER, Hans S, Wiser RS: In vitro studies on the mechanism of macrophage migration inhibition in tuberculin sensitivity. J Immunol 101:1004, 1968.

Lawrence HS, Landy M (eds): Mediators of Cellular Immunity. New York, Academic Press, 1969.

Likhite V, Sehon A: Migration inhibition and cell-mediated immunity: a review. Rev Can Biol 30:135, 1971.

Pekarek J, Krecj J: Survey of the methodologic approaches to studying delayed hypersensitivity in vitro. J Immunol Methods 6:1, 1974.

Salvin SB, Nishio J: In vitro cell reactions in delayed hypersensitivity. J Immunol 103:138, 1969.

Wagner H, Rollinghoff M, Nossal GJV: T-cell-mediated immune responses induced in vitro: a probe for allograft and tumor immunity. Transplant Rev 17:3, 1973.

Waksman BH: Studies on cellular lysis in tuberculin sensitivity. Annu Rev Tuberc 68:746, 1953.

Waksman BH, Namba Y: On soluble mediators of immunologic regulation. Cell Immunol 21:161, 1976.

Ward PA, Remold HG, David JR: Leukotactic factor produced by sensitized lymphocytes. Science 163:1079, 1969.

Wunderlich JR, Canty TG: Cell mediated immunity induced in vitro. Nature 228:62, 1970.

Cytotoxic
Lymphocytes

Berke G, Amos GB: Mechanism of lymphocyte-mediated cytolysis: the LMC cycle and its role in transplantation immunity. Transplant Rev 17:71, 1973.

Biberfield P, Holm G, Perlmann P: Morphologic observations on lymphocyte peripolesis and cytotoxic action in vitro. Exp Cell Res 52:672, 1968.

Brunner KT, Mauel J, Rudolf H, Chapuis B: Studies of allograft immunity in mice. I. Induction, development and in vitro assay of cellular immunity. Immunology 18:501, 1970.

Canty TG, Wunderlich JR: Quantitative in vitro assay of cytotoxic cellular immunity. J Nat Cancer Inst 45:761, 1970.

Chism SE, Burton RC, Grail DL, Bell PM, Warner NL: In vitro induction of tumor specific immunity. VI. Analysis of specificity of immune response by cellular competitive inhibition. Limitations and advantages of the technique. J Immunol Methods 16:254, 1977.

Flax MH: Experimental allergic thyroiditis in the guinea pig. II. Morphologic studies on the development of the disease. Lab Invest 12:199, 1971.

Goldstein P, Smith ET: Mechanism of T-cell-mediated cytolysis: the lethal hit stage. Contemp Top Immunol 7:273, 1977.

Granger GA: Mechanisms of lymphocyte-induced cell and tissue destruction in vitro. Am J Pathol 59:469, 1970.

Hayry P, Defendi V: Mixed lymphocyte cultures produce effector cells: model of in vitro allograft rejection. Science 168:133, 1970.

Hellstrom I, Hellstrom KE, Sjogren HO, Warner G: Demonstration of cell-mediated immunity to human neoplasms of various histologic types. Int J Cancer 7:1, 1971.

Hellstrom KE, Hellstrom I: Lymphocyte-mediated cytotoxicity and blocking activity to tumor antigens. Adv Immunol 18:209, 1974.

Henkart PA: Mechanism of lymphocyte mediated cytotoxicity. Annu Rev Immunol 3:31, 1985.

Henney CS: On the mechanism of T-cell mediated cytolysis. Transplant Rev 17:37, 1973.

Henney CS: T cell mediated cytolysis: an overview of some current issues. Contemp Top Immunol 7:245, 1977.

Hodes RJ, Handwerger BS, Terry WD: Synergy between subpopulations of mouse spleen cells in the in vitro germination of cell-mediated cytotoxicity. J Exp Med 140:1646, 1974.

Lohmann-Matthew ML, Fisher H: T cell cytotoxicity and amplification of the cytotoxic reaction by macrophages. Transplant Rev 17:150, 1973.

Martz E: Mechanisms of specific tumor cell lysis by alloimmune T lymphocytes: resolution and characterization of discrete steps in the cellular interaction. Contemp Top Immunol 7:301, 1977.

Moller G (ed): Mechanism of action of cytotoxic T cells. Immunol Rev 72:1983.

Nabholz M, MacDonald HR: Cytotoxic T lymphocytes. Annu Rev Immunol 11:273, 1983.

Perlmann P, Holm G: Cytotoxic effects of lymphoid cells in vitro. Adv Immunol 11:117, 1970.

Perlmann P, Perlmann H, Wigzell H: Lymphocyte-mediated cytoxicity in vitro. Induction and inhibition by humoral antibody and nature of effector cells. Transplant Rev 13:91, 1972.

Plata F, Cerottini J-C, Brunner KT: Primary and secondary in vitro generation of cytolytic T lymphocytes in the murine sarcoma virus system. Eur J Immunol 5:227, 1975.

Podack ER, Koningsburg PJ: Cytotoxic T cell granules. J Exp Med 160:695, 1984.

Rosenau W, Moon HD: Lysis of homologous cells by sensitized lymphocytes in tissue culture. J Nat Cancer Inst 27:471, 1961.

Ruddle NH: Lymphotoxic redux. Immunol Today 6:156, 1985.

Takasugi M, Klein E: A microassay for cell-mediated immunity. Transplantation 9:219, 1970.

Taylor HE, Culling CFA: Cytopathic effect in vitro of sensitized homologous and heterologous spleen cells on fibroblasts. Lab Invest 12:884–894, 1963.

Williams TW, Granger GA: Lymphocyte in vitro cytotoxicity: mechanism of lymphotoxic-induced target cell destruction. J Immunol 102:911, 1969.

Wilson DB: Quantitative studies on the behavior of sensitized lymphocytes in vitro. I. Relationship of the degree of destruction of homologous target cells to the number of lymphocytes and to the time of contact in culture and consideration of the effect of isoimmune serum. J Exp Med 122:143, 1975.

Winn HJ: Immune mechanisms in homotransplantation. II. Quantitative assay of the immunologic activity of lymphoid cells stimulated by tumor homografts. J Immunol 86:228, 1961.

Antibody-Dependent Cell-Mediated Cytotoxicity

Balch CM, Ades EW, Loken MR, Shope SL: Human "null" cells mediating antibody-dependent cellular cytotoxicity express T lymphocyte differentiation antigens. J Immunol 124:1845, 1980.

Herlin D, Herlin M, Steplewski Z, Koprowski H: Monoclonal antibodies in cell-mediated cytotoxicity against human melanoma and colorectal carcinoma. Eur J Immunol 9:657, 1979.

Kay AD, Bonnard CD, West WH, Herberman RB: A functional compression of human Fc receptor-bearing lymphocytes active in natural cytotoxicity and antibody dependent cellular cytotoxicity. J Immunol 118:2058, 1977.

Parrillo JE, Fauci AS: Apparent direct cellular cytotoxicity mediated via cellular antibody. Multiple Fc receptor bearing effector cell populations mediating cytophilic antibody induced cytotoxicity. Immunology 33:839, 1977.

Payne CM, Linde A, Kibler R, et al: Surface features of human natural killer cells and antibody dependent cytotoxic cells. J Cell Sci 77:27, 1985.

Perlmann P, Holm G: Cytotoxic effects of lymphoid cells in vitro. Adv Immunol 11:117, 1969.

Perlmann P, Perlmann H, Biberfeld P: Specifically cytotoxic lymphocytes produced by preincubation with antibody complexed target cells. J Immunol 108:558, 1972.

Perlmann P, Perlmann H, Muller-Eberhard HJ, Manni JA: Cytotoxic effects of leukocytes triggered by complement bound to target cells. Science 163:937, 1969.

Takasugi J, Koide Y, Takasugi M: Reconstitution of natural cell-mediated cytotoxicity with specific antibodies. Eur J Immunol 7:887, 1977.

Van Boxel JA, Paul WE, Green I, Frank M: Antibody-dependent lymphoid cell-mediated cytotoxicity: role of complement. J Immunol 112:398, 1974.

Natural Killer Cells

Granger GA, Kolb WB: Lymphocyte in vitro cytotoxicity: mechanisms of immune and nonimmune small lymphocyte-mediated target L cell destruction. J Immunol 101:111, 1968.

Herberman RB (ed): NK Cells and Other Natural Effector Cells. Orlando, Fla., Academic Press, 1982.

Herberman RB, Nunn ME, Lavrin DH: Natural cytotoxic reactivity of mouse lymphoid cells against syngeneic and allogeneic tumors. Int J Cancer 16:216, 1975.

Herberman RN, Reynolds CW, Ortaldo J: Mechanisms of cytotoxicity by natural killer cells. Annu Rev Immunol 4:651, 1986.

Moller G (ed): Natural Killer Cells. Immunol Rev 44, 1979.

Ortaldo JR, Herberman RB: Heterogeneity of natural killer cells. Annu Rev Immunol 2:359, 1985.

Takasugi M, Koide Y, Akira D, Ramseyer A: Specificities in natural cell mediated cytotoxicity by the cross-competitive assay. Int J Cancer 19:291, 1977.

Takasugi M, Mickey MR, Terasaki PI: Reactivity of lymphocytes from normal persons on cultured tumor cells. Cancer Res 33:2898, 1973.

Macrophage Activation

Adams DO, Hamilton TA: The cell biology of macrophage activation. Annu Rev Immunol 2:283, 1984.

Gotoff SP, Vizral IF, Malecki TJ: Macrophage aggregation in vitro. Transplantation 10:443, 1970.

Hibbs JB, Remington JS, Stewart CC: Modulation of immunity and host resistance by microorganisms. Pharmacol Ther 8:37, 1980.

Keller R: Mechanisms by which activated normal macrophages destroy syngeneic rat tumor cells in vitro. Immunology 27:285, 1974.

Mackaness GB: Resistance to intracellular infection. J Infect Dis 123:439, 1971.

Mackaness GB, Blanden RV: Cellular immunity. Drug Allergy 11:89, 1967.

Mooney J, Waksman BH: Activation of normal rabbit macrophage monolayers by supernatants of antigen stimulated macrophages. J Immunol 105:1138, 1970.

Nathan CF, Karnovsky ML, David JR: Alterations of macrophage functions by mediators from lymphocytes. J Exp Med 133:1356, 1971.

Nelson DS (ed): Immunology of the Macrophage. New York, Academic Press, 1976.

Raffel S: Types of acquired immunity to infectious diseases. Annu Rev Microbiol 3:221, 1949.

9 | The Major Histocompatibility Complex and the Immunoglobulin Gene Superfamily

The major histocompatibility complex (MHC) is a series of genes that code for protein molecules responsible for cell–cell recognition. The MHC of mammalian species contains three groups of genes: class I, class II, and class III. Class I and class II genes code for cell surface recognition molecules, and class III codes for some complement components (the complement system is presented in Chapter 12). Class I and II region products control recognition of self and nonself; T cells not only recognize antigens but also have receptors that recognize the MHC products of other cell types from the same individual as self, and the products of cells from other individuals as nonself (foreign). All nucleated cells express class I MHC antigens on their surface. Class II antigens are expressed on some cells (B cells, macrophages) but not on others (most parenchymal cells do not express class II MHC). Class II markers may appear on some activated cells, that is, activated T cells, or may be induced to higher levels in some class II marker–expressing cells, that is, macrophages under the influence of interferon. The MHC is part of the immunoglobulin supergene family, which also codes for the recognition molecules of T and B cells for antigens.

Self–Nonself Recognition

The ability of cells to recognize other cells as self or from another genetically different individual (nonself) is an important property in maintaining the integrity of tissue and organ structure. As discussed in Chapter 1, primitive organisms have the ability to distinguish cells of the same species from cells of different species through cell surface glycoprotein molecules. During mammalian embryogenesis, developing tissues must have means of interacting with some cell types and avoiding interaction with other cell types. The major histocompatibility system also prevents an individual from being invaded by cells from another individual. For example, transplants from one

169

individual generally cannot survive in another individual, because of histocompatibility differences. Histocompatibility differences between the mother and fetus during gestation may provide a mechanism preventing the mother from being invaded by fetal tissues and the fetus from being invaded by maternal cells.

Major histocompatibility complex products also play a major regulatory role in the immune response. Histocompatibility similarities are required for cellular cooperation in induction of the immune response and provide a mechanism to ensure that T cells and B cells of a given individual can recognize each other for cooperation, yet bear immunoglobin supergene receptors that recognize foreign structures at the same time (see Chaper 10). Class I products determine to a large extent the specificity of graft rejection, whereas class II region products control cell interactions during induction of immunity.

Although we do not know why 80 different variations of class I MHC antigens are carried in the human population (see below), such diversity might prove advantageous in avoiding a catastrophic viral infection that might destroy the entire population. Instead, the diversity of tissue types could ensure that no single infectious agent could evade the immunity of all individuals with widely different tissue types. Class I MHC antigens are commonly recognized by cytolytic T cells specific for virally infected cells. Even if one tissue type were associated with a poor immune response to the infection, only a small percentage of the population would be lost, and the infection could be contained by the immunity of the rest of the population.

Genetics of Tissue Transplantation

The ability of the immune system to recognize tissue from a different individual of the same species as foreign is determined by tissue antigens controlled largely by MHC class I products. If solid tissue, such as a donor kidney, from one individual of a species is transplanated to a second, genetically different individual of the same species, a characteristic reaction termed *allograft* (homograft) rejection is observed. If transplantation occurs from one part of the body to another in the same individual *(autograft)* or between two genetically identical individuals *(synograft* or *isograft)*, for example between monozygotic twins or between individual animals of an inbred strain, this reaction does not take place. If transplantation is made between individuals of different species *(xenograft)*, a more brisk and intense rejection may result.

The genetic control of transplantation antigens as demonstrated by the behavior of skin grafts among inbred strains of

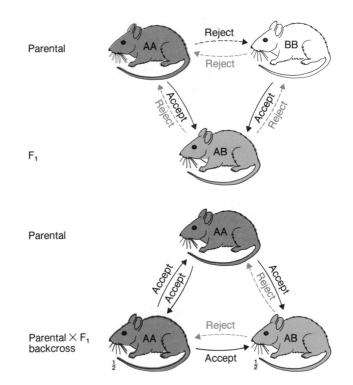

Figure 9-1. Genetics of transplantation. The behavior of skin grafts between two inbred mouse strains differing at a major histocompatibility locus (H-2) and the behavior of grafts to and from various hybrids and backcrosses to one of the parental strains are illustrated. Arrows indicate a graft from a given donor to a given recipient. Rejection occurs when the donor contains a specificity not present in the recipient. Capital letters indicate specificities present in inbred parental strains and designated progeny. Dotted lines indicate rejection of graft; solid lines, acceptance.

mice and their hybrid offspring is illustrated in Figure 9-1. MHC genes controlling transplantation antigens are usually inherited according to codominant Mendelian rules. Grafts between the homozygous parental strains are rapidly rejected. Since the F_1 contains both specificities of each parental strain, F_1 hybrids will accept grafts from each parental strain. However, grafts from F_1 mice will be rejected by each parental strain, as the F_1 carries the MHC products of the other parental strain. The results of a parental – F_1 backcross (mating of F_1 mice to one of the parental strains) are indicated at the bottom of Figure 9-1. Half these offspring will be identical to the parental strain and half to the F_1, and thus transplants to and from these mice will behave accordingly. Through the thorough study of the behavior of grafts among different strains of mice and their offspring and the correlation of this with the serologically identifiable lymphocyte antigens, the transplantation genetics and histocompatibility loci of the mouse have been identified.

Genetic Control of the Immune Response

The ability to produce an immune response is controlled by class II region gene products. The function of MHC gene products in induction of antibody formation has been delineated by studies in genetic low responder mice. Mice of the same strain or MHC type will show the same magnitude of response (high, intermediate, or low) to selected T-dependent antigens. Low responder mice generally produce very low levels of antibodies to some antigens and do not convert from an IgM (low primary response) to an IgG response after stimulation by antigen. However, low responder animals of a given MHC class II–controlled antigen can produce normal amounts of antibody if the antigen is complexed to an immunogenic carrier. Therefore, low responder animals have B cells that can recognize and produce antibody to the antigen. This implies that the B cells of low responders are functionally intact, but lack T cell help. Low responder strains also have low T cell proliferative responses to antigens, supporting the conclusion that genetic unresponsiveness is due to a specific defect in T cells. Class II region genes are linked to, but are different from, the class I genes responsible for tissue graft rejection.

The function of MHC genes in T and B cell interactions was determined by passive transfer experiments. If cells from different MHC thymus donors are transferred to nude mice (congenitally athymic, T cell deficient), the recipient nude mouse is able to respond to T-dependent antigens only when the MHC types of the thymus cell donor and the B cells in the recipient nude mouse are the same (Fig. 9-2). The B cells of the

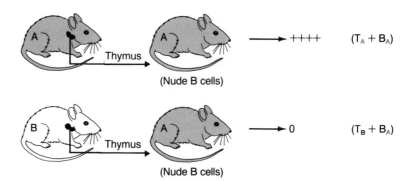

Figure 9-2. MHC restriction of T cell–B cell cooperation. In this experimental model, the capacity of nude mice, which lack T cell functions, to become immunized to a T-dependent antigen is restored by thymus cells from major histocompatibility complex (MHC)-identical donors, but not by thymus cells from MHC-different donors. If strain A thymus cells are transferred to another strain A nude mouse, an immune response may be induced; if strain B thymus cells, which differ in the MHC, are transferred to a strain A recipient, no response can be generated. Thus, in order for T and B cells to cooperate during induction of antibody production, they must share some MHC-controlled structures.

recipient must match the MHC of the thymus donor to be helped by the T cells. If they do not match, the B cell cannot respond to T cell help. Similarly, in irradiated F_1 recipients of mixtures of mature parental cells, a T-dependent antigen stimulates a response in the F_1 recipients only when the transferred parental T and B cells have the same MHC type (Fig. 9-3).

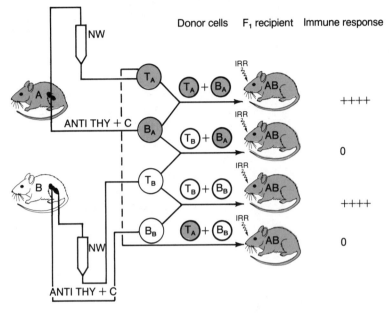

Figure 9-3. MHC control of antibody production in F_1 mice reconstituted with mixtures of parental T and B cells. The ability of F_1 (A + B) irradiated recipients to respond to T-dependent antigens is determined by MHC matching of donor T and B cells. Parental T cells are obtained by passage over nylon wool columns that retain B cells. Parental B cells are isolated by treatment with anti-T cell serum and complement (B cells survive, T cells are killed). Only when irradiated F_1 recipients are reconstituted with T and B cells of the same parental MHC type are the F_1 recipients able to mount an immune response.

Macrophage Restriction

Evidence for a macrophage–T cell MHC restriction comes from studies using inbred guinea pigs of strains 2 and 13 (Fig. 9-4). The system of analysis involves antigen-induced T cell

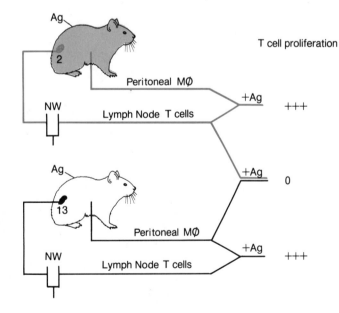

Figure 9-4. Demonstration of macrophage–T cell histocompatibility restriction in induction of immune responses in the guinea pig. Guinea pigs of strains 2 and 13 are immunized. Macrophages are obtained from peritoneal cells, and T cells from lymph node cells are passed over nylon wool columns. A proliferative immune response may be induced by antigen in vitro only when the macrophages and T cells match at the MHC.

proliferation (blast transformation). In order for antigen to induce transformation of T cells, histocompatible macrophages must be present. Mixtures of peritoneal exudate macrophages (glass adherent) and lymph node T cells (fractionated over nylon wool columns) from the same strain after immunization with antigen respond to antigen in vitro by blast transformation, whereas mixtures of macrophages and T cells from different strains do not. The compatible macrophages can be pulsed with antigen, washed, and then added to T cells. From this, a good response can be obtained. The conclusion is that the macrophage processes antigen and must be histocompatible with T cells to present the antigen to them. Macrophages must express a class II (MHC) product, and the class II product may actually function as an antigen-binding structure of macrophages that is recognized in turn by T cells that react with both antigen and the class II molecule (see below).

A simplified representation of the most likely relationship of macrophage–T helper–B cell collaboration and MHC restriction is shown in Figure 9-5. In this model, the macrophage

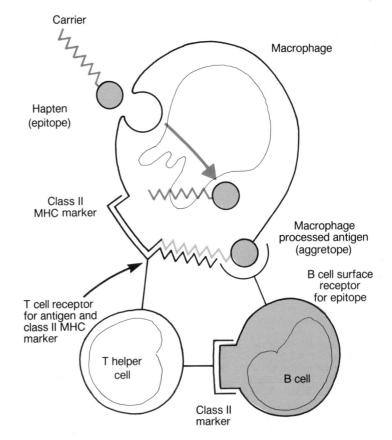

Figure 9-5. Class II region–determined recognition interaction of T cells, B cells, and macrophages during induction of antibody formation. Class II restriction requires that the T helper cell be able to recognize class II markers on macrophages. The same T cell receptor reacts with antigen and class II MHC marker on the macrophage during T cell activation and on the B cell when providing T helper function. Dual specificity (antigen and MHC marker) comes from the same pair of T cell receptor α and β chains (see Chapter 10).

and the B cell bear class II determinants and the T helper cell has receptors for these. In addition, the T cell has a receptor for antigens on the carrier, and the B cell a receptor for hapten determinants. The macrophages process antigen after phagocytosis and partial digestion by lysosomal proteases into peptide fragments 10–20 amino acids long and then present the antigenic fragments to T cells in association with class II MHC determinants. The T helper cell must be able to recognize carrier and class II markers on both the macrophage and the B cell. When each of these requirements is fulfilled, the B cell will be stimulated to proliferate, which greatly increases the number of cells capable of synthesizing specific antibody. These then differentiate into plasma cells, which secrete large amounts of antibody. The nature of the stimulating signals is presented below. A similar model employing class II receptors on T suppressor cells and class II MHC markers on macrophages and B cells may be operative in induction of T suppressor activity, which turns off antibody production (see Chapter 10).

The requirement for class II region recognition for induction of antibody responses may serve to focus T helper effects on appropriate cells, such as macrophages and B cells. During induction of immunity, T helper cells would not be useful reacting with other cell types such as heart and kidney. The presence of class II antigens on macrophages and B cells assures that T helpers will act on these cells. In addition, since T helper cells react with class II markers in the context of antigen, specific T helper cells are activated in the presence of antigen and the specific cells required for an antibody response.

The principles of self recognition by immune competent cells must be taken into consideration in attempts to reconstitute humans with immune deficiency diseases. Thus in bone marrow or thymus transplantation, the donor cells must share some histocompatibility antigen specificities with the recipient. If not, the appropriate cellular reactions required to generate an effective immune response may not be able to take place.

Structure of the Major Histocompatibility Gene Complex

In recent years extensive studies of the mouse and human have led to a much better understanding of the genetic control of immune reactions and the major histocompability complex. Since much more is known about the MHC of the mouse than that of the human, the characteristics of the mouse MHC are described in detail and compared with those of the human MHC. The MHC has been localized to the H-2 gene complex in mouse chromosome 17 and the HLA complex in human chromosome 6.

The Mouse MHC (H-2)

The pioneering work of Little, Gorer, Snell, and others who used serological methods and congenic mice has led to the current understanding of this chromosomal region in the mouse. The structure of the MHC region has been determined largely by analysis of congenic mice. Snell produced congenic mice by repeated backcrossing of selected progeny with the parental strain to the point that the genetic background of the inbred mice was identical to that of the parent except for MHC traits. As a first step (see Fig. 9-1), inbred mice of strain A and strain B are mated to produce an (A × B)F$_1$. The first backcross of the F$_1$ with parent A can be expected to produce half of the progeny with MHC phenotype (A × B). These were selected for B-type MHC based on rejection of their skin grafted onto the A parent strain. The selected mice are again mated with parent A and tested by skin grafting. This process of backcrosses and selection is repeated 20 times. During all those generations, the random assortment of chromosomes will dilute out all of the unselected chromosomes coming from the B parent. In addition, crossing over between pairs of chromosome 17 will result in a segment of chromosome 17 copying the selected trait (B phenotype at the MHC), whereas the rest of chromosome 17 will come from the A strain.

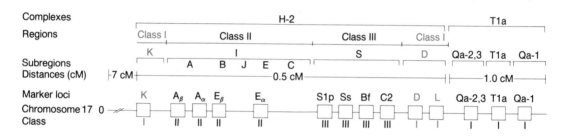

Figure 9-6. Fine-structure map of the mouse major histocompatibility complex. The mouse major histocompatibility (H-2) complex is located on chromosome 17 and contains genetic regions that control a variety of immune reactions. The H-2K and H-2D regions control the expression of tissue antigens that are recognized by immune allograft rejection. The I region controls various immune responses. The classic depiction of the I region is shown, although only genes for the A and E regions have been confirmed by gene cloning. The S1 region controls the serum concentration of components of complement. Qa1 and Qa2,3 control some erythrocytic alloantigens, and Tla the thymus-leukemia (TL) antigens. One centimorgan (CM) is equivalent to a 1% recombination frequency per generation.

Class I Genes (H-2K and H-2D)

Although the map of the mouse MHC complex is changing rapidly because of new information being collected, it may be schematically recorded as shown in Figure 9-6. The major histocompatibility antigens responsible for graft rejection (allogeneic or within-species transplantation antigens) are controlled by the class I genetic regions, H-2K and H-2D. Class I regions code for cell surface antigens that serve as targets for antibody- or cell-mediated immune reactions. H-2K and H-2D specificities also play a major role in recognition of an individual's own tissue cells. During viral infections the viral antigens expressed on infected cells are recognized by cytotoxic T cells in association with class I MHC markers. The infected cells are recognized as "altered self" and lysed by T effector lymphocytes.

Class II Genes (the "I Region")

Using congenic mice, it was found that matching of class I genes was neither necessary nor sufficient for T cell – B cell cooperation; matching for a subregion of the class II region (the "I region") was required for a mixture of T and B cells to respond to immunization with T-dependent antigens. The I region (immune response region) codes for recognition structures that control interactions of macrophages, T cells, and B cells or the respective factors produced by these cells (see Chapter 10 for details). The I region has been divided into at least five subregions, A, B, J, E, and C, which are delineated in recombinant strains of mice and by genetic crossovers that have occurred within the MHC region and result in different patterns of immune responses to a variety of antigens. However, it seems likely that only the I-A and I-E subregions actually produce gene products that function as class II MHC markers.

The A subregion of class II controls the extent of antibody formation to a variety of T-dependent antigens, including various synthetic amino acid polymers such as poly(Tyr, Glu, Ala, Lys) as well as some larger protein molecules such as ovalbumin and lysozyme. The E region controls the levels of antibody production to an additional series of natural proteins such as pigeon cytochrome *c* and synthetic polypeptides such as poly(Glu, Lys, Phe). The E region shows genetic complementation in effect by collaboration with the A region as follows: two genetic low responder strains with different A and E regions may produce F_1's that are high responders. This seemingly paradoxical result is explained by the A region of one parental strain and the E region of the other parental strain complementing each other by each producing one of the subunits of the I-E molecule. Together these subunits form a functional I-E molecule so that a high immune response may be generated. The I region class II genes code for cell surface products, Aα, Aβ, Eα, and Eβ, that are present mainly on B cells and macrophages (see below). Some are, however, also present on T cells. These molecules determine the compatibility of lymphoid cell interactions in induction of immune responses.

Class III Genes

The class III genes, located in the S region, encode for components of the complement system. S/p and Ss encode for different forms of C_4, C_2 for C_2, and Bf for factor B (see Chapter 12).

The Human MHC (HLA)

The human MHC is called HLA, because the serologically defined markers were first found on lymphocytes (human lymphocyte antigens). Understanding of the role of the HLA

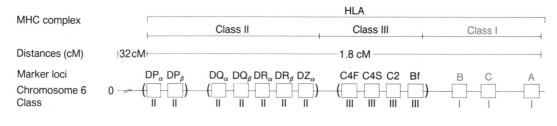

Figure 9-7. Proposed map of the human major histocompatibility (HLA) gene complex. The genes for HLA antigenic specificity are located on the sixth human chromosome in the relative order shown. There is room in this complex for many other genes. Each gene contains information for one specificity in each series.

complex in human immune responses is still incomplete. A map of the HLA complex is shown in Figure 9-7. The HLA gene complex is located on chromosome 6. Three class I genes code for transplantation antigens A, B, and C; the class II genes are DP, DQ, DR, and DZ, and the class III products are complement components C_2, C_4, and Bf. The organization of the human MHC differs from that of the mouse, but the function and the products appear analogous. In the human MHC the class I, II, and III gene regions are uninterrupted, whereas in the mouse MHC the class I gene (K) is separated from the other class I gene (D) by class II and III genes. Class I genes code for antigenic determinants present on all nucleated cells and are detected serologically (SD-defined determinants). Class II genes code for determinants recognized by mixed lymphocyte reactions (lymphocyte-defined or LD determinants). The class II gene products are now also detected serologically. Class II antigens are found primarily on B cells and macrophages, including tissue macrophages such as Kupffer cells of the liver, glial cells in the brain, and Langerhans cells in the epidermis.

The production of linked MHC specificities has given rise to the term *haplotype,* that is, specificities controlled by linked loci (see Fig. 9-15). Also present on the human chromosome 6 are genes for some red blood cell antigens. The role of class I genes in controlling human immune responses is less well understood than in the mouse. There is suggestive evidence that the antibody titers to diphtheria and measles may be MHC linked. The association of certain diseases, such as alkylosing spondylitis and uveitis, with the HLA-B27 specificity and the practical application of the relationship of HLA antigens to graft rejection are presented below.

MHC Products and the Cell Surface

Class I

Class I MHC gene products are glycoproteins of approximate MW 45,000 that are nonconvalently bound to a MW 12,000, 96-amino-acid peptide termed β_2-microglobulin. The orientation of the MHC class I molecule and β_2-microglobulin in the cell membrane is illustrated in Figure 9-8. The class I compo-

Figure 9-8. Structure of transplantation (class I) antigen. The heavy chain consists of 340 amino acids with three extracellular domains of approximately 90 residues each, a transmembrane segment of 40 amino acids, and an intracellular peptide of 30 residues. Two of the outer domains (α_2 and α_3) have intrachain disulfide bonds (forming 60-residue loops with considerable homology with Ig). Allotypic specificites are located in the α_1 and α_2 domains; α_3 is relatively invariant. β_2-Microglobulin is folded into the α_3 domain and is also invariant. The location of a variable domain at the carboxy end of the molecule with three or four invariant domains at the amino terminal is similar to the immunoglobulin heavy chain and suggests an origin from a common ancestral gene.

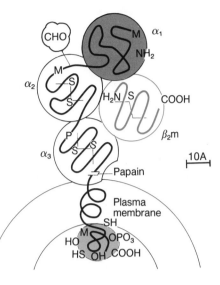

Cytoplasm

nent is referred to as the heavy chain and the β_2-microglobulin as the light chain. The heavy chain structure is organized with three exposed domains, α_1, α_2, and α_3, which extend from the cell surface and are attached to a hydrophobic transmembrane domain and a short cytoplasmic "anchor" segment within the cell. Each of the external domains contains about 90 amino acids, the transmembrane domain about 40 amino acids, and the cytoplasmic domain 30 amino acids. The light chain (β_2-microglobulin) is about the same size as one of the α external domains of the heavy chain. Each domain is immunoglobulin-like, consisting of 90 amino acids in a folded β pleated sheet structure held together by a disulfide bond at the ends, giving a plane-like surface that can be used to build a macromolecule. The β_2 chain folds with the α_3 domain of the heavy chain, and the α_1 and α_2 domains also pair.

The β_2-microglobulin gene is located on a chromosome different from that containing the MHC. Its structure is essentially invariant, whereas that of the heavy chains varies extensively from one individual to another because of differences in amino acid sequences of the external domains. The polymorphism of the heavy chain is contributed primarily by the α_1 domain and to a lesser degree by the α_2 domain. The homology between the MHC gene products and the immunoglobulins raises the possibility that the genes have a common evolutionary origin (see below).

Class I genes are organized into eight coding regions (exons) separated by seven intervening sequences (introns). The different coding regions each code for different structural domains, including the external domains (Fig. 9-9) and the

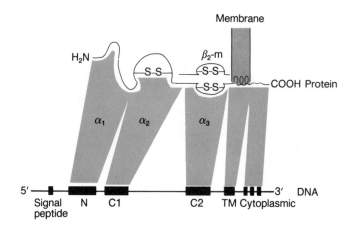

Figure 9-9. Schematic representation of class I genes and their product. Class I MHC determinants are controlled by α_1 (N) and α_2 (C1) domains. The α_3 (C2) domain associates with β_2-microglobulin and can be exchanged between different H-2 alleles or genes without affecting epitopes recognized by alloreactive or H-2 restricted CTL. (Modified from Forman et al.: Immunol Rev 81:203, 1984.)

transmembrane domain. Three small exons code for the cytoplasmic domain. The enormous degree of variation in the sequences of the class I molecules allows between 8 and 49 different versions (alleles) of each genetic locus. Expression of the class I genes is codominant. Each individual F_1 mouse expresses KAβ, KBβ, DAβ, and DBβ on all cells. The total number of combinations is the product of the number of alleles of these three loci, and is increased further by having two MHC genes at each locus (one on each sixth chromosome). Thus it is not surprising that matching between two unrelated individuals for a tissue graft is an extremely rare occurrence.

Other class I genes are also located within the MHC region of mice. Most of these are in the Qa and Tla regions; the functions of the Qa and Tla gene products are not clearly defined as yet. The product of the D or the HLA-A, B, C genes becomes inserted in the cell membrane where the extracellular domains are recognized as transplantation antigen.

Class II

The products of the class II genes are less well characterized. In the mouse the class II gene product (Ia) consists of two polypeptide chains (α and β, Fig. 9-10). The α chain has a molecular

Figure 9-10. A model of the class II MHC molecule. The α and β chains are divided into two external domains (α_1 and α_2 or β_1 and β_2), a transmembrane domain, and a cytoplasmic domain. The cysteine residues that participate in disulfide bridge formation are indicated by S, and the glycosylation sites on the external domains are indicated by CHO.

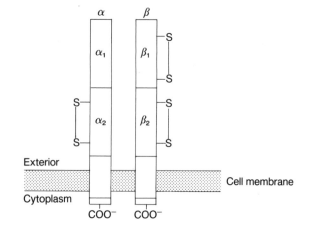

weight of 33,000, and the β chain 29,000. A third chain of MW 33,000 is invariant and is associated with the $\alpha\beta$ heterodimer before it is expressed on the cell surface. It may have an important role in transport of the heterodimer to the cell surface. Each class II polypeptide contains two external domains of 90 amino acids, a transmembrane domain of about 30 amino acids, and a cytoplasmic domain of 10–15 amino acids.

A genetic map of the class II region of the mouse is shown in Figure 9-11. The Aα, Aβ and Eβ genes are in the I-A subregion,

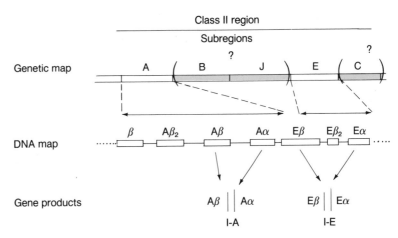

Figure 9-11. Genetic map of the class II region of the mouse based on recombination, with a DNA map based on molecular biology.

and the Eα gene is in the I-E region. These are codominantly expressed. β and Aβ2 are pseudogenes that are not expressed. Products of the B, J, and C regions have not been clearly identified. Based on functional studies, it has been postulated that a suppressor factor, I-J, is produced by genes in the J region, but there does not appear to be room on the chromosome for such a gene on the basis of recombinant DNA mapping of the class II region. Most recombinations within this region have occurred at a "hot spot" in or near the E gene. Since genetic distance is based on recombination frequency, this "hot spot" may have exaggerated the apparent distance between the I-A and I-E loci. DNA mapping shows them to be much closer, leaving little or no space for postulated B and J regions.

The gene products of the different alleles of the same locus on each chromosome can combine to form a new I-A marker. Thus in an (H-2^a × H-2^b)F$_1$ heterozygous mouse, the Aα chain of the "a" haplotype combines with either the Aβ chain of the "a" type or the Aβ chain of the "b" type. In the latter case, the A$^a\alpha$–A$^b\beta$ molecule is a hybrid determinant that can be recognized by some T cells in the F$_1$ mouse. This is yet another mechanism for increasing the diversity of class II markers recognized by T cells.

A map of the human class II region is shown in Figure 9-12. Much less is known about the human class II region than about that of the mouse. Mouse I-A and I-E molecules are homologous to the

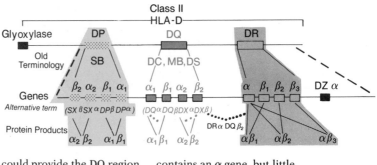

Figure 9-12. A schematic map of the human class II region. The numbers in front of α or β, such as 2α or 1α, identify different genes. The DQ region contains two α genes and two β genes that could provide the DQ region gene product. In the DR region there is one nonpolymorphic α gene and three β genes. The DP region contains two α and two β genes and the DZ region contains an α gene, but little else is known about this subregion. (See Immunology Today, March 1985, for additional information.)

human DQ and DR molecules; analogs to the DP and DZ products have not been identified in the mouse. If one can assume two α and two β chains per subregion for the four class II allelic subregion genes in the human, then up to four different products can be expressed for each class II subregion, or 16 different class II products per cell in a heterozygous individual. This provides great variability in the markers that lymphoid cells can use to identify self from nonself.

Class III

Class III gene products are complement components C2 and C4 of the classical pathway and factor B of the alternate pathway (see Chapter 12). These components are functionally related in that they are each involved in activation of the third component of complement (C3). The significance of their linkage with the MHC is not known.

Figure 9-13. Similarities in structure of lymphoid cell surface receptors: Thy 1, MHC class I, MHC class II, IgM, and T cell receptor. Receptors contain extracellular, transmembrane, and cytoplasmic domains. Thy 1 is a common T cell differentiation antigen of the mouse that is roughly analogous to CD3 in the human.

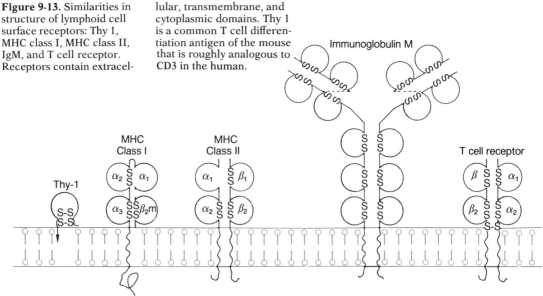

Comparison of Cell Surface Molecules of Lymphocytes

A comparison of the structure of lymphocyte cell surface receptors is illustrated in Figure 9-13. Similarities in structure and sequence homologies among the polypeptide chains in various domains suggest a common evolutionary origin of these molecules (Fig. 9-14).

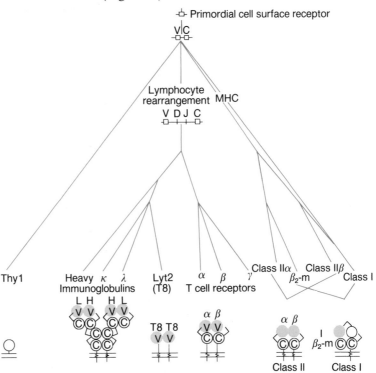

Figure 9-14. A schematic representation of the evolution of the immunoglobulin gene superfamily. V and C denote V- and C-like homology units, respectively. The open circles for the MHC molecules do not exhibit significant sequence similarity with the immunoglobulin homology units, although they are of similar length. The Thy 1 homology unit does exhibit sequence similarity, although it is not easily classified as V or C and may have diverged prior to the V–C divergence. The horizontally paired homology units represent probable domain structures apart from those hypothesized for the CD8 molecule. (Modified from Hood L, Kronenberg M, Hunkapiller T: T cell antigen receptor and the immunoglobulin supergene family. Cell 40:225–229, 1985.)

The MHC and Tissue Transplantation

Historically, the major importance of the identification of the products of the MHC involved their role in human tissue transplantation. Transplants between identical twins are not rejected, whereas rejection occurs where there are differences at the MHC. Tissue grafts from one genetically different individual to another (allografts) require suppression of the immune response if the graft is to survive.

Donor–Recipient Matching in Human Transplantation

Although immunosupression has prolonged human graft survival, the results are frequently not satisfactory. Better tissue matching of recipient and donor combined with less vigorous immunosuppression might be the most advantageous approach. Extensive serological testing is now done in attempts to match donor and recipient histocompatibility antigens, but the results have not been as productive as expected. Complementary DNA probes for human MHC genes will provide better tissue-typing results.

Histocompatibility antigens are those cellular determinants specific for each individual of a species that are responsible for immune rejection when attempts are made to transfer or transplant cellular material from one individual of the same species to another. Identical twins are the only known human individuals who share all histocompatibility antigens. Perhaps the most familiar example of histocompatibility antigens is the ABO blood group system. The A and B antigens are found not only on erythrocytes but also on other tissue cells. Therefore, no attempt to transfer solid organs from one individual to another should be made across a known AB blood group difference. However, other histocompatibility antigens are obviously important, because matching of the ABO or other erythrocyte antigen systems between donor and recipient is not enough to provide a compatible relation.

During the 1960s many attempts were made to develop tests for histocompatibility antigens and matching tests for potential donors and recipients. Tests that have been used to select organ donors include the mixed lymphocyte culture reaction (MLR) and the analysis and matching of histocompatibility antigens by serologic tests. The in vitro systems are not only useful for matching donors and recipients of grafts but provide a means of evaluating immunologic recognition and its significance.

Figure 9-15. Mixed lymphocyte reaction (MLR). The degree of stimulation in an MLR correlates to the degree of histocompatibility difference between the lymphocyte donors. This is a two-way test (a cross-match test), because the lymphocytes of each donor interact with each other. The test can be made one-way by preventing the response of one set of lymphocytes, the organ donor's, by treatment with radiation or an antimetabolite such as mitomycin C. This gives an estimate of the rejection response of a potential recipient (living cells) against the cells of a potential organ donor (the treated cells). Stimulation is measured by an increase in DNA synthesis, occurring 5–7 days after interaction in culture, that is not seen when the cells of only one individual are cultured (control). The ability to store lymphocytes in vitro in liquid nitrogen freezers permits tissue typing even when a given donor is no longer living.

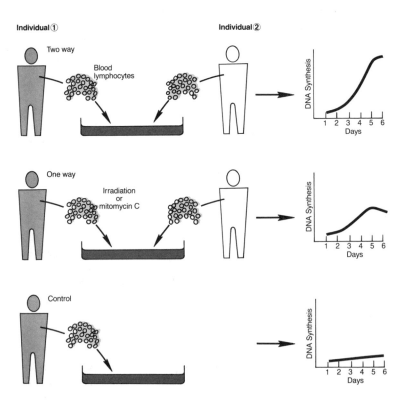

Mixed Lymphocyte Reactions

The mixed lymphocyte reaction (MLR) test is based on the observation that cultures of mixtures of lymphocytes from two genetically different individuals produce transformed immature blast cells that synthesize DNA (Fig. 9-15).

Although it was first suspected that MLR reactions depended upon the class I A, B, and C antigens defined by humoral antibodies (see below), it is now known that the extent of a mixed lymphocyte reaction is dependent not upon class I differences but upon the class II gene products. The cell that responds in the MLR is a T cell. The stimulator cell containing the antigen to which the responding T cell reacts is a macrophage or B cell. The class II antigens detected serologically are present on macrophages and B cells, but not on T cells. Class I specificities may stimulate mixed lymphocyte reactions weakly or increase class II–induced reactions, but for practical purposes MLR is considered to be the result of class II differences. A second aspect of the MLR is the generation of cytotoxic T lymphocytes (CTL) that react specifically with the class I region markers of the stimulator cells. These cells are generated from a subset of precursor T cells different from the cells that proliferate in the MLR. The killing is directed to class I MHC markers (see Chapter 10). Thus the MLR proliferation response depends upon class II products; the cytotoxicity response upon class I products (Fig. 9-16).

Serologically Defined Histocompatibility Antigens

In addition to the antigens detected by the MLR, there are serologically defined cell membrane components that are recognized during allograft rejection and are directly related to the rejection reaction. The identification of these histocompatibility antigens in the laboratory depends upon the serologic (antibody-mediated) recognition of MHC products on lymphocytes. Most tissue antigens appear to be shared by lymphocytes and solid tissue. The identification of a given antigen on a lymphocyte can be determined by the ability of an antiserum to react with the antigen, activating complement and causing the death of the lymphocytes.

Antihistocompatibility antisera that reacted with lymphocytes were recognized as long as 50 years ago, but the significance of such antibodies with respect to histocompatibility was not apparent until more recently. Antibodies in human sera to human lymphocytes are found in patients with certain diseases, in multiparous women, and in patients receiving multiple blood transfusions. In retrospect these latter situations were found to be caused by genetically controlled differences in MHC specificities among human individuals (allotypy). In the 1950s, the reaction patterns of such antisera with lymphocytes from a number of different individuals were revealed. For instance, some antisera reacted with lymphocytes from essentially the same donors in a panel (e.g., 20 of 50 donors), whereas

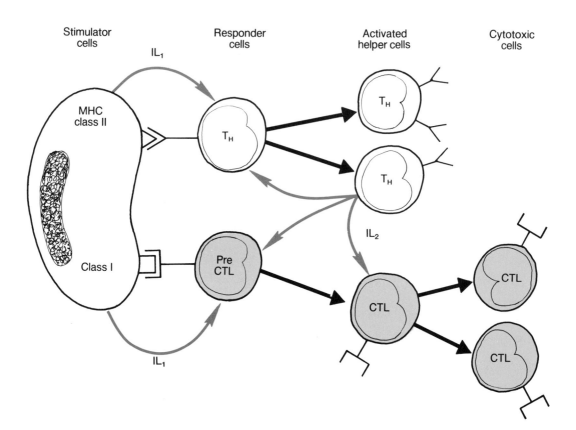

Figure 9-16. Interaction of T helper/inducer T cells and precursors of CTL during generation of CTL responsible for graft rejection. T_H cells are stimulated by reaction with class II MHC products to proliferate and produce IL2. IL2 acts on CTL precursors activated by reaction with class I MHC product to support proliferation and differentiation of CTL.

other antisera reacted with lymphocytes of different donors. The reaction patterns observed were extremely complicated and, it seemed, unresolvable. However, in the early 1960s Van Rood introduced computer analysis of the reaction patterns, a method that was soon adopted by others. This resulted in resolution of the reaction patterns of many different antisera. In the mid-1960s, a number of individuals who had been testing such antisera held a series of conferences at which many of the problems involving detection techniques and reaction patterns were compared. The result was an example of the contribution that can be made to scientific understanding by unselfish cooperation of different investigators.

Genetics of Human Histocompatibility Antigens

It is now generally accepted that human histocompatibility antigens, comprising over 50 different specificities, are controlled by the MHC. The serologic identification of MHC gene products using conventional sera from multiparous women, as well as monoclonal antibodies, has resulted in the identification of 23 A, 49 B, 8 C, 19 DW, 16 DR, 3 DQ, and 6 DP specificities (Table 9-1). Historically, typing has involved mainly A, B, and D antigens. An example of the inheritance of HLA-A, -B, and -D types is shown in Figure 9-17.

Table 9-1. Complete Listing of Recognized HLA Specificities

A	B		C	D	DR	DQ	DP
A1	B5	Bw47	Cw1	Dw1	DR1	DQw1	DPw1
A2	B7	Bw48	Cw2	Dw2	DR2	DQw2	DPw2
A3	B8	B49(21)	Cw3	Dw3	DR3	DQw3	DPw3
A9	B12	Bw50(21)	Cw4	Dw4	DR4		DPw4
A10	B13	B51(5)	Cw5	Dw5	DR5		DPw5
A11	B14	Bw52(5)	Cw6	Dw6	DRw6		DPw6
Aw19	B15	Bw53	Cw7	Dw7	DR7		
A23(9)	B16	Bw54(w22)	Cw8	Dw8	DRw8		
A24(9)	B17	Bw55(w22)		Dw9	DRw9		
A25(10)	B18	Bw56(w22)		Dw10	DRw10		
A26(10)	B21	Bw57(17)		Dw11(w7)	DRw11(5)		
A28	Bw4	Bw58(17)		Dw12	DRw12(5)		
A29(w19)	Bw6	Bw59		Dw13	DRw13(w6)		
A30(w19)	Bw22	Bw60(40)		Dw14	DRw14(w6)		
A31(w19)	B27	Bw61(40)		Dw15			
A32(w19)	B35	Bw62(15)		Dw16	DRw52		
Aw33(w19)	B37	Bw63(15)		Dw17(w7)	DRw53		
Aw34(10)	B38(16)	Bw64(14)		Dw18(w6)			
Aw36	B39(16)	Bw65(14)		Dw19(w6)			
Aw43	B40	Bw67					
Aw66(10)	Bw41	Bw70					
Aw68(28)	B44(12)	Bw71(w70)					
Aw69(28)	B45(12)	Bw72(w70)					
	B45(12)	Bw73					
	Bw46						

Antigens followed by a number in parentheses are recognized as splits of the antigen in parentheses; for example, A23 is a split of A9.

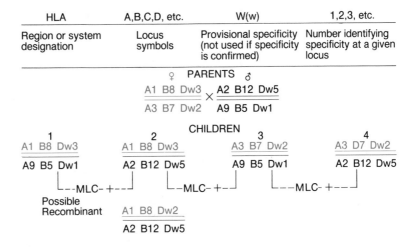

HLA	A,B,C,D, etc.	W(w)	1,2,3, etc.
Region or system designation	Locus symbols	Provisional specificity (not used if specificity is confirmed)	Number identifying specificity at a given locus

Figure 9-17. Inheritance of HLA-A, -B, and -D types. Genetically linked HLA-A, -B, and -D types are inherited as a unit on one chromosome (haplotype). The haplotype is written on one line (A1 B8 Dw3). From a given pair of parents only four haplotype combinations are possible. Thus in a family of five or more siblings, at least one pair must have identical HLA types unless a recombination of chromosomes has occurred. The recombination listed has a crossover between B and D. The identification of crossover frequencies permits a relative localization of HLA regions in the HLA supergene. MLC indicates a positive mixed lymphocyte culture reaction because of HLA-D difference. (Modified from Bodmer WF, et al.: Proc R Soc Lond [Biol] 202:93, 1978.)

The distribution of MHC genes within a family dictates that only four combinations of HLA antigens occur among siblings unless recombination occurs. Each parent has two MHC haplotypes, each made up of four HLA antigens. If the haplotypes are designated AB for one parent and CD for the other parent, the four possible haplotype combinations in their children are AC, AD, BC, and BD. Thus, in a family of five children of the same parents, two of the children will have an identical match for all HLA markers. The likelihood of crossing over between two parental chromosomes given a recombinant haplotype (part from each parental haplotype) is about 1% and is a function of the distance along the chromosome occupied by the MHC region. Such an individual would have no chance of finding an MHC matched sibling.

HLA Testing and Graft Survival

It was once thought that the HLA antigens could provide a means of identifying individuals who had similar or identical tissue antigens and who would not reject tissue grafts. Using skin grafts, it was observed that grafts between identical twins would survive indefinitely; grafts between unrelated HLA-nonidentical individuals are usually rejected within about 10 days. Grafts between HLA-matched unrelated individuals lasted only slightly longer than those between HLA-nonidentical unrelated individuals, whereas grafts between HLA-identical siblings survived 20 to 40 days. Clearly more than HLA antigen matching is required to select a histocompatible donor. At least two other factors must be considered: other HLA loci and minor histocompatibility loci (non-HLA antigens).

The existence of HLA antigens in other loci is possible. The presence of additional HLA loci adds an additional variable to the problem of tissue matching (see above). Since standard tissue typing can take into account only detectable specificities, matches presently classified as identical indicate identity only at the known HLA loci, so that nonidentity at another locus might explain some of the lack of correlation of matching to graft survival.

Transplantation studies in mice have resulted in the concept of strong and weak histocompatibility antigens. At least 11 histocompatibility systems have been identified in the mouse. The MHC system is termed the *strong* histocompatibility system because organ grafts between individual mice differing in antigenic specificities controlled by the MHC evoke strong rejection reactions. If organ donor and recipient are matched for the MHC but differ in one of the other systems, rejection is not as rapid or as severe. Therefore, these histocompatibility antigen systems are called *weak*. It is apparent that weak histocompatibility systems are also present in humans, but they remain to be defined. The evidence regarding weak histocompatibility antigens indicates that differences in these systems can be more readily overcome by immunosuppressive therapy than can differences in strong histocompatibility antigens.

The clinical experience in regard to HLA matching and renal and other tissue graft survival has been disappointing. Some representative data are presented in Figure 9-18. The

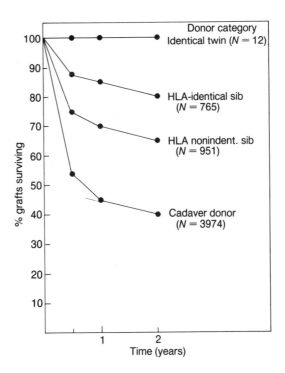

Figure 9-18. Survival times of kidney allografts among people of different genetic relationships, ranging from identical twins to unrelated individuals (cadaver donors). (From Hildemann WH: Tissue Antigens 22:1–6, 1983.)

survival of grafts reflects the histocompatibility differences (MHC and others) as well as other factors (complicating diseases, infection, etc.). The difference in survival of renal grafts between identical twins and HLA-identical siblings probably reflects non-MHC differences and indicates that non-MHC differences contribute to 15% of transplant failures. The difference between HLA-identical siblings and HLA-nonidentical siblings at 1 year suggests that MHC differences also contribute 15% to transplant failure.

Additive effects of MHC plus non-MHC alloantigens probably account in large part for the 60% failure rate in unmatched cadaver donors. At this time there appears to be little correlation between HLA-A and -B matching and graft survival. There does appear to be some correlation between HLA-DR matching and renal graft survival in North America, but not in Europe. Thus HLA typing has had decreasing influence on transplantation programs, whereas controlled immunosuppression has received greater emphasis.

Human MHC and Disease Associations

Certain HLA phenotypes are found associated with some human diseases. Of particular interest are immune-related diseases (Table 9-2), such as ankylosing spondylitis, Reiter's disease, and acute anterior uveitis, which are strongly associated with HLA-B27. The HLA-B27 specificity may be linked to an immune response (IR)–type gene that influences the response to an infectious agent or degree of inflammation in rheumatoid diseases. Reiter's disease consists of an infectious urethritis followed by arthritis, uveitis, and chronic skin lesions indistinguishable from psoriasis. The incidence of urethritis is not influenced by HLA-B27, but the incidence of the subsequent arthritis and skin lesions is. In addition, a small number of individuals may develop arthritis following intestinal infection with *Yersinia enterocolitica*. Again, the incidence of infection is not related to HLA type, but the incidence of arthritis is much higher in individuals with HLA-B27. In these diseases the finding of a B27 marker may aid diagnosis. Although the data are not as convincing, HLA-B8 and HLA-Bw15 are associated with systemic lupus erythematosus, and HLA-B13 with pemphigus. Thus, there may be an inherited tendency to produce an immunopathologic response to infections or inflammatory stimuli in certain individuals. The finding that the inheritance of some of these tendencies is linked to HLA specificities could assist in identification of new infectious agents or pathogenic mechanisms associated with rheumatoid disease.

In one instance a specific molecular defect has been described for a class I association. Individuals with congenital

Table 9-2. HLA and Disease Associations

Disease	Number of Studies	HLA SD Antigen	Frequency in Patients (%)	Frequency in Controls (%)	Average Relative Risk
Ankylosing spondylitis	5	B27	90	7	141.0
Reiter's disease	3	B27	76	6	46.6
Acute anterior uveitis	2	B27	55	8	16.7
	6	B13	18	4	5.0
Psoriasis	6	Bw17	29	8	5.0
	4	Bw16	15	5	2.9
Graves' disease	1	B8	47	21	3.3
Celiac disease	6	B8	78	24	10.4
Dermatitis herpetiformis	3	B8	62	27	4.5
Myasthenia gravis	5	B8	52	24	4.6
Systemic lupus erythematosus	2	Bw15	33	8	5.1
Multiple sclerosis	4	A3	36	25	1.7
		B7	36	25	1.5
Acute lymphatic leukemia	7	A2	63	37	1.7
	8	Bw35	25	16	1.6
Hodgkin's disease	7	A1	39	32	1.3
	7	B8	26	22	1.3
Chronic hepatitis	1	B8	68	18	9.5
Ragweed hay fever, Ra5 sensitivity	1	B7	50	19	4.0

adrenal hyperplasia have a deletion of the 21-hydroxylase gene that also deletes a portion of the class III region associated with C4 as well as a part of the neighboring HLA-B class I subregion. This deletion converts the HLA-B13 gene into the rare HLA-Bw47 that is always associated with the disease.

Summary

The major histocompatibility complex (MHC) is a series of linked genes on chromosome 6 of humans and chromosome 17 of the mouse. Class I region genes control the expression of tissue antigens responsible for graft rejection; class II region genes code for the lymphoid cell surface markers that are required for self recognition between cells and cooperation in the induction of the immune response; and class III region genes code for some of the components of complement. Histocompatibility antigens are complex cell surface structures that are recognized as foreign by one individual of a species when exposed to tissue of another individual of that species (allografts). Immune response antigens are controlled by the class II genes and determine the ability of T lymphocytes of a given individual to recognize and cooperate with macrophages and B cells of the same class II type in the response to foreign antigen. Understanding the human MHC is important for tissue matching prior to organ grafting and for determining the genetic susceptibility to certain diseases.

References

Self–Nonself Recognition

Burnet FM: The Clonal Selection Theory of Acquired Immunity. London, Cambridge University Press, 1959.

Burnet FM: The Integrity of the Body: A Discussion of Modern Immunological Ideas. Cambridge, Harvard University Press, 1962.

Burnet FM: Multiple polymorphism in relation to histocompatibility antigens. Nature 245:359, 1973.

Cohen IR, Welerle H: Regulation of autosensitization. The immune activation and specific inhibition of self recognizing thymus derived lymphocytes. J Exp Med 137:224, 1973.

Dorf ME (ed): The Role of the Major Histocompatibility Complex in Immunobiology. New York, Garland/STM Press, 1985.

Gotze D (ed): The Major Histocompatibility System in Man and Animals. New York, Springer-Verlag, 1977.

Jerne NK: The somatic generation of immune recognition. Eur J Immunol 1:1, 1971.

Hoffman GW: A theory of regulation and self–nonself discrimination. Eur J Immunol 5:638, 1975.

Klein E: Parental variants. Transplant Proc 3:1167, 1971.

Klein J: Biology of the Mouse Histocompatibility-2 Complex. New York, Springer-Verlag, 1975.

Ohno S: The original function of MHC antigens as the general plasma membrane anchorage site organogenesis-directing proteins. Immunol Rev 33:59, 1977.

Reigmann J, Miller RG: Polymorphism and gene function. Rev Comp Immunol 7:403, 1983.

Thorsby E: Biological function of HLA. Tissue Antigens 11:321, 1978.

Zinkernagel RM: Thymus and lymphohemopoietic cells: their role in T cell maturation, in selection of T cell H_2 restriction-specificity and H_2 linked Ir gene control. Immunol Rev 42:224, 1978.

Zinkernagel RM: Major transplantation antigens in host response to infection. Hosp Pract 13:83, 1978.

Genetics of Tissue Transplantation

Amos DB: Genetic aspects of human HL-A transplantation antigens. Fed Proc 29:2018, 1970.

Bach FH (ed): Immunobiology of Transplantation. New York, Grune & Stratton, 1974.

Bodmer WF, Jones EA, Barnstable CJ, Bodmer JG: Genetics of HLA: the major human histocompatibility system. Proc R Soc Lond [Biol] 202:93, 1978.

Howard JG, Michie JG: Transplantation immunology. *In* Cruickshank R (ed): Modern Trends in Immunology. London, Whitefriars, 1963.

Klein J (ed): The Biology of the Mouse Histocompability 2 Complex. New York, Springer-Verlag, 1975.

Klein J, Figueroa F, Nagy Z: Genetics of the major histocompatibility complex: the final act. Annu Rev Immunol 1:119, 1983.

Merrill JP: Human tissue transplantation. Adv Immunol 7:276, 1967.

Moller G (ed): Genetic and Biological Aspects of Histocompatibility Antigens. Transplant Rev 15, 1973.

Snell GD: Histocompatibility genes of the mouse. II. Production and analysis of isogenic resistant lines. J Nat Cancer Inst 21:843, 877, 1958.

Snell GD, Stimpfiing JH: Genetics of tissue transplantation. *In* Green EL (ed): Biology of the Laboratory Mouse, 2nd ed. New York, McGraw–Hill, 1966.

Staats J: Standardized nomenclature for inbred strains of mice: sixth listing. Cancer Res 36:4333, 1976.

Genetic Control of Immune Reactions

Bechtol KB, Freed JB, Herzenberg LA, McDevitt HO: Genetic control of the antibody response to poly-L-(Tyr, Glu)–poly-D, L-Ala–poly-L-Lys in $C_3H \leftrightarrow$ CWB tetraparental mice. J Exp Med 140:1660, 1974.

Benacerraf B: Role of MHC gene products in immune regulation. Science 212:1229, 1981.

Benacerraf B, McDevitt HO: The histocompatibility linked immune response gene. Science 175:273, 1972.

Bevin MJ, Hunig T: T cells respond preferentially to antigens that are similar to self. Proc Nat Acad Sci USA 78:1843, 1981.

Bluestein HG, Green I, Benacerraf B: Specific immune response genes of the guinea pig. I. Dominant genetic control of immune responsiveness to copolymers of L-glutamic acid and L-alanine and L-glutamic acid and L-tyrosine. J Exp Med 134:458, 1971.

Gasser DL, Silbers WK: Genetic determinants of immunologic responsiveness. Adv Immunol 18:1, 1974.

Green I, Paul WE, Benacerraf B: A study of the passive transfer of delayed hypersensitivity to DNP-poly-L-lysine and DNP-GL in responder and nonresponder guinea pigs. J Exp Med 126:959, 1967.

Haverkorn MJ, Hofmann B, Masurel N, Van Rood JJ: HLA linked genetic control of immune response in man. Transplant Rev 22: 120, 1975.

Heber-Katz E, Wilson D: Collaboration of allogeneic T and B lympholymphocytes in the primary antibody response to sheep erythrocytes in vitro. J Exp Med 142:928, 1976.

Kantor FS, Ojeda A, Benacerraf B: Studies on artificial antigens. I. Antigenicity of DNP-poly-lysine and DNP-copolymer of lysine and glutamic acid in guinea pigs. J Exp Med 117:55, 1963.

Kappler JW, Marrack PC: Helper T cells recognize antigen and macrophage components simultaneously. Nature 262:797, 1976.

Katz DH, Benacerraf B (eds): The Role of Products of the Histocompatibility Gene Complex in Immune Responses. New York, Academic Press, 1976.

Kindred B, Shreffler DC: H-2 dependence of cooperation between T and B cells in vivo. J Immunol 109:940, 1972.

McDevitt HO (ed): Ir Genes and Ia Antigens. New York, Academic Press, 1978.

McDevitt HO, Benacerraf B: Genetic control of specific immune responses. Adv Immunol 11:31, 1969.

Moller G (ed): Conditions for T cell activation. Immunol Rev 35, 1977.

Moller G (ed): Ir genes and T lymphocytes. Immunol Rev 38:1, 1978.

Rosenthal AS, Shevach EM: Functions of macrophages in antigen recognition by guinea pig T lymphocytes. I. Requirement for histocompatibility macrophages and lymphocytes. J Exp Med 138:1194–1212, 1974.

Sasportes M, Fradelizi D, Nunez-Roldan A, Wollman E, Giannopoulos Z, Dausset J: Analysis of stimulating products involved in primary and secondary allogeneic proliferation in man: I, II, and III. Immunogenetics 6:29, 43, 55, 1978.

Schwartz RH: T-lymphocyte recognition of antigen in association with gene products of the major histocompatibility complex. Annu Rev Immunol 3:237, 1985.

Shreffler DC, David CS: The H-2 major histocompatibility complex and the I immune response region: genetic variation, function and organization. Adv Immunol 20:125, 1975.

Thomas DW, Yamashita U, Shevach EM: The role of Ia antigens in T cell activation. Immunol Rev 35:97, 1977.

Unanue ER: The regulatory role of macrophages in antigenic stimulation. Adv Immunol 15:95, 1972.

Von Boehmer H, Hudson L, Sprent J: Collaboration of histoincompatible T and B lymphocytes using cells from tetraparental bone marrow chimeras. J Exp Med 142:989, 1975.

MHC T Cell Killing Restriction

Berke G, Amos GB: Mechanism of lymphocyte-mediated cytolysis: the LMC cycle and its role in transplantation immunity. Transplant Rev 17:71, 1973.

Germain R, Dorf M, Benacerraf B: Inhibition of T lymphocyte mediated tumor-specific lysis by alloantisera directed against the H₂ serologic specificities. J Exp Med 142:1023, 1975.

Klein J: Genetics of cell mediated lymphocytotoxicity in the mouse. Semin Immunopathol 1:31, 1978.

Matzinger P, Bevan MJ: Induction of H-2–restricted cytotoxic T cells: in vivo induction has the appearance of being unrestricted. Cell Immunol 33:92–100, 1977.

Moller G (ed): MHC restriction of anti-viral immunity. Immunol Rev 58, 1981.

Moller G (ed): Mechanism of action of cytotoxic T cells. Immunol Rev 72, 1983.

Shearer GM, Schmitt-Verhulst A-M: Major histocompatibility complex restricted cell-mediated immunity. Adv Immunol 25:55, 1977.

Zinkernagel R: Virus specific T-cell–mediated cytotoxicity across the H-2 barrier to virus altered alloantigen. Nature 261:139, 1976.

Zinkernagel RM, Althage A, Cooper S, Callahan G, Klein J: In irradiation chimeras, K or D region of the chimeric host, not of the donor lymphocytes, determines immune responsiveness of anti-viral cytotoxic T cell. J Exp Med 148:805, 1978.

Zinkernagel RM, Callahan GN, Althaga A, Cooper S, Klein DA, Klein J: On the thymus in the differentiation of "H-2 self-recognition" by T cells: evidence for dual recognition. J Exp Med 147:882, 1978.

Zinkernagel RM, Doherty PC: H₂ compatibility requirement for T-cell–mediated lysis of target cells infected with lymphocytic choriomeningitis virus. J Exp Med 141:1427, 1975.

MHC Genes

Amos DB: The evolution of the supergene: observation on the major histocompatibility complex. *In* Zalesk MB, Abeyounis CJ, Kano K (eds), Immunobiology of the Major Histocompatibility Complex. Basel, Karger, 1981.

Clark SS, Forman J: Allogeneic and association recognition determinants of H-2 molecules. Transplant Proc 15:2090, 1983.

Germain RN, Malissen B: Analysis of the expression and function of class-II major histocompatibility complex molecules by DNA mediated transfer. Annu Rev Immunol 4:28, 1986.

Gonwa T, Peterlin BM, Stobo JD: Human Ir genes: structure and function. Adv Immunol 34:71, 1983.

Hansen TH, et al.: The immunogenetics of the mouse major histocompatibility gene complex. Annu Rev Genet 18:99, 1984.

Hood L, Steinmetz M, Malissen B: Genes of the major histocompatibility complex of the mouse. Annu Rev Immunol 1:529, 1983.

Klein J, Figueroa F, Nagy Z: Genetics of the major histocompatibility complex: the final act. Annu Rev Immunol 1:119, 1983.

Lew AM, et al.: Class I genes and molecules: an update. Immunology 57:3, 1986.

Mengle-Gaw L, McDevitt HO: Genetics and expression of mouse Ia antigens. Annu Rev Immunol 3:363, 1985.

Nathenson SG, et al: Murine major histocompatibility complex class-I mutants: molecular analysis and structure–function implications. Annu Rev Immunol 4:471, 1986.

Steinmetz M, Hood L: Genes of the major histocompatibility complex in mouse and man. Science 222:727, 1983.

MHC Products

Algranati ID, Milstein C, Ziegler A: Studies on biosynthesis, assembly and expression of human major transplantation antigens. Eur J Biochem 103:197, 1980.

Crumpton MJ, Snary D, Walsh FS, Barnstable CJ, Goodfellow PN, Jones EA, Bodmer WF: Molecular structure of the gene products of the human HLA system: isolation and characterization of HLA-A, -B, -C and Ia antigen. Proc R Soc Lond [Biol] 202:159, 1978.

Ferrone S, Allison JP, Pellegrino MA: Human DR (Ia-like) antigens: biological and molecular profile. Contemp Top Mol Immunol 7:239, 1978.

Frelinger JA, Shreffler DC: The major histocompatibility complexes. *In* Benacerraf B (ed): Immunogenetics and Immunodeficiency. Baltimore, University Park Press, 1975, p81.

Grey HM, Kubo RT, Colon SM, Poulik MD, Cresswell P, Springer T, Turner M, Strominger JL: The small subunit of HL-A antigens is β_2 macroglobulin. J Exp Med 138:1608, 1973.

Henriksen O, Appella E, Smith DF, Tanigaki N, Pressman D: Comparative chemical analysis of the alloantigenic fragment of HL-A antigens. J Biol Chem 251:4214, 1976.

Hood L, Kronenberg M, Hunkapiller T: T cell antigen receptors and the immunoglobulin supergene family. Cell 40:225, 1985.

Kaufman JF, et al: The class II murine major histocompatibility complex. Cell 36:1, 1984.

Moller G (ed): MHC and MLS Determinants. Immunol Rev 60, 1981.

Moller G (ed): Structure and Function of HLA-DR. Immunol Rev 66, 1982.

Nathenson SG: Biochemical properties of histocompatibility antigens. Annu Rev Genet 4:69, 1970.

Nathenson SG, et al.: Murine major histocompatibility complex class I mutants: molecular analysis and structure function relationship. Annu Rev Immunol 4:47, 1986.

Norcross MA, Kanehisa M: The predicted structure of the Ia β1 domains: a hypothesis for the structural basis of major histocompatibility complex–restricted T-cell recognition of antigens. Scand J Immunol 21:511, 1985.

Peterson PA, Rask L, Lindblom JB: Highly purified papain-solubilized HL-A antigens contain β-2-microglobulin. Proc Nat Acad Sci USA 71:35, 1974.

Reisfeld RA: Isolation and serological evaluation of HL-A antigens solubilized from cultured human lymphoid cells. *In* Korn ED (ed): Methods in Membrane Biology. New York, Plenum, 1974, p143.

Reisfeld RA, Pellegrino MA, Ferrone S, Kahan BD: Chemical and molecular nature of HL-A antigens. Transplant Proc 5:447, 1973.

Strominger JL, Ferguson W, Fuks A, Giphart M, Kaufman J, Mann D, Orr H, Parham P, Robb R, Terhorst C: Isolation and structure of HLA antigens. Birth Defects 14:235, 1978.

Walford RL, Waters H, Smith GS: Human transplantation antigens. Fed Proc 29:2011, 1970.

Walker LE, Reisfeld RA: Human histocompatibility antigens: isolation and chemical characterization. J Immunol Methods 49:R25, 1982.

MHC and Organ Transplantation

Albert ED, Baver MP, Mayr WR (eds): Histocompatibility Testing 1984. New York, Springer-Verlag, 1984.

Albert E, Gotze D: The major histocompatibility system in man. *In* Gotze E (ed): Histocompatibility Antigens. Berlin, Springer-Verlag, 1978, p7.

Albrechtsen D, Bratlie A, Nousianinen H, Solheim BG, Winther N, Thorsby E: Serological typing of HLA-D: predictive value in mixed lymphocyte cultures (MLC). Immunogenetics 6:91, 1978.

Amos DB: Genetic and antigenetic aspects of human histocompatibility system. Adv Immunol 10:251, 1969.

Amos DB, Kostyu DD: HLA – a central immunological agency of man. Adv Hum Genet 10:137, 1980.

Bach FH: Transplantation: pairing of donor and recipient. Science 168:1170, 1970.

Bodmer J, Bodmer W: Histocompatibility 1984. Immunol Today 5:251, 1984.

Bodmer WF (ed): The HLA system. Br Med Bull 34, 1978.

Bodmer WF, Bodmer J, Batchelor R, Festenstein H, Morris P: Joint Report from the Seventh International Histocompatibility Workshop in Histocompatibility Testing 1977. Copenhagen, Munksgaard, 1978.

Cheigh JB, Chami J, Stenzl KH, Riggio RR, Saal S, Mouradian JA, Fotino M, Stubenbord WT, Rubel AL: Renal transplantation between HLA identical siblings: comparison with transplants from HLA semi-identical donors. N Engl J Med 296:1030, 1977.

Dausset J: The major histocompatibility complex in man. Science 213: 1469, 1981.

Ferrone S, Curtoni ES, Gorini S: HLA Antigens in Clinical Medicine and Biology. New York, Garland/STM Press, 1983.

Gray I, Russell PS: Donor selection in human organ transplantation. Lancet 2:863, 1963.

Morris PJ: Histocompatibility in organ transplantation in man. *In* Joachim HL (ed): Pathobiology Annual 1973. New York, Appleton–Century–Crofts, 1973.

Myburgh JA, Shapiro M, Maier G, Myers AM: HL-A and cadaver kidney transplantation. 7 years experience of Johannesburg General Hospital. S Afr Med J 50:1279, 1976.

Rappaport FT, Converse JM, Billingham RE: Recent advances in clinical and experimental transplantation. JAMA 27:2835, 1977.

Russell PS, Monaco AP: The biology of tissue transplantation. N Engl J Med 271:502, 553, 610, 664, 718, 776, 1964.

Salvatierra O, Feduska NS, Cochrum KC, Najarian JS, Kountz SL, Belzer FO: The impact of 1,000 renal transplants of one center. Ann Surg 186:424, 1977.

Simmons RL, Van Hook EJ, Yunis EJ, Noreen H, Kjellstrano CM, Condie RM, Mauer SM, Buselmeier TJ, Najarian JS: 100 sibling kidney transplants followed 2 to $7\frac{1}{2}$ years: a multifactorial analysis. Ann Surg 185:196, 1977.

Teraski PI, Mickey MR, Singal DP, Mitalli KK, Patel R: Serotyping for transplantation. XX. Selection of recipients for cadaver donor transplants. N Engl J Med 279:1101, 1968.

Thorsby E: The human major histocompatibility system. Transplant Rev 18:51, 1974.

Thorsby E: Histocompatibility antigens: immunogenetics and role of matching in clinical renal transplantation. Ann Clin Res 13:190, 1981.

Wilson RE, Henry L, Merrill JP: A model system for determining histocompatibility in man. J Clin Invest 52:1497, 1963.

Van Rood JJ, Eernisse JG: The detection of transplantation antigens in leukocytes. Prog Surg 7:217, 1967.

HLA and Disease Susceptibility

Arnett FC: HLA and genetic predisposition to lupus erythematosus and other dermatologic disorders. J Am Acad Dermatol 13:472, 1985.

Braun WE: HLA and Disease: A Comprehensive Review. Boca Raton, Fla., CRC Press, 1979.

Brewerton DA: HLA-B27 and the inheritance of susceptibility to rheumatic disease. Arthritis Hematol 19:656, 1976.

Brewerton DA, Caffrey M, Hart FD, James DCO, Nichols A, Sturrock RD: Ankylosing spondylitis and HL-A27. Lancet 1:904, 1973.

Brewerton DA, Caffrey M, Nichols A, Walters D, James DCO: Acute anterior uveitis and HL-A27. Lancet 2:994, 1973.

Brewerton DA, Caffrey M, Nichols A, Walters D, Oates JK, James DCO: Reiter's disease and HL-A27. Lancet 2:996, 1963.

Calin A: HLA-B27: To type or not to type. Ann Intern Med 92:208, 1980.

Calin A, Fries JF: An "experimental" epidemic of Reiter's syndrome revisited. Ann Intern Med 84:564, 1976.

Fitzmann SE: HLA patterns and disease association. JAMA 236:2305, 1976.

McDevitt HO: The HLA system and its relation to disease. Hosp Pract 20:57, 1985.

McMichael A, McDevitt HO: The association between the HLA system and disease. Prog Med Genet 2:39, 1977.

Morris PJ: Histocompatibility systems, immune response and disease in man. *In* Cooper MD, Warner NL (eds): Contemporary Topics in Immunobiology, Vol 3. New York, Plenum, 1974, p141.

Noer RN: An "experimental" epidemic of Reiter's syndrome. J Am Med Assoc 197(7):117, 1966.

Rachelefsky GS, Terasaki PI, Katz R, Steim ER: Increased prevalence of W27 in juvenile rheumatoid arthritis. N Engl J Med 290:892, 1974.

Sasazuki T, McDevitt HO: The association between genes in the major histocompatibility complex and disease susceptibility. Annu Rev Med 28:425, 1977.

Schaller JG, Hansen JA: HLA relationship to disease. Hosp Pract 16:41, 1981.

Tiilikainen A: On the way to understanding the pathogenesis of HLA associated diseases. Med Biol 58:53, 1980.

Zinkernagel RM: Association between major histocompatibility antigens and susceptibility to disease. Annu Rev Microbiol 33:201, 1979.

10 | The Immune Response

During an immune response to an immunogen, a series of cellular changes occurs in the responding animal that results in the production of serum antibody or specifically sensitized T cells. In addition to the "positive" effects of immunity, that is, the production of protective antibody or sensitized cells, immune responses are also controlled or limited so that overproduction of a particular antibody or population of sensitized cells does not occur. In this chapter, an overview of the cell interactions during induction of immunity and control of the response is presented.

Cellular Interactions in the Induction of Antibody Formation

T Cell–B Cell Collaboration

At least three distinct cell types are required for maximal antibody production to most antigens: T cells, B cells, and macrophages (Fig. 10-1). Macrophages in most instances (or other antigen-presenting cells) are required for stimulation of T helper cells; T helper cells produce growth and differentiation factors for B cells; and B cells are precursors that differentiate into antibody-producing and -secreting plasma cells. The necessity for T cells and B cells to cooperate during antibody formation was first demonstrated by passive transfer of thymus, bone marrow, and spleen cells to irradiated mice, followed by antigen challenge (Fig. 10-2). Mixtures of thymus and bone marrow cells were effective, whereas thymus or bone marrow cells alone were not. Cell suspensions from the spleen include both T and B cells, so that transfer of spleen cells alone was effective. In vitro studies using mixtures of purified cell populations also demonstrated that mixtures of T cells and B cells are required for induction of antibody formation.

Accessory Functions of Macrophages during Induction of Immune Responses

In addition to T and B cell collaboration during induction of antibody formation, there is a requirement for antigen processing by macrophages or other cell types (Fig. 10-3). Macrophages do not recognize antigens specifically but enhance T

199

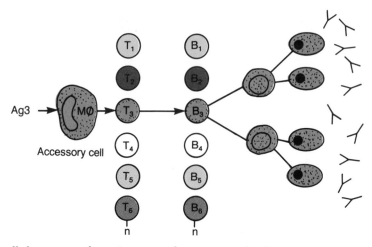

Figure 10-1. Simplified three-cell-population cooperation in induction of antibody formation: macrophages, T cells, and B cells. Macrophages do not recognize antigen specifi- cally but process the antigen and present it to T and/or B cells. Specific antigen recognition (in this case, antigen 3) occurs at the level of T and B cells, by selection of cells with specific cell surface receptors for the an- tigen, T_3 and B_3. T cells help stimulate B cells to proliferate and differentiate into plasma cells that synthesize and secrete spe- cific antibody.

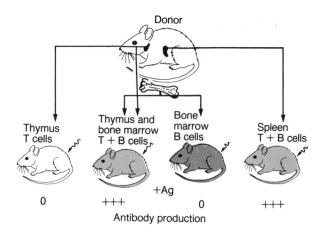

Figure 10-2. Thymus–bone marrow collaboration in induction of antibody formation. The demonstra- tion of the requirement of two cell types (T and B cells) in induction of antibody was accomplished by Henry Claman. Cells from the spleen, thymus, and bone marrow were passively transferred separately or admixed before being transferred into irradiated recipients. The recipient was then challenged with antigen. The doses of radia- tion used were high enough to eliminate T and B cell functions in the recipient animal. Splenic cells alone produced high responses, whereas bone marrow or thymus cells alone produced no response. On the other hand, mixtures of thymus and bone marrow cells were capable of producing a strong response. The role of the macrophage was not identified in these experi- ments, because macrophages are relatively radioresistant and are functionally active in the irradiated recipients. Some antigens are "T indepen- dent" and can stimulate B cells without T cell help (see below).

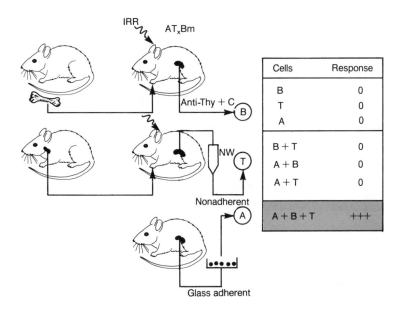

Cells	Response
B	0
T	0
A	0
B + T	0
A + B	0
A + T	0
A + B + T	+++

Figure 10-3. Demonstration of the requirement of "accessory" macrophages for induction of antibody formation in vitro. In this experimental model, B cells are obtained from the spleens of adult mice that have been injected with bone marrow cells from a normal adult donor following thymectomy and radiation treatment (ATxBm). T cells are obtained from the spleens of mice previously injected with thymus cells of a normal donor following radiation. Accessory cells (A) are obtained from the spleen cells of normal mice that are allowed to adhere to a glass surface. Nonadherent cells include T and B cells, whereas the adherent population is composed mainly of macrophages. Any one, or mixture of two, of these cell populations is not able to respond optimally to antigen stimulation in vitro. However, a mixture of the three cell populations does respond.

cell–B cell collaboration via antigen presentation. Such cellular cooperation experiments require the proper proportions of T cells, B cells, and accessory macrophages. For instance, too few or too many accessory cells may result in suboptimal conditions for antibody production.

Macrophage–T Cell–B Cell Cooperation

A model of the cellular interactions in induction of antibody formation is illustrated in Figure 10-4. An immunogen is first processed by a macrophage. The macrophage does not have a specific receptor for the antigen, although some macrophages may carry specific receptors transferred from T or B cells (cytophilic antibody). The macrophages concentrate or process the immunogen and facilitate T and B cell interactions. Analysis of peptide molecules that react with and activate T helper cells to proliferate has suggested that stimulating antigenic peptides contain two domains: an *epitope* that reacts with the paratope of the T cell receptor and an *aggretope* that reacts with an antigen-presenting class II MHC molecule. The epitope is

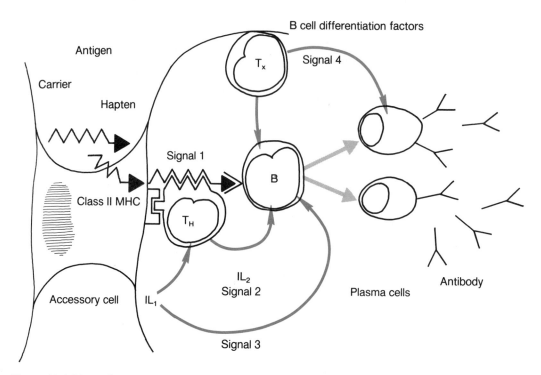

Figure 10-4. Macrophage–T cell–B cell cooperation in induction of antibody formation to haptens. Macrophages process the antigen nonspecifically and provide activation signals to T and B cells. T cells recognize the immunogenic carrier molecule in association with class II MHC markers (see Chapter 9), whereas B cells recognize the hapten. The reaction of the B cell with the hapten in the presence of the reaction of the T cell with the carrier along with the macrophage provides the required set of signals for B cell stimulation. It is postulated that at least three signals are required to stimulate B cells: one signal supplied by the antigen (hapten), one by the macrophage, and one by the T cell. Further signals are required to induce differentiation of B cells (see Fig. 10-5). During induction of these responses, antibodies to the carrier antigen are also produced (i.e., B cells to the carrier as well as to the hapten are stimulated), as are memory B cells.

the classic hydrophilic antigenic determinant; the aggretope is a hydrophobic domain that has affinity for the lipid bilayer of the antigen-presenting cell. Macrophages *process* the antigen, presumably by inserting the hydrophobic aggretope domains of the antigen into membrane structures containing the class II (I-A) molecules. This processed antigen then reacts with T cell receptors that recognize both the epitope and the class II marker of the processed antigen (see Fig. 10-12). The subject of activation of T cell subsets is presented in more detail below. T helper cells are activated by reaction with antigen and interleukin 1 (IL1), a factor produced by activated macrophages, and, in turn, produce interleukin 2 (IL2).

B cells are activated by a combination of signals, one specific (reaction of B cells with antigen) and others antigenically nonspecific (macrophage or T cell mediation). Activated lymphoid cells produce and secrete factors that are critical for the activation of proliferation and differentiation of cells in the immune response. These factors are termed *interleukins*. The properties of interleukins are presented in more detail below. For activation of B cells, T helper cells are activated by reaction with antigen processed by macrophages in association with class II MHC restriction elements. IL2 produced by activated T cells acts as a "second" signal for B cell activation and further T cell activation. Once the B cell is "turned on," it passes through a series of maturation divisions, resulting in the appearance of antibody-producing plasma cells. Continued presence of antigen in some form may be required to complete the proliferation–maturation phase. In addition, a number of B cell proliferation and differentiation factors are required to achieve full B cell expansion and differentiation into antibody-secreting cells (see below).

B cells may be stimulated in the absence of macrophages or T cells by "thymus-independent" antigens or B cell mitogens. Thymus-independent antigens stimulate B cells directly, are usually polymeric, and are believed to activate B cells by extensive cross-linking of surface receptors for antigen. T-independent antigens bypass the two or three signal mechanisms required for thymus-dependent antigens. Such antigens may be able to stimulate the specific antigen receptor of the B cells as well as stimulate proliferation, that is, be immunogens as well as mitogens.

Proliferation and Differentiation of Activated B Cells

Factors secreted by lymphoid cells during induction of an immune response appear to play a major role in proliferation and differentiation of activated B cells. A current model is presented in Figure 10-5. This model is based largely on in vitro studies. The model incorporates a combination of specific and nonspecific signals involving T cells, accessory cells, and B cells. Different T cell populations in the T helper series may be active at different stages of B cell activation and differentiation, or one T cell population may mature and acquire another function as the immune response proceeds. Both activation and differentiation of B cells require specific recognition of antigen provided through macrophage–T helper cell–B cell interaction and the effect of up to 10 or more B cell growth and differentiation factors released by lymphoid cells (interleukins).

B Cell Growth and Differentiation Factors

A partial listing of soluble factors secreted by activated T helper cells that act on B cells to support proliferation and/or differentiation is given in Table 10-1. These factors are studied by adding supernates of T cell cultures activated by antigen or

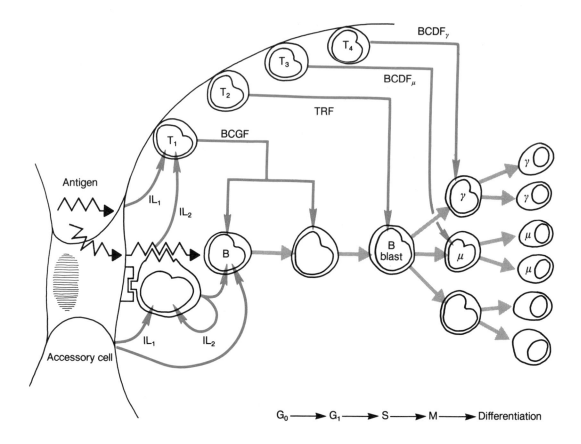

$$G_0 \longrightarrow G_1 \longrightarrow S \longrightarrow M \longrightarrow \text{Differentiation}$$

Figure 10-5. Scheme for activation and differentiation of B cells during induction of antibody formation. In this scheme T_H cells recognize antigen and class II self recognition markers on accessory cells that have processed the antigen. The macrophage accessory cell is stimulated to release interleukin 1 (IL1). IL1 acts on other T helper cells (T_1, T_2, T_3, and T_4), which have also reacted with antigen. IL1-activated helper T cells produce a second interleukin (IL2). IL1 acts on other T helper cells (T_1–T_4) that have been activated by antigen so that there are more receptors on these cells for IL2. IL2 also acts on the cells that produce it to stimulate the further activation of the cell (autocrine effect). T helper cells activated by IL2 stimulate proliferation of B cells that have been activated by specific cell surface reaction with antigen presented by the accessory cell and the action of IL1 and IL2. The activated B cells are then further stimulated to proliferate, through the action of B cell growth factors (BCGF), or to differentiate into antibody secreting plasma cells, by B cell differentiation factors (BCDF). These factors are also produced by T helper cells that have in turn been activated by reaction with antigen, IL1, and IL2.

mitogens, or supernates of T cell lines, to B cells in vitro. Because the in vitro culture conditions are selected to emphasize the effects of different culture supernates, it is not clear whether or not the effects noted in vitro have a physiological significance in vivo. In general these factors increase the proliferation or immunoglobulin (antibody) synthesis of B cell cultures activated by mitogens or by antigens and T helper cells.

Table 10-1. B Cell Growth and Differentiation Factors

Name	Function
BCGF I	Stimulates activated B cells to proliferate
BCGF II (T cell replacing factor)	Stimulates activated B cells to proliferate
BCDF	Differentiation of B cells
BCDF μ	Differentiation of μ-producing B cells
Isotype (Ig class) specific BCDF ϵ, δ, α	Induce isotype specific B cell line ϵ, δ, or α
LBCDF	Induces terminal differentiation of B cells
Interferon	Synergizes with interleukin 1 and 2
Interleukin 2	Synergizes with interleukin 1
Interleukin 4 (BSF1)	Stimulates activated cells

BCGF, B cell growth factor; BCDF, B cell differentiation factor.

Cellular Interactions in the Induction of Immune T Cells

As discussed in Chapter 8, in addition to providing help for T-dependent antibody production, T cells have many other major functions. These include suppressor cells (T_S), which serve to limit or control immune responses, T cytotoxic cells (CTL or T_K), which are capable in vitro of lysing target cells to which they are sensitized, and T_D cells, which mediate delayed hypersensitivity (DTH) in vivo through reaction with specific antigen and release of lymphokines. These functional subpopulations of T cells bear different cell surface markers (see Chapter 4).

T Cell–T Cell Cooperation

Functional T cell subpopulations are activated by a complicated set of interactions. Our present understanding of these cellular interactions depends upon separating lymphocyte subpopulations on the basis of surface markers and reconstituting function by mixing back together different cells. The functional subpopulations include helper/inducer cells capable of helping the expansion of B cells and their differentiation into antibody-secreting plasma cells, as well as other T inducer cells capable of expanding T cell precursors and stimulating them to differentiate into functionally mature T cells. These mature effector cells include CTL and DTH T cells as well as T_S cells. The T_S cells can function as a negative feedback arm to turn off inducer function or precursor responses. Experimentally, it takes an inducer cell plus a precursor cell in culture to generate an effector CTL, just as it requires a helper cell plus a B cell to generate antibody-producing plasma cells from B cells. Some of these inducer or suppressor interactions require direct cell-to-cell contact, whereas others are regulated via soluble factors released into the culture medium. Some of these factors (such as IL2) have been purified to homogeneity, cloned by recombinant methods, and found to bind to specific receptors on the surface of precursor cells. A diagram of the interactions is provided in Figure 10-6. It must be stressed that this scheme is based on in vitro systems that are subject to different interpretations.

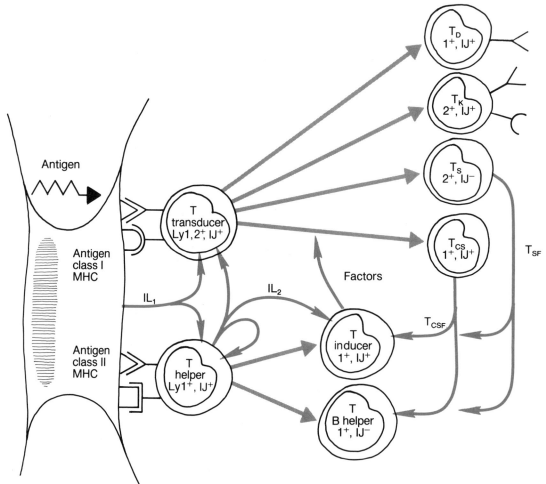

Figure 10-6. Hypothetical scheme of T cell interactions during an immune response in mice. This scheme is based on a composite of data from different systems. T cells are stimulated by antigen plus class II MHC markers on accessory cells to differentiate into the *inducer* series, or are stimulated by antigen plus class I MHC markers to differentiate into the *transducer* series. The inducer cells are capable of helping in the expansion of transducer precursor cells and the subsequent maturation into effector cells, such as CTL, DTH cells, or suppressor T cells. These inducer T cells may work through a soluble factor (IL2) or through direct cell-to-cell contact, which shows MHC restriction. The inducer cells may differentiate into functional T helper cells, aiding in the expansion of specific B cells in response to antigen. As with B cell specificities, the precursor T cells are already committed to a single specificity by rearrangement of V region genes of the T cell receptor for antigen. It is the critical role of the inducer T cells to stimulate clonal expansion of specific clones after selection by antigen.

Table 10-2. Interleukins Involved in T Cell Interactions of Mice

Name	Molecular Weight	Source	Target Cell	MHC Restriction	Function
Interleukin 1 (lymphocyte-activating factor)	15,000	Activated accessory macrophage	T cells, many other cells	None	Enhances T cell proliferation, IL2 production, B cell activation
Interleukin 2 (T cell growth factor)	30,000–35,000	Activated T cells	Activated T cells	None	Stimulates T cell proliferation and differentiation of activated T cells, binds to a specific receptor that is expressed after activation
Interleukin 3	40,000	Activated T cells	Activated T cells	None	Induces 20α-hydroxysteroid dehydrogenase in spleen cells, stimulates differentiation of activated T cells
Interleukin 4 (BSF1)	20,000	Cultured thymocytes	T and activated B cells	None	Stimulates resting T cells, anti-Ig activated B cells
Interferon α	25,000	T cells	NK cells	None	Stimulates IL1 production and NK activity, suppresses growth of certain viruses
Interferon γ (immune interferon)	20,000–25,000	T cells	T cells, NK cells	None	Stimulates NK and TK activity, enhances B cell differentiation (see Table 10-4)
T suppressor factor	70,000, single chain	T cells	T_S cells	Class I, V_H, antigen	Inhibits T helper cells

Data from Smith KA: Annu Rev Immunol 2:319, 1984; Howard M, Paul W: Annu Rev Immunol 1:307, 1983; Green DR, et al: Annu Rev Immunol 1:439, 1983; Robb RJ: Immunol Today 5:203, 1984; Ihle JN, et al, *in* Lymphokines and Thymic Hormones, New York, Raven Press, 1981; Kishimoto T: Annu Rev Immunol 3:133, 1985.

Interleukins

Interleukins are produced by cells that are activated during immune responses, and are critical for induction, maintenance and control of an immune response. The major factors are interleukin 1 (IL1) and interleukin 2 (IL2). Interleukin 1 was first called *lymphocyte-activating factor* because of its ability to induce resting T cells to proliferate. IL1 is produced by macrophages activated either by nonspecific activators, such as latex beads and phorbol esters, or by reaction with products of mitogen-stimulated T cells or T cells that have reacted with antigen and class II MHC associated antigen on macrophages (macrophage activating factors). IL1 in turn acts on T helper/inducer cells that have reacted with antigen to stimulate the production of IL2. IL2 stimulates the proliferation of T cells that have been "activated" by reaction with IL1 and antigen. Such "activated" cells have increased IL2 receptors that can be demonstrated by the monoclonal antibody anti-TAC. The IL2 receptor is a cell surface glycoprotein of molecular weight 55,000 with a high affinity for IL2 binding. T cell subpopulations activated by antigen, IL1, and IL2 may produce a number of B cell growth and differentiation factors (see below). IL1 may also activate B cells that have reacted with antigen and T helper cells, but the evidence for this is not conclusive. Other interleukins and their putative actions are listed in Table 10-2.

Interferons

The term *interferon* is used for a family of proteins produced by virus-infected cells that interfere with virus replication. *Viral interference* refers to the phenomenon in which infection of cells with one virus inhibits multiplication in the cells of a second virus. Interferon production may also be stimulated by treating cells with synthetic polyribonucleotides or by activating lymphocytes (primarily T cells) with antigens or mitogens. The three major interferons are listed in Table 10-3. Interferons

Table 10-3. Interferon Nomenclature

New	Old
IFN - α	Type I, leukocyte, pH 2 stable
IFN - β	Type I, fibroblast, pH 2 stable
IFN - γ	Type II, immune, pH 2 labile

produced by cultured cell lines or by recombinant DNA in bacteria are now available in industrial quantities.

Interferons act at the cell surface via receptors and inhibit translation of viral mRNA by stimulation of protein kinase (which phosphorylates initiation factor) and of a ribonuclease that destroys viral mRNA. As noted above, immune interferon (IFN - γ) or type II interferon is produced by activated T cells and may have a more important immunoregulatory role than IFN-α or IFN-β. IFN-γ may be produced by either helper or suppressor T cells, after stimulation by antigens or mitogens, and is also produced by activated NK cells. IFN-γ is a single polypeptide chain of MW 20,000–25,000 depending on the degree of glycosylation, and has a number of activities in immune responses (Table 10-4). At present there is interest in the appli-

Table 10-4. Some Activities of IFN-γ

Inhibits growth of normal and neoplastic cells

Synergizes with lymphotoxins

Induces proliferation and differentiation of NK/K and T_K (CTL)

Increases Class I and Class II MHC antigen expression in different cell types including macrophages, endothelial cells, and tumor cells

Increases expression of Fc receptor of myelomonocytic cells

Induces differentiation of myeloid cells and activates macrophages

Synergizes with BCDF to stimulate B cell differentiation and increase Ig production by B cells

Data from Trinchieri and Perussia: Immunol Today 6:131, 1985.

cation of interferons for treatment of cancer and/or virus infections, but the results of extensive clinical trials have been disappointing (see Chapter 29).

MHC Restriction of T_K Cytotoxicity

As presented in Chapter 8, CTL (T_K) can recognize and kill foreign cells, such as those provided by xeno- or allografts, and cells bearing "foreign antigens," such as tumor antigens or viral antigens. However, the recognition and killing of autologous cells that bear foreign antigens, such as virus-infected cells, also require self recognition. The CTL receptor for foreign antigen also carries specificity for self class I MHC markers. If an individual becomes infected with a virus that produces a cell surface antigen or develops a tumor that expresses a tumor antigen, the altered cells may be rejected by CTL that recognize both the new cell surface antigens and the self markers of the infected cells (see Figure 10-6).

MHC Antigens and T Cell Killing

The relationship of mouse MHC antigens to the specificity of virus cytotoxicity may be demonstrated using in vitro systems for killing of virus-infected target cells. Cytotoxic T cells from mice immunized to virus are cytotoxic for target cells containing the viral antigen only if the cells also have the same MHC type as the killer cells. Thus, cytotoxic spleen lymphocytes obtained from a virus immune donor of strain A will kill other virus-infected target cells of strain A origin, but not of strain B origin, and vice versa. CTL from (A × B)F_1 donors will kill both A and B infected targets, but not those of another strain (Fig. 10-7). Cloned CTL from (A × B)F_1 immune donors will kill either the A or the B infected cells, but not both, because each clone has a single receptor specificity for class I MHC markers. Interestingly some CTL clones are specific for hybrid MHC markers formed in the F_1 and not in either A or B parental

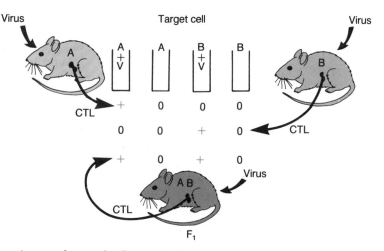

Figure 10-7. Histocompatibility restriction of cell-mediated cytotoxicity. Sensitized T cytotoxic cells of mice of a given MHC (histocompatibility) type are capable of lysing only virus-infected target cells that also have the same MHC type. +, Lysis of target cells; O, no lysis.

strains, such as $A_\alpha^A A_\beta^B$ or $A_\alpha^B A_\beta^A$. Antisera to MHC class I mouse H-2D or H-2K regions will inhibit killing of target cells by CTL by blocking the H-2K or H-2D determinants on the target cell. Presumably these antisera block the self recognition required for lysis of tumor target cells by immune specific T cytotoxic cells.

Mechanism of MHC Restriction of Cytotoxicity

The mechanisms of MHC-restricted antigen recognition by CTL are not clearly understood. Three concepts have been offered: dual recognition; composite single receptor; and single receptor, altered self (Fig. 10-8). According to the dual recognition

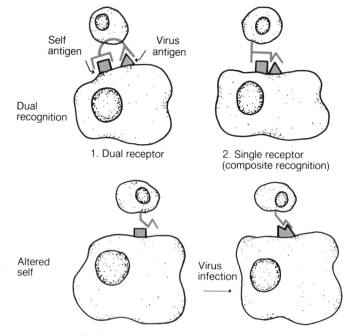

Figure 10-8. Self recognition in target cell killing. T cytotoxic cells must be able to recognize self markers as well as foreign antigens in order to kill the target cell. Several possible models of this recognition have been proposed: (1) Dual receptor: The killer cell possesses two separate receptors, one for self, another for the foreign antigen. (2) Composite single receptor: There is a single T cell receptor that can recognize both self and foreign antigen. (3) Altered self: There is a single receptor that can recognize an altered self cell surface marker. Model 2 appears most likely on the basis of DNA transfection (see text), but model 3 is also possible.

hypothesis, two receptors are required for cell killing, one reacting with self class I MHC and the other with the foreign (virus) antigen. Reaction of both receptors with the target cell is required for cell killing. The composite single receptor hypothesis postulates a single receptor that recognizes both viral antigen (epitope) and class I MHC aggretope. The altered self hypothesis defines a single receptor that recognizes the viral antigen (epitope) as part of an MHC cell surface complex; the viral antigen is incorporated into the cell surface as part of or associated with the class I MHC cell surface molecules (aggretope). The virus–self interaction results in a structure recognized by the reacting cell that is not provided by either virus or self alone. Evidence supporting each model is available.

Recently, a single receptor with dual specificity has been confirmed, at least for some T cells. Transfer by DNA transfection of the T cell receptor alpha and beta donor genes for a known antigen and MHC specificity into a new cell gives the new cell the same antigen and MHC specificity as the donor cell. Thus, the two chains of a single T cell receptor carry the specificity for both antigen and MHC recognition (model 2 or 3, Fig. 10-8). Whether the antigen and MHC also combine to form an "altered self" complex prior to binding the T cell receptor remains controversial (model 3).

Adaptive Differentiation of Self Recognition

The ability of T cells to recognize the self class I MHC markers on target cells depends on the environment in which the CTL precursors develop (i.e., the MHC type of the thymus) and not on the genotype of the precursor cells (Fig. 10-9). Thus, if F_1

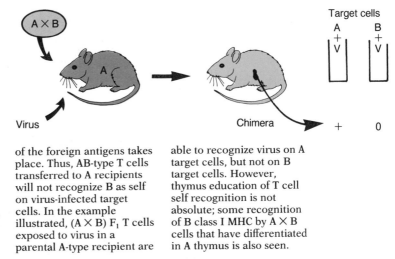

Figure 10-9. Adaptive differentiation of self recognition. The ability to recognize self on target cells is an inherited genetic property of the effector cells, but phenotypic expression is controlled by the environment in which recognition of the foreign antigens takes place. Thus, AB-type T cells transferred to A recipients will not recognize B as self on virus-infected target cells. In the example illustrated, (A × B) F_1 T cells exposed to virus in a parental A-type recipient are able to recognize virus on A target cells, but not on B target cells. However, thymus education of T cell self recognition is not absolute; some recognition of B class I MHC by A × B cells that have differentiated in A thymus is also seen.

(AB) stem cells are injected into a parental irradiated recipient (A), the T cytotoxic cells that develop in the A-type thymus are capable of killing A, but not B, virus-infected cells. If the (A × B)F_1 stem cells had matured in their own F_1 thymus, they would have acquired the ability to kill either A or B infected cells. It is postulated that the CTL develop receptors for self in the environment of the thymus. Since the A and B CTL develop in an A thymus environment, only A target cells are recognized (self A receptors but not self B receptors are produced). The epithelial cells of the thymus express class I MHC markers and may be capable of "educating" the precursors of CTL during thymic maturation to recognize self class I MHC.

MHC Restrictions in Induction of Cytotoxic T Cells

Whereas the thymus limits the range of what the T cells will see as self, the expansion of the T cell clones of a given specificity depends on the MHC type of the antigen-presenting cell. Interaction of T inducer cells with precursors of CTL is activated by infected immunogenic cells bearing class I and II MHC markers. This is the critical step in ensuring that antigen-specific CTL will be available to combat specific virus infections (see Chapter 24). Infected host cells specifically are killed; other host cells are not killed, and limitation of virus infection is achieved with minimal damage to noninfected cells.

A schematic presentation of the cellular interactions involved in generation of human CTL is given in Figure 10-10. The activation of T helper/inducer cells for CTL is restricted by antigen on the presenting cell and class II MHC products. The activation of CTL is restricted by antigen and either class I or class II MHC products.

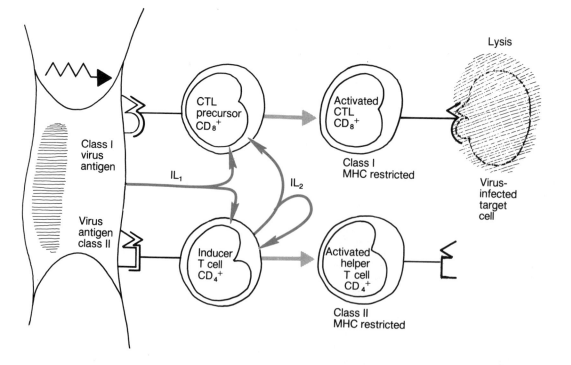

Antigen and MHC Recognition Structure of T Cells (T Cell Receptor)

The T cell surface receptor complex involved in antigen and MHC recognition is characterized in Table 10-5. The variable regions of the α- and β-chains form the antigen-binding site and

Table 10-5. Surface Structures Involved in Antigen Recognition by Human T Lymphocytes

Chains	Molecular Weight		Function
	Nonreduced	Reduced	
A. T cell receptor complex α and β	90,000	41,000–43,000 (two chains)	Dual recognition of antigen and MHC
"T$_3$ complex"—δ	23,000	23,000	Phosphorylated during cell activation
γ	20,000–23,000	20,000–23,000	Unknown
ϵ	20,000	20,000	Phosphorylated during cell activation
ζ	32,000	16 (two chains)	Unknown
B. T$_4$ (CD4)	62,000	62,000	MHC class II recognition
C. T$_8$ (CD8)	76,000	31,000 + 33,000	MHC class I recognition

also determine the MHC specificity. In the presence of antigen and MHC, the T cell is activated. This results in phosphorylation of at least two subunits of the receptor complex, the δ- and ϵ-chains. By analogy with other receptors, one of these subunits may act as a regulatory protein for another enzyme system, which generates an internal "second signal" for T cell activation. Current work focuses on the possibility that phosphodiesterase is activated, resulting in the release of diacylglycerol, which in turn activates protein kinase C. In addition, the other product of phosphodiesterase action, inositol trisphosphate, may serve to mobilize calcium stores, resulting in further activation of protein kinase C. The observed phosphorylation of some of the subunits of the T cell receptor complex may reflect the function of protein kinase C during T cell activation.

Antigen binding can be mimicked by monoclonal antibodies to the T cell receptor α- and β-chains or to the δ-chains. By immobilizing the antibodies on beads, cross-linking of receptors by the antibody is enhanced, and T cell activation by either type of antibody bound to beads is facilitated. Similarly, when

◀ **Figure 10-10.** Generation of class I MHC restricted CTL (T$_K$ cells). A T$_8$$^+$ human precursor cell is activated by reaction with antigen, MHC class I products, and IL1. Differentiation into an activated killer occurs under the influence of IL2 from T$_4$$^+$ helper cells. The cytotoxic T cells produced require reaction with both antigen and class I markers on target cells in order to effect lysis of the target cell. It should be emphasized that functions of T$_4$ (CD4) cells are MHC class II restricted and that functions of T$_8$ (CD8) cells are MHC class I restricted.

OKT$_3$ monoclonal antibody is used to modulate off the δ-chain, the other chains of the receptor complex are found to modulate as well; and when antibody to the α- and β-chains is used, the δ-chain also modulates.

Two other chains on the T cell surface, T$_4$ (CD4) and T$_8$ (CD8), are associated with the recognition of class I or class II only, without interacting with antigen at all. They are thought to work by binding nonpolymorphic (constant) determinants on class I or class II antigens of the antigen presenting cell. Whether these molecules are associated with the T cell receptor complex is not certain at this time. Ti, the T cell receptor responsible for antigen recognition, is associated strongly with T$_3$, the common T cell marker. A theoretical scheme for T cell recognition is given in Figure 10-11.

Figure 10-11. Model of antigen recognition by human T lymphocytes. Each T lymphocyte possesses two types of recognition structures. The T$_8$ and T$_4$ glycoproteins bind to nonpolymorphic regions of class I and class II MHC gene products, respectively. In contrast, T$_3$–Ti recognizes specific antigen in the context of a polymorphic MHC gene product.

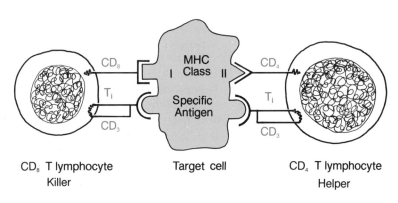

CD$_8$ T lymphocyte Killer — Target cell — CD$_4$ T lymphocyte Helper

Significance of MHC Restriction of Killing

The significance of MHC restriction of killing in human immune responses remains uncertain. It seems unlikely in humans that immune lymphocytes will be faced with viral antigens presented on histoincompatible cells. However, in vitro studies have demonstrated how recognition occurs and which surface molecules are important. Also, rejection of MHC-different grafts may occur without self recognition as part of the graft rejection mechanism. Organ grafts between an MHC-incompatible donor and recipient are rapidly rejected. It is possible that foreign MHC markers are recognized as "altered self."

Major histocompatibility complex markers may act to focus the effect of T cytotoxic cells on virus-infected cells. The function of T killer cells is to kill other cells. It is well known that cellular immune mechanisms play a major role in defense against virus infections. Since T killer cells do not bind free virus but can act only on viral antigens associated with MHC on a cell surface, MHC restriction prevents diversion of T$_K$ cells and focuses their effects on cells. Thus MHC restriction may provide an effective means of concentrating the effects of T killer cells on virus-infected cells.

It is also possible that self recognition MHC restriction of killing may play a role in recognition of neoantigens that may appear in developing or incipient tumors. Thus, altered self may be recognized and the altered tumor cells eliminated before frank cancer develops. This concept, termed *immune surveillance*, has been considered by some to play an important role in preventing tumor development (see Chapter 29).

Summary of MHC Restrictions during Activation of T Cells

A summary of MHC and antigenic restrictions in generation of immune reactive T cells is given in Table 10-6. T helper cell activation and delayed hypersensitivity effector cells are anti-

Table 10-6. Restrictions on Lymphoid Cell Activation

Function	Surface Phenotype	Restriction
T helper	CD4$^+$CD8$^-$	Class II MHC + antigen
DTH	CD4$^+$CD8$^-$	Class II MHC + antigen
CTL	CD4$^-$CD8$^+$ or CD4$^+$CD8$^-$	Class I or II MHC + antigen
Suppressor	CD4$^-$CD8$^+$	Class I MHC

gen and class II MHC restricted; CTL activities are antigen and class I or class II MHC restricted. Suppression can be class I restricted or unrestricted. Surface phenotype (CD4 or CD8) correlates mainly with MHC recognition of class II (CD4$^+$) or class I (CD8$^+$).

Considering the important regulatory role of class II restricted inducer cells (all of which are CD4$^+$), it is not surprising that a virus such as the AIDS-related virus, which infects T cells through the CD4 marker and thus selectively depletes the CD4 population, can cause the severe immune suppression and other abnormalities of lymphocyte growth seen in AIDS patients (see Chapters 26 and 28).

Lymphoid Cell Interactions in Vivo

The anatomic location of macrophage–T cell–B cell interactions in vivo is the cortex of the lymph node and the white pulp of the spleen (see Chapter 3). T and B cells may start out anatomically separated but come together during the induction of a primary antibody response. A special mechanism may exist to permit circulating T lymphocytes to lodge not only in thymus-dependent areas but also in B cell areas such as lymph node follicles or within splenic follicles, thus providing an anatomic focus for the direct cellular interaction of T and B cells (see Fig. 10-5). Lymphoid cell interactions may occur dynamically during induction of a primary immune response, as illustrated by the morphologic events that occur in the spleen leading to the production of germinal centers in the white pulp (Fig. 10-12). Labeled antigen localizes in dendritic macrophages that lie along the penicilli arterioles. These macrophages migrate to

Figure 10-12. Formation of germinal centers in the splenic white pulp following immunization. Penicilli arterioles of the spleen may be divided into three segments: the pulp arteriole, the sheathed arteriole, and the terminal arteriole. Injected antigen is taken up by dendritic macrophages located adjacent to penicilli arterioles and germinal centers formed at the bifurcation of the arteriole after migration of the periarteriolar macrophage. The antigen-localizing macrophage may serve as a nucleus around which T and B cells interact, resulting in formation of a mature germinal center. Antibody-secreting plasma cells are produced by proliferation and differentiation of B cells and migrate into the cords of the splenic red pulp.

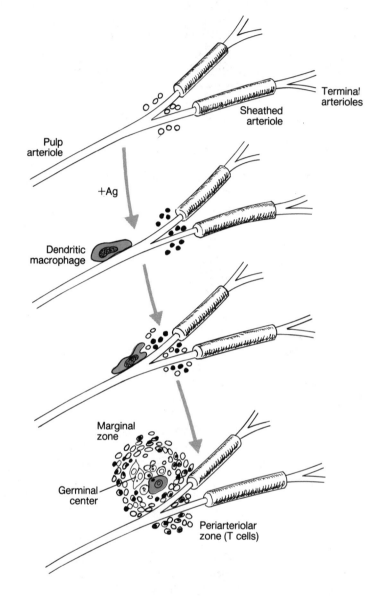

the point of bifurcation of the arteriole, where other lymphoid cells accumulate, leading to the production of a "germinal center." By 4 days after injection, antigen-containing macrophages may be observed in the periarteriolar sheath, and by 6 days, in the germinal center. It is not clear just how macrophages, T cells, and B cells migrate together during the primary antibody response in vivo, but structures such as the white pulp of the spleen may facilitate housing of different cell types, permitting cellular interactions to take place. The dendritic macrophages of lymphoid organs may act to bring together T cells and B cells, with proliferation of the B cells resulting in the formation of germinal centers.

Immune Memory

Following stimulation by antigen, the responding B and T lymphocytes undergo proliferation and differentiation, respectively, into plasma cells that synthesize and secrete antibody (humoral immunity) or into T lymphocytes (specifically sensitized cells) that have the ability to react directly and specifically with antigen (cellular immunity). In addition, long-lived cell lines with the ability to react upon second contact with the original antigen by a more rapid and increased proliferation and differentiation are also produced for both T cell and B cell function (memory cells or antigen-primed cells). A second contact with the same or a closely related antigen stimulates a more rapid reaction, with the production of a greater specific immune response. This anamnestic, or secondary, response is believed to be the result of the memory cells elicited by the preceding antigenic stimulation. Memory is expressed by both T and B cells. In certain situations where two different but related antigens share some antigenic determinants in common but also have determinants that are unique for each antigen, exposure to the second related antigen (after previous exposure to the other antigen) results in an anamnestic response both to the shared determinants and to the unique determinants of the first antigen even though the second antigen does not contain such determinants ("original antigenic sin").

The antibody formed as a result of the secondary response differs not only in quantity but also in quality from that formed as a result of the primary response. There are two main differences: the immunoglobulin class of antibody produced and the strength of binding to the antigen (avidity). The initial antibody is of the IgM class; that of the secondary response is usually IgG.

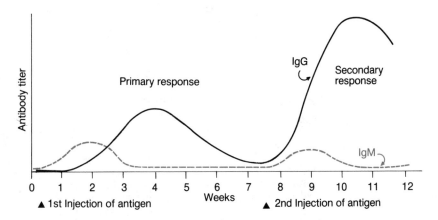

Figure 10-13. Primary and secondary antibody responses. Serum levels of IgM and IgG after primary (Day 0) and secondary (Week 8) immunization with the same antigen. In a primary response, IgM antibody precedes IgG antibody. In a secondary response, IgM and IgG both appear early and the IgG response is much greater. Not only is the titer of the IgG antibody elevated to a much higher titer more rapidly during a secondary response as compared with the primary response, but the avidity of the secondary response antibody is also much higher.

A secondary response usually results in more antibody with stronger binding affinity for the immunizing antigen than the primary response. However, a number of variables, such as antigen dose, route of exposure, and length of time between the primary and secondary immunizations, determine the nature of a secondary response.

Control of Antibody Production

Regulatory mechanisms are important in controlling the size, nature, and duration of an immune response. If the response were not controlled, antigen stimulation of proliferation would lead to an overgrowth of body tissues similar to that seen with lymphoid tumors, such as multiple myeloma (plasma cells), lymphoma, or leukemia. Following primary or secondary immunization, there is a burst of antibody production that peaks in a few days. Serum antibody titers then fall off gradually owing to a decreasing number of antibody producing cells and catabolism of the antibody formed. Further antibody formation occurs at a very low rate and may eventually be undetectable if no reexposure to the antigen occurs. After a primary immunization, there is a refractory period during which reinjection of antigen will not produce a further increase in the immune response. The number of antibody-forming cells produced and the serum titer of antibody formed upon secondary immunization is directly related to the time between the first and second immunizations with the same antigen (Fig. 10-14). The extent of

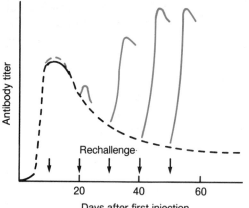

Figure 10-14. Relationship between the magnitude of a secondary antibody response and the interval between first and second exposure to an antigen. The magnitude of an antibody response to a second exposure to the same antigen depends upon the time between the first and second exposures. Although a secondary response is usually greater than the primary, there is a refractory period during the primary response when exposure to a second antigen has little effect. ---, primary response; —, secondary response. The arrows indicate the time of the second injection of antigen.

antibody production by B cells is regulated by at least three possible mechanisms: a humoral antibody feedback mechanism, T suppressor action, and idiotype control networks (Fig. 10-15).

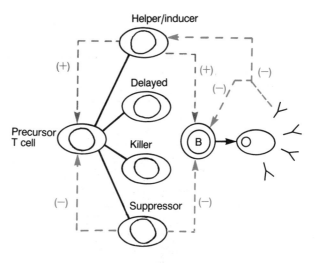

Figure 10-15. Immune response control mechanisms. T helper and T suppressor cells act on both T and B cell generating systems to control the extent of an immune response. T helper cells collaborate with B cells during the induction of T cell–dependent antibody responses, and with T inducer cells for the development of effector T cell populations, such as T_D, T_K, and T_S cells. T suppressor cells act on both B cells and T cells to limit the development of antibody-producing cells or T effector cells. In addition, immunoglobulin antibody inhibits antibody production by action on T and/or B cells, possibly through an idiotype network.

Feedback Inhibition by Passive Antibody

Passive administered specific antibody can suppress the induction of an immune response to the specific antigen without affecting responses to other antigens. The mechanism of action of the specific antibody in this situation is unknown, but the observation supports the concept that specific antibody inhibits further production of antibody of the same specificity by a feedback control system. Continued antibody production most likely requires the steady recruitment of antigen-reactive B cells to differentiate into antibody-secreting plasma cells. The presence of specific antibody may block antigenic stimulation of most of the reactive B cells.

T Suppressor Cells

During induction of an immune response, T_S cell activity is also stimulated, and it is likely these cells play a critical role in limiting the extent of antibody production. T_S cells are believed to act by mediation of a suppressor factor (T_sF) on T helper cells or on B cell differentiation (see above). During a primary or secondary immune response, T_H cells dominate during the inductive and productive phases, but T_S cells dominate during a refractory period following a primary immune response. This dominance is short-lived. Thus, a secondary injection of antigen shortly after a primary response may produce little or no additional reaction, whereas a secondary injection given weeks later will produce a rapid and extensive secondary response (see Fig. 10-14). The loss of suppression may be due to a decline in T_s cells or to the development of contrasuppressor cells, which counteract the effect of suppressor cells. However, the role and existence of contrasuppressor cells are controversial.

Idiotype Networks

The essence of the idiotype network as hypothesized by Niels Jerne is shown in Figure 10-16. Jerne postulated that each anti-

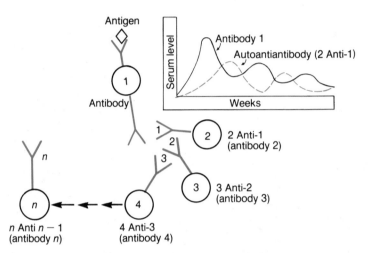

Figure 10-16. The network theory. The network theory postulates a circular set of antibodies to idiotypes (receptors) that interact to limit immune responses. It is further postulated that for each antibody produced, an anti-idiotype response is also produced. Thus if an antigen stimulates a B cell receptor (idiotype), the antibody produced will stimulate an anti-idiotype. This anti-idiotype, in turn, will stimulate a second anti-idiotype. Such a system provides a step-down mechanism to turn off the ongoing response. Thus the 2 anti-1 idiotype turns off the 1 anti-antigen; the 3 anti-2 turns off the 2 anti-1; etc. It is postulated that each step requires less anti-idiotype, so that eventually the system absorbs the stimulus and restores the series of anti-idiotype responses to "normal levels." In this manner a "dynamic equilibrium" is maintained. The inset depicts the cyclic appearance of primary antibody (solid line) and auto-anti-idiotype (2 anti-1) to this antibody following immunization.

body is itself looked upon by the immune system as an antigen with unique determinants (idiotype). Antibody produced in response to a foreign antigen elicits an anti-idiotypic antibody, which serves to control the further production of more idiotype-containing antibody. Anti-idiotypic antibodies have been demonstrated to appear in a cyclic manner following an antibody response, and the levels fluctuate immensely with the levels of the original antibody (idiotype). However, the exact mechanism whereby anti-idiotype controls the production of idiotype is not known.

The Immune System–Nervous System Relation

Several circumstantial observations have linked the extent of an immune response to control by the nervous system. These observations are:

1. There are sympathetic nerve fibers in lymphoid organs.
2. Lymphocytes have receptors for sympathetic mediators (norepinephrine, epinephrine).
3. Sympathectomy increases the density of β-adrenergic receptors on T and B lymphocytes and increases antibody responses by spleen cells.
4. Diminished norepinephrine levels are found in rat spleen during the primary immune response.
5. Stress, which increases sympathetic mediators (norepinephrine), decreases immune response.
6. Experimental animals may be "conditioned" to exhibit lower-than-normal immune responses by taste aversion learning.

These findings suggest that sympathetic–parasympathetic balance can affect the immune response and perhaps the immune response can be influenced by the central nervous system. Sympathetic dominance decreases immune responsiveness. Further understanding of the potential of this controlling mechanism is anticipated with intense interest.

Theories of Antigen Recognition

Historically, two mechanisms of specific induction of an immune response have been proposed: instructive and selective (Fig. 10-17).

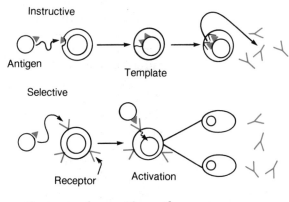

Figure 10-17. Theories of antigen recognition. Two major theories of antigen recognition have been proposed: instructive and selective. The instructive theory implies that the antigen in some way supplies specific structural information to the responding cell. Selective theories hold that the responding cells already contain in their genome the information required to produce specific antibody. The antigen reacts with specific receptors on the cell surface (preformed antibody) and thus selects a population of cells with the specific receptor to proliferate and differentiate into antibody-secreting cells.

Instructive

Instructive theories of antibody formation are included for historical interest only, as they are no longer considered plausible. Instructive theories state that antigen serves as a template upon which antibody molecules are folded to impose an antigen combining site. This theory was in vogue in the early part of the twentieth century and was supported by the findings of Linus Pauling, who denatured antibody and then tried to recover activity by renaturation of the antibody. He was unable to do so in the absence of antigen. It is now known that the tertiary structure of antibody can be destroyed by breaking the disulfide bonds of the molecule, but when these bonds are rejoined correctly, the antigen-binding activity of the antibody is restored even in the absence of antigen. The primary structure of a protein determines the folding of the molecules (tertiary structure), and therefore the antigen-binding specificity of an antibody must be dictated by the amino acid sequence of the antibody molecule. Most immunologists now agree that instructive theories are no longer tenable in the light of our present knowledge of molecular biology. Instead of "instructing" the cell regarding the structure of the antibody to be produced, the role of antigen is now known to be selecting cells already expressing a receptor for the antigen.

Selective

Selective theories state that the coding for antibody specificity is genetically determined and already present in the responding cell; contact of the cell with antigen serves to stimulate the expression of the preexisting potential. There are two variations of selective theories: germ line and somatic mutation. The germ line selective theory postulates that vertebrates have a separate gene for each polypeptide chain that has developed with evolution of the species. The somatic mutation theory postulates that the evolution of immune cells occurs within the lifetime of the individual by mutation or modulation of a much smaller number of inherited cistrons.

Germ Line

In 1900, Paul Ehrlich presented his side-chain theory, in which he stated that all cells, not just lymphoid cells, had a variety of side chains (termed *haptophores*) that had evolved in the germ line. These side chains normally functioned as receptors for metabolites, but could also react with antigens. As a result of reaction with antigen, there was a compensatory synthesis of new side chains. This synthesis resulted in an excess of side chains, so that many were released into the circulation and became detectable as antibodies.

In 1955, Jerne postulated the natural selection theory, which took into account some of the information that had accumulated during the preceding 50 years. Jerne postulated that the production of specific antigen receptor molecules by lymphoid cells was random. The number of antigenic specificities that each of these receptor molecules would recognize was finite and dictated by the genome of the individual. Receptor molecules were released from the cells (natural antibody), and antigen served to select the specific circulating receptors with which it reacted (natural selection). The receptor that had reacted with antigen was then carried back to the cell with the potential to produce antibody, and the antigen–receptor molecule complex in some way stimulated the cell to proliferate, differentiate, and produce more receptor molecules (antibody). Szilard, in 1960, postulated that there was a separate gene that coded for each antibody and that the complete array of genes required for all antibodies was present in each potentially reacting cell. Antigen served to induce cell differentiation, fix the specificity of the reacting cell, and stimulate production of antibody. Both Jerne and Szilard said that the precursor of the antibody-producing cell was omnipotent and could generate separate cells that collectively recognize all immunogens.

Somatic

Burnet was the first to postulate that the immune potential was the result of somatic mutation. He reasoned that the immune response to a specific antigen originated in a few omnipotent stem cells that were highly mutable. During somatic development, individual precursor cells that had the capacity to respond to one or a very limited number of antigens were differentiated. Upon contact with the specific antigen, these precursors were stimulated to proliferate, and the progeny constituted a clone of cells producing the specific antibody (clonal selection). Burnet's clonal selection theory stimulated a vast amount of important research. A number of workers have extended Burnet's theory and have implicated various genetic mechanisms as occurring during somatic development to explain the amino acid structure of immunoglobulins. However, somatic mutation on a random basis as a means of creating the diversity needed for recognition of many different antigens implies uncontrolled production of information with a high rate of nonsense mutations (wastage). Recent observations suggest that somatic mutation occurs mainly during the maturation of an ongoing antibody response and may result in antibodies of high affinity during the secondary response.

* * *

The most pressing questions to be examined by any theory are: (1) How does an immunologically reactive cell recognize antigen? (2) How does this recognition stimulate antibody production? (3) How does an individual develop the capacity to recognize so many different antigenic specificities (generation of diversity)?

Immunologically reactive cells recognize antigens by means of specific receptor molecules present on their surface. The process whereby this reaction of antigen with a reactive or precursor cell stimulates the cell to proliferate is related to the ability of the antigen to activate the cell through reaction with cell surface receptors, and is incompletely understood. Generation of diversity may occur by germ line evolution or by somatic mutation. Each reactive cell has the capacity to recognize one or very few antigens (i.e., is restricted). There must be a very active selective mechanism capable of finding the rare T or B cell specific for each antigen. It is known that each differentiated antibody-producing plasma cell is restricted to producing antibody of one specificity and immunoglobulin of one type, but the potential of the recognition cell or precursor cell is not clearly defined. It is possible that restriction may occur during differentiation of a given cell line by rearrangement of receptor genes. There is evidence the unrearranged Ig genes may be expressed in very early B cell differentiation. V_H-to-VDJ rearrangement in a heavy chain gene enhances Ig secretion in mature cells.

Summary

Antigen recognition leading to an immune response involves different functional cell populations (Fig. 10-18). Immunogens

Figure 10-18. Cellular interactions in the immune response. The immune response involves the interaction and differentiation of a number of different cell populations from immature precursor cells to mature effector cells. During the early steps of development, precursor cells acquire specificity through gene rearrangement and production of specific receptors. Antigen specifically selects receptor cells at a later step and selectively stimulates the appropriate cells to proliferate and differentiate into functional effector cells. Controlling mechanisms are also activated that turn off the proliferation of reactive cells and limit the extent of the response. (For details see Summary.)

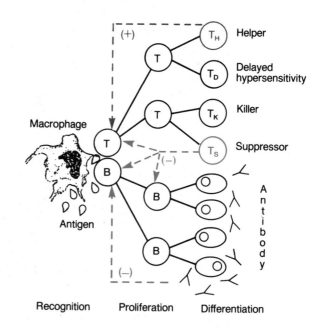

are processed by macrophages that present the antigen to specifically reactive T and B cells. Antigen processing by macrophages results in association of the antigen with class II MHC gene products (I-A). T cells recognize antigen and I-A simultaneously, so that most immune responses are class II MHC restricted. Activated macrophages produce interleukin 1, which activates T cells in the presence of antigen. In turn, activated T helper/inducer cells secrete interleukin 2, which supports proliferation of activated T and B cells. B cells are stimulated by antigen and other T cell factors (interleukins) to proliferate and differentiate into plasma cells, which secrete specific immunoglobulin antibodies. T cells proliferate and differentiate into at least four functional populations: helper/inducer cells (T_H), cells that effect delayed hypersensitivity reactions (T_D), cytotoxic killer cells (T_K), and suppressor cells (T_S). T_H cells cooperate with B cells during induction of antibody formation, and T_S cells provide a mechanism for limiting the extent of an immune response. Another T cell population, T contrasuppressor cells, may modulate the effect of T suppressor cells in mice, but such an activity in humans is controversial. In addition, T and B memory cell populations are produced that permit the primed individual to respond more rapidly to a second exposure of the same antigen. Thus, immunization results in the establishment of a new state of awareness in the responding individual via the generation of a complex of new cell populations. The immune response provides not only specifically sensitized cells and immunoglobulin antibody but also an inherent control system that limits the extent of the response. It is now generally accepted that the germ line receptor genes provide the basic structures needed to encode for antigen receptors and that further diversity may be added by somatic mutation.

References

Cell Interactions in the Induction of Antibody Formation

Altman A, Katz DH: The biology of monoclonal lymphokines secreted by T cell lines and hybridomas. Adv Immunol 33:73, 1982.

Dinarello CA: An update on human interleukin-1: from molecular biology to clinical relevance. J Clin Immunol 5:287, 1985.

Durum SK, Schmidt JA, Oppenheim JJ: Interleukin 1: an immunological perspective. Annu Rev Immunol 3:263, 1985.

Henry C, Trefts PE: Helper activity in vitro to a defined determinant. Eur J Immunol 4:824, 1974.

Katz DH: Lymphocyte Differentiation, Recognition, and Regulation. New York, Academic Press, 1977.

Makela O, Cross A, Kosunen TV (eds): Cell Interactions and Receptor Antibodies in Immune Responses. New York, Academic Press, 1971.

Miller JFAP, Basten A, Sprent J, Cheers C: Interaction between lymphocytes in immune response. Cell Immunol 2:469, 1971.

Miller JFAP, Mitchell FG: Cell to cell interaction in the immune response. I. Hemolysin forming cells in neonatally thymectomized mice reconstituted with thymus or thoracic duct lymphocytes. J Exp Med 128:801, 1968.

Mitchison NA: The carrier effect in the secondary response to hapten – protein conjugates. II. Cellular cooperation. Eur J Immunol 1:18, 1971.

Moller G (ed): Role of macrophages in the immune response. Transplant Rev 40, 1978.

Moller G (ed): Interleukins and lymphocyte activation. Immunol Rev 63, 1982.

Moiser DE, Coppleson LW: A three-cell interaction required for the induction of the primary response in vitro. Proc Nat Acad Sci USA 61:542, 1968.

Mosier DE, Johnson BM, Paul WE, McMaster PRB: Cellular requirements for the primary in vitro antibody response to DNP-Ficoll. J Exp Med 139:1354, 1974.

Nelson DS (ed): Immunobiology of the Macrophage. New York, Academic Press, 1976.

Rosenthal AS: Regulation of the immune response: role of the macrophage. N Engl J Med 303:1153, 1980.

Schwartz RS, Ryder RJW, Gottlieb BAA: Macrophages and antibody synthesis. Prog Allergy 14:81, 1970.

Sercarz EE, Metzger DW: Epitope specific and idiotype specific cellular interactions in a model protein antigen system. Springer Semin Immunopathol 3:145, 1980.

Shevach EM, Rosenthal AS: Function of macrophages in antigen recognition by guinea pig T lymphocytes. II. Role of the macrophage in the regulation of genetic control of the immune response. J Exp Med 138:1213, 1974.

Singer A, Hodes RJ: Mechanisms of T-cell B-cell interaction. Annu Rev Immunol 1:211, 1983.

Taylor RB, Iverson GM: Hapten competition and the nature of cell cooperation in the antibody response. Proc R Soc Lond [Biol] 176:393–418, 1971.

Unanue ER: Cooperation between mononuclear phagocytes and lymphocytes in immunity. N Engl J Med 303:977, 1980.

Weinbaum FI, Butchko GM, Lerman S, Thorbecke GJ, Nisonoff A: Comparison of cross-reactivities between albumins of various species at the level of antibody and helper T cells—studies in mice. J Immunol 113:257, 1974.

B Cell Differentiation

Aarden LA, et al: Revised nomenclature for antigen non-specific T cell proliferation and helper factors. Mol Immunol 17:641, 1980.

Abney E, et al: Sequential expression of immunoglobulin on developing B lymphocytes: a systematic survey that suggests a model for the generation of immunoglobulin isotype diversity. J Immunol 120:2041, 1978.

Byers VS, Sercarz EE: The X–Y–Z scheme of immunocyte maturation. IV. The exhaustion of memory cells. J Exp Med 127:307, 1968.

Cantor H, Boyse EA: Lymphocytes as models for the study of mammalian cellular differentiation. Immunol Rev 33:105, 1976.

Cebra JJ, Komisar JL, Schweitzer PA: C_H isotype "switching" during normal B-cell development. Annu Rev Immunol 2:493, 1984.

Dutton RW: Separate signals for the initiation of proliferation and differentiation in the B cell response to antigen. Transplant Rev 23:66, 1975.

Gearing AJH, Johnstone AP, Thorpe R: Production and assay of the interleukins. J Immunol Methods 83:1, 1985.

Hamaoka T, Ohno S: Regulation of B cell differentiation: interactions factors and corresponding receptors. Annu Rev Immunol 4:167, 1986.

Hanleyhyde JM, Lynch RG: The physiology of B cells as studied with tumor models. Annu Rev Immunol 4:621, 1986.

Howard M, Paul WE: Regulation of B-cell growth and differentiation by soluble factors. Annu Rev Immunol 1:307, 1983.

Kishimoto T: Factors affecting B-cell growth and differentiation. Annu Rev Immunol 3:133, 1985.

Makinodan T, Albright JF: Proliferative and differentiative manifestations of cellular immune potential. Prog Allergy 10:1, 1967.

Mather EL, et al: Mode of regulation of immunoglobulin μ- and γ-chain expression varies during B-lymphocyte maturation. Cell 36:329, 1984.

Melchers F, Anderson J: Factors controlling the B cell cycle. Annu Rev Immunol 4:13, 1986.

Moller G (ed): Effects of Anti-Immunoglobulin Sera on B Lymphocyte Function. Immunol Rev 52, 1980.

Moller G (ed): B Cell Differentiation Antigens. Immunol Rev 69, 1983.

Moller G (ed): B Cell Growth and Differentiation Factors. Immunol Rev 78, 1984.

Rajewsky K, Takemori T: Genetics, expression and function of idiotypes. Annu Rev Immunol 1:569, 1983.

Robertson SM, et al: Antiarsenate antibody response: A model for studying antibody diversity. Fed Proc 41:2502, 1982.

Sell S: Development of restriction in the expression of immunoglobulin specificities by lymphoid cells. Transplant Rev 5:19, 1970.

Vitetta ES, Uhr JW: Immunoglobulin-receptors revisited: a model for the differentiation of bone marrow lymphocytes is discussed. Science 189:964, 1975.

Waldemann TA, Broder S: Polyclonal B-cell activators in the study of the regulation of immunoglobulin synthesis in humans. Adv Immunol 32:1, 1982.

Wall R, Kuehl M: Biosynthesis and regulation of immunoglobulins. Annu Rev Immunol 1:499, 1983.

Whitlock C, et al: In vitro analysis of murine B cell development. Annu Rev Immunol 3:213, 1985.

Yancopoulos CP, Alt FW: Regulation of the assembly and expression of variable region genes. Annu Rev Immunol 4:339, 1986.

T Cell Activation and Differentiation

Ashwell JD, et al: Can resting B cells present antigen to T cells? Fed Proc 44:2475, 1985.

Atassi MZ, et al: Immune recognition of serum albumin. XIV. Cross reactivity of T lymphocyte proliferation of subdomains 3, 6 and 9 of bovine serum albumin. Mol Immunol 19:313, 1982.

Barth RK, et al: The murine T cell receptor uses a limited repertoire of expressed V_β gene segments. Nature 316:517, 1985.

Binz H, Wigzell H: Antigen binding idiotypic T-lymphocyte receptors. Contemp Top Immunobiol 7:113, 1977.

Cantor H, Asofsky R: Synergy among lymphoid cells mediating the graft-versus-host syndrome. II. Synergy in G. v H. reactions produced by Balb/c lymphoid cells of differing anatomic origin. J Exp Med 131:235, 1970.

Cantrell PA, Smith KA: The interleukin-2 T-cell system: a new cell growth model. Science 224:1312, 1984.

Fitch FT: Cell clones and T cell receptors. Microbiol Rev 50:50, 1986.

Goodman JW, et al: The complexity of structures involved in T-cell activation. Annu Rev Immunol 1:465, 1983.

Grey HM, Chesnut R: Antigen processing and presentation to T cells. Immunol Today 6:101, 1985.

Kreiger JI, et al: Antigen presentation by spleen B cells: Resting B cells are ineffective, whereas activated B cells are effective accessory cells for T cell responses. J Immunol 135:2937, 1985.

Leskowitz S, Jones VE, Zak SJ: Immunochemical study of antigenic specificity in delayed hypersensitivity. V. Immunization with monovalent low molecular weight conjugates. J Exp Med 123:229, 1966.

Marchalonis JJ: Lymphocyte surface immunoglobulins: molecular properties and functions as receptors for antigens are discussed. Science 190:20, 1975.

McNamara M, Gleason K, Kohler H: T cell helper circuits. Immunol Rev 79:87, 1984.

Moller G (ed): Lymphocyte activation by mitogens. Transplant Rev 11, 1972.

Moller G (ed): Interleukins and lymphocyte activation. Immunol Rev 63, 1982.

Paul WE: Functional specificity of antigen-binding receptors of lymphocytes. Transplant Rev 5:130–166, 1970.

Paul WE, Benacerraf B: Functional specificity of thymus-dependent lymphocytes: a relationship between the specificity of T lymphocytes and their function is proposed. Science 195:1293, 1977.

Robb RJ: Interleukin 2: the molecule and its function. Immunol Today 5:203, 1984.

Tigelaar RE, Asofsky R: Synergy among lymphoid cells mediating the graft-versus-host response. V. Derivation by migration in lethally irradiated recipients of two interacting subpopulations of thymus derived cells from normal spleen. J Exp Med 137:239, 1973.

Weiss A, et al: The role of the T3/antigen receptor complex in T cell activation. Annu Rev Immunol 4:593, 1986.

Cellular Reactions in Vivo

Gutman GA, Weissman IL: Lymphoid tissue architecture: experimental analysis of the origin and distribution of T-cells and B-cells. Immunology 23:465, 1972.

Humphrey JG, Frank MM: The localization of non-microbial antigens in the draining lymph nodes of tolerant, normal and primed rabbits. Immunology 13:87, 1967.

Mitchell J: Lymphocyte circulation in the spleen. Marginal zone bridging channels and their possible role in cell traffic. Immunology 24:93, 1973.

Moller G (ed): Accessory cells in the immune response. Immunol Rev 53, 1980.

Nossal GJV, Ada GL: Antigens, Lymphoid Cells and the Immune Response. New York, Academic Press, 1971.

Nossal GJV, Ada GL, Austin CM: Antigens in immunity. IV. Cellular localization of ^{125}I-labeled flagella in lymph nodes. Aust J Exp Biol Med Sci 42:311, 1964.

Parrott DM, DeSousa MA: Thymus dependent and thymus independent populations, origin, migratory patterns and lifespan. Clin Exp Immunol 8:663, 1971.

Sertl K: Dendritic cells with antigen-presenting capacity reside in airway epithelium, lung parenchyma and visceral pleura. J Exp Med 163:436, 1986.

Silveira NPA, Mendes NF, Tolnai MEA: Tissue localization of two populations of human lymphocytes distinguished by membrane receptors. J Immunol 108:1456, 1972.

Stingl G, et al: Analogous functions of macrophages and Langerhans cells in the initiation of the immune response. J Invest Dermatol 71:59, 1978.

Tew JG, Mandel TE, Burgess AW: Retention of intact HSA for prolonged periods in the popliteal nodes of specifically immunized mice. Cell Immunol 45:207, 1979.

White RG: Functional recognition of immunologically competent cells by means of fluorescent antibody technique. *In* Wolstenholme GEW, Knight J (eds): The Immunologically Competent Cell. London, Churchill, 1963.

White RG, French VI, Stark JM: Germinal center formation and antigen localization in Malpighian bodies of the chicken spleen. *In* Cottier H (ed): Germinal Centers in Immune Responses. Berlin, Springer, 1966, pp131–142.

MHC Restriction of Cell Interactions

Cone RE: Molecular basis for T cell recognition of antigen. Prog Allergy 29:182, 1981.

Feeney AJ, et al: T helper cells required for the in vitro primary antibodies response to SRBC are neither SRBC-specific nor MHC restricted. J Mol Cell Immunol 1:211, 1984.

Haskins K, Kappler J, Marrack P: The major histocompatibility complex–restricted antigen receptor on T cells. Annu Rev Immunol 2:51, 1984.

Katz DH, Hamaoka T, Dorf ME, Benacerraf B: Cell interactions between histoincompatible T and B lymphocytes. The H-2 gene complex determines successful physiologic lymphocyte interactions. Proc Nat Acad Sci USA 70:2624–2628, 1973.

Malissen B, et al: Gene transfer of H_2 class II genes: antigen presentation by mouse fibroblast and hamster B cell lines. Cell 36:319, 1984.

Moller G (ed): Acquisition of the T cell repertoire. Immunol Rev 42, 1978.

Moller G (ed): Structure and function of HLA-DR. Immunol Rev 66, 1982.

Nagy Z, et al: Ia antigens as restriction molecules in Ir gene controlled T-cell proliferation. Immunol Rev 60:59, 1981.

Rosenthal AS, Shevach EM: Function of macrophages in antigen recognition by guinea pig T lymphocytes. I. Requirement for histocompatible macrophages and lymphocytes. J Exp Med 138:1194, 1974.

Santos GW: Adoptive transfer of immunologically competent cells. III. Comparative ability of allogenic and syngeneic spleen cells to produce a primary antibody response in the cyclophosphamide treated mouse. J Immunol 97:587, 1966.

Schrader SW: Mechanism of activation of the bone marrow–derived lymphocyte. III. A distinction between a macrophage-produced triggering signal and the amplifying affect on triggered B lymphocytes of allogeneic interaction. J Exp Med 138:1466, 1973.

Schwartz RH: T lymphocyte recognition of antigen in association with gene products of the major histocompatibility complex. Annu Rev Immunol 3:237, 1985.

Shih WH, et al: Analysis of histocompatibility requirements for proliferation and helper T cell activity. T cell population depleted of alloreactive cells by negative selection. J Exp Med 152:1311, 1980.

Singer A, Hathcock KS, Hodes RJ: Cellular and genetic control of antibody responses. V. Helper T cell recognition of H-2 determinants on accessory cells but not on B cells. J Exp Med 149:1208, 1979.

Zinkernagel RM, et al: On the thymus in the differentiation of "H-2 self-recognition" by T cells. Evidence for dual recognition. J Exp Med 147:882, 1978.

Control of Immune Response

See Chapter 11.

Asherson GL, Colizzi V, Zembala M: An overview of T-suppressor cell circuits. Annu Rev Immunol 4:37, 1986.

Dorf ME, Benacerraf B: Suppressor cells and immunoregulation. Annu Rev Immunol 2:127, 1984.

Gershon RK, et al: Suppressor T cells. J Immunol 108:586, 1972.

Gershon RK, et al: Contrasuppression: A normal immunoregulatory activity. J Exp Med 153:1533, 1981.

Green DR, Flood PM, Gershon R: Immunoregulatory T-cell pathways. Annu Rev Immunol 1:439,1983.

Greene MI, et al: Regulation of immunity to the azobenzenearsonate hapten. Adv Immunol 32:253, 1982.

Hamaoka T, Yoshizawa M, Yamamoto H, Kuroki M, Kitagawa M: Regulatory functions of hapten-reactive helper and suppressor T lymphocytes. II. Selective reactivation of hapten-reactive suppressor T cells by hapten-nonimmunogenic copolymers of C-amino acids, and its applications to the study of suppressor T-cell effect on helper T-cell development. J Exp Med 146:91, 1977.

Hausman PB, Sherr DH, Dorf ME: Anti-idiotypic B cells are required for induction of suppressor T cells. J Immunol 136:48, 1986.

Herzenberg LA, Tokuhisa T, Hayakawa K: Epitope specific regulation. Annu Rev Immunol 1:609, 1983.

Ishizaka K: Regulation of IgE synthesis. Annu Rev Immunol 2:159, 1984.

Jerne NK: The immune system: A network of V domains. Harvey Lect 70:93, 1975.

Katz DH: The allogeneic effect on immune responses: model for regulatory influences of T lymphocytes on the immune system. Transplant Rev 12:141, 1972.

Moller G (ed): Suppressor T lymphocytes. Transplant Rev 26, 1975.

Moller G (ed): Regulation of the immune response by antibodies against the immunogen. Immunol Rev 49, 1980.

Moller G (ed): Idiotype networks. Immunol Rev 79, 1984.

Rowley DA, Fitch FW, Stuart FP, Kohler H, Cosenza H: Specific suppression of immune responses. Science 181:1133, 1973.

Sterzl J: Factors and methods for the control of the immune response. *In* Rose N, et al (eds): International Convocation on Immunology. New York, Karger, 1969, p81.

Uhr JW, Moller G: Regulatory effect of antibody on the immune response. Adv Immunol 8:81, 1968.

Unanue EF: The regulatory role of macrophages in antigenic stimulation. Adv Immunol 15:95, 1972.

Unanue EF: The regulatory role of macrophages in antigenic stimulation. Part two: Symbiotic relationship between lymphocytes and macrophages. Adv Immunol 31:1, 1981.

Immune Memory

Bandilla KK, McDuffie FC, Gleich GJ: Immunoglobulin classes of antibodies produced in the primary and secondary responses in man. Clin Exp Immunol 5:627, 1969.

Celada F: Quantitative studies of the adaptive immunological memory in mice. II. Linear transmission of memory. J Exp Med 125:199, 1967.

Cerottini J-C, Trnka Z: The role of persisting antigen in the development of immunological memory. Int Arch Allergy 38:37, 1970.

Dutton DW, Eady JD: An in vitro system for the study of the mechanism of antigen stimulation in the secondary response. Immunology 7:40, 1964.

Fecsik AI, Butler WT, Coons AH: Studies on antibody production. XI. Variation in the secondary response as a function of the length of interval between the two antigenic stimuli. J Exp Med 12:1041, 1964.

Hege JS, Cole LJ: Antibody plaque-forming cells: kinetics of primary and secondary responses. J Immunol 96:559, 1966.

Jerne NK, et al: Plaque forming cells: methodology and theory. Transplant Rev 18:130, 1974.

Mason DW, Gowans J-L: Subpopulations of B lymphocytes and the carriage of immunological memory. Ann Inst Pasteur Ser C 127:657, 1976.

Nossal GJV, Austin CM, Ada GL: Antigens in immunity. VII. Analysis of immunological memory. Immunology 9:333, 1965.

Ovary Z, Benacerraf B: Immunological specificity of the secondary response with dinitrophenylated proteins. Proc Soc Exp Biol Med 114:72–76, 1963.

Paul WE, Siskind GW, Benacerraf B, Ovary Z: Secondary antibody responses in haptenic systems: cell population selection by antigen. J Immunol 99:760, 1967.

Sell S, Park AH, Nordin AA: Immunoglobulin classes of mouse antibody forming cells. I. Localized hemolysis-in-agar plaque forming cells belonging to five immunoglobulin classes. J Immunol 104:483, 1970.

Tada T, Takemori T, Okumura K, Nonaka M, Tokuhisa T: Two distinct types of helper T cells involved in the secondary response: independent and synergistic effects of Ia$^-$ and Ia$^+$ helper T cells. J Exp Med 147:446, 1978.

Takaoki M: Transition in the character of immunological memory in mice after immunization. II. Memory in T and B cell populations. Jpn J Microbiol 20:475, 1976.

Tew JG, Mandel TE: The maintenance and regulation of serum antibody levels: evidence indicating a role for antigen in lymphoid follicles. J Immunol 120:1063, 1978.

Weigle WO: Cyclical production of antibody as a regulatory mechanism in the immune response. Adv Immunol 21:87, 1975.

The Immune System–Nervous System Relation

Adler R: Psychoneuroimmunology. Orlando, Fla., Academic Press, 1981.

Blalock JE, Bost KL, Smith EM: Neuroendocrine peptide hormones and their receptors in the immune system: production, processing and action. J Neuroimmunol 10:31, 1985.

Cohen N, Adler R: Antibodies and learning: a new dimension. In Sternberg CM, Lefkovits I (eds): The Immune System. Basel, Karger, 1981, p51.

Hall NR, et al: Immunoregulatory peptides and the central nervous system. Springer Semin Immunopathol 8:153, 1985.

Kerza-Kwiatecki AP: First international workshop on neuroimmunomodulation (NIM). J Neuroimmunol 10:9, 1985.

Livnat S, et al: Involvement of peripheral and central catecholamine systems in neuroimmune interactions. J Neuroimmunol 10:5, 1985.

Roszman TL, Brooks WH: Neural modulation of immune function. J Neuroimmunol 10:59, 1985.

Wybran J: Enkephalins and endorphins as modifiers of the immune system present and future. Fed Proc 44:92, 1985.

Theories of Antibody Formation

Burnet FM: Enzyme, Antigen, and Virus. London, Cambridge University Press, 1956.

Burnet FM: The Clonal Selection Theory of Acquired Immunity. London, Cambridge University Press, 1959.

Burnet FM: The Integrity of the Body: A Discussion of Modern Immunological Ideas. Cambridge, Harvard University Press, 1962.

Bretcher PA, Cohn M: A theory of self–non self discrimination. Science 189:1042, 1970.

Dreyer WJ, Bennett JC: The molecular basis of antibody formation: A paradox. Proc Nat Acad Sci USA 54:864, 1965.

Ehrlich P: An immunity with special reference to cell life. Proc Soc Lond [Biol] 66:424, 1900.

Finch LR: γ-Globulin operon: a hypothesis for the mechanism of the specific response in antibody synthesis. Nature 201:1288, 1964.

Habe E: Recovery of antigenic specificity of denaturation and complete reduction of disulphides in a papain fragment of antibody. Proc Nat Acad Sci USA 52:1099, 1964.

Haurowitz F: Antibody formation and the coding problem. Nature 205:847, 1965.

Hood L, Talmadge DW: Mechanisms of antibody diversity: germ line basis for variability. Science 168:325, 1970.

Jerne NK: The natural selection theory of antibody formation. Proc Nat Acad Sci USA 41:849, 1955.

Jerne NK: The somatic generation of immune recognition. Eur J Immunol 1:1, 1971.

Landsteiner K: The specificity of serological reactions, 2nd ed. Cambridge, Harvard University Press, 1945.

Lederberg IS: Genes and antibodies. Science 129:1649, 1959.

Pauling LA: A theory of the structure and process of formation of antibodies. J Am Chem Soc 62:2643, 1940.

Perlmann GE, Diringer R: The structure of proteins. Annu Rev Biochem 29:151, 1960.

Schweet R, Owen RD: Concepts of protein synthesis in relation to antibody formation. J Cell Physiol (Suppl) 50(1):199, 1957.

Smith T: Active immunity produced by so-called balanced or neutral mixtures of diphtheria toxin and anti-toxin. J Exp Med 11:241, 1909.

Smithies O, Poulik MD: Initiation of protein synthesis at an unusual position in an immunoglobulin gene. Science 175:187, 1972.

Szilard L: The molecular basis of antibody formation. Proc Nat Acad Sci USA 46:293, 1960.

Talmadge DW, Perlman DS: The antibody response: a model based on the antagonistic actions of antigen. J Theor Biol 5:321, 1963.

11 | Immune Tolerance and Autoimmunity

The exposure of a responsive individual to a potential immunogen may result in an immune response or it may not. It is critical that an individual respond to foreign antigens for protection, but not to self antigens. Thus, exposure to foreign antigens should elicit immunity; exposure to self antigens should not. The lack of an immune response to a specific antigen when responses to other antigens are retained is termed *immune tolerance*. Tolerance is a specific example of the effect of control mechanisms on the immune response. Tolerance has been one of the most controversial areas in immunology and remains a phenomenon that must be explained by any theories of immunity. Sir MacFarlane Burnet first postulated immune tolerance to explain why an individual does not normally make an immune response to his own tissues, although his macromolecules may be immunogenic when they are given to a different individual. He further explained immune tolerance as a means of recognition of "self" and "nonself." He considered the mechanism of immune self recognition as not innate, but a process of maturation; that is, tolerance is acquired somatically. Loss of tolerance to self antigens would lead to the production of autoantibodies and autoimmune disease; thus the other side of the tolerance coin is autoimmunity (see below).

Natural Tolerance

Natural tolerance was postulated to develop during fetal life, when the individual does not yet have the capacity to produce an immune response. Contact with antigens at this time would affect the maturation of the immune system so that recognition of antigen and reaction of immune mechanisms to the antigen would not develop. Under usual conditions during intrauterine embryonic development the fetus contacts only its own antigens and therefore develops immune tolerance to them. However, Burnet predicted that if a foreign antigen were presented to the fetus before or during maturation of its immune system,

235

specific immune tolerance could be produced to this antigen as well.

Burnet's theories were largely stimulated by Ray Owen's demonstration of tolerance to foreign antigens in dizygotic twins of cattle. Such twins are genetically different, but have a common circulation during fetal life so that there is a continuous exchange of proteins and blood cells. When mature, these twins tolerate and do not manifest an immune response to each other's antigens, although they display normal immunity to antigens that are foreign to both. Since Owen's observation, many other instances of immune tolerance to foreign antigens have been produced in experimental animals. Sir Peter Medawar demonstrated that if a potential foreign immunogen is introduced into an animal early in its life, instead of producing antibody or sensitized cells the animal develops specific immune tolerance to it. Upon second contact with the same antigen at an age when an immune response would be expected, the tolerant animal does not respond.

The successful induction of neonatal tolerance was demonstrated for foreign cells by Rupert Billingham. States of tolerance can be most easily induced in fetal and neonatal animals until a few days after birth. This is known as the "window" of tolerance induction. A few days after birth, exposure to an antigen no longer induces tolerance. At the same time it is known that in some circumstances the fetal animal can make an immune response to many antigens. As is discussed below, the induction of tolerance or immunity depends on a number of variables, but in general tolerance is much more readily induced in fetal than in adult animals. The induction of tolerance to self antigens is believed to take place during maturation of lymphoid cells, in both the fetus and the adult. In this chapter some of the characteristics of tolerance are described, and then the hypothetical mechanisms of tolerance and autoimmunity, as well as the breaking of tolerance, are presented. A single mechanism does not explain all the characteristics of the different states of tolerance. Different mechanisms may be responsible for different tolerance phenomena. Immune tolerance to nonself antigens is called *acquired* tolerance, in contrast to the developmental phenomenon of natural tolerance to self antigens.

Acquired Tolerance

A number of factors determine the type and extent of an immune response, because of activation of negative or positive arms of the immune response control system (see Chapter 10). Some of the factors include the age and immune status of the responding animal, the properties of the antigen (e.g., molecular weight, number of repeating units, solubility), the antigen dose and route of exposure, the genetic makeup of the responding animal, and the number of previous exposures to the same antigen or structurally related antigens. Because of these variables, a given individual may produce different amounts of different classes of antibody and different degrees of cellular reactivity or suppressor activity to the same antigen. Tolerance may be instituted in an adult animal by contact with antigen after exposure to systemic immunosuppressive events, such as the administration of irradiation or large doses of antimetabolic agents. An antigen that induces tolerance is called a tolerogen; the same antigen presented in different circumstances may stimulate an immune response (immunogen). A strong immunogen is by definition a poor tolerogen and vice versa. Some of the characteristics of the acquired tolerant state that have been discovered from experimental work are the following:

1. Tolerance is most easily induced by antigens that are closely related to those of the host; induction of the tolerant state becomes more difficult as the complexity and the number of antigenic determinants of the antigen increase. In other words, the ability to induce acquired tolerance to a given antigen is inversely related to the degree of immunogenicity of the antigen (Table 11-1).

Table 11-1. Relation of Degree of Immunogenicity to Source and Complexity of Antigen

Complexity of Antigen	Autogeneic (Same Individual)	Syngeneic (Genetically Identical Individual)	Allogeneic (Different Individual, Same Species)	Xenogeneic (Different Species)
Serum proteins	0	0	±[b]	++
Altered serum proteins[a]	+	+	+	++
Erythrocytes	0	0	++	++++
Tissue grafts	0	0	+++	+++++

0, no response; ±, inconsistent response, + weak response, ++ through +++++, rough indication of degree of immunogenicity.
[a] Denatured or conjugated with haptens.
[b] An immune response may occur to some serum proteins (see Allotypes, Chapter 6).

2. Tolerance is of finite duration, and the duration of the tolerant state depends upon the continued presence of antigen. Newborn rabbits made tolerant to an antigen so that no immune response can be elicited at 4 months of age may have an immune response to the same antigen at 12 months of age. If such animals are given repeated doses of the antigen, they remain tolerant at 12 months of age.
3. Either very high or very low doses of antigen may induce tolerance to an antigen that will elicit an antibody response when an intermediate dose is used (high- and low-dose tolerance).
4. The state of tolerance may be terminated by injection of

antigens that contain antigenic determinants (specificities) in common with the antigen to which the individual is tolerant but also contain antigenic determinants to which the same individual is not tolerant.

5. Both T cells and B cells may be made tolerant (Fig. 11-1). T

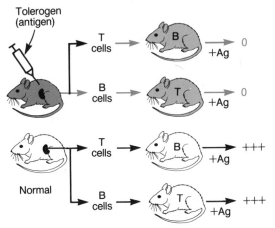

Figure 11-1. Demonstration of tolerance in T and B cells. Spleen cells from mice tolerant to a specific antigen are separated into T cells (nylon wool passage) and B cells (survive antithymocyte treatment). The T cells are injected into B cell mice (adult thymectomized, irradiated, and restored with

Donors

normal bone marrow cells) and the B cells into T cell mice (irradiated and restored with normal thymus cells). Upon challenge with antigen (Ag), neither reconstituted mouse responds. However, injection of T or B cells from normal mice into B or T cell animals results in a

Recipients

responding animal. In addition, challenge with an antigen unrelated to the tolerogen results in an immune response to this second antigen. Similar results are obtained in vitro, when T or B cells from a tolerant animal are mixed with B or T cells from a normal animal.

cells are made tolerant for long periods of time by low doses of antigen, whereas B cells require higher doses of antigen. Tolerance of either T or B cells leads to tolerance in the animal. However, the B cells "recover" or are replaced by new B cells after a relatively short time, whereas T cells may remain tolerant for longer periods. B cells are more easily made tolerant early in development, at the stage when surface IgM first appears, than at later stages of maturation.

6. Transfer of cells from a tolerant donor to a normal syngeneic host may confer specific tolerance in the recipient. This effect is not produced if the T cells of the donor are killed prior to transfer. Cells transferred from a tolerant donor animal to an irradiated host (e.g., an animal whose own immune system has been destroyed) restore the general immune responsive state of the irradiated animal, except that tolerance to the specific antigen to which the original donor of the cells was tolerant is also transferred (adoptive tolerance).

The breaking of self tolerance by related antigens can be explained by a two-cell system (Fig. 11-2). Antigens that cross-

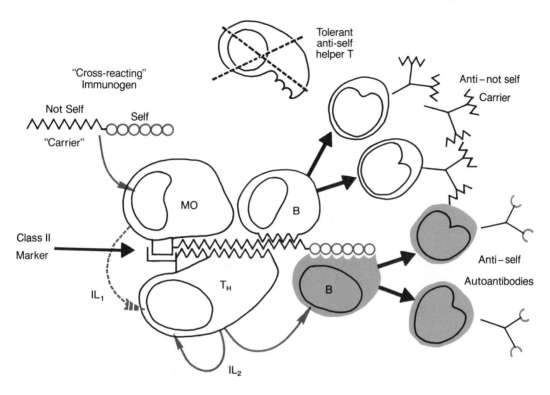

Figure 11-2. Interplay of T and B cells in "breaking" of B cell tolerance to self antigens. The immunogen contains two types of determinants: one set of foreign (nonself) determinants and one set of self determinants. T and B cells, each required for maximum primary antibody responses, contain individual cells or populations of cells that separately recognize these different determinants. Both T and B cells can become tolerant to these antigens, but experimental data show that T cells are made tolerant for much longer periods. Thus, recovery of responsiveness of B cells to self antigens may occur rapidly. However, T cells are needed to provide helper function to B cells for antibody production to occur. If an immunogen contains both self and foreign antigens, T cells specific for the foreign determinant can provide helper function for both self and foreign antigens to B cells. Thus, antibodies to both self and foreign antigens are produced.

react (i.e., contain some determinants in common) with the antigen used to induce tolerance are processed by the antigen-presenting macrophage and presented to cells that specifically recognize the foreign immunogenic epitopes of the antigen. These recognition cells are able to induce a response in self reacting responsive precursor lines that have recovered from the tolerant state. The recovery of cells from a tolerant state may result from the ongoing development from uncommitted stem cells of cells with the ability to react with the specific antigen, the resynthesis of receptor sites by cells whose sites have been blocked or destroyed, or the removal of some block to the development of a potentially reactive cell. T cells and B cells may become tolerant or lose tolerance as a result of different mechanisms.

Mechanisms of Tolerance

Tolerance may involve either positive or negative control systems entailing the interaction of cells during induction of an immune response. For many years the explanation of tolerance was based on the clonal selection of Burnet. Although this theory may still explain some types of tolerance, more recent studies have identified tolerant situations that require a different explanation. In general, tolerance may be explained by clonal deletion/anergy or by complex immunoregulatory systems involving suppressor T cells or antibody inhibition pathways. Six general mechanisms of immune tolerance are presented: clonal elimination/anergy, suppressor T cells, natural suppressor cells, blocking antibody, idiotype network, and antigen catabolism (processing).

Clonal Elimination/ Clonal Anergy

The clonal selection theory of Burnet postulates that the ability of an individual to recognize an immunogen lies in individual reactive cells or cell lines (clones) (Fig. 11-3). Upon contact with the antigen, the cells with the capacity to recognize the antigen are stimulated to multiply and differentiate. The property of antigen recognition is restricted in the sense that each reactive cell recognizes only one antigen. In fetal life or in special situations in adults, contact of the reacting cell with antigen causes the elimination of this cell and, therefore, loss of the ability of the individual to make an immune response to that antigen (tolerance). The death or loss of immunologically reactive precursor cells upon contact of these cells with the individual's own tissues in fetal life results in the establishment of natural tolerance. In adult animals, the establishment of acquired tolerance may be preceded by a brief period of antibody production. This is explained by antigen-driven differentiation leading to depletion of antigen recognition cells (exhaustive differentiation). The clonal selection theory of tolerance is unable to explain the observation that tolerance is often easily broken. Such experiments indicate that acquired tolerance depends not on the loss of immunologically reactive precursor cells but on an altered reactivity of cells that can be redirected to immune responsiveness by certain procedures. Thus, acquired tolerance is most likely due not to the elimination or failure of development of specifically reactive cells but to blocking of expression or temporary inactivation of cells required for a specific response, that is, *clonal anergy.*

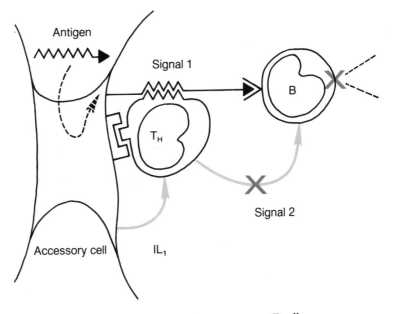

Figure 11-3. Clonal elimination or anergy. In this model of tolerance the responding immune cells are either eliminated or rendered inert. As depicted in this figure, B cells require at least two signals to be stimulated to proliferate. Signal 1 is provided by contact with antigen and signal 2 by factors (IL2, BCGF, etc.) produced by T helper cells. If the B cell receives the antigenic first signal in the absence of the second signal, it may be made tolerant. B cells are most easily made tolerant when they are in an immature (surface IgM only) IgD negative state. A similar mechanism may function if thymocytes or pre-T cells contact self antigens in the thymus while in an immature state. T cells require contact with antigen (signal 1), activation by IL1 (signal 2), and autostimulation by IL1 (signal 3). If T cells make contact with antigen without processing by macrophages or in the absence of IL1 or IL2 production, it is possible that elimination rather than stimulation may occur.

Suppressor Cells

The first clues to the presence of suppressor T cells came with the observations of Richard Gershon concerning the effects of transfer of normal or immune cells to tolerant hosts and of tolerant cells to normal hosts of the same MHC type. Gershon found that tolerance could be passively transferred using T cells from tolerant animals. This phenomenon was termed *infectious tolerance* and strongly implied a role for suppressor T cells in the induction and maintenance of tolerance (Fig. 11-4).

A number of additional findings support a role for suppressor T cells in controlling the response of B cells: (1) An increase in antibody production may be obtained after thymectomy. (2) Thymocytes from rats treated with antigen 48 hours previously, when transferred to syngeneic recipients, may specifically suppress the response of the recipients to the same antigen. (3) Anti-T cell treatment of young NZB mice increases the antibody response to certain antigens, but this effect is not seen in older NZB mice who may have lost their suppressor T

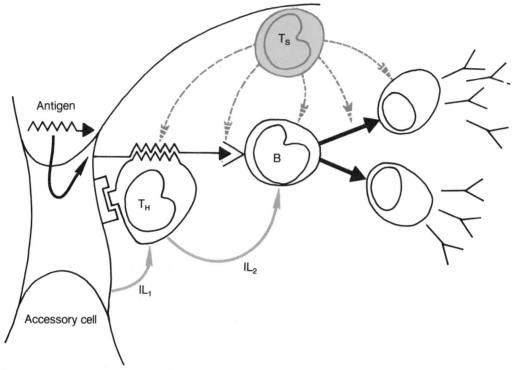

Figure 11-4. T suppressor cells and tolerance. During an immune response, T helper/inducer cells activate not only B cells but also T suppressor cells. T suppressor cells produce an antigen-specific factor that can act at the T_H or B cell level to inhibit the immune response to that antigen only.

cell population and thus become prone to development of certain "autoallergic" diseases. (4) Lymphocytes from mice with chronic suppression of a given immunoglobulin allotype suppress expression of that allotype on normal cells in vitro or upon passive transfer into a normal host. (5) Lymphocytes stimulated by certain mitogens, such as concanavalin A, inhibit the immune response of normal cells. (6) Removal of the bursa of Fabricius in chickens may lead to the appearance of T cells that suppress IgA- or IgG-bearing B cells. Each of these observations supports the concept that a certain population of T cells controls the response of B cells. The mechanism through which T cells suppress the response of B cells is unclear. Suppressor T cells may prevent presentation of antigen, block the function of T helper cells, inhibit proliferation of B cells, or block the differentiation of B cells to antibody-secreting plasma cells.

Suppressor T cells may also limit the activity of other T cells. The part of the T cell population that exerts a suppressor effect is probably about 10% to 20%. Certain T cells inhibit mixed lymphocyte reactions and the blastogenic response to mitogens such as phytohemagglutinin or to specific antigens. In addition, treatment of recipient rats with antithymocyte serum (ATS) may increase the severity of a graft versus host reaction produced upon transfer of thymus cells. Since the graft versus host reaction is T cell mediated, the ATS may depress suppressor T cells of the host that control the graft versus host cells. Therefore, suppressor T cells may function in the tolerant animal and may be the primary mechanism for preventing antibody production by B cells or cellular immunologic reaction by other T cells. When the suppressor T cells are specific for a given antigen, the immune response to other antigens may be normal in animals rendered tolerant by this mechanism.

In a mouse model, Ig class–specific T_S cells that act only on B cells for IgE have also been identified. After immunization with antigen in complete Freund's adjuvant, a population of T_S cells in the spleen (pass through nylon wool, killed by anti-Thy + C) inhibits the production of IgE by primed B cells, but does not affect IgG production to the same antigen. These T_S cells produce a soluble factor when exposed to specific antigen that acts only on B cells of the IgE class (Fig. 11-5). This model,

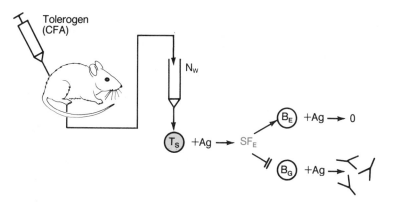

Figure 11-5. Demonstration of suppressor T cell factor specific for IgE antibody. T suppressor cells obtained by passage over nylon wool of spleen cells from animals immunized with antigen in complete Freund's adjuvant produce a suppressor factor (SF$_e$) that specifically inhibits B cells from making IgE antibody when the B cells are reexposed to the same antigen, but has no effect on B cells having the capacity to make IgG antibody to the same antigen.

if applicable to man, could have far-reaching implications in regard to specific immunotherapy for IgE-mediated allergic reactions (see also Chapter 18).

The properties of a population of suppressor cells known as *natural* suppressor cells are listed in Table 11-2. Natural suppressor cells are active upon T cell–mediated reactions primarily to MHC alloantigens, but are not antigen specific. Such cells could be responsible for both neonatal tolerance and tolerance in immunosuppressed adults. These cells are null cells in the large granular lymphocyte population. In irradiated adults, there seems to be a short-lived reappearance of natural

Table 11-2. Properties of Natural Suppressor Cells

Found in fetal and neonatal animals
Disappear a few days after birth
Activity demonstrable in irradiated adults
Not induced by antigen
Not antigen specific
Suppress:
   Mixed lymphocyte reactions
   Generation of T_K cells
   Graft versus host reactions
Have neither T nor B markers
Are large granular lymphocytes
Do not suppress B cells

suppressor cells and, later, the presence of an antigen-specific T suppressor cell that can be induced upon exposure to antigen shortly after irradiation. This latter T suppressor cell may be important in prolonging suppression to host (recipient) tissue and modifying graft versus host disease if allogeneic cells such as bone marrow cells are transferred to an adult after irradiation.

Blocking Antibody

Earlier, it was pointed out that specific antibody may act through a feedback mechanism to limit the production of specific antibody and to control the extent of an immune response. During the induction of tolerance, a phase of antibody production sometimes occurs prior to the establishment of the tolerant state. It is tenuous to postulate that such blocking antibody can induce tolerance, as it is impossible to induce adoptive tolerance by passive transfer with antiserum.

However, the extent of an immune response might be limited by feedback inhibition of antibody production (see Chapter 10). Conflicting evidence exists regarding whether this inhibition acts on accessory macrophages, T cells, B cells, or some interaction step (Fig. 11-6). It has been suggested that the immunological activities of T cells can be blocked by antigen–antibody complexes. Although there is little concrete evidence to support this, it is possible that antigen–antibody complexes could bind to the surface receptors of helper T cells in such a way as to block reaction with free antigen and prevent helper function. Such blocking effects of antibody–antigen complexes have been postulated as preventing tumor and tissue graft rejection.

Idiotype Network

Each antibody variable region itself might be the antigen recognized by a series of autoantibodies that suppress the specific immune response (auto-anti-idiotype network) (Fig. 11-7). T cells as well as specific antibodies may have idiotypic determinants and may be subject to regulation by anti-idiotypes. Anti-idiotype sera are able to block T cell functions in some

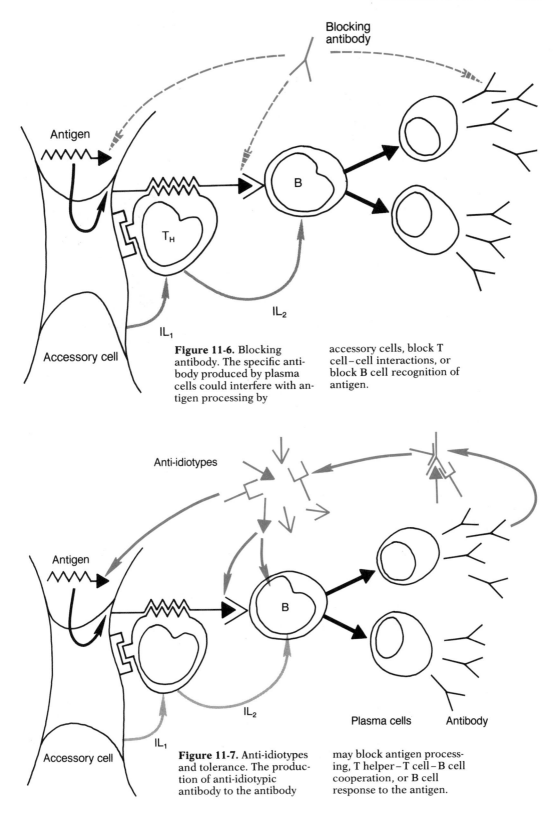

Figure 11-6. Blocking antibody. The specific antibody produced by plasma cells could interfere with antigen processing by accessory cells, block T cell–cell interactions, or block B cell recognition of antigen.

Figure 11-7. Anti-idiotypes and tolerance. The production of anti-idiotypic antibody to the antibody may block antigen processing, T helper–T cell–B cell cooperation, or B cell response to the antigen.

experimental systems. It is postulated that the presence of small amounts of such anti-idiotypes (undetectable by most techniques) is responsible for maintenance of self tolerance in some systems. (See also Chapter 10.)

Antigen Catabolism

The tolerant state may be established because of the inability of the affected animal to metabolize the antigen properly for antigen presentation, so that the stimulation necessary for a specific immune response is not made available (Fig. 11-8). Such

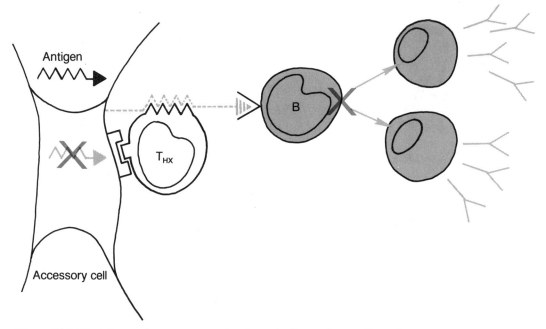

Figure 11-8. The tolerogenic effect of unprocessed antigen. If B cells or T cells are exposed directly to unprocessed antigens in the absence of antigen-presenting cells, class II MHC, or IL1, they may not respond to the specific antigens. Tolerance could be broken when the antigen processing mechanism is mature.

ineffective antigen processing could be due to a failure of the macrophage to process the antigen to immunogenic peptides expressed in association with class II MHC markers.

Tolerance may be a function of the cell type that first contacts the antigen. According to this concept, the induction of an immune response requires the processing of antigen by macrophages, which prepares the antigen for recognition by specific immunologically reactive T and/or B cells. Direct interaction of the unprocessed antigen with the specific reactive cells may result in the loss of the ability of these cells to be immunologically stimulated (tolerance). The processing of immunogen by macrophages is an immunologically nonspecific event, but the loss of recognition by specifically reactive lymphocytes results in antigen-specific tolerance.

Summary

There is no single explanation for all of the natural and experimental phenomena that are grouped under the umbrella of tolerance. Different mechanisms may explain different phenomena, or more than one mechanism may be operative in a given situation. Different cells with the capacity to respond to a specific antigen (immunologically competent cells) may undergo induction upon contact with the antigen: this may result in immunity (antibody-producing plasma cells or sensitized lymphocytes), immune memory, or tolerance. The outcome depends on the dose and type of antigen and on the state of the potentially responding individual. It is also possible that some reactive cells are killed by reaction with tolerogen or that an immunogen may be presented in a nonimmunogenic manner, causing tolerance. However, tolerance is best considered as an active process involving the production of tolerant cells that cannot respond to an immunogen, suppressor cells, or antibodies that inhibit potentially responding cells.

Split Tolerance and Immune Deviation

Split tolerance refers to the lack of response to an antigen as measured by one type of effector mechanism, while another effector arm is quite active. In some human infectious diseases, individuals may demonstrate high antibody titers but little or no cellular immunity (and vice versa) to the antigens of the infecting agent. In leprosy and chronic mucocutaneous candidiasis, good cellular response with low or no antibody responses is associated with effective protective immunity, whereas high antibody titers and low cellular responses are associated with progressive infection (see Chapter 24).

Immune deviation refers to the changing of one type of immune response to another. Effective therapy for leprosy is associated with a change from hormonal to cellular immunity. Therapy for IgE-mediated allergic reactions may be effected by changing the predominant antibody response from one immunoglobulin class (IgE) to another (IgG) by repeated antigenic challenge (see Chapter 18).

Immune Paralysis

An effect similar to tolerance may be induced by injection of moderate amounts of nondegradable antigen (Felton's immunological paralysis) (Fig. 11-9). In such cases, antibody-producing cells may be identified if they are removed from the animal, but secreted antibody is rapidly bound to the circulating antigen. Usually antigens bound to antibody (complexes) are taken up by macrophages (phagocytosis), and both antigen and antibody are degraded. With an undegradable antigen, only the antibody is destroyed and the antigen is released so that it may again combine with antibody. Thus, any antibody formed is removed rapidly by antigen so that circulating antibody is not detectable. This "paralysis" of antibody by antigen has been likened to a treadmill.

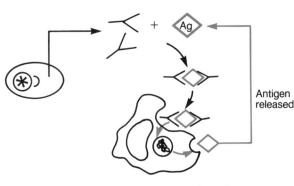

Antigen
released

Figure 11-9. Immune paralysis. *Immune paralysis refers to the consumption of antibody by poorly degradable antigens. The antibodies produced after injection of such an antigen* react with the antigen to form antibody–antigen complexes. These complexes are taken up by the reticuloendothelial system (macrophages), where the antibody is catabolized but the antigen is released into the circulation system. In this manner, the antigen continues to react with and remove antibody so that titers of circulating antibody may not be demonstrable.

Desensitization

Therapeutic "hyposensitization" may involve tolerance, immune deviation, or *desensitization*. Desensitization is a temporary state of unresponsiveness in an already immunized animal, induced by relatively large doses of degradable antigen administered in such a way as to be relatively innocuous. Desensitization occurs as a result of combination between antigen and antibody; the specific antibody or sensitized cells are exhausted by reaction with the specific antigen. This is similar to the effect observed in immunological paralysis. However, since the antigen is degradable, resynthesis of antibody or re-formation of sensitized cells will result in the desensitized state being overcome, usually in a few days, with restoration of the immune state of the treated individual. The duration of the desensitized state depends on the rate at which the desensitized individual is producing the specific antibody or specifically sensitized cells and on the amount of antigen used for desensitization. Desensitization must be differentiated from clinical hyposensitization, which most likely is dependent upon a different mechanism. (See atopic or anaphylactic reactions in Chapter 18.)

Tolerance and Immunity

Immune tolerance may be a more common or more natural state than immune reactivity. An individual is likely to be presented with small amounts of antigen (everyday contact with nonpathogenic organisms) or very high and continued doses of antigen (an individual's own serum proteins), in a manner more conducive to the production of tolerance than to the production of active immunity. The immunologist has worked most often in dose ranges likely to result in active immunity and commonly uses nonspecific adjuvants to enhance immune responses. These adjuvants generally have the effect of mobilizing lymphoid cells and concentrating reactive cells at the site of antigen deposition; a similar effect would occur in the case of an infection with an organism capable of producing an inflammatory response. The role of tolerance or lack of tolerance is important in the understanding of autoimmune diseases and transplantation.

Autoimmunity

Specific immune tolerant states provide mechanisms whereby an immune response to self antigens, *autoimmunity*, is prevented. Thus, establishment of tolerance to self antigens could be considered the natural state for self antigens. Autoimmunity may then be defined as a loss of tolerance to self antigens. With recognition of the destructive power of the immune system when directed to specific antigens, it becomes obvious that an immune response to one's own antigens could be disastrous. At the end of the last century Paul Ehrlich coined the term *horror autotoxicus* for such circumstances. However, we now know that autoimmune responses are in fact quite common. Autoantibodies can be found in many normal individuals and increase in frequency with aging. In the 1960s Pierre Grabar hypothesized that autoantibodies might be important for reacting with and causing the elimination of defective or denatured molecules. Antibody-excess immune complexes are cleared rapidly by the reticuloendothelial system (see Chapter 12). Thus autoantibodies could act as carrier molecules to clear the body of effete molecules.

The reality of the situation actually lies somewhere between horror autotoxicus and garbage collection. We now know that many diseases are attributable to an autoimmune response, whereas, on the other hand, many otherwise healthy individuals may have detectable autoantibodies in their blood. The ability to induce tolerance is related to two major factors: the degree of complexity of the antigen and the amount of antigen present (see Table 11-1). The relationship of concentration of serum proteins to the incidence of autoantibodies (B cells) or autoreactive T cells to these proteins as seen by William Weigle is illustrated in Figure 11-10. As shown, autoreactivity to some determinants such as IgG idiotypes occurs naturally and may be physiological. Autoantibodies are found to a variety of other serum proteins less frequently. Autoreactive T cells occur much less frequently and may be associated with tissue lesions (thyroglobulin—thyroiditis; myelin basic protein—encephalomyelitis). Polyclonal activation of B cells may result in a number of autoantibodies. In most instances, these are of low avidity and are not associated with tissue lesions (see below).

Autoantibodies and Autoallergic Disease

A number of antibodies to tissue or serum antigens have been observed in the sera of human patients with certain diseases

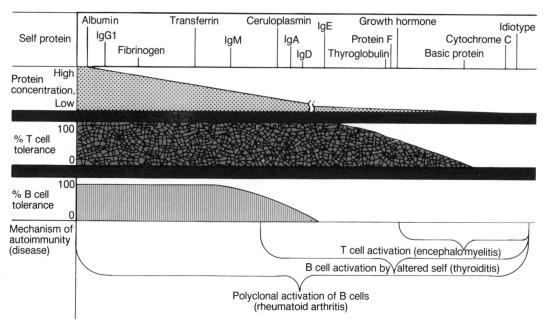

Figure 11-10. Theoretical relationship between serum protein concentration and degree of T and B cell tolerance.

(Table 11-3). Several examples are considered now; others are discussed in much greater detail in later chapters dealing with immunopathology (see Chapters 14–21).

Autoantibodies to cardiac muscle may be demonstrated in some patients following myocardial infarction. The induction of these antibodies may be due to alteration of myocardial antigens secondary to necrosis; the antibodies found react (? cross-react) with normal myocardial antigens. It is not likely that these antibodies play a role in the original infarction, but they have been implicated in the postinfarction syndrome, and autoantibodies to the conductive tissue of the heart (Purkinje's fibers) may be responsible for chronic heart block. Henry Kaplan has shown that there are antigens of group A streptococci that cross-react with cardiac tissue. The occurrence of this type of antibody suggests that an appropriate streptococcal infection may break tolerance to normal cardiac tissue antigens (see Fig. 11-2), with the resulting autoallergic reaction and production of rheumatic fever (see Chapter 17). Autoantibodies are also found after cardiopulmonary bypass perfusion or massive blood transfusion.

The significance of most autoantibodies is unknown. In some cases, but certainly not all, a pathogenic function has been convincingly demonstrated. Antinuclear antibody in lupus erythematosus, rheumatoid factor in rheumatoid arthritis, antiacetylcholine receptor in myasthenia gravis, anti-

Table 11-3. Some Human Diseases in Which Serum Antibodies to Serum or Tissue Antigens Have Been Found by Various Methods

Disease	Antigen	Method of Antibody Detection
Addison's disease, idiopathic	Adrenal	CF, F
Dermatitis, chronic	Dermis	F, A
Glomerulonephritis, poststreptococcal	Kidney	CF, F, H, A
Other kidney diseases	Kidney	F, A
Viral hepatitis	Liver, spleen, smooth muscle	CF, F, H, A, P
Cirrhosis of liver	Liver, spleen, kidney	CF, F, H, A
Lung diseases (emphysema, asthma, tuberculosis)	Lung	CF, GC, P
Lupus erythematosus	Liver, spleen, kidney, muscle, platelets, blood cells, nucleoprotein, RNA, DNA, histone	CF, F, A
Multiple sclerosis	Brain or white matter	CF, tissue culture demyelination
Carcinomatous neuropathy	Neurons	F, CF (gray, white)
Other CNS diseases (cerebrovascular accident)	Brain	CF
Myasthenia gravis	Muscle, thymus, thyroid	CF, F, H, GC
Myocardial infarction	Heart	H, P
Orchitis, infertility	Sperm	A
Pancreatitis, chronic cystic fibrosis	Pancreas glandular epithelium	P, H
Pernicious anemia	Intrinsic factor, parietal cell microsomes	CF, F, inhibition
Atrophic gastritis	Gastric mucosa	
Rheumatic fever	Heart, muscle, joint	CF, F, H, GC P, H, A
Rheumatoid arthritis	Heart, muscle, joint, subcutaneous nodules, aggregated γ-globulin	
Scleroderma, dermatomyositis	Kidney, muscle, joint, cell nuclei	F
Sjögren's syndrome	Salivary gland, liver, kidney, thyroid cell nuclei	CF, P, F, H
Syphilis	Wassermann antigen	CF, A
Thyroiditis, myxedema, thyrotoxicosis	Thyroglobulin, globular epithelium, gastric mucosa cell nuclei	P, CF, H, F
Ulcerative colitis	Mucosal glands, mucus	CF, F, H, P
Uveal injury	Uveal pigment	CF

A, agglutination of other antigen-coated particles; CF, complement fixation; CNS, central nervous system; F, fluorescent antibody fixation; GC, antiglobulin consumption; H, hemagglutination, passive; P, precipitation.

(Modified from Waksman, BH: Medicine, 41:93, 1963. Copyright 1962, The Williams & Wilkins Co.)

erythrocyte antibody in autoallergic hemolytic anemia, and antiheart antibody in rheumatic fever are almost certainly significant in the etiology of these autoallergic diseases. Other autoantibodies are characteristic of a specific disease entity and are useful diagnostic aids but are without obvious roles in causation of the disease. Antibodies that bind to hepatocytic mitochrondria may be detected by the fluorescent antibody technique in the sera of patients with primary biliary cirrhosis and chronic active hepatitis, but not in the sera of patients with other forms of cirrhosis or extrahepatic biliary obstruction. One is left with the explanation that many autoantibodies are more likely to be the result than the cause of tissue alteration or breakdown.

Criteria for Identification of Autoimmunity

There are certain characteristics, ideally identifiable in all immune responses, that should be sought in diseases of suspected autoimmune etiology. These include (1) a well-defined immunizing event (infection, immunization, vaccination), (2) a latent period (usually 6–14 days), (3) a secondary response (a more rapid and more intense reaction on second exposure to the antigen), (4) an ability to transfer the sensitive state with cells or serum from an affected individual to a normal individual, (5) a specific depression of the sensitive state by large amounts of antigen (desensitization), (6) identification and isolation of the antigen in a pure form, and (7) chemical characterization of the antigen. All, or even a few, of these criteria can rarely, if ever, be established for human diseases. The criteria are most closely approximated in certain blood dyscrasias such as autoimmune hemolytic anemia. However, these criteria can be met in experimental models that mimic human diseases (see Chapters 14–21 for specific examples).

Presumptive findings consistent with, but not strong evidence for, an allergic mechanism in disease states include (1) a morphologic picture consistent with known allergic reactions; (2) demonstration of specific antibody or of a positive delayed skin reaction; (3) depression of complement during some stage of the disease; (4) beneficial effect of agents known to inhibit some portion of an allergic reaction (steroids, radiation, cyclosporine); (5) identification of a reasonable experimental model in animals that mimics the human disease; (6) association with other possible autoallergic diseases; and (7) increased familial susceptibility to the same disease or other autoallergic diseases.

Theories of Autoimmunization

1. The tissues involved in autoallergic diseases are derived from ectoderm or endoderm and are regarded as foreign by the immune apparatus, which is mesodermal. These autoantigens are substances that are absent or sequestered during

the immune neutral period of development and, therefore, fail to induce tolerance like other body antigens. Blood–tissue barriers normally prevent these antigens from reaching the circulation and the immune apparatus. When viral infection, injury, or other episodes cause breakdown of blood–tissue barriers and release of these sequestered antigens into circulation, an allergic reaction may occur.

2. Viral infections or other events cause alteration of tissue substances not normally antigenic, so that they are recognized as antigen by the immune system. This hypothesis has received experimental support. William Weigle has been able to break tolerance using chemically modified antigens. By immunizing animals with aqueous homologous thyroglobulin to which arsenilic or sulfanilic acid haptens had been coupled, he was able to induce experimental autoallergic inflammation of the thyroid; the supposition is that tolerance to autologous proteins can be broken by antigenically modified proteins of the same class.

3. T helper cells may be stimulated to activate previously inactivated B cells (cross-reactive autoimmunity).

4. The function of suppressor cells may be lost. Suppressor cells may prevent other immunologically competent cells from responding to self antigens. Presentation of the antigen in a particular manner may circumvent suppressor cell activity. Suppressor cells are short-lived and may become less numerous with aging, permitting other cells to respond to self antigens. The incidence of autoallergic diseases and autoantibodies increases with age, presumably because atrophy of the thymus with aging results in a failure in the ability of the thymus to produce new T suppressor cells.

5. B cells may be nonspecifically activated by B cell mitogens that lead to *polyclonal activation,* that is, a nonspecific increase in immunoglobulin molecules of different specificities or IgG classes. Some of the immunoglobulins produced may react with self antigens. In this manner polyclonal activation may result in autoantibody production.

6. According to the clonal selection theory of Burnet (see above) an alteration, not in the tissue in which the lesion appears but in the cells of the immune system, leads to autoimmunity. Because of an unknown mechanism, some immunologically competent cells, which do not normally react against tissues of the same animal, go out of control and recognize normal tissue substances as antigens.

7. The effects of blocking antibodies or the idiotype network may be lost. These effects appear to be cyclic. Thus the extent of an immune response may be held at a low level by the idiotype network. However, an antigenic exposure may affect one or some of the members of the anti-idiotypic reac-

tants in the network, permitting an autoimmune response to become manifested. Wavering of control is a possible explanation for the frequent cyclic remissions and relapses that are common occurrences in diseases caused by autoimmunity.

8. A recently suggested mechanism is the induction of class II MHC expression on cells normally not expressing class II MHC, permitting antigen presentation and induction of an immune response.

A summary of B cell control mechanisms in autoantibody responses and B cell proliferation responses that could progress to lymphoma is given in Figure 11-11.

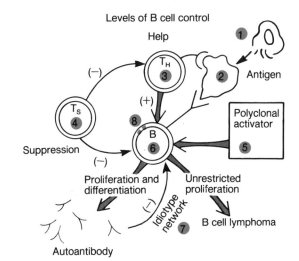

Figure 11-11. Control of B cells: autoantibody production and B cell lymphoma. Loss of control of B cells may occur at a number of possible sites: (1) Sequestered antigens may be released into the circulation and become available for immunization. (2) Alteration of self antigens or unusual antigen presentation (i.e., associated with viral infections) may lead to stimulation of B cells and breaking of tolerance to self antigens. (3) Increased T_H (helper) activity may occur, resulting in inappropriate stimulation of normal B cells. (4) A loss of suppressor activity (T_S) could result in increased T_H activity or B cell proliferation. (5) Polyclonal activators (bacterial endotoxins, etc.) may bypass control mechanisms and activate B cells directly to produce antibodies nonspecifically. (6) An inherent (somatic) change may occur in a B cell, resulting in loss of tolerance due to production of a new reactive clone. (7) Fluctuations in idiotype network antibodies may permit greater production of previously suppressed autoantibodies. (8) Expression of class II MHC (IA) on cells not normally expressing class II MHC, leading to antigen presentation and induction of an immune response.

Summary

Immune tolerance is the specific loss of the ability to produce an immune response to a given antigen; normal responses to other antigens remain intact. Some possible mechanisms of tolerance are:

1. Clonal elimination/anergy: elimination or inactivation in the tolerant animal of the cells responsible for recognizing and responding to the given antigen.

2. Suppressor cells: active inhibition of reactive cells present in the animal by specific suppressor cells.
3. Blocking antibody: reaction of potentially responding cells blocked by specific antibody or antibody–antigen complexes.
4. Network theory: anti-idiotype antibodies that act on the surface of cells are boosted by rising levels of idiotype-containing antibodies.
5. Immunogen processing: Immunogen reaches the potentially responding cells in an unprocessed form, rendering them nonreactive. Unprocessed antigen may induce suppressor cells.

Normally an individual develops tolerance to his own antigens during development (natural tolerance). A loss of natural tolerance is believed to be responsible for autoimmune diseases. However, many normal individuals have demonstrable autoantibodies without evidence of disease. Breaking of tolerance to self antigens may have a normal function or may cause disease.

References

Tolerance

Neonatal

Auerbach R, Clark S: Immunological tolerance: transmission from mother to offspring. Science 189:84, 1975.

Billingham RE, Brent L: Acquired tolerance of foreign cells in newborn animals. Proc R Soc B 146:28, 1956.

Boyden SV: Natural antibodies and the immune response. Adv Immunol 5:1, 1965.

Burnet FM, Fenner F: The Production of Antibodies. Melbourne, Macmillan, 1949.

Hasek M, Langerova A, Hraba T: Transplantation immunity and tolerance. Adv Immunol 1:1, 1961.

Howard JC, Michie D: Induction of transplantation immunity in newborn mice. Transplant Bull 29:91, 1962.

Hraba T: Mechanisms and role of immunological tolerance. *In* Kallos P, Goodman HC, Hasek M, Inderbitzen T (eds): Monographs in Allergy. Basel, Karger, 1968.

Medawar PB: Actively acquired tolerance of foreign cells. Nature 172:603, 1953.

Moller G (ed): Transplantation Tolerance. Immunol Rev 46, 1979.

Owen RD: Immunogenetic consequence of vascular anastomoses between bovine twins. Science 102:400, 1945.

Streilein JW: Neonatal tolerance: towards an immunogenetic definition of self. Immunol Rev 46:125, 1979.

Triplett EL: On the mechanism of immunologic self recognition. J Immunol 89:505, 1962.

Weigle WO: Immunological unresponsiveness. Adv Immunol 16:61, 1973.

Clonal Elimination/ Anergy

Basten A, Miller JFAP, Sprent J, Cheers C: Cell-to-cell interaction in the immune response. X. T cell-dependent suppression in tolerant mice. J Exp Med 140:199, 1974.

Benjamin DC: Neonatally induced tolerance to HcG: duration in B cells and absence of specific suppressor cells. J Immunol 119:311, 1977.

Burnet FM: The Clonal Selection Theory of Acquired Immunity. London, Cambridge University Press, 1959.

Burnet FM: The Integrity of the Body: A Discussion of Modern Immunological Ideas. Cambridge, Harvard University Press, 1962.

Chiller JM, Habicht GS, Weigle WO: Cellular sites of immunologic unresponsiveness. Proc Nat Acad Sci USA 65:551, 1970.

Chiller JM, Rombard CG, Weigle WO: Induction of immunological tolerance in neonatal and adult rabbits. Cell Immunol 8:28, 1973.

Dresser DW, Mitchison NA: The mechanism of immunological paralysis. Adv Immunol 8:128, 1968.

Mitchison NA: Induction of immunological paralysis with two zones of dosage. Proc R Soc Land [Biol] 161:275, 1966.

Moller G (ed): Mechanism of B cell tolerance. Immunol Rev 43, 1979.

Nossal GJV: Cellular mechanisms of immunological tolerance. Ann Rev Immunol 1:33, 1983.

Nossal GJV, Pike BL: Evidence for the clonal abortion theory of B lymphocyte tolerance. J Exp Med 141:904, 1975.

Parks E, Weigle WO: Current perspectives on the cellular mechanisms of tolerance induction. Clin Exp Immunol 39:257, 1980.

Scibienski RJ, et al: Active and inactive states of immunologic unresponsiveness. J Immunol 113:45, 1974.

Weigle WO: Termination of acquired immunological tolerance to protein antigens following immunization with altered protein antigens. J Exp Med 116:913, 1962.

Suppressor Cells

Argyris BF: Adoptive tolerance: transfer of the tolerant state. J Immunol 90:29, 1963.

Argyris BF: Adoptive tolerance transferred by bone marrow, spleen, lymph node or thymus cells. J Immunol 96:273, 1966.

Baker PJ, Stashak PW, Ambsbaugh DF, Prescott B: Regulation of the antibody response to type III pneumococcal polysaccharide. II. Mode of action of thymic-derived suppressor cells. J Immunol 112:404, 1974.

Baker PJ, Stashak PW, Ambsbaugh DR, Prescott B, Barth RF: Evidence for the existence of two functionally distinct types of cells which regulate the antibody response to type III pneumococcal polysaccharide. J Immunol 105:1581, 1970.

Benjamin DC: Evidence for specific suppression in the maintenance of immunologic tolerance. J Exp Med 141:635, 1975.

Cantor H, Asofsky R: Paradoxical effect of anti-thymocyte serum on the thymus. Nature 243:39, 1973.

Dorf ME, Benacerraf B: Suppressor cells and immunoregulation. Annu Rev Immunol 2:126, 1984.

Dutton RW: Inhibitory and stimulatory effects of Concanavalin A on the response of mouse spleen cell suspensions to antigen. II. Evidence for separate stimulatory and inhibitory cells. J Exp Med 138:1496, 1973.

Gershon R, Cohan P, Hencin R, Liebhaber SA: Suppressor T cells. J Immunol 108:586, 1972.

Gershon R, Kondo K: Cell interactions in the induction of tolerance: the role of thymic lymphocytes. Immunology 18:723, 1970.

Gershon R, Kondo K: Infectious immunological tolerance. Immunology 21:903, 1971.

Green DR, Flood PM, Gershon R: Immunoregulatory T-cell pathways. Annu Rev Immunol 1:439, 1983.

Ha T-Y, Waksman BH, Treffers HP: The thymic suppressor cell. I. Separation of subpopulations with suppressor activity. J Exp Med 139:13–23, 1974.

Kerbel RS, Eidinger D: Enhanced immune responsiveness to a thymus-independent antigen early after adult thymectomy: evidence for short-lived inhibitory thymus-derived cells. Eur J Immunol 2:114–118, 1972.

Moller G (ed): Unresponsiveness to Haptenionated Self Molecules. Immunol Rev 50, 1980.

Okumura K, Tada T: Regulation of homocytotropic antibody formation in the rat. VI. Inhibitory effect of thymocytes on the homocytotropic antibody response. J Immunol 107:1682–1689, 1971.

Scibienski RS: Active and inactive states of immunologic unresponsiveness. J Immunol 113:45, 1974.

Strober S: Natural suppressor cells, neonatal tolerance and total lymphoid irradiation: exploring obscure relationships. Annu Rev Immunol 2:219, 1984.

Weber G, Kolsch E: Transfer of low zone tolerance to normal syngeneic mice by θ positive cells. Eur J Immunol 3:767, 1973.

Blocking Antibody

Bansal SC, et al: Cell-mediated immunity and blocking serum activity to tolerated allografts in rats. J Exp Med 137:590, 1973.

Brent L, et al.: Attempts to demonstrate an in vivo role for serum blocking factors in tolerant mice. Transplantation 14:382, 1972.

Gorczynski R, Kontiainen S, Mitchison NA, Tigelar RE: Antigen–antibody complexes as blocking factors on the T lymphocyte surface. *In* Edelman GM (ed): Cellular Selection and Regulation in the Immune Response. New York, Raven Press, 1974, p143.

Hasek M, et al: Attempts to compare the effectiveness of blocking factors and enhancing antibodies in vivo and vitro. Transplantation 20:95, 1975.

Hellstrom I, Hellstrom KE, Allison AC: Neonatally induced tolerance may be mediated by serum borne factors. Nature 230:49, 1971.

Moller G (ed): Regulation of the immune response by antibodies against the immunogen. Immunol Rev 49:1980.

Voisin GA: Immunologic facilitation: a broadening of the concept of the enhancement phenomenon. Prog Allergy 5:328, 1971.

Wright PW, et al: In vitro reactivity in allograft tolerance. Persistence of cell mediated cytotoxicity and serum blocking activity in highly tolerant rats. Transplantation 19:437, 1975.

Idiotype Network

Cazenave PA: Idiotype–antiidiotype regulation of antibody synthesis in rabbits. Proc Nat Acad Sci USA 74:5122, 1977.

Cerny J, Kelsoe G: Priority of the anti-idiotypic response after antigen administration: artifact or integrating network mechanism. Immunol Today 5:61, 1984.

Herzenberg LA, Tokuhisa K, Hayakawa K: Epitope-specific regulation. Annu Rev Immunol 1:609, 1983.

Hoffman GW: A theory of regulation and self–nonself discrimination. Eur J Immunol 5:638, 1975.

Jerne NK: Towards a network theory of the immune system. Ann Immunol (Inst Pasteur) Ser C125:373, 1974.

Jerne NK: The immune system: a web of V domains. Harvey Lect 70:93, 1975.

Kelsoe G, Reth M, Rajewsky K: Control of idiotype expression by monoclonal antiidiotope bearing antibody. Immunol Rev 52:75, 1980.

Kohler H, Muller S, Bona C: Internal antigen and immune network. Proc Soc Exp Biol Med 178:189, 1985.

Moller G (ed): Idiotype Networks. Immunol Rev 79, 1984.

Moller G (ed): Idiotypes on T Cells and B Cells. Immunol Rev 27, 1975.

Nisonoff A, Bangasser SA: Immunological suppression of idiotypic specificities. Transplant Rev 27:100, 1975.

Paul WE, Bona C: Regulatory idiotopes and immune networks. A hypothesis. Immunol Today 3:9, 1982.

Rajewsky K: Symmetry and asymmetry in idiotypic interactions. Ann Immunol (Inst Pasteur) 1340:133, 1983.

Rajewsky K, Takemori T: Genetics expression and function of idiotypes. Annu Rev Immunol 1:569, 1983.

Rodkey LS: Studies of idiotypic antibodies: production and characterization of auto-antiidiotypic antisera. J Exp Med 139:712, 1974.

Antigen Processing

Ada GL, Nossal GJV, Pye J: Antigens in immunity. XI. The uptake of antigen in animals previously rendered immunologically tolerant. Aust J Exp Biol Med Sci 43:337, 1965.

Ada GL, Parish CR: Low zone tolerance to bacterial flagellin in adult rats. A possible role for antigen localized in lymphoid follicles. Proc Nat Acad Sci USA 61:556, 1968.

Aldo-Benson M, Borel Y: The tolerant cell: direct evidence for receptor blockade by tolerogen. J Immunol 112:1793, 1974.

Garvey J, Eitzman DV, Smith RI: The distribution of S^{35} labeled bovine serum albumin in newborn and immunologically tolerant adult rats. J Exp Med 112:533, 1960.

Humphrey JH: The fate of antigen. Proc R Soc Lond [Biol] 146:34, 1956.

Kripke ML: Immunological unresponsiveness induced by ultraviolet irradiation. Immunol Rev 80:87, 1984.

Moller G (ed): Role of macrophages in the immune response. Immunol Rev 40, 1978.

Schwartz RS, Ryder RJW, Gottlieb BAA: Macrophages and antibody synthesis. Prog Allergy 14:81, 1970.

Unanue ER: The regulatory role of macrophages in antigenic stimulation. Part two. Symbiotic relationship between lymphocytes and macrophages. Adv Immunol 31:1, 1981.

Split Tolerance

See Chapters 18 and 24.

Ishizaka K: Cellular events in the IgE antibody response. Adv Immunol 23:1, 1976.

Ishizaka K: Regulation of IgE synthesis. Annu Rev Immunol 2:259, 1984.

Ishizaka K, Ishizaka T: Mechanisms of reaginic hypersensitivity and IgE antibody response. Immunol Rev 41:109, 1978.

Katz DH: The allergic phenotype: manifestation of "allergic breakthrough" and imbalance in normal "damping" of IgE antibody production. Immunol Rev 41:77, 1978.

Lee WY, Sehon AN: Suppression of reaginic antibodies. Immunol Rev 41:200, 1978.

Rogers TJ, Balish E: Immunity to candida albicans. Microbiol Rev 44:660, 1980.

Turk JL, Bryceson ADM: Immunological phenomena in leprosy and related diseases. Adv Immunol 13:209, 1971.

Immune Paralysis

Felton LD: The significance of antigen in animal tissue. J Immunol 61:107, 1949.

Halliday WJ: Immunological paralysis of mice with pneumococcal polysaccharide antigens. Bacteriol Rev 35:267, 1971.

Autoimmunity

See Chapter 20.

Battisto JR, Claman HN (eds): Immunological Tolerance to Self and Not-self. Ann NY Acad Sci 392, 1982.

Grabar D: Autoantibodies and the physiologic role of immunoglobulin. Immunol Today 4:337, 1983.

Moller G (ed): Autoimmunity and Self–Nonself Discrimination. Immunol Rev 31:1976.

Smith HR, Steinberg AD: Autoimmunity: a perspective. Annu Rev Immunol 1:175, 1983.

12 | Inflammation

Inflammation is the primary process through which the body repairs tissue damage and defends itself against infection (see Chapter 1). Inflammation may be initiated by either immune or nonimmune pathways, but both pathways employ similar effector mechanisms. Activation of immune pathways is initiated by a specific reaction of immunoglobulin antibody or sensitized T lymphocytes with antigen. The in vivo effects of immune activation are determined by amplification mechanisms that are also components of nonimmune inflammatory processes. These amplification mechanisms, rather than the specific immune reaction alone, are largely responsible for the tissue lesions actually observed. Nonimmune inflammation is initiated by release of bacterial products or components of dying tissue cells.

The function of inflammation is to deliver plasma and cellular components of the blood to extravascular tissues. The extravasation of plasma fluid into tissue (edema) causes dilution of toxic materials and increases lymphatic flow. Phagocytic blood cells infiltrate inflamed tissued and destroy bacteria. At late stages, fibrosis walls off foci of infection. As a physiological response to injury, inflammation clears and restores damaged tissue; as a pathologic process, inflammation produces tissue damage (lesions). General inflammatory mechanisms are described here; their pathogenic effects in mediating immune-activated lesions are presented under the different immunopathologic mechanisms discussed in chapters that follow in Part II of this text.

The Process of Inflammation

The phases of inflammation are given in Table 12-1. The following sequence of events occurs during an inflammatory response: (1) increased blood flow (vasodilation) preceded by transient vasoconstriction, (2) increased vascular permeability leading to edema (vasopermeability), (3) infiltration by poly-

261

Table 12-1. Phases of Inflammation: Neurologic, Vascular, Cellular

Initiating event	→	Acute vascular response (minutes)	→	Acute cellular response (hours)	→	Chronic cellular response (days)	→	Scarring or resolution (weeks)
Trauma, necrosis, infection	→	Vasodilation, increased vasopermeability (hyperemia, edema)	→	Neutrophil infiltrate (pus)	→	Mononuclear cell infiltrate[a]	→	Fibrosis or clearing

[a] Lymphocytes, macrophages, and plasma cells.

morphonuclear neutrophils, (4) infiltration by lymphocytes and macrophages (chronic inflammation), leading to (5) resolution (restoration of normal structure) or (6) scarring (filling in of areas of tissue destruction by fibroblasts and collagen) (see Fig. 12-1). The first three events are considered *acute* inflammation; the latter three stages, *chronic* inflammation.

Inflammation is initiated by trauma, tissue necrosis (death), infection, or immune reactions. The immediate response is a temporary vasoconstriction causing blanching of the skin. The mechanism for this is not well understood, but is believed to be mediated by the sympathetic nervous system. Vasoconstriction is followed within seconds by the acute vascular response resulting in increased blood flow (hyperemia) and edema. If there has been only mild injury, such as is caused by stroking the skin, the inflammatory process may be limited to this phase only. However, if there is sufficient cell death or infection the acute cellular phase will follow. Changes in blood flow lead to margination of neutrophils next to endothelial cells, followed by emigration of neutrophils into the adjacent tissue. Contraction of endothelial cells causes leakage (diapedesis) of red blood cells, which progresses to hemorrhage if necrosis of endothelial cells occurs. Exposure of fibrinogen and fibronectin provides sites for platelet aggregation and activation. Alterations in the viscosity of the blood and the electrostatic charge of plasma may aggregate red cells into stacks like pancakes (rouleau formation) as the normal negative repelling charge of the erythrocytes is lost. Depending on the degree of injury or infection, the acute cellular phase may be sufficient to clear the tissue. However, it is usually necessary for the chronic cellular infiltrate of lymphocytes and macrophages to effect removal of tissue debris or dead bacteria. The macrophage is the major player in this process. If damage is sufficient to result in loss of normal tissue, fibroblastic proliferation and scarring will occur.

The gross manifestations of the acute vascular response (the *triple response*) may be evoked by scratching the skin. The triple response proceeds as follows:

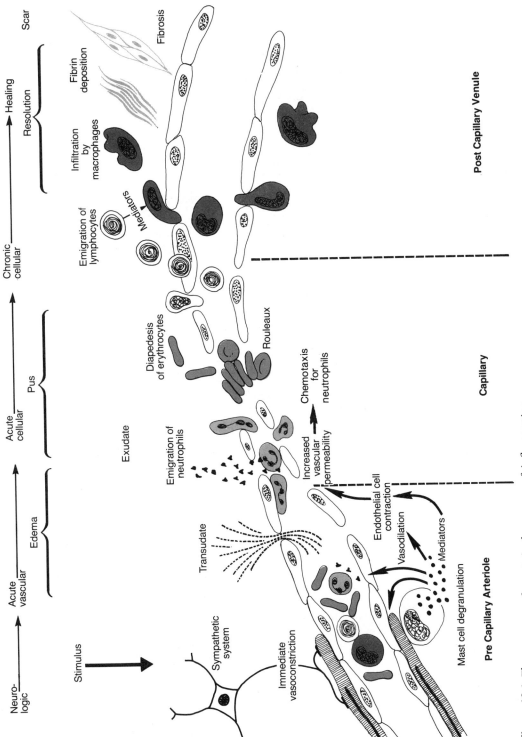

Figure 12-1. The sequence of events in the process of inflammation.

1. 3–50 seconds: thin red line (vasodilation of capillaries)
2. 30–60 seconds: flush (vasodilation of arterioles)
3. 1–5 minutes: wheal (increased vascular permeability, edema)

The term *wheal* refers to pale, soft, swollen areas on the skin caused by leakage of fluid from capillaries. Some individuals react to skin stroking by marked wheal formation, such that words may actually be written on the skin by whealing (dermatographism).

The ancient Greeks, who recognized the four classic cardinal signs of inflammation (Fig. 12-2), considered inflammation

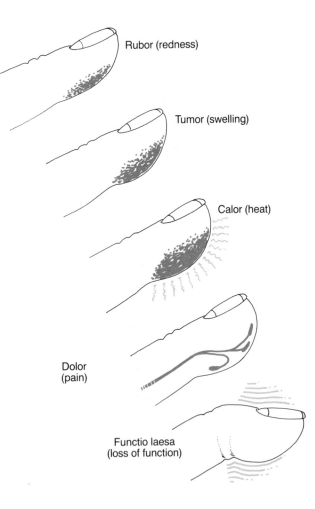

Figure 12-2. The five cardinal signs of inflammation.

Rubor (redness)

Tumor (swelling)

Calor (heat)

Dolor (pain)

Functio laesa (loss of function)

to be a disease. Later the fifth sign, loss of function, was added by the great German pathologist Rudolf Virchow. Increased blood flow is manifested grossly by redness (*rubor*) and increased local temperature (*calor*). The increased blood flow delivers serum factors and blood cells to the tissue. The increase in vascular permeability permits exudation of plasma from the capillaries or postcapillary venules into the tissue, causing edema and increase in tissue mass (*tumor*). Tissue swelling and chemical mediators act on nerve endings to produce pain (*dolor*). Swelling and pain lead to loss of function (*functio laesa*).

Chemical mediators are signaling molecules that act on smooth muscle cells, endothelial cells, or white blood cells to induce, maintain, or limit inflammation. The agents that act first in the sequence affect smooth muscle cells of precapillary arterioles to produce dilation and increased blood flow. Increased vascular permeability occurs in two phases: early (within minutes) and late (6 – 12 hours). The early phase is mediated by histamine and serotonin, whereas several other mediators contribute to the later phase. Late-phase mediators are derived from a variety of sources including arachidonic acid metabolites, breakdown products of the coagulation system (fibrin split products), peptides formed from blood or tissue proteins (bradykinin), and activated complement components, as well as factors released from bacteria, necrotic tissue, neutrophils (inflammatory peptides), lymphocytes (lymphokines), and monocytes (monokines). The generation of these factors and their effects will be presented in more detail below.

Histologically, the essential feature of acute inflammation is infiltration of the tissue by neutrophils. Neutrophils are believed to pass through gaps in capillary endothelium and are attracted to sites of inflammation by chemotactic factors. Tissue necrosis is caused by release of proteolytic enzymes into the tissue from the lysosomes of the neutrophils. Neutrophilic infiltrate is followed by infiltration by mononuclear (round) cells (i.e., lymphocytes and macrophages). Macrophages, although they move less rapidly than neutrophils, are also attracted by chemotactic mediators and are activated to phagocytose and digest necrotic tissue or inflammatory products, including effete neutrophils that have become damaged in the inflammatory process. If tissue damage is not extensive, the inflammation will be limited by controlling factors such as enzyme inhibitors and oxygen scavengers. Macrophages will then clear the inflamed area, and the tissue will return to normal (*resolution*). However, if tissue damage is extensive or the initiating stimulus persists, then mediators of chronic inflammation are activated. If tissue damage is significant or the organ has limited ability to regenerate, resolution cannot be achieved and the damaged tissue will be replaced by fibroblastic proliferation and collagen deposition (*fibrous scar*). If extensive, fibrous scarring may lead to a compromise in normal function. The fibrotic process may include proliferation of both fibroblasts and endothelial cells (capillaries), which forms granulation tissue, so named because grossly it has the appearance of small granules like sand. If the inflamed tissue contains material that is difficult for macrophages to digest (such as silica or complex lipids), a particular form of chronic inflammation, *granulomatous* (like granulation tissue), takes place (see Chapter 19). The process of inflammation is modified by infection, immune products, tissue death (necrosis), and foreign bodies. Examples of the lesions of different stages of inflammation in different tissue are given later in this chapter.

Some terms used to describe various manifestations of the inflammatory process are listed in Table 12-2. The manifesta-

Table 12-2. Definitions of Terms Used to Describe Manifestations of Inflammation

---

Hyperemia: increased blood in tissue, caused by vasodilation.

Edema: excess fluid in tissues, caused by increased vascular permeability.

Transudate: physiologic, low-protein-concentration edema fluid, containing albumin; specific gravity less than 1.012; cleared by lymphatics.

Exudate: pathologic, high-protein edema fluid containing immunoglobulins and macroglobulin; specific gravity greater than 1.02.

Pus: exudate rich in white cells and necrotic debris, caused by emigration of neutrophils and release of enzymes.

Fibrinoid necrosis: enzymatic digestion of tissue resulting in an appearance like fibrin; example: fibrinoid necrosis of vessels in vasculitis.

TYPES OF EXUDATE

Serous: thin fluid (like transudate).

Fibrinous: stringy, containing fibrin.

Suppurative: pus (neutrophils and necrotic debris).

Hemorrhagic: bloody (vascular necrosis).

Fibrous: healed exudate, scar, adhesions.

TYPES OF LESIONS

Ulcer: surface erosion.

Abscess: cavity filled with pus.

Cellulitis: diffuse inflammatory infiltrate in tissue.

Pseudomembrane: fibrinous or necrotic layer on epithelial surface.

Catarrhal: excess mucus production.

---

tions of inflammation depend upon the severity and location of the reaction as well as the nature of the inflammatory stimulus. Systemic effects of inflammation include fever and increased numbers of white blood cells (leukocytosis). Fever is caused by increase in the metabolic rate of muscular tissue secondary to effects of *pyrogens* released from damaged tissue that act on the hypothalamus. Leukocytosis is caused by increased production and release of white cells from the bone marrow.

The Cells of Acute Inflammation

The cellular players in the process of acute inflammation include mast cells, neutrophils, platelets and eosinophils, which act in sequence. They are activated by a variety of chemical processes and, in turn, produce and release a number of chemical mediators. Most of the manifestations of the acute vascular response are the result of chemical mediators released from mast cells.

Mast Cells

Mast cells contain granules with a variety of biologically active agents (Table 12-3), which, when released extracellularly (de-

Table 12-3. Mast Cell Mediators

Mediator	Structure/Chemistry	Source	Effects
Histamine	β-Imidazolylethylamine	Mast cells, basophils	Vasodilation; increase vascular permeability (venules), mucus production
Serotonin	5-Hydroxytryptamine	Mast cells (rodent), platelets, cells of enterochromaffin system	Vasodilation; increase vascular permeability (venules)
Neutrophil chemotactic factor	MW > 750,000	Mast cells	Chemotaxis of neutrophils
Eosinophil chemotactic factor A	Tetrapeptide	Mast cells	Chemotaxis of eosinophils
Vasoactive intestinal peptide	28-Amino-acid peptide	Mast cells, neutrophils, cutaneous nerves	Vasodilation; potentiate edema produced by bradykinin and C5a des-Arg
Thromboxane A_2		Arachidonic acid (cyclooxygenase pathway)	Vasoconstriction, bronchoconstriction, platelet aggregation
Prostaglandin E_2 (or D_2)		Arachidonic acid (cyclooxygenase pathway)	Vasodilation; potentiate permeability effects of histamine and bradykinin; increase permeability when acting with leukotactic agent; potentiate leukotriene effect; hyperalgesia
Leukotriene B_4		Arachidonic acid (lipoxygenase pathway)	Chemotaxis of neutrophils; increase vascular permeability in the presence of PGE_2
Leukotriene D_4		Arachidonic acid (lipoxygenase pathway)	Increase vascular permeability
Platelet-activating factor	Acetylated glycerol ether phosphocholine	Basophils, neutrophils, monocytes, macrophages	Release of mediators from platelets, neutrophil aggregation, neutrophil secretion, superoxide production by neutrophils; increase vascular permeability

granulation), cause contraction of endothelial cells, thus open-ing up vessel walls to permit egress of antibodies, complement, or inflammatory cells into tissue spaces. Mast cells were ob-served by early histologists to be filled with cellular material (the granules). The term *mast cell* was applied to indicate that these cells appeared to be stuffed as if by overeating (German *Mast*, "forced fattening"). The cellular granules contain biolog-ically active agents produced by the mast cell, which are re-leased upon activation of the cells. Mast cells are usually located adjacent to small arterioles and in submucosal tissues where released vasoactive mediators would be expected to be most active in causing relaxation of smooth muscle cells and dilatation of arterioles. In classic anaphylactic reactions, mast cells are degranulated by reaction of antigen with IgE antibody that adheres to the surface of mast cells because of a specific configuration of the Fc part of the antibody molecules. Mast cells have receptors for IgE that are composed of two chains, α and β. The α chain (MW 50,000) extends from the cell surface and is believed to combine with IgE. Upon reaction of antigen with IgE antibody on the surface of the mast cells, a complex cellular activation mechanism causes the mast cells to release the pharmacologically active agents contained in cytoplasmic granules (Fig. 12-3).

Figure 12-3. Postulated steps in mast cell degranula-tion. (1) Binding of antigen (allergen), crosslinking two IgE molecules on mast cell surface. (2) Dimerization of IgE receptors: α, MW 50,000, attached to IgE; β, MW 30,000. (3) Activation of phospholipase C; action of phospholipase C on membrane phosphatidylino-sitol-4,5-biphosphate to form inositoltriphosphate and diacylglycerol. (4) Activation of protein kinase C. (5) Mobilization of intracellular Ca^{++}. (7) Enlargement of granules by protein kinases. (8) Activation of phospholi-pase A_2 with formation of lysolecithin and arachidonic acid. (9) Lysolecithin acts as "fusogen" causing granule to fuse with membrane and release contents. (10) Activation of granules de-pendent on levels of cAMP and cGMP, which in turn are regulated by α and β ad-renergic receptors. (11) Release of histamine and membrane phospholipids (arachidonic acid).

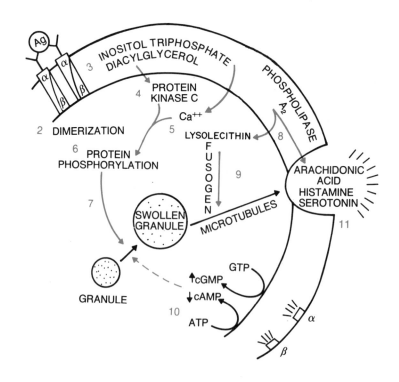

The pharmacologically active agents of mast cells are the chemical mediators of atopic or anaphylactic hypersensitivity. The effects of their release are described in more detail in Chapter 17. The major effects of mast cell mediators are listed in Figure 12-4. The major early events in inflammation—

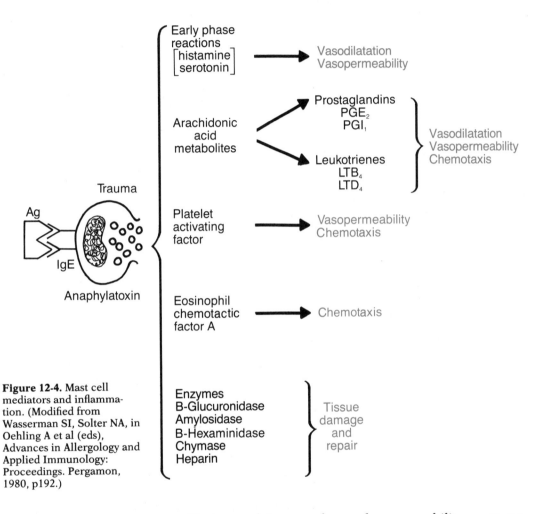

Figure 12-4. Mast cell mediators and inflammation. (Modified from Wasserman SI, Solter NA, in Oehling A et al (eds), Advances in Allergology and Applied Immunology: Proceedings. Pergamon, 1980, p192.)

vasodilation and increased vascular permeability—are mediated by the immediate degranulation of mast cells and the release of histamine and serotonin. Later vascular events, occurring 6–12 hours after initiation of inflammation, are mediated by prostaglandins and leukotrienes produced as a result of metabolism of phospholipids from membrane-like material released from mast cell granules (see below). Chemotaxis of neutrophils and eosinophils is affected by leukotrienes as well as by platelet-activating factor. Enzymes activated by solubilization of granular material may also contribute to tissue damage and/or repair.

Histamine

Histamine is the major preformed mast cell mediator. Injection of histamine into the skin produces the typical wheal and flare reaction of the immediate acute vascular response. Histamine causes endothelial cell contraction and vasodilation leading to edema (wheal) and redness (flare). Histamine is formed from the amino acid L-histidine by the action of the enzyme L-histidine decarboxylase, found in the cytoplasm of mast cells and basophils. The biologic effects of histamine are mediated by two distinct sets of receptors, H_1 and H_2 (Table 12-4). Effects

Table 12-4. H_1- and H_2-Dependent Actions of Histamine

H_1 Receptor–Mediated	H_2 Receptor–Mediated	H_1 and H_2
Increased cGMP	Increased cAMP	Vasodilation (hypotension)
Smooth-muscle constriction (bronchi)	Smooth muscle dilation (vascular)	Flush
Increased vascular permeability	Gastric-acid secretion	Headache
Pruritus	Mucous secretion	
Prostaglandin generation	Inhibition of basophil histamine release	
	Inhibition of lymphokine release	
	Inhibition of neutrophil enzyme release	
	Inhibition of eosinophil migration	
	Inhibition of T-lymphocyte–mediated cytotoxicity	
Antagonized by "classical" antihistamines	Antagonized by cimetidine	

Modified from Metcalfe DD, Kaliner M: Mast cells and basophils, in Oppenheim JJ, Rosenstreich DL, Potter M (eds), Cellular Functions in Immunity and Inflammation. New York, Elsevier, 1981.

mediated through H_1 receptors are the classic acute vascular inflammatory events. Anti-inflammatory effects, as well as vasodilation, are mediated through H_2 receptors. Thus, histamine may activate acute vascular effects, yet inhibit acute cellular inflammation. Acute cellular inflammation is mediated by products of arachidonic acid.

Arachidonic Acid Metabolites

Major mediators of inflammation are the metabolic derivatives of arachidonic acid. Arachidonic acid is derived from membrane phospholipids that are broken down by phospholipases. In the human, membrane phospholipids are released from mast cells during the early phase of acute inflammation but may also be derived from other cell membranes. The metabolism of arachidonic acid is believed to occur mainly in macrophages, but metabolites may also be synthesized by most, if not all, cells that take part in an inflammatory response, including the mast cell. Metabolism of arachidonic acid occurs via two major pathways: the cyclooxygenase pathway and the lipoxygenase pathway (Fig. 12-5). The cyclooxygenase pathway gives rise to prostaglandins; the lipoxygenase pathway to leukotrienes.

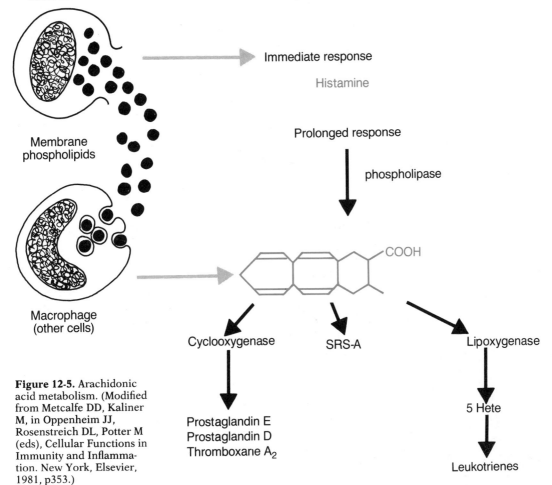

Mast cell

Membrane
phospholipids

Macrophage
(other cells)

Immediate response

Histamine

Prolonged response

phospholipase

COOH

Cyclooxygenase   SRS-A   Lipoxygenase

Prostaglandin E
Prostaglandin D
Thromboxane A$_2$

5 Hete

Leukotrienes

Figure 12-5. Arachidonic acid metabolism. (Modified from Metcalfe DD, Kaliner M, in Oppenheim JJ, Rosenstreich DL, Potter M (eds), Cellular Functions in Immunity and Inflammation. New York, Elsevier, 1981, p353.)

Prostaglandins. The prostaglandins are derived by oxidation of prostanoic acid (cyclooxygenation).

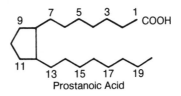

Prostanoic Acid

The numerical subscript in each prostaglandin (PG) refers to the number of unsaturated bonds. PGE$_1$ has one unsaturated bond at the 13–14 position; PGE$_2$ has two unsaturated bonds, at the 5–6 and at the 13–14 positions. The letter designations refer to the position of bonds in the ring structure:

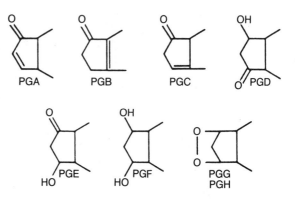

Prostaglandins were originally identified in seminal fluid and were believed to be produced by the prostate. It is now known that other tissue cells, particularly mast cells, are the major source of prostaglandins. Prostaglandins are prominent in anaphylactic reactions (see Chapter 18). The most active components are PGE_2 and PGD_2, which produce vasodilation, increase vascular permeability, and cause hyperalgesia (increased sensitivity to pain). The primary source for thromboxane A_2 is the platelet. Thromboxane A_2 is also produced by the cyclooxygenase pathway and is active in vasoconstriction, bronchoconstriction, and platelet aggregation. These metabolites are rapidly metabolized to inactive forms (PGE_1, PGD_1, and thromboxane B_2) by further oxygenation. The nonsteroidal anti-inflammatory drugs (NSAID), such as aspirin, act to inhibit cyclooxygenase and block formation of these inflammatory mediators.

Leukotrienes. The products of the lipoxygenase pathway are called leukotrienes. They are generated by leukocytes and mast cells. Again the subscript denotes the number of double bonds. The activity of leukotrienes C_4, D_4, and E_4 is believed to be responsible for a factor previously called *slow reacting substance of anaphylaxis* (SRS-A); that of leukotriene B_4 is chemotactic for eosinophils (*eosinophilic chemotactic factor of anaphylaxis*, ECFA) and neutrophils. Although prostaglandins are responsible for some of the late vascular effects of anaphylaxis, they may also modulate anaphylaxis by increasing cyclic nucleotide levels of mast cells and inhibiting histamine release.

Polymorphonuclear Neutrophils

Neutrophilic polymorphonuclear leukocytes are the major cellular component of the acute inflammatory reaction. Neutrophils are characterized by numerous cytoplasmic granules that contain highly destructive hydrolytic enzymes (Table 12-5). At

Table 12-5. Antimicrobial Systems in Neutrophils

Oxygen Dependent	Oxygen Independent
Myeloperoxidase	Lysozyme
Superoxide anion (O_2^-)	Lactoferrin
Hydroxyl radical (OH^-)	Cationic proteins
Singlet oxygen ($^1O_2$)	Neutral proteases
Hydrogen peroxide	Acid hydrolases

least three cytoplasmic granules are identifiable: specific granules (lactoferrin, etc.), azurophilic granules (lysosomes containing acid hydrolases and other enzymes), and a third granule compartment containing gelatinase. Neutrophils may be attracted to sites of inflammation by a number of chemotactic factors (Table 12-6). Neutrophils have cell surface receptors for

Table 12-6. Chemotactic Factors for Neutrophils

Complement
  C_5a
  C_5a des-Arg
Kallikrein
Fibrinopeptide B
f-Met tripeptides
Collagen peptides
Transfer factor (lymphokine)
Neutrophil chemotactic factors of:
  Fibroblasts
  Macrophages (interleukin 1)
  Lymphocytes
Platelet-activating factor
Leukotriene B_4

some of these factors, such as activated fragments of complement (see below) and formylmethionyl tripeptides. Acute inflammatory reactions need not be initiated by immune mechanisms and are frequently associated with bacterial infections (such as staphylococcal and streptococcal infections) or traumatic tissue injury. In these situations neutrophils are attracted into sites of inflammation by chemotactic factors released by the infecting organism (f-Met peptides) or by products of damaged tissue, such as fibronectin, fibrin or collagen degradation products, or factors produced by other inflammatory cells. In immune complex reactions, neutrophils are attracted by formation of activated complement components (see below) following antibody–antigen reaction in tissues. Upon attraction to sites of inflammation, neutrophils attempt to engulf and digest complexes consisting of bacteria coated with antibody and complement. However, phagocytosis by neutrophils is usually accompanied by release of the lysosomal enzymes from these cells into the tissue spaces, particularly if the antigen is difficult for the polymorphonuclear neutrophil to ingest. The lysosomal acid hydrolases cause local tissue digestion at the site of the reactions. The characteristic lesion is fibrinoid necrosis —areas of acellular digested tissue that look like fibrin but lack any fibrillar appearance. Reactive oxygen metabolites (Table 12-5), primarily involved in bacterial killing, may also damage infiltrating neutrophils and adjacent tissues, resulting in the formation of pus.

Complement

The complement system consists of a set of up to 20 serum proteins that form a controlled sequence for production of activated molecules (Table 12-7). The complete activation sequence occurs on the surface of cells and involves a series of molecular interactions during which fragments as well as new multimolecular complexes with biologic activity are formed. Activation of the complement system via the classic sequence is initiated by antibody–antigen reactions, whereas an alternate pathway may be activated by certain bacterial products. Activated components mediate a variety of tissue responses, including cell lysis, chemotaxis of neutrophils and monocytes, enhancement of phagocytosis, and increased vascular permeability. These activated components also interact with other accessory systems, including the coagulation and fibrinolytic systems, to amplify and/or limit the acute inflammatory reaction. The major functions of activated complement fragments are to open blood vessels and to attract and activate polymorphonuclear neutrophils.

Classical Pathway

A simplified diagrammatic representation of the *classical pathway* for complement activation is shown in Figure 12-6, and the sequence described in detail in Table 12-8. The first component of complement, C1, has the capacity to bind and be activated by antibody molecules that have been altered in their Fc region by reaction with antigen. The Ig classes that are active in fixing complement are IgG and IgM. One molecule of IgM is capable of activating C1, whereas two molecules of IgG reacting close together are required. Activation of C1 may take place in a fluid phase, as when antibody reacts with soluble antigens in the bloodstream; or activation may occur on the surface of cells, as is the case when antierythrocyte antibody reacts with a red cell. In order for two IgG molecules to achieve close enough apposition on a red cell to activate C1, approximately 600 to 1000 molecules must bind to the cell, whereas only one IgM molecule is required.

The components of the classical pathway leading to cell lysis are C1 through C9. In the activation sequence occurring at the cell surface, C1 functions as a recognition unit, C2–C4 as an activation unit, and C5–C9 as a membrane attack unit. When C1 attaches to antibody, it becomes activated as an enzyme (C1 esterase), which cleaves C4 and C2 into two fragments each

Table 12-7. Complement Components

Component	Function	Molecular Weight	Number of Polypeptide Chains	Serum Concentration (μg/ml)	Site of Synthesis
CLASSICAL PATHWAY					
C1q	Recognition	400,000	18	200	Small intestine epithelium
C1r	Enzyme	160,000	2	—	Small intestine epithelium
C1s	Enzyme	80,000	1	120	Small intestine epithelium
C2	Activation	115,000	1	30	Macrophages
C3	Activation	180,000	2	1,200	Macrophages
C4	Activation	210,000	3	400	Liver epithelium
C5	Attack	180,000	2	75	Macrophages
C6	Attack	128,000	1	60	Liver
C7	Attack	150,000	3	60	—
C8	Attack	150,000	3	15	—
C9	Attack	75,000	1	Trace	Liver
ALTERNATE PATHWAY					
Properdin		190,000	4	20	Macrophages
Factor B	C3 Activator	100,000	1	225	Macrophages
Factor D	C3 Coactivator	25,000	4	Trace	Macrophages
C3	Activation	210,000	3	400	Macrophages

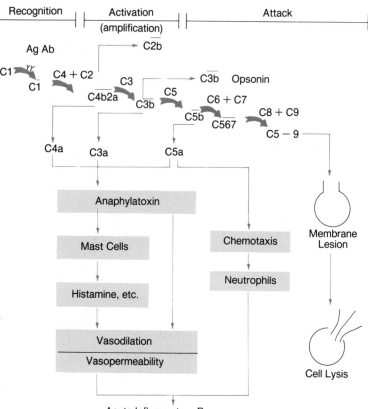

Figure 12-6. Classical pathway of complement activation. Following reaction of antibody with antigen, a cascade reaction of complement components is activated. C1 functions as a recognition unit for the altered Fc of two IgG or one IgM molecule(s); C2 and C4, as an activation unit leading to cleavage of C3. C3 fragments have a number of biological activities: C3a anaphylatoxin, and C3b is recognized by receptors on macrophages (opsonin). C3b also joins with fragments of C4 and C2 to form C3 convertase, which cleaves C5. C5 then reacts with C6 through C9 to form a membrane attack unit that produces a lesion in cell membranes, through which intracellular components may escape (lysis).

(C4a and C4b, C2a and C2b). One of the fragments of C4 (C4b) and one of the C2 fragments (C2a) join together and bind to new sites on the cell surface. Other fragments, C4a and C2b, are released into the fluid phase. C4a has weak anaphylatoxic activity, whereas C2b is converted by plasmin into a C2b kinin-like molecule believed to be responsible for the lesions of hereditary angioedema (see below). The complex of C4b2a forms an enzyme, C3 convertase, which binds and cleaves C3 into C3a and C3b. C3b binds to new sites on the cell surface. As activated C1 can cleave many molecules of C4 and C2 and the C4b2a complex can cleave many molecules of C3, these serve as amplification steps. C3a is released into the fluid phase, where it functions as anaphylatoxin. Phagocytic cells have receptors for C3b; C3b serves as an opsonin (enhances phagocytosis). In addition C3b forms a trimolecular complex with C4b2a (C4b2a3b) that is able to cleave C5 into C5a and C5b (C5 convertase). C5a is released into the fluid phase and C5b binds to the cell surface. C5a is a polypeptide of MW 15,000 with the most potent chemotactic and anaphylatoxic activity of any chemical mediator. C4a and C3a do not have chemotactic activity. In tissues C5a is rapidly broken down to C5a des-Arg by

Table 12-8. Sequence and Mechanism of Immune Hemolysis

Reaction	Biochemical Event
$E + A \rightarrow EA$	Reaction of erythrocyte and antierythrocyte antibody.
$EA + C1 \rightarrow EAC1q^*$	C1q attaches to antibody at a site on Fc portion of Ig antibody bound to the cell.
$C1r \rightarrow \overline{C1r}$	Bound C1q* converts C1r to active form by cleavage of C1r.
$C1s \rightarrow \overline{C1s}$	$\overline{C1r}$ activates C1s by cleavage of C1s.
$C4 \rightarrow \overline{C4a} + C4b^*$ $C2 \rightarrow C2a^* + \overline{C2b}$	$\overline{C1s}$ cleaves C4 into $\overline{C4a}$ and C4b* and C2 into C2a* and $\overline{C2b}$; plasmin acts on C_2b to produce C_2b kinin; $\overline{C4a}$ has weak anaphylatoxin activity.
$C4b^* + C2a^* \rightarrow \overline{C4b2a}$	C4b* and C2a* combine to form C3 convertase.
$C3 \rightarrow \overline{C3a} + C3b^*$	$\overline{C4b2a}$ cleaves C3 into $\overline{C3a}$ and C3b*; $\overline{C3a}$ (anaphylatoxin) causes smooth muscle contraction and degranulation of mast cells.
$C3b^* + C4b2a \rightarrow \overline{C4b2a3b}$	C3b* binds to activated bimolecular complex of $\overline{C4b2a}$ to form a trimolecular complex, C5 convertase, that is a specific enzyme for C5. Macrophages have receptors for C3b, so that C3b acts as opsonin.
$C5 \rightarrow \overline{C5a} + C5b^*$	C5 is cleaved into $\overline{C5a}$ and C5b* by C5 convertase; $\overline{C5a}$ has anaphylactic and strong chemotactic activity for polymorphonuclear neutrophils.
$\overline{C5b}^* + C6789 \rightarrow \overline{C5b.9}$	C5b* reacts with other complement components to produce a macromolecular complex that has the ability to alter cell membrane permeability. $\overline{C8}$ is most likely the active component, with $\overline{C9}$ increasing efficiency of $\overline{C8}$ and producing maximal cell lysis.

E, erythrocyte; A, antibody to erythrocyte.
$\overline{C1}$, $\overline{C4}$, etc.: a line above the C number indicates the activated form of the component.
C4a, C4b, etc.: the lower-case letters indicate cleavage products of the parent complement molecule.
C4b*, C2a*: the asterisk indicates a cleavage product that contains an active binding site for other complement components.

cleavage of the amino-terminal arginine. C5 des-Arg is inactive as anaphylatoxin but retains potent chemotactic activity for neutrophils in the presence of whole serum. Anaphylatoxins C5a and C3a (and, weakly, C4a) produce direct contraction of smooth muscle. Addition of these complement fragments will produce contraction of intestine, uterine, tracheal, or other smooth muscle in vitro (Schultz–Dale test), followed by a refractory period termed *tachyphylaxis* that is specific for C3a or C5a (i.e., C3a desensitizes the muscle to further stimulation by C3a but not by C5a). This suggests separate, distinct receptors for C3a and C5a on smooth muscle. In addition, anaphylactic complement fragments induce the release of histamine from mast cells via receptors for C3a and C5a on the mast cell. C5a induces acute inflammation if activated in tissue by soluble antibody–antigen complexes (toxic complex reactions). C5b binds to the cell surface, where it reacts with the remaining complement components, C6–C9, to produce a multimolecular complex that is capable of inserting itself into the cell membrane, forming a channel that permits release of the cytoplasm (lysis).

Alternate Pathway

The complement cascade may be activated by another set of proteins similar to C4, C2, C1, and C3; this is called the *alternate pathway*. A more detailed schematic representation of both the classical and alternate pathways of complement activation is shown in Figure 12-7. The alternate pathway is activated by

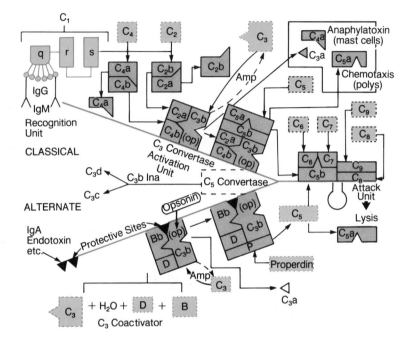

Figure 12-7. Details of the classical and alternate pathways of complement activation. For description, see text.

materials such as bacterial lipopolysaccharide (endotoxin), yeasts (zymosan), or IgA antibody. Three factors—initiating factor, factor B, and factor D—interact in a manner similar to that of the first three complement components of the classical pathway, producing a complex of activated B (Bb) and D that functions as a C3 convertase. A trimolecular complex of Bb, D, and C3b is then formed that is stabilized by the addition of another component, properdin. This complex functions as C5 convertase in activation of C5 and the remaining components of the attack unit.

Regulation and Amplification Mechanisms in the Complement System

Regulation of the complement system is accomplished by a set of inactivators. Complement activation occurs at low levels normally at all times as well as at high levels during inflammation. If left uncontrolled, the cascade of activation could result in serious damage to normal tissue. A number of inactivators of complement have been identified, which act on different stages of complement activation (Table 12-9). Included are C1q inhibitor, C1 esterase inhibitor, the C3 esterase inhibitor system, a membrane activation complex (MAC) inhibitor that competes with cell membrane sites for C5–9, and serum carboxypepti-

Table 12-9. Regulatory Components of the Complement System

C1q inhibitor	Inactivates C1q binding
C1 esterase inhibitor	Inactivates esterase activity
C3 convertase inhibitor system	Inactivates C3 convertase
MAC inhibitor	Competes with cell surface for C5–9
Serum carboxypeptidase N	Inactivates anaphylatoxin

dase N, which inactivates anaphylatoxin (C5a). A deficiency of the C1 esterase inhibitor is found in hereditary angioedema (see also Chapter 18). These patients exhibit massive acute transient swelling of areas of the skin, the bronchi, or the gastrointestinal tract, associated with depressed serum levels of C4 and C2 because of an inability to inactivate C1 esterase. This reaction results in the continued formation of C4 and C2 fragments, particularly C2b; C2b is converted by plasmin to a molecule with kinin-like activity. The C2b–kinin causes contraction of endothelial cells and edema. The reaction continues for approximately 24 hours, which is essentially the biological life of C1 esterase in the absence of C1 esterase inhibitor.

The C3 esterase inhibitor system consists of at least six different components (Table 12-10). The major inactivator is

Table 12-10. Regulatory Proteins of Complement C3 Convertase

Regulator	Properties	Function	Deficiency State
CR1 (C3b/C4b receptor)	MW 160,000–250,000 Cell membrane of neutrophils, macrophages, and erythrocytes	Binds C3b and C4b; promotes phagocytosis and degranulation; cofactor for C3b inactivator; increases decay of C4b2a and C3bBb (C3 convertases)	Hemolytic anemias, chronic granulomatous disease
Factor H	MW 150,000–160,000 Serum glycoprotein	Cofactor for C3b INH; binds C3b, increases decay of C3bBb in the alternative pathway	Low C3, recurrent infections, C3 detectable on erythrocytes
C4-binding protein	MW 540,000–590,000 Serum protein	Binds C4b; cofactor for C3b INH; increases decay of C4b2a	
Decay-activating factor (DAF)	MW 70,000 Cell membrane glycoprotein	Binds C3bBb or C4b2a; increases decay of C3 convertase of both classical and alternative pathway	Paroxysmal nocturnal hemoglobulinuria (lysis of RBC)
JP45-70	MW 45,000–70,000 Membrane	Binds C3b; inactivates C3 convertase (preferential for classical pathway)	
C3b inactivator (C3b INH)	Serine protease endopeptidase	Inactivates C3b by cleavage of α chain; requires cofactors	Low C3, recurrent infections, angioedema

C3b inactivator (C3b INH). C3b INH is an enzyme that cleaves the α chain of C3b to C3bi, then further cleaves C3bi to C3c and C3d. A number of cofactors are involved for the classical and alternate pathways of formation of C3 convertase. CR1, C4bp, and DAF displace C2a from C4b, whereas CR1, factor H, and DAF displace Bb from C3b. This displacement results in decay of C3 convertase and permits cleavage of the C3b by C3b INH. CR1, C4bp, and factor H are closely linked genetically, but are not linked to the MHC complex. Two other complement receptors are CR2 and CR3. CR2 is the binding site for C3d on B cells. The function of this receptor is not known, but it also functions as the binding site for Epstein–Barr virus on B cells. CR3 is a receptor for C3bi on phagocytic cells. Individuals with decreased CR3 receptors have defects in neutrophil functions and increased bacterial infections.

Activation of complement components is an essential feature of cytotoxic and immune complex reactions and may play a role in initiating some delayed cellular reactions, as well. The fixation of complement to a cell surface by action of antibody or via the alternate pathway is responsible for cytolytic reactions. Opsonization is activated because of coating by C3b (or C4b), and lysis of cells by formation of the membrane attack complex C5–9. The chemotactic effect of C5a attracts polymorphonuclear leukocytes and is largely responsible for the participation of these cells in immune complex reactions. The anaphylatoxic effects of C3a and C5a cause separation of endothelial cells. This serves to open vascular barriers to inflammatory cells so that neutrophils, lymphocytes, and macrophages may emigrate from the blood and induce inflammation in tissues.

Platelets

The role of platelets in inflammation is not well understood. Platelets contain heparin and serotonin, so that release of these mediators may contribute to the acute vascular phase of inflammation. Platelets also produce oxygen radicals, which may cause tissue damage. However, the major role of platelets is to block damaged vessel walls and prevent hemorrhage.

Platelets react at sites of vascular damage via a receptor for a triplet peptide, arginine-glycine-asparagine (Arg-Gly-Asp), present in fibrin, fibronectin, and vitronectin. At sites of vascular damage the extracellular matrix proteins fibronectin and vitronectin are exposed, and fibrin is formed through activation of the clotting system (see below). Platelets bind to these molecules, forming clumps of platelets that plug up leaks in the vascular system.

The Coagulation System

Any significant inflammation will result in activation of the coagulation system; several components of this system may serve as inflammatory mediators (Fig. 12-8). The coagulation

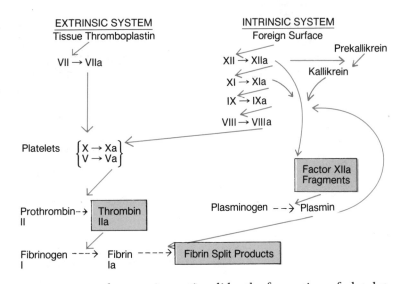

Figure 12-8. The coagulation system and inflammation.

system responds to various stimuli by the formation of platelet plugs and insoluble protein aggregates (fibrin) formed from soluble precursors. Fibrin forms clots that serve to stop bleeding following injury to blood vessels. The fibrinolytic system is activated soon after clot formation in order to limit the extent of fibrin deposition and to initiate dissolution of fibrin so that circulation can be restored to injured tissues. Fibrin may also act as a scaffold for the ingrowth of fibroblasts and capillaries to initiate repair. If fibrin formed intravascularly is not cleared, multiple areas of tissue necrosis (infarcts) may occur. This is known as disseminated intravascular coagulation (see Shwartzman Reaction below). The kinin system increases vascular permeability in areas of inflammation and may be activated by intermediate products of the coagulation cascade.

Roman numerals designate the major components of the coagulation system; a Roman numeral followed by the letter *a* indicates the active fragment of that factor. Coagulation products active in inflammation are fragments of Hageman factor (XIIa) and of thrombin (IIa), and fibrin split products. The coagulation system consists of three major parts: the extrinsic system, the intrinsic system, and the common thrombin–fibrin pathway. The extrinsic system is activated by the action of tissue thromboplastin on factor VII. The intrinsic system involves activation of a series of components beginning with factor XII (Hageman factor). The common pathway is the activation of factors X and V on platelets with the subsequent formation of thrombin and fibrin. Kallikrein, activated factor XI, and plasmin can all act to cleave activated factor XII to produce fragments that initiate fibrinolysis and kinin release, as well as generate a plasma factor that enhances vascular permeability. Activated factor XII converts prekallikrein to kallikrein (see The Kinin System below), so that activation of the intrinsic coagulation system also generates inflammatory mediators.

The Kinin System

Peptides that are active as mediators of inflammation may be generated from a number of cells and tissue products. Of these the most active is the kinin system. The components of this system are generated by the cleavage of plasma proteins into active peptides by proteolytic enzymes of the kallikrein system or trypsin. Kallikreins are small proteolytic enzymes found in tissues (particularly glandular organs) and in plasma, that act on large molecules such as kininogens to produce active peptides. Kallikreins are activated from prekallikreins by the action of activated factor XII (Hageman factor) of the intrinsic coagulation system.

Prekallikrein in plasma exists as a single polypeptide chain with an intrachain disulfide bond. There is also a tissue form, which is slightly different. Activated factor XII (XIIa) cleaves polypeptide chain to form an active two-chain disulfide-linked kallikrein molecule.

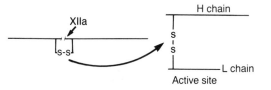

Kallikrein, factor XIIa, factor XI, and trypsin act on kininogens to produce biologically active fragments (see Fig. 12-9). The active peptides are kallidin and bradykinin. Kallidin is a

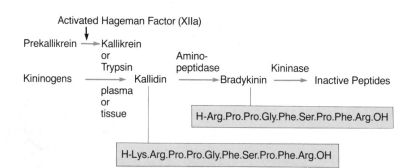

Figure 12-9. The kinin system.

decapeptide and bradykinin is a nanopeptide formed by cleavage of the amino-terminal lysine from kallidin. These mediators, particularly bradykinin, are highly active in stimulating vasodilation and increased vascular permeability but are rapidly catabolized by kininases into inactive peptides.

Eosinophils

Polymorphonuclear eosinophils are distinguished by the affinity of their cytoplasmic granules for acidic dyes such as eosin, resulting in an intense red staining. This staining is primarily due to the presence of a major basic protein (MBP) that binds acid dyes. Eosinophils are found predominantly in two types of inflammation: allergy and parasitic worm infections. Some chemotactic factors for eosinophils are listed in Table 12-11. These factors are derived from inflammatory cells, complement, or worm extracts. Eosinophils contain many of the same lysosomal enzymes as neutrophils, but appear to function quite differently by limiting or controlling the extent of inflamma-

Table 12-11. Chemotactic Factors for Eosinophils

Factor	Origin
Histamine	Mast cells
Eosinophilic chemotactic factor A	Mast cells
Neutrophil peptides	Neutrophils
Eosinophil stimulator promoter	Lymphocytes
C5a	Complement
Worm extracts	*Ascaris*

tion. Injection of eosinophils into sites of inflammation induced by histamine, serotonin, or bradykinin effectively diminishes the inflammation. Antibody–antigen complexes are phagocytosed and deactivated by eosinophils. The major basic protein appears to inhibit the action of heparin. These products are uniquely equipped to inactivate inflammatory mediators of mast cells (Table 12-12). In addition, eosinophils are cytotoxic to schistosome larvae through an antibody-dependent cell-mediated mechanism.

Table 12-12. Eosinophil Modulating Factors for Mast Cell Products

Mast Cell Product	Eosinophil Product
Histamine	Histaminase
SRS-A (leukotrienes)	Arylsulfatase
Heparin	MBP
(Chemotactic factors)	Esterase

Interrelationships of Inflammatory Cells and Systems in Acute Inflammation

A composite of inflammatory mechanisms and interrelationships is illustrated in Figure 12-10. The complement, kinin, coagulation, and mast cell systems as well as bacterial products contribute to vasodilation, increased vascular permeability, and chemotaxis of the primary cellular mediator of acute inflammation, the neutrophil. The neutrophil and its lysosomal enzymes are responsible for killing microorganisms, on the one hand, or causing tissue necrosis, on the other hand.

Products of the complement, kinin, coagulation, and mast cell systems produce vasoactive and chemotactic mediators of acute inflammation. The major mediators are highlighted by boxes in Figure 12-10.

The anaphylactic peptides C3a and C5a are the major in-

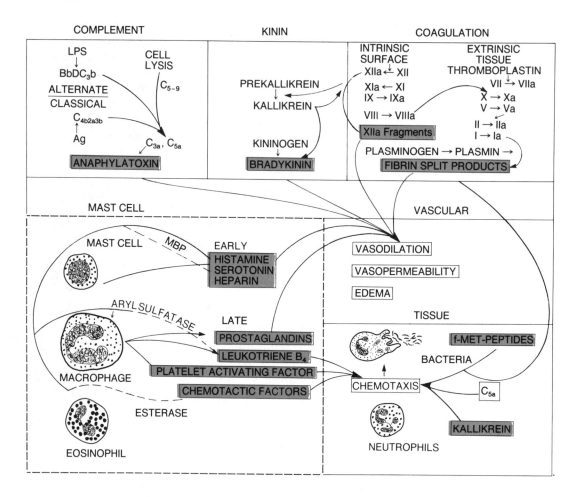

COMPLEMENT   KININ   COAGULATION

Figure 12-10. Interrelationships of inflammatory cells and systems in acute inflammation.

flammatory mediators derived from complement. Cells destroyed by the activation of complement may contribute indirectly through release of intracellular contents that may cause further tissue destruction (enzymes) or activate the extrinsic coagulation system. Activation of the intrinsic coagulation system produces a series of active fragments. Activated factor XII (Hageman factor) contributes to generation of three inflammatory mediators: bradykinin, Hageman factor fragments, and fibrin split products. Mast cells contribute directly by release of mediators such as histamine and serotonin and indirectly by providing arachidonic acid precursors for generation of leukotrienes, prostaglandins, and other factors. These systems act to increase blood flow and vascular permeability, leading to edema, in addition to attracting polymorphonuclear neutrophils and eosinophils to sites of inflammation. Neutrophils destroy infecting organisms by phagocytosis and digestion but also release lysosomal enzymes that may produce tissue damage. Eosinophils are believed to modulate inflammatory reactions by deactivating mast cell mediators.

Adult Respiratory Distress Syndrome

The adult respiratory distress syndrome (ARDS) is the result of diffuse damage to the alveolar epithelium and capillary endothelium of the lung (alveolar wall). This causes increased capillary permeability, interstitial and intraalveolar edema, fibrin exudation, and hyaline membrane formation. ARDS is an increasingly frequent cause of death in patients with diffuse respiratory infections, burns, oxygen toxicity, or narcotic overdose or who undergo open cardiac surgery.

The etiology of ARDS is not precisely defined but is thought to involve shock, oxygen toxicity, complement activation, bacterial products, or a combination of these. In oxygen toxicity associated with artificially assisted respiration, free radicals injure endothelium, causing increased permeability, and epithelium, inducing alveolar edema. Complement activation generates C5a, which induces leukocyte aggregation and activation in the lung. Alveolar cell injury causes loss of surfactant and collapse of air spaces. The role of the different acute inflammatory mechanisms in ARDS is not clear at this time, but most likely involves multiple mediators and may be potentiated by a failure of inactivation mechanisms.

The Cells of Chronic Inflammation

The cells of chronic inflammation are lymphocytes, macrophages, and plasma cells. To contrast these with the cells of acute inflammation (*polymorphonuclear* cells), the cells of chronic inflammation collectively are termed *mononuclear* cells. The function of lymphocytes and macrophages in chronic inflammation is presented here; plasma cells are also present in many forms of chronic inflammation and represent antibody producing cells resulting from stimulation of B cells by antigens.

Lymphocytes

Lymphocytes are prominent in chronic inflammation and are the immune-specific effector cells of delayed hypersensitivity. The immune-specific effects of lymphocytes are presented in detail in Chapter 19, and in vitro effects are discussed in Chapter 8. In immune-specific inflammation, lymphocytes are activated by specific reaction with antigen to release lymphokines responsible for delayed hypersensitivity. In nonimmune chronic inflammation, it is not clear what attracts lymphocytes to sites of inflammation. Lymphocytes do not respond chemotactically to factors that attract other white blood cells. Lymphocytes activated by antigen secrete a number of biologically active inflammatory mediators (Table 12-13). The major function of these mediators appears to be the attraction and activation of macrophages, but other functions such as increasing vascular permeability, killing target cells, and controlling lymphocyte proliferation have been attributed to lymphokines.

Table 12-13. Lymphokines

Factor	MW	Produced by	Effect
Migration inhibitory factor	15,000–70,000	Activated TD cells	Inhibits migration of macrophages
Macrophage activating factor	35,000–55,000	Activated TD cells	Increases lysosomes in macrophages; increases phagocytic activity
Macrophage chemotactic factor	12,500	1. Activated TD cells 2. Lysates of PMNs 3. Ag-Ab complexes (complement)	Attracts macrophages; gradient chemotaxis
Lymphotoxin	Multiple (10,000–200,000)	Activated TK or NK cells	Causes lysis of target cells
Lymphocyte stimulating factor	85,000	Activated TD cells	Stimulates proliferation of lymphocytes
Proliferation inhibitory factor	70,000	Activated TD cells	Inhibits proliferation of lymphocytes
Aggregation factor		Activated TD cells	Causes lymphocytes and macrophages to adhere together
Interferon	20,000–25,000	Activated TD cells	Inhibits growth of viruses; activates NK cells
Lymphocyte-permeability Factor	12,000	Lymph node cells	Increases vascular permeability
Transfer factor	10,000	Activated TD cells	Induces antigen-specific delayed hypersensitivity after passive transfer
Skin reactive factor	10,000	Activated TD cells	Induces inflammation upon injection into skin
Cytophilic antibody	160,000	Plasma cells	Binds to macrophages; stimulates phagocytosis of specific antigen
Leukocyte inhibitory factor	68,000	Activated T cells	Inhibits neutrophil mobility
Osteoclast activating factor	17,000	T and B cells	Stimulates osteoclasts to absorb bone

Figure 12-11. Phagocytosis: stages of intracellular digestion and different kinds of lysosomes. Foreign material is ingested into a phagosome. Phagosome fuses with primary lysosome (formed by Golgi body), which contains enzymes to digest ingested material. Resulting fusion vacuole is termed a secondary lysosome. When digestion is ended, some material may remain in residual body, or be eliminated from cell by cell defecation.

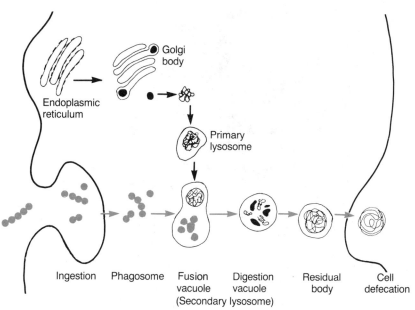

Macrophages

Macrophages (see Chapter 2) play an important role in chronic inflammation in general, and in delayed hypersensitivity reactions in particular. Macrophages usually infiltrate sites of inflammation several hours after polymorphonuclear cells. The main function of macrophages is to phagocytose damaged tissue components, microorganisms, or other cells (Fig. 12-11). In this manner, by the action of potent macrophage lysosomal enzymes, the macrophage clears the tissue of the products of inflammation and sets the stage for resolution of the inflammatory process. In delayed hypersensitivity reactions, macrophages are attracted and activated by *lymphokines* produced by reaction of antigen with specifically sensitized lymphocytes (T_D cells) (see Table 12-13). Delayed hypersensitivity reactions are presented in more detail in Chapter 19.

Phagocytosis

The stages of phagocytosis are illustrated in Figure 12-12. Coating of bacteria by complement or antibody enhances phagocytosis, although phagocytosis certainly occurs in the absence of antibody and complement. Cell surface aggregation of receptors precedes invagination of the cell membrane. Ingestion of material is accompanied by ion fluxes (positive ions entering cell) and superoxide formation. After formation of a phagocytic vacuole, fusion with enzyme containing lysosomes (phagolysosome) and digestion of phagocytosed material occurs.

Products of Macrophages

The products of macrophages that are important for consideration in inflammation are (1) the cytoplasmic constituents re-

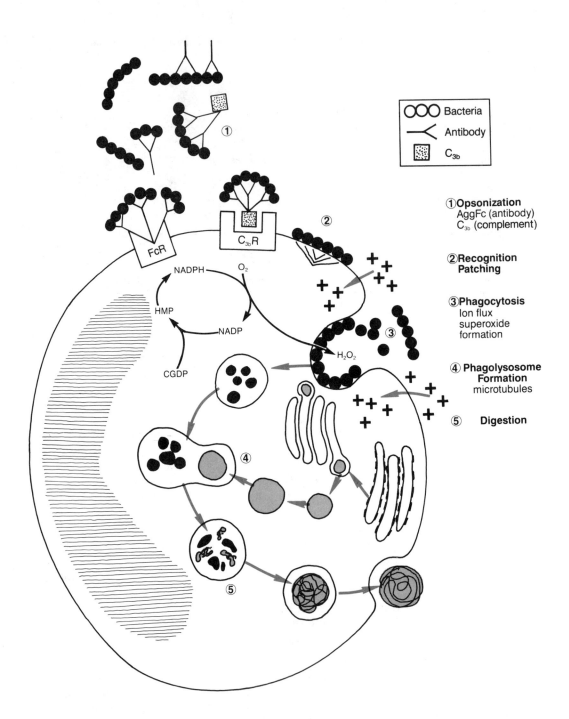

Bacteria

Antibody

C₃b

①Opsonization
AggFc (antibody)
C₃b (complement)

**②Recognition
Patching**

③Phagocytosis
Ion flux
superoxide
formation

**④ Phagolysosome
Formation**
microtubules

⑤ Digestion

Figure 12-12. Schematic drawing of steps in phagocytosis: (1) opsonization —aggregated Fc of antibody, formation of C3b; (2) recognition through receptors and patching; (3) ingestion—cation influx stimulates transduction of hexose monophosphate shunt and conversion of O₂ to H₂O₂; (4) fusion of lysosome and phagosome to form phagolysosome involving microtubules; (5) digestion of bacteria in phagolysosome.

Table 12-14. Cellular, Cell Surface, and Secreted Products of Macrophages

I. CELLULAR	
Peroxidase (RER)	Aminopeptidase
5' nucleotidase	Alkaline phosphatase

II. CELL SURFACE RECEPTORS	
Fc receptor I (IgG$_2$a)	High-density lipoprotein
Fc receptor II (IgG$_2$b)	Lactoferrin
IgM	Insulin
C3b	Fibrinogen
Lymphokines	Asialoglycoprotein
Protein aggregates (nonspecific)	f-Met-Leu-Phe
Fibronectin	

III. SECRETED BIOLOGICALLY ACTIVE PRODUCTS OF MACROPHAGES	
Hydrolytic enzymes	Cell stimulatory proteins
Lysosomal hydrolases	Colony-stimulating factor
Neutral proteases	Interleukin 1
Collagenase	Interferon
Plasminogen activator	Tumor necrosis factor
Elastase	Osteoclast activating factor
Lysozyme	Others
Arginase	Complement components
	(C2, C3, C4, C5, factor B)
	Oxygen intermediates
	α_2 macroglobulin
	Prostaglandins

sponsible for cellular metabolism and the degradation of phagocytosed material, (2) the cell surface receptors that contribute to phagocytosis, and (3) the secreted products that may cause tissue damage (Table 12-14). Depending on the nature of the inflammatory stimulus, the macrophage functions to clear necrotic tissue and to eradicate invading organisms, leading to resolution of the acute inflammatory response or, if the organism persists, to initiate a chronic or prolonged defensive reaction, granulomatous inflammation (discussed in Chapter 21). Macrophages may also release products to stimulate specific immune functions to aid in the defense against persistent microorganisms.

The importance of macrophages in inflammation was emphasized by Eli Metchnikoff almost 100 years ago. Macrophages are attracted to sites of inflammation by a number of chemotactic factors (see Table 12-15). The most potent are those derived from activated lymphocytes (lymphokines), but factors may also be derived from other cell types. In addition, macrophages are attracted by C5a and by f-Met peptides. Thus macrophages are attracted to sites of acute inflammation both by products of immune specific activation of lymphocytes and by products of nonimmune cells. In addition, lymphocytes activated by non-

Table 12-15. Growth-Stimulating, Chemotactic, and Activation Factors Acting on Macrophages

Substance	Physicochemical Characteristics (MW)	Source	Functional Properties
Macrophage colony-stimulating factor (CSF)	70,000	Fibroblasts	Macrophage colony formation from bone marrow cells. Also induces macrophage secretion
Macrophage growth factor (MGF)	Same as CSF	Fibroblasts, activated T lymphocytes	Acts on promonocytes
Factor inducing monocytosis (FIM)	18,000–23,000	Unknown	Increases macrophages in blood
Leukocyte-derived chemotactic factor (LDCF)	12,000	Activated T lymphocytes	Chemotactic for macrophages
Plasminogen activator inducer (IPA)		Activated T lymphocytes	Stimulates plasminogen activator secretion
Macrophage stimulatory protein (MSP)	100,000	Unknown	Increases spreading and phagocytosis
Factor Bb	65,000	Alternate complement pathway	Increases spreading and phagocytosis; inhibits migration
Macrophage activating factor (MAF)	50,000–60,000	Activated T lymphocytes	Increases macrophage tumoricidal and microbicidal function
Migration inhibitory factor (MIF)	25,000–60,000	Activated T lymphocytes	Inhibits migration
Soluble immune response suppressor (SIRS)	Similar to MIF	Activated T lymphocytes	
Interferon	Several MW species	Fibroblasts, activated T lymphocytes	Both Types I and II activate macrophages
Macrophage aggregating factor	>100,000	Activated T lymphocytes	Distinct from MIF. Causes clumping of macrophages in vivo and in vitro; may be fibronectin
C5a	15,000	Complement activation	Chemotactic
f-Met peptides	Tripeptides	Bacteria	Chemotactic
Phorbol esters		Tumor promotors	Activate macrophage secretion
LPS (endotoxin)		Bacteria	Activates macrophages

Modified from Rosenstreich DL: The macrophage, in Oppenheim JJ, Rosenstreich DL, Potter M (eds), Cellular Functions in Immunity and Inflammation. New York, Elsevier, 1981, p 140.

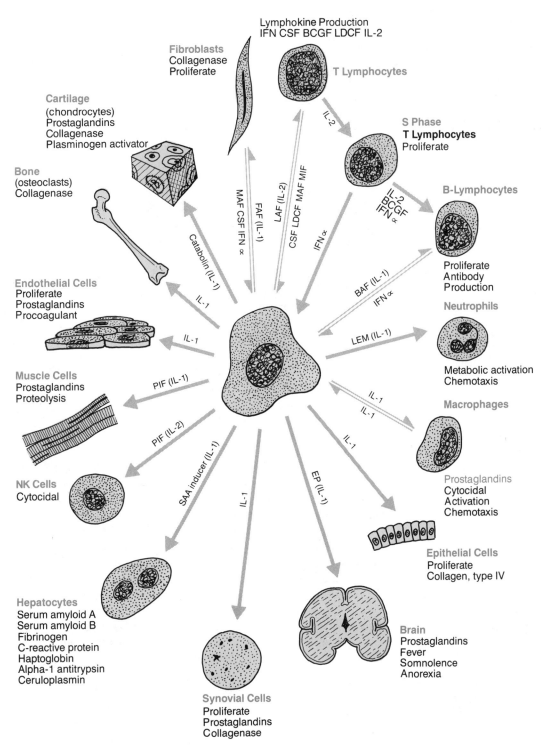

Figure 12-13. Effects of IL1 on target cells and tissues. The diagram shows bidirectional interactions between macrophages and lymphoid cells or fibroblasts mediated by IL1 and other cytokines, and the activities of target cells known to be augmented by IL1. IFN, interferon; CSF, colony stimulating factor; BCGF, B cell growth factor; LDCF, lymphocyte-derived chemotactic factor; SAA, serum amyloid A; PIF, proteolysis-inducing factor; EP, endogenous pyrogen.

immune specific mitogens, such as endotoxin (lipopolysaccharide, LPS) or other bacterial products, will produce lymphokines active on macrophages. Activated macrophages have an increased capacity for phagocytosis and an increased capacity to digest phagocytosed objects and, in addition, secrete factors (monokines) active in inflammation and immune reactions (see Table 12-14). Activated macrophages have changes in lysosomal enzyme content: a decrease in 5' nucleotidase and an increase in aminopeptidase and alkaline phosphatase as well as an increase in adenosine triphosphate and in production of superoxide anion and hydrogen peroxide. There is also an increase in activity of cell surface receptors on macrophages, in particular for Fc of immunoglobulin and for C3b.

Interleukin 1

A major macrophage mediator (monokine) is interleukin 1 (IL1). This mediator has a large number of biological effects (Fig. 12-13). Active investigation has led to the conclusion that the activities attributed to interleukin 1 may, in fact, be caused by more than one mediator.

Origin and Development of Macrophages

Macrophages are derived from bone marrow cells and are stimulated to mature to activated effector cells by a number of factors. These factors are listed in Table 12-15, and the stages of action of the factors given in Figure 12-14.

Phagocytic Deficiencies

In some cases, either because of the nature of the phagocytosed material or because of an insufficiency in lysosomal hydrolases, ingested particles or organisms are not killed and digested. Some organisms (e.g., *Histoplasma capsulatum*) have the ability to survive phagocytosis and reproduce within phagocytes. Infection with such an agent may result in the presence of large numbers of viable organisms in the cytoplasm of phagocytic cells. Some inorganic particles (e.g., silica) cannot be digested, remain in phagocytic cells, and eventually cause destruction of the phagocyte (phagocytic suicide), tissue damage and fibrosis, and increased susceptibility to certain infections. Certain human diseases are characterized by abnormalities in phagocytosis (phagocytic dysfunction). Such phagocytic deficiencies are usually associated with susceptibility to infections. These diseases are presented in more detail in Chapter 24.

Activated Macrophages

An acquired cellular resistance to microbial infection may be observed in an infected host whose mononuclear phagocytes have an increased capacity for destroying infected organisms (i.e., the host has activated macrophages). Macrophage activation may occur by increasing the number of lysosomes per cell, by increasing the amount of hydrolytic enzymes in each lysosome, or by increasing the number of phagocytes available. Once such an increased capacity has been established, it is

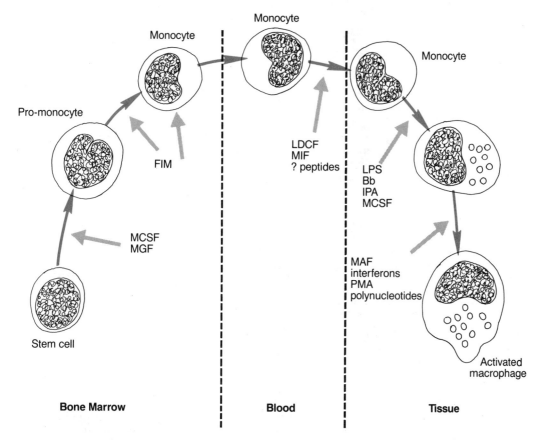

Figure 12-14. Postulated stages in development and activation of macrophages. The proliferation and differentiation of monocytes are stimulated by factors that act on bone marrow precursors. Monocytes are released into the peripheral blood and are attracted to sites of inflammation by inflammatory mediators, where they are stimulated by other factors to become activated for increased phagocytosis and secretion.

active against infections caused by unrelated organisms. A number of agents have been found that cause activation of macrophages. These include bacillus Calmette-Guérin (BCG), *Listeria monocytogenes*, toxoplasma, endotoxin, levamisole, and polynucleotides (Fig. 12-15). A considerable interest in the role of this phenomenon in enhancing tumor immunity has developed because of the possibility of limiting tumor growth with activated macrophages (see Chapter 29). This type of cellular immunity has been termed *immune phagocytosis,* even though this "immunity" is nonspecific.

The Reticuloendothelial System

The reticuloendothelial system (RES) is a multiorgan collection of cells whose primary common functional capacity is phagocytosis. Two general types of phagocytes are recognized — wandering and fixed. The wandering cells are the monocytes of the peripheral blood. These cells may be found in other

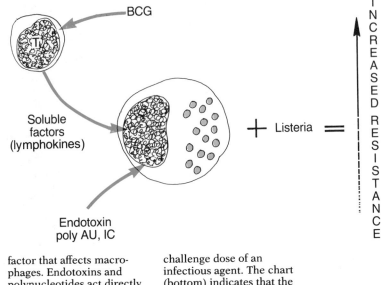

Figure 12-15. Nonspecific macrophage activation. Macrophages may acquire an increased capacity to destroy infective organisms or target cells after treatment with a variety of agents. Bacillus Calmette-Guérin acts upon T cells, which produce a soluble factor that affects macrophages. Endotoxins and polynucleotides act directly on macrophages. The mechanism of action of these agents is not understood, but as a result of macrophage activation, an experimental animal will resist a normally infectious challenge dose of an infectious agent. The chart (bottom) indicates that the dose of *Listeria monocytogenes* required to kill an experimental animal is significantly higher after treatment of the animals with BCG.

organs, for example in the sinusoids of lymphoid organs or the connective tissue (stroma) of many organs, where they may be only temporary residents. The fixed cells (histiocytes) are permanent residents in these tissue locations. Histiocytes may be found in liver (Kupffer cells or sinusoid-lining cells), spleen (sinusoid-lining cells, reticular cells, dendritic macrophages), lymph nodes, connective tissue, brain (microglia), bone marrow, adrenals, thymus, and lungs (alveolar macrophages). If particles such as carbon or vital dyes are injected into the blood, the Kupffer cells of the liver and the phagocytic cells of the spleen ingest most of them; if the particles are inhaled, the pulmonary alveolar macrophages ingest them; if they are injected into connective tissue, the local phagocytes ingest them; if the particles are injected into the brain, the microglia destroy them. All these cells have in common the ability to ingest foreign materials.

Phagocytic Index

Measurement of the phagocytic capacity of an animal may be accomplished by determining the rate of disappearance of stable, inert, uniform particles such as gelatin-stabilized carbon particles. Upon intravenous injection of such particles, about 90% are taken up by the liver, most of the remainder by the spleen. Carbon clearance is measured after saturation of the clearing mechanism, because a dose of particles lower than the saturation dose is cleared during the first few passages of the blood through the liver. Determination of carbon clearance under these conditions primarily measures liver blood flow. If a dose large enough to saturate the reticuloendothelial system is given, a two-stage elimination occurs: (1) a rapid clearance as the particle-laden blood first passes through the liver and spleen, and (2) a slower clearance, which occurs upon recirculation through the previously saturated reticuloendothelial system. The slope of this second curve is the *phagocytic index*. It measures regeneration of phagocytic capacity after saturation.

The clearance of particles from the blood by the reticuloendothelial system follows first-order reaction kinetics:

reactant $\rightarrow$ product

or

particles in blood $\rightarrow$ ingestion by RES

The change in concentration of the particles in the blood over a given time is related to the concentration at the start of the experiment, as follows:

$$dC/dt + KC_0.$$

This becomes:

$$C_t = C_0 10^{-Kt}$$

where
C_t = concentration at time t,
C_0 = initial concentration,
t = time,
K = constant (phagocytic index).

Solving for K:

$$K = \frac{\log C_1 - \log C_2}{t_2 - t_1}$$

After injection of a dose of carbon particles sufficient to saturate the reticuloendothelial system, the concentration of carbon in the blood at a given time is determined (C_1, t_1). After a period of several hours, the animal is bled and the concentration of carbon again determined (C_2, t_2). K, the phagocytic index, can then be determined from the formula given above.

Stimulation of the Reticuloendothelial System

A number of agents may affect the phagocytic index. Products of microorganisms, such as the cell wall of yeast (zymosan), bacterial endotoxins, extracts of *Mycobacterium tuberculosis*, living and killed organisms, simple lipids such as triglycerides, and hormones such as estrogen, have all been shown to increase carbon clearance. The ability of some organisms such as *Salmonella typhimurium* to increase phagocytic activity results in increased resistance of the host to other infecting microorganisms (see Activated Macrophages, above). Antibody to a given organism or particle may increase the capacity of the host to phagocytose antibody-coated particles (opsonin). The mechanisms of action of agents that stimulate phagocytic clearance are not clear.

Blockade of the Reticuloendothelial System

Phagocytic clearance may be depressed by overloading the reticuloendothelial system. Thus, a saturating dose of carbon may decrease the clearance of a second dose of carbon. Blockade of the reticuloendothelial system with fibrin results in a decreased clearance of fibrin formed after blockade (see above). Agents that blockade the system have similar properties. Colloidal carbon blockades the system for a second dose of carbon or for similar agents but does not affect the clearance of chromic phosphate. This suggests different phagocytic receptors for different particles.

Shwartzman Reaction

The Shwartzman reaction is not an immune reaction but an alteration in factors affecting intravascular coagulation and reticuloendothelial clearance.

Local Shwartzman Reaction

The local Shwartzman reaction is a lesion confined to a prepared tissue site (usually skin) and is a two-stage reaction. The tissue site is prepared by the local injection of an agent (gram-negative endotoxin) that causes accumulation of polymorphonuclear leukocytes. It is believed that the granulocytes then condition the site by releasing lysosomal acid hydrolases that damage small vessels, setting up the site for reaction to a provoking agent. A mild inflammatory reaction may serve as a preparative event. Provocation is accomplished by injection into the prepared site of agents that initiate intravascular coagulation (gram-negative endotoxins, antigen–antibody complexes, starch). The lesion is caused by intravascular clotting with localization of platelets, granulocytes, and fibrin at the site of preparation, forming white cell thrombi that lead to necrosis of vessel walls and hemorrhage. The administration of nitrogen mustard (decreased granulocytes) or vasodilators inhibits the reaction, whereas agents that block the reticuloendothelial system (e.g., carbon) increase the intensity of the reaction. Specific immunization is not necessary. Although immune reactions may serve as either a preparatory or provocative event, nonimmune reactions are also effective.

Generalized Shwartzman Reaction (Disseminated Intravascular Coagulation)

The classic generalized Shwartzman reaction is elicited by giving a young rabbit two intravascular injections of endotoxin 24 hours apart (Fig. 12-16). After the first injection, a few fibrin thrombi are found in vessels of liver, lungs, kidney, and spleen capillaries. Following the second injection, many more thrombi are found. Bilateral renal cortical necrosis and splenic hemorrhage and necrosis are prominent. The fibrin thrombi do

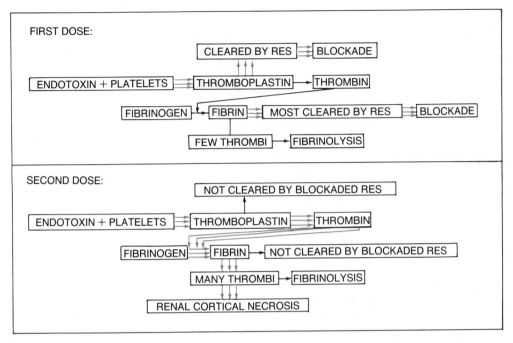

Figure 12-16. Mechanism of generalized Shwartzman reaction induced by endotoxin. Classic generalized Shwartzman reaction is elicited by giving rabbits two doses of endotoxin 24 hours apart. Primary effect of first (preparatory) dose of endotoxin is to cause release of platelet thromboplastin. Most of this thromboplastin is cleared by reticuloendothelial system (RES). Some thrombin triggers conversion of fibrinogen to fibrin, but again most of this fibrin is cleared by reticuloendothelial system. If an animal is examined after one dose of endotoxin (preparative dose), a few fibrin thrombi are found in vessels of liver, lungs, and spleen. These thrombi appear to be quickly removed by fibrinolysis, with no damage to treated rabbit. However, because of action of reticuloendothelial system in clearing thromboplastin and fibrin, blockade of reticuloendothelial system occurs. This blockade permits second dose of endotoxin to produce severe intravascular coagulation. Second dose (provocative dose) initiates same release of platelet thromboplastin as first dose, but with reticuloendothelial system blockaded, this thromboplastin is not cleared; most goes on to form thrombin and initiate conversion of fibrinogen to fibrin. This fibrin cannot be cleared by the blockaded reticuloendothelial system and most becomes lodged in capillaries, capillaries of renal glomeruli in particular. Fibrinolytic system is not capable of overcoming large amounts of fibrin formed in a short period of time. End result may be fatal renal cortical necrosis.

not contain clumps of platelets or leukocytes. In human disease, the generalized Shwartzman reaction develops as an acute and frequently fatal complication of an underlying disease, such as infection. This is called disseminated intravascular coagulation. It is triggered by one or more episodes of intravascular clotting leading to the formation of multiple fibrin or fibrin-like thrombi that lodge in small vessels. Such thrombi are prominent in the kidney or adrenal glands and cause necrosis and/or hemorrhage. Three steps appear to be necessary:

1. Intravascular clotting with fibrin formation.
2. Deposition of fibrin in small vessels. In order for this to happen, at least one, and usually all, of the following condi-

tions must apply: depression of reticuloendothelial clearance of altered fibrinogen; decrease in blood flow through affected organs; liberation of enzymes by granulocytes, which help precipitate fibrin.

3. Once deposited, the fibrin is not removed by fibrinolysis.

Agents that cause blockade of reticuloendothelial clearance (thorotrast, carbon, endotoxin, cortisone) serve as priming agents, and agents that activate intravascular clotting (endotoxin, antigen–antibody complexes, synthetic acid polysaccharides) serve as provoking agents.

Endotoxin Shock

Endotoxin shock is different from the Shwartzman reaction in that no preparative injection is necessary; shock can be induced in any species (the Shwartzman reaction occurs only in man and rabbit); shock occurs with equal intensity at any age (young rabbits are much more sensitive than old rabbits to the Shwartzman reaction); thrombi are not prominent in endotoxic shock, which features hemorrhage and necrosis, and cortisone enhances the Shwartzman reaction but does not affect endotoxic shock. Endotoxin may function by activation of complement components causing vasodilation and increased vascular permeability.

The Shwartzman Reaction and Pregnancy

A single injection of endotoxin in pregnant rabbits produces a generalized Shwartzman reaction. Bilateral renal cortical necrosis has been reported in septicemia following induced abortion in humans. Clinical evidence indicates that bilateral renal cortical necrosis in this circumstance represents a human equivalent of the generalized Shwartzman reaction due to endotoxemia during pregnancy. Pregnancy serves as the preparative step, because fibrinolytic activity and reticuloendothelial clearance are decreased during pregnancy. The occurrence of gram-negative septicemia during delivery or abortion serves as the provocative step, leading to hypotension and intravascular clotting. In addition, intravascular dissemination of amniotic fluid during delivery may activate fibrin formation. This may be followed by thrombocytopenia and hemorrhage or a typical generalized Shwartzman reaction with bilateral renal cortical necrosis. Fibrin occurs within glomerular capillary loops within 48 hours of the provocation. Hemorrhagic necrosis of the adrenals and/or renal cortical necrosis may occur 60 hours to 40 days later. However, most episodes of pregnancy-associated Shwartzman reaction do not progress to fatal renal cortical necrosis.

Review of Inflammatory Mediators

A summary of the role of different mediators at different stages of the inflammatory process is given in Figure 12-17. The early vascular stages are largely caused by mast cell mediators. In some instances products of the coagulation, kinin, and comple-

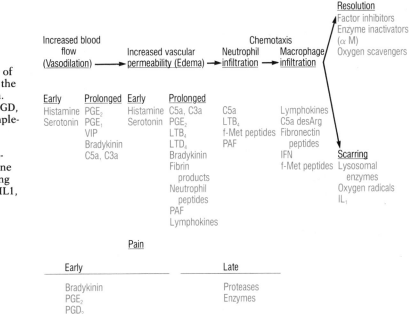

Figure 12-17. Summary of the role of mediators in the process of inflammation. PGE, prostaglandin E; PGD, prostaglandin D; C, complement components; VIP, vasoactive intestinal polypeptide; LTB, leukotriene B; LTD, leukotriene D; PAF, platelet-activating factor; IFN, interferon; IL1, interleukin 1.

ment systems may be active. The acute cellular stage is mediated by complement, leukotrienes, or bacterial or tissue products. The chronic cellular stage is influenced mainly by lymphokines. The outcome of the inflammatory process depends largely on the degree of injury and is effected mainly by macrophages, which either clear the inflamed tissue or set the stage for fibroblast proliferation and scarring. Because of the difficulty in studying this complex process, which can really only be duplicated in vivo, the precise action of the various mediators is not well understood.

Manifestations of Inflammation in Tissues

Examples of morphologic manifestations of different stages of inflammation in tissues include four different organs in which inflammation is initiated by different etiologies: (1) vessels — vasculitis induced by antigen–antibody reaction or inflammatory mediators; (2) lung — pneumonia induced by infection; (3) heart — myocardial infarction induced by blockage of blood flow (coronary thrombus), and (4) kidney — glomerulonephritis induced by antibody–antigen reaction and activation of complement (Table 12-16).

The initiating event is different, but the subsequent sequence of events is similar. Acute inflammation is first manifested in vessels by increased blood flow (congestion) and increased vascular permeability (edema). Chemotactic factors attract and activate polymorphonuclear neutrophils. If enzyme release from neutrophils occurs in the vessel walls, fibrinoid (fibrin-resembling) necrosis is seen. This is followed by lymphocyte and macrophage infiltration. If resolution does not

Table 12-16. Manifestations of Inflammation in Tissue

Organ	Etiology	Inciting Event	Acute	Subacute	Chronic
			Stages of Inflammation		
Vessel (vasculitis)	Multiple	Multiple; cell injury, infection	Increased blood flow and vasopermeability (edema) — Poly infiltrate (pus) — Mononuclear cells — *Necrosis* — Hemorrhage		Resolution / Scarring
Lung (pneumonia)	Infection	Release of bacterial products	Edema, congestion — Poly infiltrate — Macrophages — Hemorrhage — *Necrosis* — Fibroblast proliferation		Resolution / Scarring
Heart (infarct)	Disturbance of flow	Necrosis of myocardial cells	Edema, congestion — Poly infiltrate — Macrophage — Fibroblast proliferation		Scarring
Kidney (glomerulonephritis)	Immune inflammation	Deposition of Ag-Ab complexes, activation of complement	Increased glomerular permeability (proteinuria) — Poly infiltrate — mononuclear infiltrate — *Necrosis* — Hematuria — Epithelial proliferation		Resolution / Scarring (uremia)

occur, subendothelial fibroblastic proliferation leads to narrowing of the vessel wall (endarteritis) and eventually to infarction of tissue. In the lung, congestion and edema due to increased blood flow and vascular permeability are followed by polymorphonuclear infiltration, and then macrophage infiltration, fibroblast proliferation, and scarring (organizing pneumonia). In myocardial infarction, necrosis of myocardial cells is seen first. Release of cytoplasm from necrotic cells produces vasodilation and endothelial cell contraction (increased vascular permeability — edema), and chemotaxis for polymorphonuclear cells. This is followed by macrophage infiltration, fibroblast and capillary proliferation (granulation tissue), and scarring. In the renal glomerulus the sequence of events is initiated by activation of complement following deposition of antibody – antigen complexes in the basement membrane. This produces changes in the endothelial cells and basement membrane that result in leakage of protein in the urine (proteinuria, the equivalent of edema in other organs) and chemotaxis of polymorphonuclear neutrophils. Enzymes released by polymorphonuclear cells cause destruction of the basement membrane, and red cells pass into the urine (hematuria, the equivalent of hemorrhage in other tissues). Subacute glomerular inflammation is manifested by proliferation of epithelial cells and continued thickening of the basement membrane (membranoproliferative glomerulonephritis). The major consequence of the inflammatory process changes from increased glomerular permeability (proteinuria, hematuria) to decreased filtration as the basement membrane becomes thickened (uremia). As in other organs, chronic inflammation is manifested by fibrosis and scarring. Thus, in each organ the process of inflammation is essentially the same, leading to resolution or scarring through similar stages.

Summary

Inflammation is the process of delivery of proteins and cells to sites of tissue damage or infection and their activation at these sites. The process proceeds from acute, subacute, and chronic stages to resolution or scarring. Tissue lesions and extent of reaction are determined by inflammatory mechanisms mediated by serum protein or cellular systems. The serum protein systems include complement, coagulation, fibrinolysis, and kinin; the cellular systems include polymorphonuclear leukocytes, mast cells (or basophils), platelets, eosinophils, lymphocytes, macrophages, and the reticuloendothelial system. Each of these systems has a homeostatic function and is controlled by interrelated feedback mechanisms. Excessive or inadequate activation of these systems may have serious effects. Manifestions of the stages of inflammation in different tissues are similar even though the inflammatory process is initiated by different events (infections, tissue necrosis, antibody – antigen reaction).

References

General

Braunsteiner R, Zuker-Franklin D (eds): The Physiology and Pathology of Leukocytes. New York, Grune & Stratton, 1962.

Florey HW (ed): General Pathology, 4th ed. Philadelphia, Saunders, 1970.

Hunter J: A Treatise on the Blood, Inflammation and Gun Shot Wounds, Vol I. London, G. Nicoll, 1974.

Larsen CL, Henson PM: Mediators of inflammation. Annu Rev Immunol 1:335, 1983.

Lepow IH, Ward PA (eds): Inflammation: Mechanisms and Control. New York, Academic Press, 1972.

Movat HZ (ed): Inflammation, Immunity and Hypersensitivity. New York, Harper & Row, 1971.

McCutcheon M: Chemotaxis in leukocytes. Physiol Rev 26:319, 1946.

Oppenheim JJ, Rosenstreich DL, Potter M: Cellular Functions in Immunity and Inflammation. New York, Elsevier, 1981.

Spector WG, Willoughby DA: The inflammatory response. Bacteriol Rev 27:117, 1963.

Suter E, Ramseier H: Cellular reactions in infection. Adv Immunol 4:117, 1964.

Thomas L, Uhr JW, Grant L (eds): International Symposium on Injury, Inflammation and Immunity. Baltimore, Williams & Wilkins, 1964.

Zweifach BW, Grant L, McClusky RT (eds): The Inflammatory Response, Vol 3. New York, Academic Press, 1974.

Van Arman CG (ed): White Cells in Inflammation. Springfield, Ill., Thomas, 1974.

Mast Cells

Anderson P, Slorach SA, Uvnas B: Sequential exocytosis of storage granules during antigen-induced histamine release from sensitized rat mast cells in vitro. An electron microscopic study. Acta Physiol Scand 88:359, 1973.

Austen KF, Orange RP: Bronchial asthma: the possible role of the chemical mediators of immediate hypersensitivity in the pathogenesis of subacute and chronic disease. Annu Rev Resp Dis 112:423, 1975.

Bach MK: Mediators of anaphylaxis and inflammation. Annu Rev Microbiol 36:371, 1982.

Benditt BR, Lagunoff D: The mast cell: its structure and function. Prog Allergy 8:195, 1964.

Bennich H, Johansson SGO: Structure and function of human immunoglobulin E. Adv Immunol 13:1, 1971.

Berridge MJ: The molecular basis of communication within the cell. Sci Am 253:142, 1985.

Chakrin L, Bailey D: Leukotrienes. Orlando, Fla., Academic Press, 1984.

Davis P, Bailey PJ, Goldenberg MM, Ford-Hutchinson AW: The role of arachidonic acid oxygenation products in pain and inflammation. Annu Rev Immunol 2:335, 1983.

Dvorak HF, Dvorak AM: Basophils, mast cells, and cellular immunity in animals and man. Hum Pathol 3:454, 1972.

Ishizaka K, Ishizaka T, Hornbrook MH: Physico-chemical properties of human reaginic antibody. IV. Presence of a unique immunoglobulin as a cause of reaginic activity. J Immunol 97:75, 1966.

Metcalf DD, Kaliner M, Donlon MA: The mast cell. CRC Crit Rev Immunol 3:24, 1981.

Mota I: Mast cells and anaphylaxis. Ann NY Acad Sci 103:264, 1963.

Paton WDM: The release of histamine. Prog Allergy 5:79, 1958.

Uvnas B: Mechanism of histamine release in mast cells. Ann NY Acad Sci 103:278, 1963.

Wasserman SI: The human lung mast cell. Environ Health Perspect 55:259, 1984.

Neutrophils

Becker EL: Enzyme activation and the mechanism of neutrophil chemotaxis. Antibiot Chemother 19:409, 1974.

Boyden S: The chemotactic effect of mixtures of antibody and antigen on polymorphonuclear leucocytes. J Exp Med 115:453, 1962.

Cochrane CG: Immunologic tissue injury mediated by neutrophilic leukocytes. Adv Immunol 9:97, 1968.

Fantone JC, Ward PA: Role of oxygen-derived free radicals and metabolites and leukocyte-dependent inflammatory reactions. Am J Pathol 107:397, 1982.

Goldstein IM: Polymorphonuclear leukocyte lysosomes and immune tissue injury. Prog Allergy 20:301, 1976.

Naccache PH, Shaafi RI: Granulocyte activation: biochemical events associated with the mobilization of calcium. Surv Immunol Res 3:288, 1984.

Schiffmann E, Corcoran BA, Wahl SA: N-formylmethyl peptides as chemoattractants for leukocytes. Proc Nat Acad Sci USA 72:1059, 1975.

Spicer SS, Hardin JH: Ultrastructure, cytochemistry, and function of neutrophil leukocyte granules. Lab Invest 20:488, 1969.

Zigmond SH: Chemotaxis by polymorphonuclear leukocytes. J Cell Biol 77:269, 1978.

Complement

Cochrane CG, Ward PA: The role of complement in lesions induced by immunologic reactions. *In* Grabar P, Miesher P (eds): Immunology, Vol IV. Basel, Schwabe, 1966.

Cohen S: The requirement for the association of two adjacent rabbit γ-G antibody molecules in the fixation of complement by immune complexes. J Immunol 100:407, 1968.

Gewurz H, Shin HJ, Mergenhagen SE: Interactions of the complement system with endotoxic lipopolysaccharide: consumption of each of the six terminal complement components. J Exp Med 128:1049, 1968.

Gotze O, Muller-Eberhard HJ: Lysis of erythrocytes by complement in the absence of antibody. J Exp Med 132:898, 1970.

Gotze O, Muller-Eberhard HJ: The alternative pathway of complement activation. Adv Immunol 24:11, 1976.

Hirsch RL: The complement system. Its importance in the host response to viral infection. Microbiol Rev 46:71, 1982.

Hugli TE: Structure and functions of the anaphylatoxins. Springer Semin Immunopathol 7:93, 1984.

Humphrey JH, Dourmashkin RR: The lesions in cell membranes caused by complement. Adv Immunol 11: 75, 1969.

Johnson BJ: Complement: a host defense mechanism ready for pharmacological manipulation. J Pharmacol Sci 66:1367, 1977.

May JE, Frank MM: A new complement-mediated cytolytic mechanism — the C1 bypass activation pathway. Proc Nat Acad Sci USA 70:649, 1973.

Mayer MA: Membrane damage by complement. Johns Hopkins Med J 148:243, 1981.

Muller-Eberhard HJ: Chemistry and reaction mechanisms of complement. Adv Immunol 8:1, 1968.

Muller-Eberhard HJ: Complement. Annu Rev Biochem 38:389, 1969.

Pangburn MK, Muller-Eberhard HJ: The alternative pathway of complement activation. Springer Semin Immunopathol 7:163, 1984.

Rapp HJ, Borsos T: Complement research: fundamental and applied. JAMA 198:1347, 1966.

Reid KBM: Application of molecular cloning to studies on the complement system. Immunology 55:185, 1985.

Rosenberg LT: Complement. Annu Rev Microbiol 19:285, 1965.

Seeman P: Ultrastructure of membrane lesions in immune lysis, osmotic lysis and drug induced lysis. Fed Proc 33:2116, 1974.

Verroust PJ, Wilson CB, Cooper NR, Edgington TS, Dixon FJ: Glomerular complement components in human glomerulonephritis. J Clin Invest 53:77, 1974.

Wurz L: Properdin system and immunity. II. Interaction of the properdin system with polysaccharides. Science 122:545, 1955.

Coagulation

Pensky J, Kinz CF, Todd EW, Wedgwood RJ, Boyer JT, Lepow IH: Properties of highly purified human endotoxin. J Immunol 100:142, 1968.

Ratnoff O: The interrelationship of clotting factors and immunologic mechanisms. *In* Good RA, Fisher DW (eds): Immunology. Stanford, Sinauer, 1971, p 35.

Rodriguez-Erdmann F: Bleeding due to increased intravascular blood coagulation. N Engl J Med 273: 1370, 1966.

Sundsmo JS, Fair DS: Relationship among the complement, kinin, coagulation and fibrinolytic systems in the inflammatory reaction. Clin Physiol Biochem 1:225, 1983.

Kinin

Kaplan AP, Ghebrehiwet B, Silverberg M, Sealey JE: The intrinsic coagulation–kinin pathway, complement cascades, plasma kinin–angiotensin system and their interrelationship. CRC Crit Rev Immunol 3:75, 1981.

Schachter M: Kallikreins and kinins. Physiol Rev 49: 1969.

Silva K, Rothschild HA (eds): Bradykinin and related kinins. *In* International Symposium on Vasoactive Peptides. São Paulo, Brazil, 1967.

Spragg J: Complement, coagulation and kinin generation. *In* Sirois P,

Rola-Pleszcynski M (eds): Immunopharmacology. New York, Elseiver, 1982.

Webster ME: Kinin system. *In* Movat HZ (ed): Cellular and Humoral Mechanisms in Anaphylaxis and Allergy. New York, Karger, 1969.

Eosinophils

Beeson PB, Bass DA: The Eosinophil. Philadelphia, Saunders, 1977.

Gleich GJ, Loegering DA: The immunobiology of eosinophils. Annu Rev Immunol 2:429, 1983.

Lecks HI, Kravis LP: The allergist and the eosinophil. Pediatr Clin North Am 16:125, 1969.

Litt M: Studies in experimental eosinophilia. VI. Uptake of immune complexes by eosinophils. J Cell Biol 23:355, 1964.

Ross R, Klebanoff SJ: The eosinophilic leukocyte. Fine structural studies of changes in the uterus during the estrous cycle. J Exp Med 124:653, 1966.

Sampter M: Eosinophils: nominated but not elected. N Engl J Med 303:1175, 1980.

Lymphocytes

See Chapter 19

Cohen S: The role of cell-mediated immunity in the induction of inflammatory responses. Am J Pathol 88:502, 1977.

Ford WL, Gowans JL: The traffic of lymphocytes. Semin Hematol 6:67, 1969.

Gately MK, Mayer MM: Purification and characterization of lymphokines: an approach to the study of molecular mechanisms of cell mediated immunity. Prog Allergy 25:106, 1978.

Gowans JL, McGregor DD: The immunological activities of lymphocytes. Prog Allergy 9:1, 1965.

Oppenheim JJ, Jacobs D (eds): Leukocytes and Host Defense. Progress in Leukocyte Biology, Vol 5. New York, Liss, 1986.

Waksman BH, Namba Y: On soluble mediators of immunologic regulation. Cell Immunol 21:161, 1976.

Macrophages

Adams DO, Hamilton TA: The cell biology of macrophage activation. Surv Immunol Res 2:283, 1983.

Axline SG: Functional Biochemistry of the Macrophage. Semin Hematol 7:142, 1970.

Cohn ZA: The structure and function of monocytes and macrophages. Adv Immunol 9:163, 1968.

DeDuve C, Wattiauk R: Functions of lysosomes. Annu Rev Physiol 28:435, 1966.

Gresser I: Interferons. New York, Academic Press, 1981.

Kluger MJ, Oppenheim JJ, Powanda MC (eds): The Physiologic, Metabolic and Immunologic Activities of Interleukin 1. New York, Liss, 1985.

Mackaness GB, Blanden RV: Cellular immunity. Prog Allergy 11:89, 1967.

Murahata RI, Mitchell MS: Modulation of the immune response by BCG: a review. Yale J Biol Med 49:283, 1976.

Nelson DS: Immunobiology of the Macrophage. New York, Academic Press, 1976.

Reichard S, Kojima M (eds): Macrophage Biology. New York, Liss, 1985.

Snyderman R, Pike MC: Chemoattractant receptors on phagocytic cells. Annu Rev Immunol 2:257, 1984.

Van Furth R (ed): Mononuclear Phagocytes. Oxford, Blackwell, 1970.

Van Oss, CJ: Phagocytosis as a surface phenomenon. Annu Rev Microbiol 32:19, 1978.

Virelizier JL, Arenzanaseisdedos F: Immunological functions of macrophages and their regulation by interferons. Med Biol 63:149–159, 1985.

Reticuloendothelial System

Heller JH, Gordon AS: The reticuloendothelial system. Ann NY Acad Sci 88, 1960.

Stiffel C, Mouton D, Biozzl G: Kinetics of the phagocytic function of reticuloendothelial macrophages in vivo. *In* Van Furth R (ed): Mononuclear Phagocytes. Oxford, Blackwell, 1970, p335.

Stuart AE: The Reticuloendothelial System. Edinburgh, Livingston, 1970.

Shwartzman Reaction

Apitz KA: Study of the generalized Shwartzman phenomena. J Immunol 29:255, 1935.

Colman R, Robboy SJ, Minna JD: Disseminated intravascular coagulation: a reappraisal. Annu Rev Med 30:359, 1979.

Gilbert VE, Braude AI: Reduction of serum complement in rabbits after injection of endotoxin. J Exp Med 116:477, 1962.

Hjort PF, Rapaport SI: The Shwartzman reaction: pathologic mechanisms and clinical manifestations. Annu Rev Med 16:135, 1965.

Mori W: The Shwartzman reaction: a review including clinical manifestations and proposal for a universal or single organ third type. Histopathology 5:113, 1981.

Muller-Berghaus G: Pathophysiology of generalized intravascular coagulation. Serum Thromb Hemostasis 3:209, 1977.

Shwartzman G: Phenomena of Local Tissue Reactivity. New York, Hoeber, 1937.

13 | Immune-Mediated Inflammation

Immune Effector Mechanisms

The specificity of antibody and specifically sensitized T effector lymphocytes provides a means of directing the defensive force of inflammation directly to infecting foreign organisms. The immune response in this way provides immune effector mechanisms augmented by accessory inflammatory processes that protect us against specific infections. Six immune effector mechanisms are recognized: *inactivation or activation, cytotoxic, Arthus (immune complex), anaphylactic, delayed (cellular),* and *granulomatous* (Fig. 13-1). These effector mechanisms are activated by the reaction of antibody or sensitized cells with antigens in vivo (Fig. 13-2).

The first four types of immunopathologic mechanisms are mediated by immunoglobulin antibodies. The characteristics of the reactions not only are determined by the properties of the immunoglobulin molecules involved but also depend on the nature and tissue location of the antigen and on the accessory inflammatory systems that are called into play.

The last two mechanisms, delayed hypersensitivity and granulomatous reactions, are dependent not upon antibody but upon reaction of antigen with specifically sensitized cells (T_D lymphocytes). Delayed reactions are usually elicited by soluble degradable antigens, whereas granulomatous reactions are elicited by poorly degradable antigens.

Activation of T_D cells leads to production and release of soluble factors (lymphokines) whose function is to attract and activate macrophages. The major mechanism of tissue damage is phagocytosis and destruction of cells by macrophages. If macrophages, activated by antibody or by lymphocytes, are unable to digest the material they phagocytose, masses of macrophages collect in the tissues and lead to space-occupying lesions that eventually interfere with normal tissue function (granulomas). Granulomatous reactions are not separately classified in some systems, but produce tissue lesions that are

307

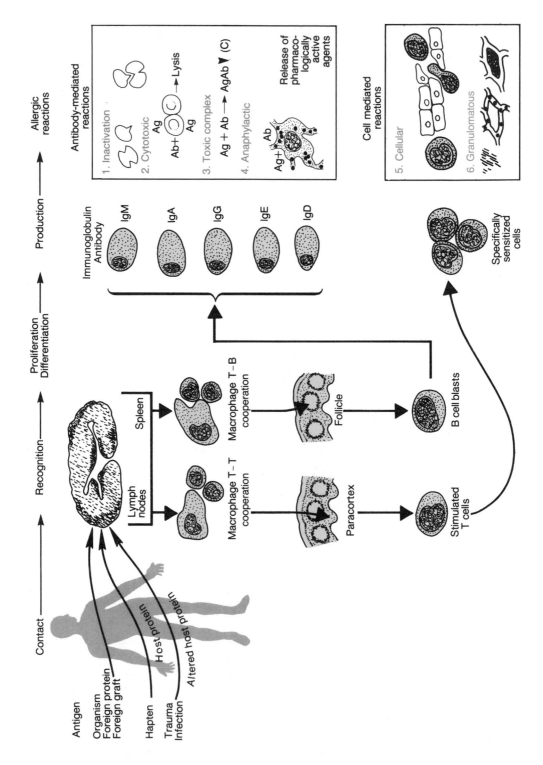

Figure 13-1. Immune response and immune effector mechanisms. Potential antigens (foreign material, haptens, or altered host material) induce immune reactivity. This reactivity is manifested by production of specifically reactive serum proteins (antibodies) or specifically modified cells (sensitized lymphocytes) ca-pable of recognizing and reacting with the antigen to which the individual is exposed. As a result of this process, the following immune effector mecha-nisms may become manifest: (1) inactivation or activation of biologically active molecules, (2) cytotoxic or cytolytic reactions, (3) anaphylactic or atopic reac-tions, (4) Arthus (immune complex) reactions, (5) delayed hypersensitivity (cellular) reactions, and (6) granulomatous reactions. Also produced is a popula-tion of cells with ability to cause more rapid and more intense response to second contact with immunizing antigen (secondary re-sponse).

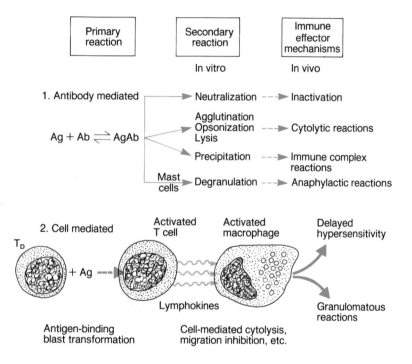

Figure 13-2. Stages of immune reactions. Primary reactions refer to binding of antigen to antibodies or cells; secondary reactions refer to various phenomena that can be measured in vitro; immune effector mechanisms are activated as a result of immune reactions in vivo.

characteristic and clearly different from delayed hypersensitiv-ity reactions.

The first four immune reactions can be transferred with antiserum, whereas DH (delayed hypersensitivity) and granu-lomatous reactions are transferrable not with antiserum but with sensitized cells. When functioning properly these mecha-nisms deliver lethal blows to foreign agents that have invaded the body, while producing little or no damage to host tissues. However, if damage is extensive or if the immune response becomes directed to host tissue, this same mechanism may cause disease.

Until the 1960s immune reactions were not classified ac-cording to mechanism, but were presented as a bewildering list of peculiar lesions. The first working classification of four major immune mechanisms was introduced by Gell and Coombs in 1963 in their classic textbook as immune mechanisms that cause disease (immunopathologic mechanisms). The classification that we will use includes six categories (Table 13-1).

Table 13-1 Classification of Immune Mechanisms

Gell and Coombs (1963)	Roitt (1971)	Sell (1972)
—	Stimulatory	Inactivation or activation
Type II	Cytotoxic	Cytotoxic or cytolytic
Type III	Immune complex	Immune complex (Arthus)
Type I	Atopic or anaphylactic	Atopic or anaphylactic
Type IV	Delayed hypersensitivity	Delayed hypersensitivity
—	—	Granulomatous

Antibody-Mediated Immune Effector Mechanisms

Inactivation or Activation

Inactivation or activation reactions occur when antibody reacts with an antigen that performs a vital function. Inactivation may occur by reaction of antibody to soluble molecules, such as bacterial toxins, or by reaction of antibody with cell surface receptors such as virus receptors. Reactions with soluble molecules produce changes in the tertiary structure of the biologically active molecule so that it no longer performs its biological function or is cleared from the circulation by the reticuloendothelial system as an immune complex. Reaction of antibody with cell surface receptors blocks or induces loss of the receptor from the cell surface by modulation.

Inactivation reactions to toxic agents, such as diphtheria or tetanus toxins, are beneficial and antibodies to virus may prevent cellular infection. In fact, this is the goal of immunization to toxoids. However, when antibody reacts with something vital for normal function, the same mechanism produces disease.

Cytotoxic or Cytolytic Reactions

Reaction of antibody with cell surface antigens results in activation of complement components and destruction of cells.

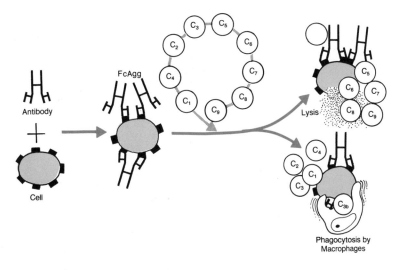

Table 13-2. Some Protective Actions of Complement

CLASSICAL COMPLEMENT PATHWAY

Components	
C14b	Viral neutralization (e.g., herpes simplex)
C14b2a3b	Viral neutralization (e.g., Newcastle disease virus, polyoma virus)
	Adherence to lymphocytes and phagocytic cells
	Enhanced phagocytosis
	Generation of lymphokines
C14b2a3d	Adherence to lymphocytes and phagocytic cells
C1-9	Lysis of cells, bacteria, and viruses
Component fragments	
C3a	Anaphylatoxin
C3b	Enhances phagocytosis (opsonin)
	Generation of lymphokines
C3e	Leukocyte mobilization
C4a	Anaphylatoxin, weak
C5a	Chemotactic factor; anaphylatoxin, strong

ALTERNATIVE COMPLEMENT PATHWAY

Cytolysis
Viral neutralization
Enhanced phagocytosis
Macrophage activation
Generation of anaphylatoxins (C3a, C5a)
Generation of chemotactic factor (C5a)

Complement components produce a realignment of membrane structures and the loss of cell membrane integrity, or the cell is coated with complement components that render the cell susceptible to phagocytosis by the reticuloendothelial system. Complement is activated by alterations in the tertiary structure of antibodies when they react with antigen. One molecule of IgM antibody reacting with a cell surface antigen is capable of activating complement and of lysing a cell, whereas two molecules of IgG antibody must react *together* to activate complement and accomplish lysis of a cell. For this reason, lytic reactions are much more effectively mediated by IgM than by IgG antibody. Other immunoglobulin classes do not fix complement and thus do not lyse cells.

Some of the protective functions of complement activation are listed in Table 13-2. Complement activation can directly inactivate viruses or bacteria and can enhance phagocytosis of infectious agents or contribute to an inflammatory response. The inflammatory activities of complement are critical for Arthus (immune complex) reactions.

Arthus (Immune Complex) Reaction

Activation of complement by reaction of antibody (usually IgG) with antigens in tissue is responsible for an inflammatory reac-

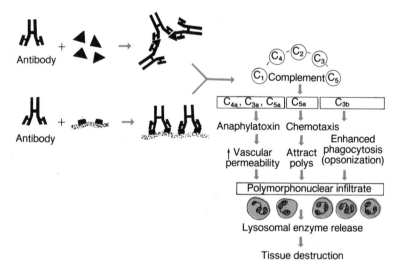

tion mediated by polymorphonuclear leukocytes. The activation of complement products C3a, C4a, and C5a can produce constriction of endothelial cells (anaphylatoxin), permitting blood components to pass into tissues. The chemotactic activity of complement fragment C5a attracts polymorphonuclear leukocytes to sites of complement activation. Damage is caused by digestion of tissue by lysosomal enzymes released from the polymorphonuclear leukocytes attracted to the tissue. Injection of antigens into the skin of animals with circulating IgG antibody results in an acute inflammatory reaction (Arthus reaction) that peaks at 6 hours and fades by 24 hours. It is characterized by perivascular necrosis and polymorphonuclear infiltration of arterioles and venules.

The protective function of immune complex reactions is to mobilize inflammatory cells at sites of acute infection. The activation of the chemotactic components of complement serves to bring polymorphonuclear cells to locations where they are needed; the released lysosomal enzymes act on infectious agents or their products, and destroy them.

Anaphylactic or Atopic Reactions

Anaphylactic or atopic reactions are initiated by pharmacologically active agents (histamine and serotonin) that are released

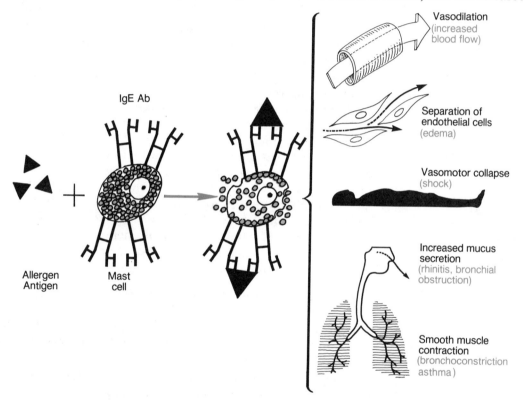

from mast cells after antibody passively bound to mast cells reacts with antigen. In addition, arachidonic acid metabolites produced by macrophages from cell membrane phospholipids released from mast cell granules contribute to later inflammatory phases of the reaction. Injection of antigen into the skin of an anaphylactically sensitive individual results in an acute reaction that peaks within 15–30 minutes and fades in 2 or 3 hours (cutaneous anaphylaxis, wheal and flare, hives). A later cellular inflammatory phase of the reaction may occur after 10–20 hours. This later phase is more evident in the biphasic bronchospastic response of the lung, where production of arachidonic metabolites by lung tissue may be more pronounced. The antibody responsible is almost always of the IgE class. Mast cells contain granules filled with pharmacological agents that act directly on smooth muscle and endothelial cells as well as cell membrane material that is metabolized to active compounds. When antigen reacts with mast cell bound IgE antibody, the cell releases the contents of its granules by a nonlytic fusion mechanism (degranulation). The released pharmacologically active agents, primarily histamine and serotonin, act on end-organ target cells to cause immediate symptoms. The membrane phospholipids are metabolized by oxidative pathways, presumably by mononuclear cells, to produce a series of biologically active compounds, leukotrienes and prostaglandins, that are responsible for later effects.

Anaphylactic or atopic reactions are elicited by reaction of antigens with IgE antibody to mast cells. The ability of IgE antibody to "fix to skin" is determined by its binding to mast cells in the skin (cytophilic antibody). The reaction can be passively transferred by injection of serum containing IgE antibody into the skin (passive cutaneous anaphylaxis). Antigen can be injected up to 45 days after injection of reaginic serum, as the antibody will remain "fixed" to mast cells in the skin. This is also referred to as the Prausnitz–Kustner reaction in honor of the authors who first described the typical reaction. Passive transfer of an Arthus reaction is demonstrable only if the antigen is injected within 24 to 48 hours after antibody, as the IgG antibody will diffuse away (it does not "fix" to mast cells).

The protective function of anaphylactic reactions is not as well understood as in other immune effector mechanisms, but several possible functions are:

Histamine and serotonin are primary mediators of increased blood flow to sites of reaction.

Anaphylactic reactions serve to open vascular endothelium, thus permitting blood-borne proteins and cells to enter inflammatory sites where they are needed.

Anaphylactic reactivity to intestinal parasites often occurs and increased intestinal motility and secretion may purge the gastrointestinal tract of them.

The acute sneezing and coughing that is part of the acute asthmatic attack may help eliminate agents in the tracheobronchial tree.

The acute reactivity may serve as a warning to avoid contact with exciting agents.

Cell-Mediated Immune Effector Mechanisms

Delayed hypersensitivity reactions are mediated by a population of specifically sensitized T lymphocytes that bear receptors for antigens. The lymphocytes that effect delayed hypersensitiv-

Delayed Hypersensitivity

ity reactions belong to a subpopulation of the T lymphocyte class: T_D cells and/or T_K cells.

The characteristic lesion of delayed hypersensitivity reactions is a perivascular mononuclear infiltrate. T_D lymphocytes reacting with antigen in tissues release lymphokines, which attract and activate macrophages. Most of the tissue damage is caused by macrophages, which have been attracted to the site of inflammation by lymphokines. T_K (killer or cytotoxic) lymphocytes may attack target cells directly. The term *delayed* is used because injection of antigen into the skin of an individual expressing delayed hypersensitivity induces an inflammatory reaction that peaks at 24 to 48 hours, in contrast to immune complex reactions, which peak at 6 hours (Arthus reactions), and cutaneous anaphylactic reactions, which peak at 15–30

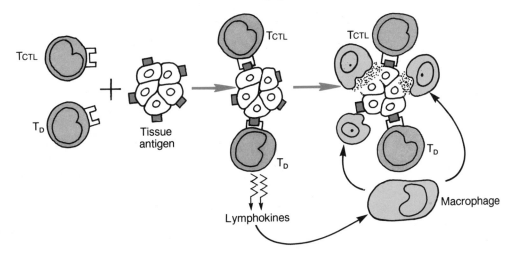

minutes. Some examples of delayed hypersensitivity reactions are tuberculin skin test, contact dermatitis (i.e., poison ivy), tissue graft rejection, virus exanthems (such as measles), and viral-associated demyelinating diseases (postinfectious encephalomyelitis, Guillain–Barré, multiple sclerosis).

Delayed skin reactions become manifest when sensitized lymphocytes react with antigen deposited into the skin. In normal skin, lymphocytes pass from venules through the dermis to lymphatics, which return these cells to the circulation. Recognition of antigen by sensitized lymphocytes (T cells) results in immobilization of lymphocytes at the site, production and release of lymphocyte mediators, and accumulation of macrophages with eventual destruction of antigen and resolution of the reaction. This results in an accumulation of cells seen at 24 to 48 hours after antigen injection. Macrophages degrade the antigen. When the antigen is destroyed, the reactive cells return via the lymphatics to the bloodstream or draining lymph nodes. In this way, specifically sensitized lymphocytes may be distributed throughout the lymphoid system following local stimulation with antigen.

The protective function of delayed hypersensitivity is directed mainly to intracellular agents, such as viruses, and to fungal and mycobacterial infections. Although delayed hypersensitivity reactions to infectious organisms may result in extensive tissue damage, the damage is a secondary effect of the immune attack on an infecting agent. It is incorrect to think, as in the past, that delayed hypersensitivity is a deleterious type of reaction. Delayed reactions are particularly important in eliminating intracellular virus infections when the viral antigens are expressed on the cell surface. It is unfortunate if the infected cell is one that performs a unique vital function, such as a neuron, because in elimination of the infected cells, irreversible tissue damage may result. The role of T_K cells in vivo remains unclear, but appears to be important in contact dermatitis, tissue graft rejection, and some autoimmune lesions.

Granulomatous Reactions A granulomatous reaction is a characteristic type of space-occupying chronic inflammatory lesion. It may be considered a

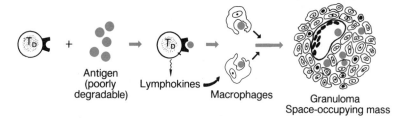

Antigen (poorly degradable)   Lymphokines   Macrophages   Granuloma Space-occupying mass

variant of delayed hypersensitivity or immune complex reaction in which the antigen is poorly catabolized and remains as a chronic irritant. Indeed, the early lesions resemble delayed hypersensitivity reactions or are associated with necrotizing vasculitis. However, instead of macrophages clearing away the antigen, there is a prolonged accumulation of macrophages and lymphocytes, which organize into granulomas. Typical granulomas consist of a ball-like mass of macrophages resembling epithelial cells (epithelioid cells) and multinucleated giant cells admixed with lymphocytes. Frequently the center of larger lesions is necrotic. Grossly this form of necrosis looks like cheese and is described as *caseous* necrosis. The major destructive mechanism is simply the occupation of organ space. The lesion may become so extensive that the normal function of the organ is impaired. Granulomas serve to isolate the infectious agent by walling off infected areas of tissue. This operates when the delayed hypersensitivity mechanism is unable to eliminate the agent. Infectious diseases in which granulomatous reactions play a major role are tuberculosis, leprosy, parasite and fungus infections, and syphilis. Granulomas occur in children who have a deficiency in macrophage digestive function (granulomatous disease of children). In these individuals, granulomas form where macrophages ingest material that cannot be degraded and large numbers of macrophages collect in the tissue.

Summary

Specific antibody and sensitized T effector lymphocytes provide mechanisms for directing protective defense mechanisms to foreign invaders. These directed immune effector mechanisms serve to focus nonimmune specific inflammatory accessory systems on the specific infectious agent. Six protective mechanisms are recognized: inactivation, cytotoxic, immune complex (Arthus), anaphylactic (atopic), delayed hypersensitivity, and granulomatous reactions. Each of these mechanisms has important protective functions, but may also cause tissue damage. Immunopathology is the study of how immune mechanisms cause disease. The role of immunopathologic mechanisms in disease is the subject of the next eight chapters.

References

(First Editions)

Bellanti JA: Immunology. Philadelphia, Saunders, 1971.

Boyd WC: Fundamentals of Immunology. New York, Interscience, 1943.

Criep LH: Clinical Immunology and Allergy. New York, Grune & Stratton, 1962.

Gell PGH, Coombs RRA: Clinical Aspects of Immunology. Oxford, Blackwell, 1963.

Humphrey JH, White RG: Immunology for Students of Medicine. Oxford, Blackwell, 1963.

Miescher PA, Muller-Eberhard HJ: Textbook of Immunopathology. New York, Grune & Stratton, 1968.

Raffel S: Immunity, Hypersensitivity, Serology. New York, Appleton–Century–Crofts, 1953.

Roitt IM: Essential Immunology. Oxford, Blackwell, 1971.

Sampter M, Alexander HL (eds): Immunological Diseases. Boston, Little, Brown, 1965.

Sell S: Immunology, Immunopathology, and Immunity. Hagerstown, Md., Harper & Row, 1972.

PART 2

IMMUNOPATHOLOGY

Immune reactions of both humoral and cellular types play critical roles in the defense of the host against infectious agents. Antibody is generally operative against bacteria or bacterial products, whereas cellular reactivity is primarily operative against viral and mycotic organisms. The protective effect of immune reactions is called *immunity* and is presented in more detail in the third part of this text. However, we increasingly recognize instances in which the immune reaction of the host produces tissue damage (disease). In the next eight chapters the role of immune effector mechanisms in causing tissue damage and disease is presented. This subject is known as *immunopathology*.

The term *immunopathology* has a double meaning: *immune* means "protected or exempt from"; *pathology* is the study of disease. Thus *immunopathology* literally means the study of the protection from disease, but in usage it means the study of how immune mechanisms cause diseases. The terms *allergy* and *hypersensitivity* are often used to denote deleterious immune reactions. *Allergy* is frequently used for a particular type of reaction (anaphylactic), and *hypersensitivity* for delayed or cellular reactivity.

In the systemic study of disease, pathogenic changes are classified according to their anatomic location. In the study of diseases due to immune mechanisms, however, more than one organ system may be involved with the same process. Because the alterations in different organ systems caused by the same process have pathologic similarities, the lesions caused by allergic reactions are best classified by the particular type of immunopathologic effector mechanism involved. These effector mechanisms also serve as the protective immune mechanisms presented later. Thus immune mechanisms represent a "double-edged sword" cutting down our enemies with one edge and causing disease with the other edge. Some examples of protective and destructive effects of immune effector mechanism are listed in the table below. These are presented in greater detail in the following chapters.

The "Double-Edged Sword" of Immune Reactions

Immune Effector Mechanism	Protective Functions: "Immunity"	Destructive Reactions: "Allergy"
Neutralization	Diphtheria, tetanus, cholera, endotoxin neutralization, blockade of virus receptors	Insulin resistance, pernicious anemia, myasthenia gravis, hyperthyroidism
Cytotoxic	Bacteriolysis, opsonization	Hemolysis, leukopenia, thrombocytopenia
Immune complex	Acute inflammation, polymorphonuclear leukocyte activition	Vasculitis, glomerulonephritis, serum sickness, rheumatoid diseases
Anaphylactic	Focal inflammation, increased vascular permeability, expulsion of intestinal parasites	Asthma, urticaria, anaphylactic shock, hay fever
Delayed hypersensitivity	Destruction of virus-infected cells, tuberculosis, syphilis, immune surveillance of cancer	Contact dermatitis, autoallergies, viral exanthems, postvaccinial encephalomyelitis
Granulomatous[a]	Leprosy, tuberculosis, helminths, fungi, isolation of organisms in granulomas	Beryllosis, sarcoidosis, tuberculosis, filariasis, schistosomiasis

[a] Granulomatous reactions, as other inflammatory lesions, may result from nonimmune stimuli as well as from an immune reaction activated by antibody or by sensitized cells. The frequent association of granulomatous reactions with delayed hypersensitivity reactions has resulted in the inclusion of granulomatous reactions as a subset of delayed hypersensitivity.

Modified from Sell S: Introduction to symposium on immunopathology: "Immune Mechanisms in Disease." Hum Pathol 9:24, 1978.

Why a "Double-Edged Sword"?

Much of what we recognize as immunopathology may result from artificial stresses put on a system that normally would not occur. The use of abnormally high doses of exogenous agents used in therapy and the delivery of these agents by unnatural routes (such as intravascularly) may produce deleterious reactions such as anaphylaxis, serum sickness, transfusion reactions, drug allergies, and graft rejections that do not occur naturally. However, there are many naturally occurring immune diseases, including autoimmune hemolytic anemias, erythroblastosis fetalis, hay fever, anaphylactic shock, polyarteritis nodosa, collagen diseases, poison ivy, and allergic granulomas. In many of these diseases infectious agents are not the primary pathogenic agent. It may thus be said that the immune response is being used for the wrong purpose, yet the very same processes that are responsible for the pathogenesis of these diseases are also essential for protective responses that are required for life.

Classification by Origin of Response and Source of Antigen

A second method of classification, based on the source of antigen and the origin of the immune response in relation to the affected individual, is presented in outline form below. When considering specific diseases, it is

---
Classification of Allergic Diseases According to Source of Antigen and Origin of Response
---

I. Endogenous immune respone to endogenous antigens
   A. Circulating antibody
      1. Autoimmune hematologic diseases
      2. Antibodies to tissue antigens in human diseases
   B. Cellular (delayed) sensitivity
      1. Experimental autoimmune diseases
      2. Human autoimmune diseases

II. Endogenous immune response to exogenous antigens
   A. Circulating antibody
      1. Anaphylactic-type reactions
      2. Atopic reactions
      3. Arthus reactions
   B. Cellular (delayed) sensitivity
      1. Tuberculin reaction
   C. Granulomatous hypersensitivity
      1. Berylliosis

III. Exogenous immune response to endogenous antigens
   A. Tranfer of maternal antibody to fetus
      1. Erythroblastosis fetalis
      2. Neonatal leukopenia; thrombocytopenia
      3. Neonatal myasthenia gravis
   B. Transfer of antibodies
      1. Reverse transfusion reaction
   C. Transfer of cells
      1. Graft versus host reaction

IV. Exogenous immune response to exogenous antigens
   A. Experimental transfer of antibody and antigens
      1. Passive anaphylaxis (Prausnitz–Kustner reaction)
      2. Passive Arthus reaction
   B. Experimental transfer of cells and antigens
      1. Tuberculin reaction
      2. Contact dermatitis

Modified from lecture notes of Frank J. Dixon, M.D.

often enlightening to determine the source of the antigen and the origin of the immune products. In the system of study followed in Part 2 of this text, immune reactions are classified according to the immune effector mechanisms.

14 | Inactivation or Activation of Biologically Active Molecules

Antibody to an enzyme, hormone, growth factor, or cell surface receptor may inactivate the biological function of these molecules. In some cases, antibody to a receptor may activate the biological function of the cells bearing the receptor. The nature of the disease caused by activation or inactivation depends on the biological function of the affected biologically active molecule.

Antibodies to biologically active molecules are produced in two general circumstances:

1. Breaking of tolerance with autoantibody production.
2. Immune response to a foreign antigen such as a therapeutically administered hormone (e.g., insulin) or drug.

Mechanisms of Antibody-Mediated Inactivation

Antibody may neutralize or inactivate biologically active molecules by several mechanisms (Fig. 14-1): direct reaction with the biologically active molecule, resulting in structural alteration of the molecule so that it is no longer active; causing increased catabolism of the antibody–antigen complex, effectively lowering the concentration of the biologically active molecules; and reaction of antibody to cell surface receptors, causing blocking (steric hindrance), modulation (endocytosis), or destruction of the receptor so that the cell is no longer able to respond to activating stimuli. Antibodies to cell surface receptors may also cause the loss of surface expression of the receptors by attracting inflammatory cells that destroy the surface receptors (antibody-dependent cell-mediated inactivation). The loss of receptor function and destruction of target cells in some diseases such as insulinitis, thyroiditis, atrophic gastritis, and myasthenia gravis are often associated with a lymphocytic infiltrate. This could be due to delayed hypersensitivity (see Chapter 18), or the autoantireceptors may effect antibody-de-

323

Figure 14-1. Inactivation or activation of biologically active molecules. Reaction of antibody with enzyme or other biologically active molecules may result in loss of biological function due to steric hindrance of binding of the activating ligand with its receptor. However, the antigenic sites of an enzyme are usually located on a different part of the molecule than the substrate binding site. Inactivation may occur by alteration of the tertiary structure of the enzyme following reaction with antibody. Increased catabolism of an enzyme–antibody complex in vivo may occur. The biological effect of neutralization depends upon the molecule neutralized. Antibodies to cell surface receptors may block or stimulate the receptor, or cause receptor modulation by endocytosis or antibody-dependent cell-mediated cytotoxicity.

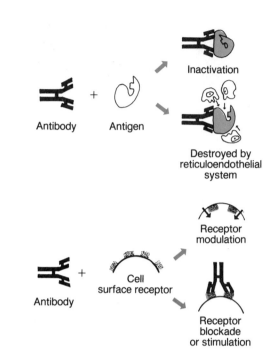

pendent cell-mediated cytotoxicity (ADCC). In some diseases, reaction of antibodies to a cell surface receptor may activate the cells (e.g., antithyroid receptor), because the antibody-binding paratope mimics the structure of the activating ligand for the receptor.

Direct Inactivation

Biologically active molecules generally have one site that is necessary for biological activity; a large portion of the molecule may not be directly involved. For example, an enzyme has an active site localized in a small area of the whole molecule. An antibody reacting with or near this active site may block the reaction of the enzyme with its substrate. However, most antibodies that inactivate enzymes react with an antigenic site quite distant from the biologically active site. Inactivation occurs by alteration of the tertiary structure of the enzyme because of its reaction with antibody. Not all such reactions result in loss of substrate binding or inactivation. In fact, classic precipitin reactions with enzymes may occur with no apparent loss of activity in the precipitated enzyme, and at least one instance has been reported in which the reaction of an inactive form of the enzyme β-D-galactosidase with an antibody results in activation of the enzyme. Presumably reaction of the antibody with the inactive form of the enzyme results in an alteration of tertiary structure so that the active site becomes available.

Not only is the site of antibody reaction important in neutralization of a biologically active molecule, but the effect of the antibody also depends on other characteristics of the antibody – antigen reaction, such as the ratio of antibody to antigen, the strength of antibody – antigen binding, and the biological properties of the antibody (e.g., complement fixation). Inactivation may be induced by the antibodies formed in one individual, whereas the antibodies formed in another individual may react with the same enzyme, but not inactivate it.

Indirect Inactivation

Antigen – antibody complexes in antibody excess or at equivalence formed in vivo are rapidly cleared by the reticuloendothelial system because of formation of aggregated Fc's of IgG (macrophages have receptors for aggregated Fc or C3b). A nonneutralizing antibody might effectively reduce the availability of an enzyme or hormone through this mechanism. However, not all antigen – antibody complexes are rapidly removed; some soluble complexes in antigen excess may continue to circulate. In some situations, binding of antibody to a serum protein may actually produce a longer half-life, because bound molecules are degraded more slowly than unbound molecules. This may lead to increased serum concentrations for the material involved but, paradoxically, a loss of biological function. The presence of such complexes may also lead to inflammatory lesions from the deposition of antibody – antigen complexes in vessels or renal glomeruli (see Chapter 16).

Receptor Loss

Antibodies may block or induce changes in cell surface receptors. Many cells respond to an activating molecule via cell surface receptors. For example, insulin, estrogen, and other hormones act through cell surface receptors. The ability of cells to respond to activating stimuli may be lost because of reaction of antibody with the receptor. Antibodies to cell surface receptors may occupy the receptor (steric hindrance) or may induce endocytosis, stripping, or structural alteration of the receptor (modulation). In addition, antibodies reacting with cell surface receptors may induce the infiltration of inflammatory cells that secondarily destroy the receptors (see Antibody-Dependent Cell-Mediated Cytotoxicity, Chapter 8). Antibodies reacting to acetylcholine receptors on the postsynaptic membrane of muscle cells are responsible for the disease myasthenia gravis (see below). Among other antireceptors that are responsible for human disease are anti-thyroid hormone receptor and anti-insulin receptor.

Examples of Antibody-Mediated Inactivation

Some specific antibodies to biologically active molecules are listed in Table 14-1.

Diabetes Mellitus

At least four different antibodies are associated with diabetes mellitus: to insulin, to insulin receptors, to islet cell cytoplasm,

Table 14-1. Diseases from Immune Neutralization or Inactivation

Disease	Antigen
Diabetes mellitus	Insulin
	Insulin receptor
	Islet cell cytoplasm
	Islet cell surface
Thyroid disease	
Hyperthyroidism	TSH[a] receptor (LATS)
Hypothyroidism	Triiodothyronine
Pernicious anemia	
Atrophic gastritis	Parietal cells
Megaloblastic anemia	Intrinsic factor
Polyendocrinopathy	Multiple (adrenal, thyroid, parathyroid, gonads, pancreas, melanocytes)
Infertility (induced)	Chorionic gonadotropin
Hemophilia, other blood diseases	Blood clotting factors (multiple)
Aplastic anemia	Erythropoietin
Chronic asthma	β-Adrenergic receptor
Myasthenia gravis	Acetylcholine receptor

[a] TSH, thyroid stimulating hormone; LATS, long-acting thyroid stimulator.

and to islet cell surface antigen. Diabetes mellitus is a general term for a heterogeneous group of diseases that have as a common denominator abnormalities in carbohydrate metabolism (Table 14-2). In most cases of diabetes mellitus, there is a defi-

Table 14-2. Immunologic Factors in Diabetes Mellitus[a]

Type	Etiologic Factor
IMMUNE	
Type Ia juvenile onset	Early, but not late, anti-islet cell antibody; HLA-DR3, DR4 associated
Type Ib juvenile onset	Both early and late islet cell antibody, associated with autoimmune endocrinopathies
Insulin resistant	Anti-insulin antibodies in response to therapy
Insulin receptor	Autoimmune insulin receptor antibodies
NONIMMUNE	
Type II maturity onset	May develop insulin resistance
Secondary	Pancreatic disease (Type III), hormonal (corticosteroid excess, etc.), drug induced.

[a] *Diabetes*, from the Greek *dia* (through) and *bainein* (to go): to go through; a siphon.

ciency in the production or utilization of insulin. Insulin is an endocrine hormone produced by beta cells in the islets of Langerhans in the pancreas. Insulin specifically reacts with many other cells of the body through cell surface receptors. Insulin acts to stimulate transport and utilization of glucose for conversion to energy or for storage as glycogen in the liver or glycosides in fat cells. Diabetes results from impaired production or decreased utilization of insulin with a resultant increase in blood glucose and related abnormalities of metabolism. Decreased insulin utilization occurs from impaired insulin secretion, loss of receptors, or presence of blocking antibodies to insulin or to the insulin receptor (Fig. 14-2). About 20% of pa-

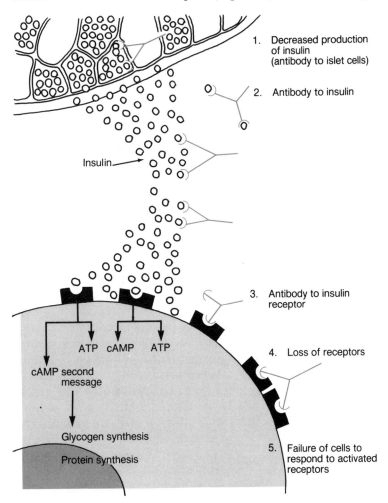

1. Decreased production of insulin (antibody to islet cells)

2. Antibody to insulin

Insulin

3. Antibody to insulin receptor

ATP cAMP ATP

cAMP second message

4. Loss of receptors

Glycogen synthesis

Protein synthesis

5. Failure of cells to respond to activated receptors

Figure 14-2. Level of abnormality in diabetes. Antibody to insulin may block insulin action and antibodies to receptors may block or modulate receptors. Many patients with loss of receptors do not have antireceptor antibodies. Inflammation of islet cells is associated with autoantibody to islet cells and precedes juvenile-onset insulin-dependent diabetes.

tients have "insulin-dependent" diabetes (i.e., the receptors are normal, but insulin availability is low); the remaining 80% have "insulin-independent" diabetes (insulin availability is normal, but the number of receptors is low). Loss of receptors may be secondary to antibody to receptors, but most patients with this form of diabetes do not have antireceptor antibodies.

Antibodies to insulin are often found in patients to whom exogenous insulin is administered. In 1938, Banting and his group observed an antibody-like neutralizer of insulin in a schizophrenic patient who had been receiving insulin shock treatment. Insulin resistance occurs in diabetic patients receiving exogenous bovine or ovine insulin for therapy. As antibodies develop, increasing doses of insulin are required. In many cases, resistance to exogenous insulin derived from one species (ox) does not hold for insulin derived from another species (pig). However, in some cases resistance may occur in insulins of a different origin because they contain some antigenic determinants in common and some that are unique. Sulfated insulin is less immunogenic than insulin lente, and highly purified insulin preparations are less immunogenic than those containing impurities. In addition, bovine insulin may be more immunogenic than porcine insulin. Production of human insulin by gene cloning techniques may provide a less immunogenic molecule, but will not completely eliminate the possibility of antibody formation. Not all anti-insulins are neutralizing, and not all insulins are neutralizable by the same antibody.

The binding of insulin by anti-insulin in vivo usually causes slowing of the disappearance of insulin from the bloodstream, that is, a longer half-life. Since insulin is a small antigen available in large amounts, insulin–anti-insulin complexes are usually not cross-linked and therefore not subject to clearance by the reticuloendothelial system (RES). Insulin bound to antibody is catabolized at the rate of the antibody (IgG) and not at the rate of insulin. Therefore, instead of reducing the half-life of insulin, antibody to insulin actually prolongs the half-life, because the bound insulin is protected from degradation by insulinase in the liver. However, the antibody-bound insulin does not have biological activity.

The amount of insulin required to overcome the antibody depends on the amount and binding affinity of the antibody, but a close correlation between antibody titers and insulin requirements is usually not seen. The insulin–anti-insulin reaction has been adapted to provide an extremely sensitive immunoassay for insulin. Acute skin reactions and systemic anaphylactic shock may also occur if insulin is injected into a sensitive individual (see Chapter 18). In addition, immune complexes of various antibody–antigen proportions may be formed. These may deposit in vessel walls or in renal glomeruli and induce immune complex reactions (see Chapter 16).

Autoantibodies to cell surface receptors for insulin have been found in patients with extreme insulin resistance. Most of these patients are female and also have a pigmented skin condition known as acanthosis nigricans. Antibodies to insulin receptors from different patients appear to recognize different antigenic determinants. These antibodies inhibit the binding of insulin to cell surface receptors, thus interfering with the biological function of insulin. At the same time, antibodies to receptors may also increase basal glucose oxidation of reactive cells, thus producing insulin-like effects in vitro. Antireceptor antibody causes patching and capping of the insulin receptor. Receptor crosslinking appears to be required for antibody induced insulin receptor activation, as Fab univalent fragments will not activate. Presumably insulin activation of the receptor is different, as insulin is univalent and cannot cross-link receptors. However, insulin reaction with receptors does cause aggregation of receptors presumably by perturbation of cytoskeletal elements. The insulin-like effect of antireceptor antibody does not seem to be significant in vivo, because patients with these antibodies usually have insulin-resistance hyperglycemia.

Autoantibodies to islet cell cytoplasm (beta cells) and/or islet cell surface antigens are associated with insulin-dependent juvenile onset diabetes mellitus. Anticytoplasmic antibodies are found in approximately 80% of newly diagnosed juvenile onset diabetes. The incidence of serum antibody drops markedly after onset of the disease so that after 1 year only about 20% of patients have detectable antibody. Acute onset juvenile diabetes is also associated with a lymphocyte infiltration of islets (lymphocytic insulitis). Juvenile diabetes shows a high relationship to certain histocompatibility types (see Chapter 9). It has been suggested that juvenile onset diabetes is a genetically controlled autoallergic reaction, perhaps triggered by a viral infection. The significance of antibodies to islet cell surface antigens is not known. Presumably, they could play an important role in the pathogenesis of the disease via an antibody-dependent cell-mediated cytotoxic mechanism.

Thyroid Disease

A number of autoantibodies to thyroid antigens are found in normal individuals (particularly with aging) as well as associated with thyroid diseases (Table 14-3). Some of these have

Table 14-3. Autoantibodies to Thyroid Antigens

Antigen	Effect of Antibody
Thyroxine and triiodothyronine	Blocks thyroid hormone action—hypothyroidism
TSH	Blocks effect of TSH—hypothyroidism
TSH receptor	Stimulates receptor—hyperthyroidism (LATS)
	Inhibits TSH binding—hypothyroidism or both
Not defined (TSH related)	Stimulates growth of thyroid cells in vitro
Cell surface antigen	Cytotoxic with lymphocytes (ADCC); associated with thyroiditis
Microsomal antigen	Cytotoxic with lymphocytes, thyroiditis
Thyroglobulin	Not clear, associated with thyroiditis
Colloid antigen	Not known, associated with thyroiditis

TSH, thyroid-stimulating hormone; LATS, long-acting thyroid stimulator; ADCC, antibody-dependent cell-mediated cytotoxicity.

biological effects and some do not. Antibodies to thyroid hormone or thyroid-stimulating hormone (TSH) may be responsible for hypothyroidism, whereas antibodies to the thyroid receptor for thyroid-stimulating hormone (TSH) may produce hyperthyroidism (Graves' disease). Transplacental transfer of antibodies to TSH receptor may cause neonatal transient hyperthyroidism. Autoallergic thyroiditis may be induced in animals by immunization with thyroid hormone. The major feature of this disease is infiltration of the thyroid gland with mononuclear cells. The disease is believed to be mediated by specific delayed hypersensitivity but could be caused by antibody-dependent cell-mediated cytotoxicity (see Delayed Hypersensitivity, Chapter 19). Circulating antibody to thyroid hormone is also produced. In humans with chronic lymphocytic thyroiditis, autoantibodies to thyroid hormones may be found and may be responsible for hypothyroidism by binding thyroxine or triiodothyronine. There is a high association of Graves' disease with HLA-DR3 (about 60%), and those patients who are HLA-DR3 positive almost never go into remission, whereas non-HLA-DR3 patients with Graves' disease frequently have remission.

Autoantibodies to thyroid stimulating hormone receptors that cause hyperthyroidism are termed long-acting thyroid stimulators (LATS). LATS has been shown to be an immunoglobin antibody that can, on the one hand, inhibit the binding of TSH to human thyroid membranes, and, on the other hand, stimulate thyroid cyclic AMP and thyroid hormone release. Animals that are immunized with hormones not only produce blocking antibodies but also may produce a thyroid-stimulating globulin. Thus, both hyperthyroidism (Graves' disease) and hypothyroidism may result from an autoallergic response. The end result depends upon the degree of tissue damage and the type and amount of autoantibody produced. A distinct population of antithyroid autoantibodies is able to stimulate cyclic AMP and promote growth of thyroid cells in vitro. This antibody is also associated with enlargement of the thyroid in Graves' disease and not with other thyroid diseases. Thus some anti-TSH receptors stimulate both production of thyroid hormone and growth of thyroid cells, whereas others stimulate only hormone production. Monoclonal antibody studies suggest that these epitopes may be part of the TSH receptor, in particular, part of the ganglioside component rather than the glycoprotein component.

Massive swelling of the extraocular muscles (Graves' ophthalmopathy) is frequently associated with hyperthyroidism. This reaction may progress rapidly and produce blindness. The cause of exophthalmus (buldging eyes) is not known. It is possible that there is cross-reactivity between the cell membrane of the eye muscles and some epitopes of the TSH receptor. Immune complexes may deposit on extraocular muscle membranes. These could produce cell damage and lymphocytic infiltration, perhaps by antibody-directed cell-mediated cytotoxicity. It is not clear why the extraocular muscles would be selectively involved, but an antibody effector mechanism could explain many of the features of Graves' ophthalmopathy.

Pernicious Anemia

Pernicious anemia is a disease in which there is an abnormality in the absorption of vitamin B_{12}. B_{12} is required for the normal maturation of bone marrow precursors, so that failure of B_{12} absorption leads to a deficit in production of mature erythrocytes and to anemia. Absorption of B_{12} requires the action of a substance known as *intrinsic factor* that is secreted by some specialized cells lining the stomach (parietal cells). Pernicious anemia is associated with two distinct antibodies. One reacts specifically with the parietal cells of the gastric mucosa. The presence of this antibody is almost invariably associated with a reduction in acid secretion, atrophic gastritis, and lymphocytic infiltration. Cellular reactions (delayed hypersensitivity) or ADCC are most likely responsible for atrophic gastritis.

The second antibody is to intrinsic factor itself. This antibody was first observed because of an acquired resistance to intrinsic factor in patients treated for pernicious anemia. Anti–intrinsic factor antibody can be demonstrated to inhibit the binding of vitamin B_{12} to intrinsic factor and is associated with abnormalities of vitamin B_{12} absorption. Two types of anti–intrinsic factor antibody have been observed: (1) blocking antibody, which prevents subsequent formation of vitamin B_{12}–intrinsic factor complexes and is associated with the presence of megaloblastic cells, and (2) binding antibody, which can be shown to bind to intrinsic factor but does not prevent bound intrinsic factor from subsequent combination with vitamin B_{12}. Intrinsic factor blocking antibody appears to play a significant role in the pathogenesis of pernicious anemia.

Polyendocrinopathy

Multiple endocrine gland insufficiency, including primary hypoadrenalism, hypothyroidism, hypogonadism, and diabetes mellitus, in a single patient is a rare but recognized syndrome. More frequently, one patient may have two primary endocrine hypofunctions, such as the combination of hypoadrenalism (Addison's disease) and hypothyroidism. The association of these diseases with circulating autoantibodies has stimulated the hypothesis that there is a loss of immune tolerance to endocrine hormones, perhaps through a depression of controlling suppressor T cells, resulting in autoallergic reactions to more than one endocrine system. Shared epitopes on different endocrine organs have been demonstrated using monoclonal antibodies. It is possible that a viral infection might stimulate such an autoallergic reaction.

Infertility

Antibodies to human chorionic gonadotropin (hCG) have been reported in patients after hCG treatment of women with hypopituitarism as well as in apparently normal individuals. These antibodies may explain the poor results of hCG therapy in some infertile women. Antibodies to hCG are able to prevent or terminate early pregnancy. Studies in Rhesus monkeys demonstrate that active immunization with hCG or passive transfer of antibodies to hCG can effectively reduce the number of conceptions or cause early abortions. Anti-hCG apparently blocks the luteotropic support of the corpus luteum and may affect the development of the placenta or fetus as well. Trials of hCG immunization for selected human populations in which more effective birth control is considered essential have been successful.

Estrogen

Women treated with oral contraceptive pills containing estrogen-like compounds may develop circulating antibody to ethyl estradiol, which may be detected either as free antibody or in the form of circulating immune complexes. These women have a higher incidence of thrombosis than do women who do not develop antibodies.

Hemophilia (Blood Clotting Factors)

The clotting system requires the interaction of up to 30 different factors. Antibodies that may inactivate these factors have been reported. Antibodies to antihemophilic globulin frequently appear in hemophiliacs, who genetically lack this globulin and are treated with infusions containing antihemophilic globulin. The hemophiliac recognizes the antihemophilic globulin as foreign. Similarly, individuals who lack other clotting components may develop antibody to the appropriate component when transfused. For reasons that are poorly understood, individuals with diseases such as lupus erythematosus, Sjögren's syndrome, tuberculosis, or hyperglobulinemia may also produce antibodies to clotting factors that complicate an already confusing clinical picture. Circulating antibodies to clotting factors have also been found in association with penicillin allergy. Finally, some individuals apparently produce circulating anticoagulants unassociated with any known disease. The exact mechanism of action of antibodies to clotting factors is poorly understood. The clinical effect depends on the particular factor or factors affected. Paradoxically some antibodies to phospholipids may promote coagulation, perhaps by activation of platelets. In severe cases, treatment with immunosuppressive drugs such as prednisone or cyclophosphamide may reduce inhibitors of blood clotting factors, but care must be exercised because of possible toxicity.

Erythropoietin

Erythropoietin is a biologically active material, produced by the kidney, that stimulates the production of erythrocytes in the bone marrow. Erythropoietic inhibitors have been identified in the plasma of patients with refractory anemia, and it is possible that these patients may have an antibody that inhibits the action of erythropoietin.

β-Adrenergic Receptor

The β-adrenergic catecholamine hormone receptor – adenylate cyclase complex functions to regulate the level of cyclic AMP in essentially all cells but in particular those involved in anaphylactic reactions, that is, mast cells and smooth muscle end organs (see Chapter 18). The "β-blockade" theory of asthma proposes that chronic asthma is related to a decrease in β-adrenergic sensitivity in bronchial smooth muscle, mucous glands, mucosal blood vessels, and mast cells. Autoantibodies to β_2 (lung) adrenergic receptors have been found in some patients with hay fever and/or asthma. Receptor blockade by β-receptor antibodies raises the level of excitability of the end organ cells, setting the stage for chronic asthma.

Myasthenia Gravis

Myasthenia gravis is characterized by muscle weakness and easy fatigability; weakness is most prominent in the muscles of the face and throat. The disorder is the result of a functional abnormality in which the conduction of nerve impulses from the motor nerve to the muscle fiber is impaired (Fig. 14-3). Patients afflicted with this disease tire very easily; usually they awake with close to normal muscular function, but this deteriorates during the day. The clinical course is punctuated with remissions and exacerbations; total incapacitation and death from respiratory failure may occur. Classical therapy includes thymectomy and the use of medication that inhibits cholinesterase. These may temporarily reverse the muscle weakness, but little can be done if the disease progresses rapidly.

Myasthenia gravis represents more than a single disease syndrome. A partial listing of some of the recognized syndromes is given in Table 14-4. Classical myasthenia gravis is

Table 14-4. Some Myasthenia Syndromes

Type	Characteristics	Pathogenesis
Neonatal	Transient	Placental transfer of maternal anti-AcChR
Adult I	Females under 40	Auto-anti-AcChR (HLA-B8, -DR3 associated)
Adult II	Males over 40	Auto-anti-AcChR (HLA-A2 associated)
Ocular	Eyes only	Unknown
Congenital	Permanent	Unknown
Drug induced (penicillamine)	Transient	Anti-AcChR (HLA-DR1 associated)
Eaton – Lambert	Adults, cancer related	Unknown
Engel's disease	Mild, nonprogressive	Unknown

associated with autoantibodies to the acetylcholine receptor; some variant syndromes have defects in neuromuscular transmission at other levels.

The following associations implicate serum antibody in myasthenia gravis.

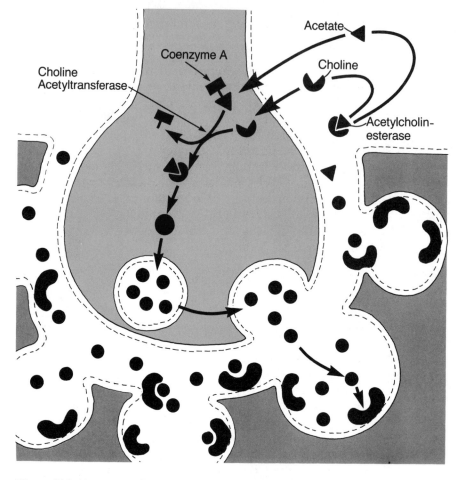

Figure 14-3. Neuromuscular transmission is mediated by acetylcholine (AcCh) released from vesicles in the neuronal axon which bind to acetylcholine receptors (AcChR) in the motor end plate. Acetylcholine is broken into choline and acetate by acetylcholinester-ase, which inactivates AcCh. AcCh is produced from acetate and choline in the motor neuron by choline acetyltransferase. Neuro-muscular transmission may be impaired by (1) de-creased production of AcCh, (2) congenital decrease in AcCh receptors, (3) increased breakdown of AcCh, or (4) action of antibodies to AcChR. (Modi-fied from Lisak RP: Myasthenia gravis: mecha-nisms and management. Hosp Pract, March:101, 1983.)

1. The serum of most myasthenics contains an antibody that binds to muscle fibers and epithelial reticular cells of the thymus. The level of this antibody does not always correlate to the severity of the disease. These muscle-binding antibod-ies could be the cause, a secondary effect of the disease, or only an associated finding.

2. Newborn infants of mothers with myasthenia gravis may exhibit a temporary muscular weakness because of placen-tal transfer of a humoral factor from mother to fetus.

3. Myasthenia is often associated with a peculiar thymic hyper-plasia in which germinal centers are formed in the medulla

of the thymus or with tumors of the thymus; thymectomy may lead to clinical improvement.

4. Myasthenia frequently occurs in patients who demonstrate other diseases of autoimmune origin, such as rheumatoid disease or endocrinopathies. A variety of autoantibodies to organs other than thymus and muscle also occur in myasthenics.

5. An experimental thymitis may be produced by immunization of experimental animals with thymus tissue, but confirmation that these animals have abnormal muscle function has not been uniformly found.

6. The muscles of myasthenics may contain focal collections of lymphocytes (lymphorrhages), suggesting ADCC.

The above associations provide circumstantial evidence supporting an autoimmune mechanism for myasthenia gravis, but they do not prove a causal relationship. Three more direct observations have essentially proven an autoallergic reaction.

1. The defect in myasthenia has been localized to the postsynaptic surface of the neuromuscular junction rather than to the presynaptic surface.

2. Experimental allergic myasthenia gravis (EAMG) has been developed in an animal model.

3. Antibodies to acetylcholine receptors have been demonstrated in the serum of patients with myasthenia gravis (MG).

Until about 10 years ago, it was generally believed that MG was the result of a presynaptic lesion. More recent evidence indicates that this is not true. Purified radiolabeled bungarotoxin binds to acetylcholine receptor (AcChR). The amount of bungarotoxin-binding sites is markedly decreased in muscle from MG patients. Thus, the decrease in neuromuscular transmission in MG is associated with decreased AcChR in the postsynaptic muscle membrane, not with a decreased production or survival of acetylcholine.

The development of an experimental model of MG has provided evidence that immune products to AcChR alter the postsynaptic AcChR sites on muscle membranes. A syndrome with features almost identical to human MG has been produced by immunizing experimental animals with AcChR from the electric eel (Fig. 14-4). AcChR-immunized animals develop precipitating antibody to AcChR, antibody to syngeneic muscle, and a flaccid paralysis that can be reversed by neostigmine, an agent that can also temporarily reverse the muscular weakness of patients with MG. Experimental allergic myasthenia gravis has also been produced by immunization with syngeneic muscle AcChR in complete Freund's adjuvant.

Antibody to AcChR may alter neuromuscular transmission in at least three ways. It may block or inhibit AcChR activ-

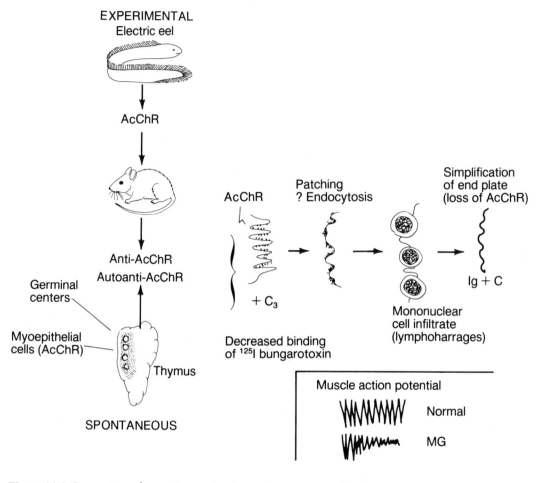

Figure 14-4. Comparison of experimental allergic and naturally occurring myasthenia gravis. Antibody to acetylcholine receptors (AcChR) may be induced in experimental animals by immunization with AcChR from the electric eel or autologous AcChR. Autoantibodies to AcChR occur spontaneously in humans with myasthenia gravis. Both experimental animals and affected humans demonstrate progressive muscle weakness, a decrease in AcChR, immunoglobulin, and complement deposition, and a mononuclear infiltrate at the neuromuscular junction. On restimulation the muscle action potential reveals a rapid decline. The thymus of affected humans may contain germinal centers not normally found in the thymus. Since the thymus contains myoepithelial cells with AcChR, it is possible that autoantibody production of AcChR occurs in the thymus.

ity, cause modulation of AcChR from muscle membranes, or fix complement and cause destruction of the postsynaptic membranes either directly or by ADCC. A simple blocking or inhibition effect seems unlikely, because anti-AcChR does not affect binding of bungarotoxin by AcChR and does not alter the end plate potential of neuromuscular junctions in vitro. A decrease in AcChR activities by modulation or immune destruction appears at this time to be more likely. The addition of immunoglobulin from myasthenic patients to mouse neuromuscular junctions produces an accelerated degradation of the AcChR receptors.

EAMG can be passively transferred with cells from immunized animals or with antibody to AcChR. In either case, there is infiltration of the motor end plate region with mononuclear inflammatory cells. Passive transfer of antibody produces an acute MG syndrome associated with lymphocytic invasion of the motor end plate. Anti-idiotypic antibodies to an anti-AcChR agonist are able to cause MG. The agonist, *trans*-3,3′-bis[α-(trimethylammonia)methyl]azonbenzene bromide (Bis Q), was conjugated to bovine serum albumin, and antibodies to Bis Q

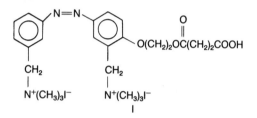

were induced in rabbits. Anti-Bis Q mimics the binding characteristic of AcChR. Immunization of rabbits with anti-Bis Q resulted in anti-anti-Bis Q, which blocked binding of AcCh to AcChR and reproduced experimental myasthenia gravis (Fig. 14-5).

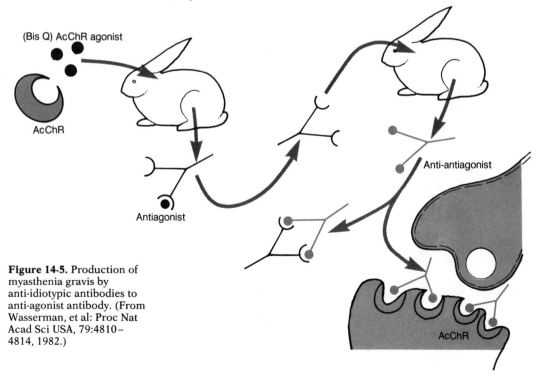

Figure 14-5. Production of myasthenia gravis by anti-idiotypic antibodies to anti-agonist antibody. (From Wasserman, et al: Proc Nat Acad Sci USA, 79:4810–4814, 1982.)

Finally, antibodies to AcChR may be demonstrated in over 90% of MG patients if highly sensitive assays are employed, although lower percentages are found using other methods. Therefore, most of the evidence supports the concept that human MG and EAMG are very similar and that the major pathogenesis of the disease is an antibody-mediated neutralization of AcChR, most likely secondary to formation of antibody–antigen complexes, leading to AcChR modulation or an inflammatory reaction. Treatment of severely myasthenic patients by plasmapheresis (to remove anti-AcChR) and immunosuppressive drugs (to suppress anti-AcChR production) has produced improved muscle reactivity in some patients. This improvement is associated with a fall in anti-AcChR titers in serum.

The primary pathogenic role of antibodies to AcChR does not explain all myasthenic syndromes (Tables 14-4). In addition to autoimmunity, genetic, infectious, and pharmacological mechanisms have been implicated. There is evidence that humoral factors produced in the thymus may be the blocking agent. The synthetic polypeptide containing amino acids 29–41 of thymopoietin is able to block neuromuscular transmission in mice, and the block is reversible by neostigmine. This same peptide is able to induce T cell differentiation. It is speculated that the neuromuscular block in MG is caused by release of thymopoietin from the thymus as a result of an autoallergic thymitis. Some support for this mechanism is provided by the observation that thymectomy early in the course of MG frequently has a beneficial effect. The presence of anti-AcChR is explained as being secondary or an epiphenomenon and not causally related to the neuromuscular block. Participation of a thymopoietin blocking mechanism in MG cannot be ruled out at this time, but most data support a more direct pathogenic role for antibody to AcChR.

Dopamine Receptor

It has been hypothesized that schizophrenia might be caused, at least in part, by autoantibodies to dopamine receptors. Antipsychotic drugs effective in the treatment of schizophrenia block dopamine receptors. Schizophrenia may be caused by overactivity of dopaminergic pathways. Dopamine receptor stimulating autoantibodies have been suggested as a possible cause for overactivity. Antiserum to brain tissue evokes epileptic activity when applied topically to the cerebral cortex of animals.

Associated with the pandemic of influenza between 1919 and 1926 was a variety of parkinsonism disorders known collectively as Von Economo's encephalitis. It has been argued that certain strains of virus may have had an affinity for dopamine receptors, resulting in selective destruction of extrapyramidal neurons.

Drugs

Antibodies to drugs may produce a number of different diseases, such as hemolytic anemias (Chapters 15) and immune complex disease (Chapter 16). Antibodies to drugs may also be used to treat drug overdoses. For instance, digoxin specific F(ab')$_2$ antibody fragments have been used to reduce digitoxin levels rapidly in cases of digitoxin poisoning. Antibody inhibition also affects other drugs such as steroids, chloramphenicol, morphine, oxytocin, and vasopressin.

Other Antibodies

Autoantibodies to vasopressin in rabbits produce diabetes insipidus. Antibodies to gluten may react with gluten bound to epithelial cells and damage intestinal epithelium by an ADCC mechanism, causing sprue or celiac disease. Passive antibodies to gastrin have been used to reduce serum gastrin levels in patients with the Zollinger–Ellison syndrome (intractable peptic ulcers caused by high gastrin levels). Sheep immunized with inhibin, a nonsteroid hormone found in ovarian follicular fluid which inhibits follicle-stimulating hormone (FSH), have an increased ovulation rate. This has resulted in increased fecundity in sheep in Australia. Autoantibodies to parathyroid hormone receptors are found in patients with secondary hyperparathyroidism. These antibodies block binding of hormone to receptors.

Ligands, Receptors, and Idiotypes

Antibodies, hormone receptors, and enzymes have important similarities. Each type of molecule is organized into functional domains consisting of a specific ligand-binding domain and a transmission domain. Reaction of the binding domain with ligand results in alteration of the transmission domain and activation of an effector system. Antibodies, hormone receptors, and enzymes are able to distinguish a series of ligands with similar structures and bind the appropriate ligand with a high affinity (Fig. 14-6). Each has epitopes specific for the binding site as well as epitopes on nonbinding portions of the molecule.

Antibodies to receptors, enzymes, or other antibodies may react with ligand (antigen)-binding site epitopes or with nonbinding epitopes (Fig. 14-7). Antibodies that react directly with the binding site may mimic the structure of the natural ligand.

Anti-idiotypes and Ligand Mimicry

The interrelationship of antibodies to ligands and receptors provides an idiotype network of related structures (Fig. 14-8). The paratope (antigen-binding site) of antibody to the ligand will mimic the receptor for the ligand. The anti-idiotype to the antiligand (anti-antiligand) will mimic the ligand. Similarly, antibody to the receptor may mimic the ligand, and anti-idiotype to the antireceptor (anti-antireceptor) may mimic the re-

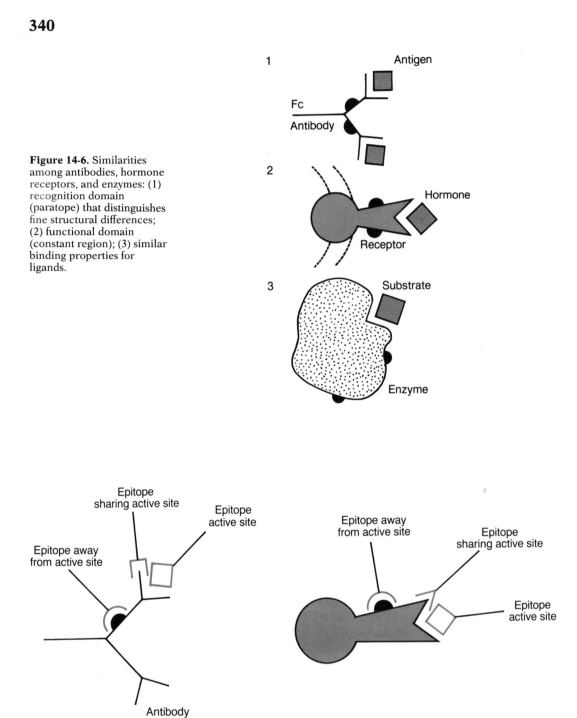

Figure 14-6. Similarities among antibodies, hormone receptors, and enzymes: (1) recognition domain (paratope) that distinguishes fine structural differences; (2) functional domain (constant region); (3) similar binding properties for ligands.

Figure 14-7. Antibodies to receptors may bind (1) the active site, (2) epitopes away from the active site, or (3) epitopes sharing part of the active site. Anti-idiotypes may react with (1) the active site of antibody, (2) epitopes away from the active site, or (3) epitopes sharing part of the active site.

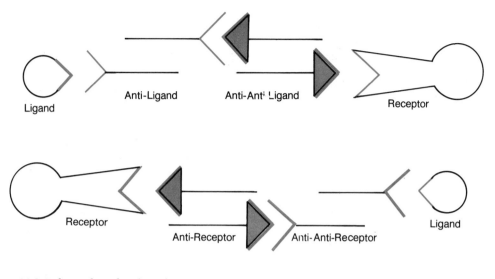

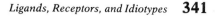

Figure 14-8. Relationship of ligand, antiligand, anti-idiotypes, receptor, anti-receptor, and anti-idiotypes. An immune response to a ligand may result in antibodies that mimic the receptor and anti-idiotypes that mimic the ligand; an immune response to the receptor may produce antibodies that mimic the ligand and anti-idiotypes that mimic the receptor.

ceptor site for the ligand. In this way a network of interactions may be completed (Fig. 14-9).

Figure 14-9. The ligand–antibody–receptor network. An immune response to a ligand may result in antibodies that mimic the receptor or the ligand (anti-antireceptor). An immune response to a receptor may produce antibodies that mimic the ligand or the receptor. In this way immune response to either ligand or receptor may produce inactivating or activating antibodies. Experimental animals immunized with insulin develop not only antibodies to insulin, but also antibodies to the insulin receptor.

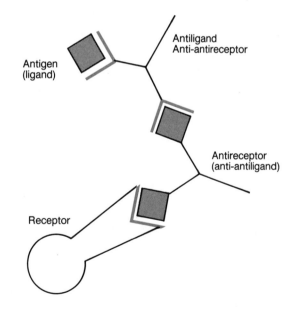

Anti-idiotypes and Disease

Some examples of molecular mimicry between biologically active ligands and anti-idiotypic antibodies to antiligands are:

1. Anti-idiotypic antibodies against anti-insulin, containing the internal image of insulin, interact with the membrane-bound insulin receptor and mimic insulin action in vitro.

2. Anti-β-adrenergic ligand anti-idiotype antibodies bind to the β-adrenergic receptor and stimulate cyclase activity.

3. Rabbits immunized with rat anti-human TSH antibodies produce anti-antibodies that inhibit the binding of TSH to the TSH receptor (Fig. 14-10).

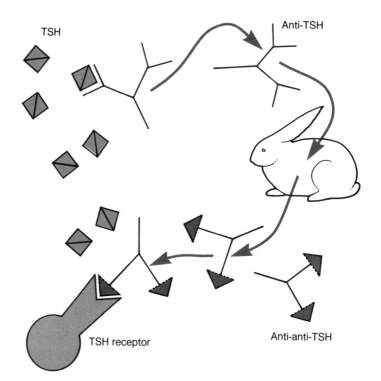

Figure 14-10. Production of TSH blocking antibodies by immunization of rabbits with anti-TSH. Anti-idiotype to anti-TSH reacts with TSH receptor and blocks TSH binding.

4. Antibodies to an agonist of the acetylcholine receptor mimic the binding characteristics of acetylcholine receptor, that is, the anti-agonist antibody binding site binds the same ligands as the receptor. An anti-idiotypic antibody to the anti-agonist causes myasthenia gravis. (See above.)

Neutralizing Antibodies: Cause and Effect

The presence of antibodies to a biologically active molecule in a patient with a given disease does not necessarily mean that the antibody actually causes the disease or is even responsible for any of the symptoms of the disease. Pierre Grabar has postulated that most autoantibodies are part of a physiological system for handling metabolic or catabolic products (transporters). Autoantibodies help in disposing of self materials, particularly if an unrelated event causes release of abnormally high amounts of tissue components. For example, massive tissue necrosis in an acute myocardial infarction releases intracellular antigens and triggers autoantibody formation. In this example, autoantibody formation occurs secondarily to cell necrosis and is not responsible for initiating this type of tissue damage. However, it has become increasingly apparent that autoantibodies either may produce disease as a primary mechanism or may cause resistance to therapy or other secondary effects. For a more encompassing discussion of autoimmunity and tolerance see Chapter 11.

Summary

Circulating antibodies to biologically active molecules may effectively inactivate or neutralize the activity of these molecules and thus produce deficiency diseases. In some instances, autoantibodies may actually stimulate increased function. Biologically active molecules that may be affected by antibodies include hormones, enzymes, growth factors, clotting factors, and cell surface receptors. Inactivation may occur by alteration of tertiary structure, blocking of active sites, or modulation of cell surface receptors. Autoantibodies to endocrine glands, hormones, or hormone receptors are the best understood examples of these activation or inactivation reactions. Antiantibodies (anti-idiotypes) formed to antibodies that react with receptors or ligands may mimic the receptor or ligand (mirror image, molecular mimicry) and function either to activate or to inactivate biological processes.

References

Mechanism of Inactivation

Cinader B (ed): Antibodies to Biologically Active Molecules. New York, Pergamon, 1967.

Melchers F, Messer W: The mechanism of activation of mutant β-galactosidase by specific antibodies. Eur J Biochem 35:380, 1973.

Rotman MB, Celada F: Antibody-mediated activation of a defective β-D-galactosidase extracted from an Escherichia coli mutant. Proc Nat Acad Sci USA 60:660, 1968.

Weigle WO: Fate and biological action of antigen–antibody complexes. Adv Immunol 1:283, 1961.

Diabetes Mellitus

Banting FG, Franks WR, Gairns S: Anti-insulin activity of serum of insulin-treated patients. Am J Psychiatry 95:562, 1938.

Berson SA, Yalow RS: Quantitative aspects of reaction between insulin and insulin-binding antibody. J Clin Invest 38:1996, 1959.

de Shazo RD, Levinson AI, Boehm T, Evans R, Ward G Jr: Severe persistent biphasic local (immediate and late) skin reactions to insulin. J Allergy Clin Immunol 59:161, 1977.

Flier JS, Kahn CR, Jarrett DB, Roth J: Characterization of antibodies to the insulin receptor. A case of insulin-resistant diabetes in man. J Clin Invest 58:1442, 1976.

Harrison LC, Kahn CR: Autoantibodies to the insulin receptor. Clinical significance and experimental application. Clin Immunol 4:107, 1985.

Jacobs S, Chang KJ, Cuatrecasas P: Antibodies to purified insulin receptor have insulin-like activity. Science 200:1283, 1978.

Kahn GR, Baird K, Flier JS, Jarrett DB: Effects of autoantibodies to the insulin receptor on isolated adipocytes. J Clin Invest 60:1106, 1977.

Little JA, Lee R, Sebriakova M, Csima A: Insulin antibodies and clinical complications in diabetes treated for five years with lente or sulfated insulin. Diabetes 26:980, 1977.

MacLaren NK: Viral and immunologic basis of beta cell failure in insulin-dependent diabetes. Am J Dis Child 131:1149, 1977.

Nerup J, Platz P, Ryder LP, Thomsen M, Svejgaard A: HLA, islet cell autoantibodies and types of diabetes mellitus. Diabetes 27:247, 1978.

Obberghen EV, Kahn CR: Autoantibodies and insulin receptor. Mol Cell Endocrinol 22:271, 1981.

Paley RG, Tunbridge RE: Dermal reactions to insulin therapy. Diabetes 1:22, 1952.

Pope CC: The immunology of insulin. Adv Immunol 5:209, 1966.

Roth J: Insulin receptor in diabetes. Hosp Pract 17:98, 1980.

Yalow RS, Berson SA: Apparent inhibition of liver insulinase activity by serum and serum fractions containing insulin-binding antibody. J Clin Invest 36:648, 1957.

Yasuna E: Generalized allergic reactions to insulin. J Allergy 12:295, 1940.

Thyroid Disease

Doniach D, Roitt IM: Autoimmunity in Hashimoto's disease and its implications. J Clin Endocrinol Metab 77:1293, 1957.

Ginsberg J, Segal D, Ehrlich RM, Walfish DG: Inappropriate triiodothyronine (T$_3$) and thyroxine (T$_4$) radioimmunoassay levels secondary to circulating thyroid hormone autoantibodies. Clin Endocrinol (Oxf) 8:133, 1978.

Heide DV, et al: Circulating immune complexes and thyroid stimulating immunoglobulins before, during and after antithyroid drug therapy in patients with Graves' disease. Lancet 1:1376, 1980.

Karlsson FA, Wibell L, Wide L: Hypothyroidism due to thyroid-hormone–binding antibodies. N Engl J Med 296:1146, 1977.

Kriss JP: Graves' ophthalmopathy: etiology and treatment. Hosp Pract 10:125, 1975.

McKenzie JM: Humoral factors in the pathogenesis of Graves' disease. Physiol Rev 48:252, 1968.

McKenzie JM, Zakarija M: LATS in Graves' disease. Recent Prog Horm Res 33:29, 1977.

Ochi Y, DeGroot LJ: Long acting thyroid stimulator of Graves' disease. N Engl J Med 278:718, 1968.

Solomon DH, Beall GN: Thyroid-stimulating activity in the serum of immunized rabbits. II. Nature of the thyroid-stimulating material. J Clin Endocrinol Metab 28:1496, 1968.

Volpé R: Autoimmune thyroid disease. Hosp Pract 19:141, 1984.

Weiner JD, VouderGaag RD: Autoimmunity and the pathogenesis of localized thyroid autonomy (Plummer's disease). Clin Endocrinol 23:635, 1985.

Zakarija M, McKenzie JM: Thyroid stimulating hormone in Graves' disease. Life Sci 32:31, 1983.

Pernicious Anemia

Glass GBJ: Gastric intrinsic factor and its function in the metabolism of B_{12}. Physiol Rev 43:529, 1963.

Goldberg LS, Bluestone R, Steihm ER, Terasaki PI, Weisbart RH: Human autoimmunity, with pernicious anemia as a model. Ann Intern Med 81:372, 1974.

Irvine WJ: Immunologic aspects of pernicious anemia. N Engl J Med 273:432, 1965.

Jeffries GH, Sleisenger MH: Studies of parietal cell antibody in pernicious anemia. J Clin Invest 44:2021, 1965.

Kawashima K: Effects of gastric antibodies on gastric secretion. II. Effects of rabbit antibodies against rat gastric mucosa and gastric juice on gastric secretion in the rat. Jap J Pharmacol 22:155–165, 1972.

Taylor KB, Roitt IM, Doniach D, Couchman KG, Shapland C: Autoimmune phenomena in pernicious anemia. Gastric antibodies. Br Med J 2:1347, 1962.

Fertility

Beaumont V, Lemort N, Beaumont JL: Oral contraception, circulating immune complexes, antiethirylestradiol antibodies and thrombosis. Am J Reprod Immunol 2:8, 1982.

Musch K, Wolf AS, Lauritzen C: Antibodies to chorionic gonadotropin in humans. Clin Chim Acta 113:95, 1981.

Nash HA, Chang CC, Tsong YY: Formulation of a potential antipregnancy vaccine based on the β-subunit of human chronic gonadotropin. J Reprod Immunol 7:151, 1985.

Talwar GP. Immunology of gonadotropin-releasing hormone. J Steroid Biochem 23: 795, 1985.

Talwar GP, et al: Anti-hCG immunization. Contraception 18:19,23,35,51,59,71,91, 1978.

Tung KSK, et al: The black mink (Mustela vison): a natural model of immunologic male infertility. J Exp Med 154:1016, 1981.

Wood DM, Liu C, Dunbar BS: Effect of alloimmunization and heteroimmunization with zonae pellucidae on fertility in rabbits. Biol Reprod 25:439, 1981.

β-Adrenergic Receptors

Courand PO, Lu BZ, Schmutz A, et al: Immunologic studies of β-adrenergic receptors. J Cell Biochem 21:187, 1983.

Guillet JG, Chanet S, Hoeberke J, Strosberg AD: Production and detection of monoclonal anti-idiotype antibodies directed against a monoclonal anti-β-adrenergic ligand antibody. J Immunol Methods 74:163, 1984.

Venter JG, Fraser CM, Harrison LC: Autoantibodies to β_2 adrenergic receptors: a possible cause of adrenergic hyporesponsiveness in allergic rhinitis asthma. Science 207:1361, 1980.

Myasthenia Gravis

Bussard EF: The clinical history and postmortem examination of five cases of myasthenia gravis. Brain 28:438, 1905.

Castleman B: Pathology of the thymus gland in myasthenia gravis. *In* Viets HR, Schwab RS (eds): Thymectomy for Myasthenia Gravis. Springfield, Ill., Thomas, 1960.

Dau P, Lindstrom JM, Cassel CK, Denys EH, Shev EE, Spitler LE: Plasmapheresis and immunosuppressive drug therapy in myasthenia gravis. N Engl J Med 297:1134, 1977.

Elias SB, Appel SH: Recent advances in myasthenia gravis. Life Sci 18:1031, 1976.

Fambrough D, Drachman D, Satyamurti S: Neuromuscular junction in myasthenia gravis: decreased acetylcholine receptors. Science 182:293, 1973.

Fenichel GM: Clinical syndrome of myasthenia in infancy and childhood. A review. Arch Neurol 35:97, 1978.

Galbraith RF, Summerskill MA, Murray J: Systemic lupus erythematosus, cirrhosis and ulcerative colitis after thymectomy for myasthenia gravis. N Engl J Med 270:229, 1964.

Goldstein G, Hoffman WW: Electrophysiological changes similar to those of myasthenia gravis in rats with experimental autoimmune thymitis. J Neurol Neurosurg Psychiatry 31:453, 1968.

Grob D (ed): Myasthenia gravis. Ann NY Acad Sci 274:1976.

Kelly RB, Hall ZW: Immunology of the neuromuscular function. *In* Brockes J (ed): Neuroimmunology. New York, Plenum, 1982.

Lennon VA, Lindstrom J, Seybold ME: Experimental autoimmune myasthenia: a model of myasthenia gravis in rats and guinea pigs. J Exp Med 141:1365, 1975.

Lindstrom JM, Einarson BL, Lennon VA, Seybold ME: Pathological mechanism in experimental autoimmune myasthenia gravis. I. Immunogenicity of syngeneic muscle acetycholine receptor and quantitative extraction of receptor and antibody–receptor complexes from muscles of rats with experimental autoimmune myasthenia gravis. J Exp Med 144:726, 1976.

Lindstrom JM, Engel AG, Seybold ME, Lennon VA, Lambert EH: Pathological mechanisms in experimental autoimmune myasthenia gravis. II. Passive transfer of experimental autoimmune myasthenia gravis in rats with anti-acetylcholine receptor antibodies. J Exp Med 144:739, 1976.

Lindstrom JM, Lennon VA, Seybold ME, Whittingham S: Experimental autoimmune myasthenia gravis and myasthenia gravis: biochemical and immunochemical aspects. Ann NY Acad Sci 274:254, 1976.

Lisak RP: Myasthenia gravis: mechanisms and management. Hosp Pract 17:101, 1983.

Osserman KE: Myasthenia Gravis. New York, Grune & Stratton, 1958.

Osterman PO, Aquilonius SM: Treatment of myasthenia gravis. Pharm Int, April: 94, 1985.

Papatestas AE, Alpert LI, Osserman KE, Osserman RS, Kark AE: Studies in myasthenia gravis: effects of thymectomy. Results on 185 patients with nonthymomatous and thymomatous myasthenia gravis, 1941–1969. Am J Med 50:465, 1971.

Patrick J, Lindstrom J: Autoimmune response to acetycholine receptor. Science 180:821, 1973.

Simpson JA: Myasthenia gravis: a new hypothesis. Scott Med J 5:419, 1960.

Stanley EF, Drachman DB: Effect of myasthenic immunoglobulin on acetylcholine receptors of intact mammalian neuromuscular junctions. Science 200:1285, 1978.

Strauss AJL, van der Geld HWR, Kemp PG Jr, Exum ED, Goodman HC: Immunological concomitants of myasthenia gravis. Ann NY Acad Sci 124:744, 1965.

Strickroot FL, Schaeffer RL, Bergo HL: Myasthenia gravis occurring in an infant born of a myasthenic mother. JAMA 120:1207, 1942.

Tarrab-Hazdi R, Aharonov A, Abramsky O, Yaar I, Fuchs S: Passive transfer of experimental autoimmune myasthenia by lymph node cells in inbred guinea pigs. J Exp Med 142:785, 1975.

van der Geld HWR, Feltkamp TEW, VanLoghem JJ, Oosterhuis HJGH, Biemond A: Multiple antibody production in myasthenia gravis. Lancet 2:373, 1963.

Vetters JM, Simpson JA, Folkard A: Experimental myasthenia gravis. Lancet 2:29, 1969.

Viets HR: Myasthenia gravis. N Engl J Med 251:97,141, 1954.

Anticoagulants

Hultin MB, Shapiro SS, Bowman HS, Gill FM, Andrews AT, Marinez J, Eyster ME, Sherwood WC: Immunosuppressive therapy of Factor VIII inhibitors. Blood 48:94, 1976.

Margolius A, Jackson DP, Ratnoff OD: Circulating anticoagulants: a study of 40 cases and a review of the literature. Medicine 40:197, 1961.

Shapiro SS, Hultin M: Acquired inhibitors to the blood coagulation factors. Semin Thromb Hemostasis 1:336, 1975.

Other Diseases

Appel GB, Holub DA: The syndrome of multiple endocrine gland deficiencies. Am J Med 61:129, 1976.

Butler VP, Chen JP: Digitoxin specific autoantibodies. Proc Nat Acad Sci USA 57:71, 1967.

Gordon AS, Cooper GW, Zanjani ED: The kidney and erythropoiesis. Semin Hematol 4:337, 1967.

Jepson JH, Lowenstein L: Panhypoplasia of the bone marrow. I. Demonstration of a plasma factor with anti-erythropoietin-like activity. Can Med Assoc J 99:99, 1968.

Levitt MD, Cooperband SR: Hyperamylasemia from the binding of serum amylase by an 11S IgA globulin. N Engl J Med 278:474, 1968.

Smolarz A, Roesch E, Lenz E, et al: Digoxin specific antibody (Fab) fragments in 34 cases of severe digitalis intoxication. Clin Toxicol 23:327, 1985.

Volpe R: The role of autoimmunity in hypoendocrine and hyperendocrine function. Ann Intern Med 87:86, 1977.

Idiotypes and Receptors

Strosberg AD: Anti-idiotype and anti-hormone receptor antibodies. Springer Semin Immunopathol 6:67, 1983.

Wasserman NH, Penn AS, Freimuth PI, et al: Anti-idiotype route to anti-acetylcholine receptor antibodies and experimental myasthenia gravis. Proc Nat Acad Sci USA 79:4810, 1982.

Yavin E, Yavin Z, Schneider MD, Kohn LD: Monoclonal antibodies to the thyrotropin receptor: implications for receptor structure and the action of autoantibodies in Graves disease. Proc Nat Acad Sci USA 78:3180, 1981.

Cause and Effect

Grabar P: Hypothesis: Auto-antibodies and immunological theories: an analytical review. Clin Immunol Immunopathol 4:453, 1975.

15 | Cytotoxic or Cytolytic Reactions

Cytotoxic or cytolytic reactions occur when antibody reacts with either an antigenic component of a cell membrane or an antigen that has become passively attached to a cell. The interaction of antigen and antibody may activate the complement system and cause death or lysis of the target cell or result in adherence of antibody-coated cells to phagocytic cells and phagocytosis via aggregated immunoglobulin Fc and/or C3b receptor binding (Fig. 15-1).

Cytotoxic or cytolytic reactions are mediated by IgM or those IgG immunoglobulin subclasses that have the capacity to activate complement. Selected IgG subclasses, for example IgG$_3$ and IgG$_1$, bind complement better than IgG$_2$ or IgG$_4$. One IgM antibody molecule reacting with a cell is sufficient to activate complement, whereas two IgG molecules in close apposition are required, so that antibodies of the IgM class are much more efficient in causing lytic reactions than antibodies of the IgG class (approximately 600 times more efficient; for more information see Chapter 12). If the number of antigen sites on a cell is low, IgG coating may not result in complement fixation. The ultimate effect depends upon the type of cell involved, antibody characteristics, number of antigen sites per cell, and amount of antibody available. The cells usually affected are red blood cells (erythrocytes), white blood cells, platelets, and vascular endothelium. The resulting diseases are hemolytic anemia, thrombocytopenia, agranulocytosis, and vascular purpura, and they are grouped together as immunohematologic diseases. An experimental model of the effects of an anti-red cell antibody is illustrated in Figure 15-2.

Immunohemato-logic Diseases

Disease conditions arising from the immune destruction of red blood cells result from loss of erythrocyte function, from the damaging effects of the released cell contents, and from toxic

349

350

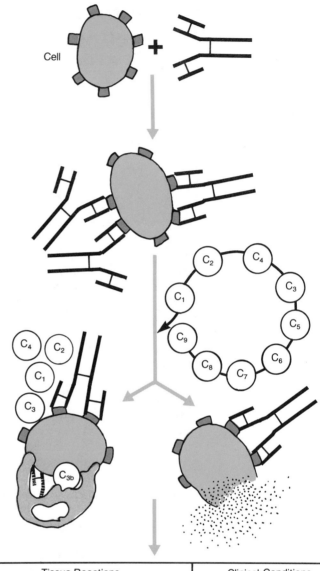

Figure 15-1. Cytotoxic or cytolytic reactions. These reactions most often affect cellular elements in intimate contact with circulating plasma, such as erythrocytes, leukocytes, platelets, or vascular endothelium. Circulating humoral antibody reacts with antigens present on cell membrane. Through action of the complement system, the integrity of cell membrane is compromised and the cell lysed. The osmotic difference in intracellular and extracellular fluids causes release of intracellular fluids or the altered cell is subject to phagocytosis. Such reactions may be observed experimentally with antibody to solid tissue cells, such as liver cells, when these cells are placed in suspension in appropriate antiserum and complement, indicating that this mechanism is not due to a peculiarity in the membranes of the affected cells but to the availability of the cell to action of antibody and complement.

Tissue Reactions	Clinical Conditions
1. ERYTHROCYTES Hemolysis	1. HEMOLYTIC ANEMIA
2. LEUKOCYTES Agranulocytosis	2. SUSCEPTIBILITY TO INFECTION
3. PLATELETS Thrombocytopenia	3. PURPURA
4. VASCULAR ENDOTHELIUM Vascular fragility	4. VASCULAR PURPURA

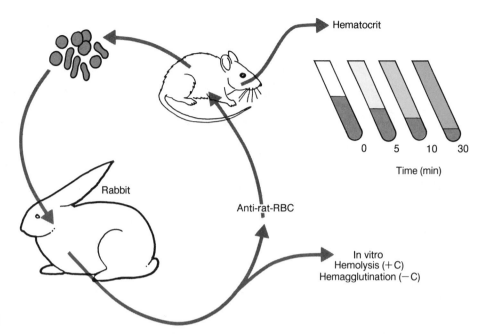

Figure 15-2. Experimental model of acute hemolytic reaction. (1) Rat RBC are used to immunize a rabbit to produce rabbit anti-rat RBC serum. (2) In vitro, this antiserum will lyse rat RBC in the presence of complement. If the antiserum is decomplemented, agglutination, but not lysis, occurs. (3) Injection of the rabbit anti-rat RBC serum into rats results in a rapid drop in the hematocrit (the hematocrit is the proportion of cells in the blood as compared with plasma) and increasing red color in the plasma due to hemoglobin released from lysed cells. Death of the infected rat occurs at doses sufficient to reduce the hematocrit below 20%. In the dead rat the organs, particularly the liver and spleen, are filled with red blood cells.

Erythrocytes (Anemia)

effects due to antigen–antibody complexes formed. These disorders include transfusion reactions, erythroblastosis fetalis, acquired autoimmune hemolytic diseases, and hemolytic reactions to drugs (Fig. 15-3).

Transfusion Reactions

A transfusion reaction occurs when circulating antibody of host origin contacts erythrocytes from an incompatible donor. The antigen is exogenous and the immune response is endogenous. Blood group antigens are genetically controlled cell surface structures present on blood cells. Some characteristics of the ABO blood group system are presented in Figure 15-4. An individual with blood type A has isoantibodies against type B erythrocytes. If this individual is transfused with type B blood, the anti-B antibodies react with B erythrocytes, causing them to agglutinate. These sensitized cells may then be lysed by complement or destroyed in the spleen. Over 14 human red blood cell antigen systems, which include over 60 different blood group factors, are known. The ABO and Rh systems are the most important to identify for the routine transfusion service, as these represent the majority of incompatibilities implicated in transfusion reactions. The other antigens are not usually of

Figure 15-3. Hemolytic reactions. Shown are four types of hemolytic reactions caused by antibody-mediated complement activation, and the source of the antibody and antigen: (I). Transfusion reactions. Erythrocytes from a donor (A⁺) that are antigenic for a recipient whose serum contains antibody to the donor's erythrocyte antigen (O anti-A) will be lysed immediately upon transfusion, resulting in release of hemoglobin and a clinical syndrome known as a transfusion reaction. Exogenous antigen–endogenous antibody. (II). Erythroblastosis fetalis. Rh⁺ fetal erythrocytes cross the placenta and stimulate the production of antibody to Rh if the mother is not Rh⁺. These antibodies will cross back through the placenta to attack fetal erythrocytes. Endogenous antigen–exogenous antibody. (III). Autoimmune hemolytic anemia. An individual becomes sensitized to the antigens of his own erythrocytes (autoantibody). Endogenous antigen–endogenous antibody. (IV). Reverse transfusion reaction. Antibodies are transfused from a donor to a recipient whose red cells contain the antigen. This passively transferred antibody causes lysis of recipient red cells. Endogenous antigen–exogenous antibody.

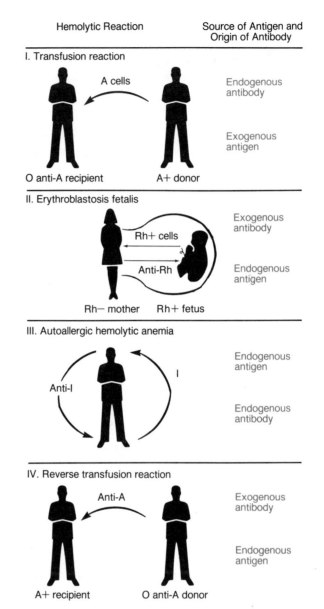

importance clinically, because of low antigenicity or low incompatibility frequency. Transfusion reactions are usually predictable from blood group typing, serum screening for antierythrocyte antibodies, or cross-matching. For blood typing, the red cells of an individual are tested in vitro for reaction with a panel of selected antisera that are known to react with given blood group antigens. For antibody screening the serum of a potential recipient is tested in vitro with red cells from two or three donors who have been antigen typed and represent all of the common red cell antibodies among them. For cross-matching, the serum from a potential recipient is mixed with the cells of a potential donor. If agglutination occurs, the donor

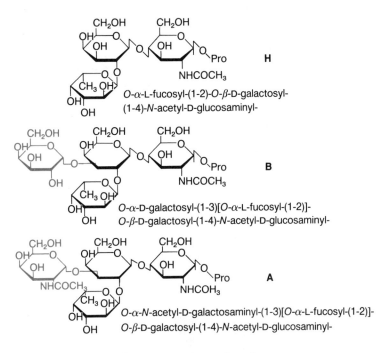

H

O-α-L-fucosyl-(1-2)-O-β-D-galactosyl-
(1-4)-N-acetyl-D-glucosaminyl-

B

O-α-D-galactosyl-(1-3)[O-α-L-fucosyl-(1-2)]-
O-β-D-galactosyl-(1-4)-N-acetyl-D-glucosaminyl-

A

O-α-N-acetyl-D-galactosaminyl-(1-3)[O-α-L-fucosyl-(1-2)]-
O-β-D-galactosyl-(1-4)-N-acetyl-D-glucosaminyl-

Figure 15-4. Chemical relations of ABO blood group system. Blood group identification depends on the presence of antigenic specificities on surfaces of red cells. Blood group characteristics are inherited according to simple Mendelian laws. ABO blood group antigens have been characterized by analysis of purified blood group substances. They contain about 85% carbohydrate and 15% amino acids. The peptide component contains 15 amino acids and is the same for each blood group substance. Antigenic specificity is determined by carbohydrate moiety. Individuals with type O blood who do not have A or B group specificity have a specificity now recognized as H, which consists of three sugar groups attached to a peptide. Addition of a fourth sugar group to the basic H structure produces A or B specificity. If additional sugar is O-α-D-galactose, specificity is B; if it is O-α-N-acetyl-D-galactose, specificity is A. Formation of H substance is controlled by a pair of alleles, H and h. H gene gives rise to production of H specificity. H-active material is converted to A- or B-active substances under the influence of the A or B gene. Rare individuals lack A, B, and H reactivity, presumably due to the inability to form normal precursor for H substance. (Modified from Watkins WM: Science 152:172, 1966.)

cells contain an antigen, the recipient has antibody to the antigen, and the donor cells cannot be used, even if there is no difference in ABO antigens or other detectable major blood groups. The potential for acute transfusion reactions due to the presence of preformed antibodies is easily recognized clinically and should be prevented by the appropriate cell typing, antibody screening, or crossmatch testing.

In some cases, delayed transfusion reactions may occur because of induction in the recipient of an immune response to transfused cells. The transfused donor cells may survive well initially, but after 3–14 days, hemolysis occurs because of the production of an antibody that was not detectable at the time of the initial crossmatch. This is most probably because of a secondary response in a patient previously primed, but could also be because of a primary antibody response. The compatibility test relies on an agglutination endpoint and may, therefore, miss low concentrations of serum antibodies. Patients who receive multiple transfusions frequently develop antibodies to minor blood group antigens. The incidence of hemolytic reactions in any given individual is related to the number of previous transfusions that have been given.

Erythroblastosis Fetalis

The Rh system of red cell antigens was first identified in 1939, and the first case of hemolytic disease of the newborn due to Rh incompatibility was reported in 1941 by Philip Levine and his co-workers. A pregnant woman's blood may lack antigens present in the fetus that are contributed by paternal genes. An Rh$^-$ mother may become sensitized to Rh$^+$ erythrocytes produced by the fetus. If the antibodies formed by the mother cross the placenta, they may destroy the fetal erythrocytes (Fig. 15-5).

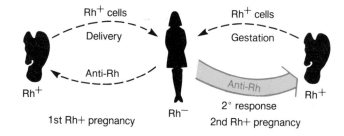

Figure 15-5. Erythroblastosis fetalis. Rh$^-$ mother carrying an Rh$^+$ fetus. During the first pregnancy, sensitization occurs. During subsequent pregnancies of a sensitized mother carrying an Rh$^+$ fetus, anti-Rh antibodies may cross the placenta and react with fetal red cells. During the first pregnancy, small numbers of Rh$^+$ fetal erythrocytes, usually insufficient for sensitization, cross the placenta. However, at delivery a substantial number of Rh$^+$ erythrocytes are released into maternal circulation. In a small percentage of Rh-incompatible pregnancies, this is sufficient to immunize the mother if the mother is not treated with passively administered anti-Rh antibody. During a second pregnancy, the small number of erythrocytes that reach the maternal circulation will induce a secondary antibody response in the mother to the Rh antigen. The maternal antibody is IgG and crosses the placenta to the fetus, where it acts on fetal erythrocytes, causing their destruction.

Destruction of fetal erythrocytes may occur by the action of antibody and complement or by an antibody-dependent cell-mediated mechanism. Thus, red blood cells (RBC) from infants with maternal anti-Rh may be coated with maternal antibody and killed by fetal lymphocytes or macrophages that react with the antibody on the RBC surface through Fc receptors.

The Rh antigenic system is a mosaic of genetically controlled specific antigenic determinants. The antigen in this situation is endogenous, and the immune response exogenous. Because of the proliferation of cells by the fetus in an attempt to make up for the destruction of fetal erythrocytes in the erythrocyte series, a characteristic morphologic picture of extremedullary hematopoiesis may be observed, giving rise to the name *erythroblastosis fetalis*. A high concentration of one hemoglobin breakdown product, bilirubin, during the immediate neonatal period may lead to brain damage (kernicterus).

Prevention of Rh Immunization. Hemolytic disease of the newborn is now largely a preventable disease. Prevention of immunization of Rh⁻ mothers carrying Rh⁺ fetuses is now commonly practiced by treating Rh⁻ mothers who have just delivered an Rh⁺ fetus with passive antibody to Rh⁺ antigens. The observation that led to such a procedure was that protection against Rh immunization occurs if the fetus contains ABO blood group antigens not present in the mother (Fig. 15-6).

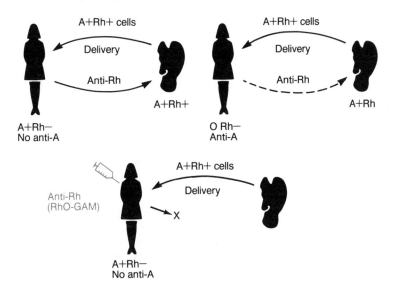

Figure 15-6. Prevention of Rh immunization by passive antibody. Top: Naturally occurring situation in which ABO and Rh incompatibility are combined; sensitization of the mother to Rh⁺ antigens is significantly more frequent than when there is an Rh incompatibility but no ABO incompatibility. The presence of antibody to A in the non-A mother prevents sensitization to the Rh⁺ antigen, whereas the mother with no anti-A becomes sensitized to the Rh system. This observation was used as a rationale for passively transferring antibody to Rh to mothers who were Rh⁻ and were carrying an Rh⁺ fetus. Bottom: Administration of anti-Rh at delivery significantly reduces the incidence of sensitization of the mother to the Rh system; erythroblastosis fetalis has thus become a preventable disease through the application of immunoprophylaxis.

Thus, if the blood of the fetus is A Rh⁺ or B Rh⁺ and the mother's blood is O Rh⁻, the mother develops anti-Rh antibodies less frequently than when the blood of the fetus is O Rh⁺ and the mother's is O Rh⁻, or when the blood of the fetus is A Rh⁺ and the mother's is A Rh⁻. The presence in the mother of antibodies to ABO group antigens on the fetal erythrocytes prevents immunization to the Rh antigens. In Rh incompatibility fetal erythrocytes usually appear in the circulation of the mother in sufficient quantity to stimulate antibody production at the time of delivery, and this is the time most Rh^- mothers first become sensitized by Rh^+ fetal cells. Because of the possibility that such sensitization could be prevented by passive transfer of anti-Rh antisera to Rh^- mothers, trials were made on Rh^- male volunteers. Passive transfer of anti-Rh serum along with Rh^+ cells prevented immunization of these volunteers. Extensive trials were made in Rh^- mothers, and the data clearly demonstrated that the incidence of Rh immunization in subsequent pregnancies can be greatly reduced by the passive transfer of anti-Rh sera (or globulin) to an Rh^- mother at the time of delivery of an Rh^+ fetus.

In addition, since sensitization may occur following spontaneous or therapeutic abortion of an Rh^+ fetus in an Rh^- mother, anti-Rh^+ globulin should also be administered after abortion of an Rh^+ fetus in an Rh^- mother. Rare cases of sensitization may still occur, as by the inadvertent transfusion of Rh^+ blood to an Rh^- woman and in a small number of instances when sensitization occurs prior to delivery. Recent studies suggest that antepartum administration of anti-Rh serum can also prevent those rare cases due to in utero sensitization of Rh^- mothers by Rh^+ babies.

Treatment of Erythroblastosis Fetalis. In cases where Rh sensitization has occurred, the affected fetus may be treated by intrauterine transfusion of Rh^- blood cells. Since the transfused blood does not have the Rh antigen, the erythrocytes will not be destroyed by maternal antibodies. However, this procedure has a high rate of complications and must be done only after amniocentesis and analysis of amniotic fluid by optical density to determine the severity of the hemolytic process. Fluoroscopic and ultrasound examination of the fetal position are required in order to place the transfusion needle in the fetal abdomen. The transfused red cells eventually transverse the peritoneum and enter the fetal circulation. In less severe cases, the patient may be followed and transfusions delayed until after birth (exchange transfusion). If the fetal age is sufficient, labor is induced, as the risks of prematurity are less than the risk of intrauterine transfusion. Exchange transfusions become mandatory to lower neonatal bilirubin if the level of bilirubin becomes high enough to cause brain damage.

One of the factors believed to be important in determining which Rh^- mothers may become sensitized (about one in six will become sensitized if not treated) is the Rh type of the grandmother. Thus if the grandmother is Rh^+, the mother Rh^-, and the fetus Rh^+, a higher incidence of erythroblastoses is seen than if both the mother and grandmother are Rh^-. This effect may be explained by initial immunization of the Rh^- mother by Rh^+ erythrocytes of the grandmother during fetal development or neonatally.

ABO Hemolytic Disease of Newborn. ABO hemolytic disease of the newborn is usually mild to minimal clinically, even if the mother's blood contains high titers of anti-A or anti-B antibodies and the fetus's blood is A, B, or AB. This may occur for three reasons: (1) anti-A and anti-B antibodies are usually IgM and therefore do not cross the placenta; (2) ABO blood group antigens are widely distributed in the fetal tissues and the placenta, so that the effect upon fetal erythrocytes of any 7 S anti-A or anti-B antibodies that may cross the placenta is diluted out in the sense that antibodies react with many other tissue sites; and (3) ABO blood group antigens are not fully developed on fetal erythrocytes. In contrast, the Rh specificity is unique for erythrocytes, and the effect of anti-Rh antibodies that cross the placenta is concentrated on the fetal erythrocytes that have fully developed Rh antigens.

Acquired Autoimmune Hemolytic Disorders

Acquired autoimmune hemolytic disorders are caused in an individual by formation of antibodies to antigens present on his/her own erythrocytes. Autoimmune hemolytic anemia must be differentiated from congenital metabolic hemolytic disorders by careful testing. The major difference between immune and congenital hemolytic diseases is that the erythrocytes are defective in the latter and do not usually survive in either the patient or a "normal" individual. In contrast, the erythrocytes are normal in patients with immune hemolytic disease and survive better in a "normal" recipient than in the patient. Therefore, congenital disease demonstrates an intracorpuscular defect; immune disease, an extracorpuscular defect. The extracorpuscular defect is an autoantibody. Two major forms of hemolytic disease caused by autoantibodies to red cells have been identified: warm antibody mediated and cold antibody mediated.

Warm Antibody Disease. This disease is almost always caused by IgG antibody that reacts with the patient's own red cells. In two-thirds of the cases, the antibody reacts with Rh determinants. The antibody may appear as an isolated phenomenon (idiopathic), but more frequently is associated with a collagen disease or with a lymphoproliferative disorder, for example, chronic lymphocytic leukemia. The patient's erythrocytes may be coated in vivo with IgG antibody, IgG and complement, or complement alone when tested by the Coombs technique. The cells containing complement alone may have IgG when tested by more sensitive techniques. The action of antibody and complement leads to destruction of the erythrocytes (hemolytic anemia), usually by alteration of the cell membrane and phagocytosis, which occurs principally in the spleen. The reticuloendothelial cells of the phagocytic organs have receptors that bind the Fc region of IgG and C3b coating red blood cells.

Frank intravascular hemolysis by the complete complement sequence may also be observed. Treatment with corticosteroids may abort life-threatening acute hemolytic episodes. Steroids are believed to have at least three possible effects on autoimmune hemolytic anemia: (1) decreased affinity of Fc receptor binding, (2) decreased phagocytic activity of the RES, and (3) decreased antibody production. Splenectomy is of some temporary value, but usually the anemia recurs even after the spleen is removed, indicating that the reticuloendothelial cells of other organs, for example, liver, can cause red cell destruction. The reason for the production of the autoantibody is not clear.

Cold Antibody Disease. Cold reacting antibodies may react not only with red cells but also with other blood cells. They are most commonly of the IgM class, but some are IgG class antibodies. Cold reactive antibodies are usually found in patients with a viral infection or a lymphoproliferative disease. Cold antibody hemolytic disease occurs in two forms: cold agglutinin disease and paroxysmal cold hemoglobinuria. In these disorders, the antierythrocytic antibody is not capable of binding to the red cell at 37°C but will do so at lower temperatures. When cells are coated by antibody in the cooler peripheral circulation and then warmed to core body temperature, complement components bind to the cell membrane and the cells are susceptible to lysis. At warm temperatures, the antibody comes off the cell so that complement may be detected on the affected cells in the absence of antibody. Hemolytic attacks occur on exposure to cold. The cold antibody binds to cells in the exposed areas of the body (skin). These cells are coated with complement and are destroyed on entering the bloodstream of warmer parts of the body.

Paroxysmal cold hemoglobinuria refers to the production of dark urine because of the presence of hemoglobin from lysed red cells. The antibody responsible was first recognized in 1904 and is referred to as Donath–Landsteiner (DL) antibody. Demonstration of the antibody requires two steps: The patient's serum is mixed with erythrocytes at 4°C; the mixture is then warmed to 37°C. Lysis occurs upon warming. This type of antibody was classically found in patients with syphilis, but may occur idiopathically or after a viral infection. The antibody is of the IgG class and the specificity is usually to blood group P.

Cold agglutinin disease is similar, but clear differences have been noted. Intense agglutination of red cells occurs in the cold, which is not the case with DL antibody. The antibody is a monoclonal or polyclonal IgM and is directed to the blood group I specificity. Mycoplasma infections have been associated with polyclonal anti-I formation, whereas monoclonal antibodies occur in lymphoproliferative diseases. Most patients with cold antibody hemolytic disease do well as long as they are kept warm and tolerate a chronic mild anemia with minimal disability. In fact, low titers of cold antibody are found in most normal adults and cause no apparent symptoms.

Hemolytic Reactions to Drugs

Hemolytic reactions to drugs may be activated by at least five mechanisms (Fig. 15-7). Many drugs adhere to red cells and function as haptens. As such, the red cell–hapten complex induces an immune response, and cytotoxic reactions to the red cell or red cell–drug complex may occur. The exact mechanism of such a drug-induced hemolytic reaction depends upon the drug involved. *Penicillin* covalently binds to red cells, and the antibody formed reacts with the penicillin bound to the cell. Immunoglobulin can be demonstrated on the surface of affected cells by the direct Coombs test. If the antibody is extracted from the red cell membrane, it will react only with cells preincubated with penicillin in an indirect Coombs test. *Quinidine* administration can result in quinidine–antibody complexes that bind loosely to red cells. Antibody–quinidine complexes can dissociate from red cell surfaces and in complex form pass from one red cell to another. Destruction of red cells occurs as an "innocent bystander" reaction. Components of complement may be demonstrated on the affected cells in the absence of detectable antibody globulin. *α-Methyl dopa* (aldomet) apparently induces alterations in lymphocytes so that the lymphocytes become "autoreactive." The antibody produced reacts with the patient's own red cells in the absence of bound drug. Normal erythrocytes are destroyed during a hemolytic drug reaction due to aldomet or quinidine, because the autoantibody of the antigen–antibody complex can bind to any red blood cell. In cases of hemolytic reactions to penicillin or quinidine, red cell destruction ceases soon after administration of the drug is stopped; α-methyl dopa hemolytic reactions may persist for as long as a year after the drug is stopped. In hemolytic reactions to quinidine and penicillin, the source of the antigen is exogenous (or a complex of exogenous hapten and host red cell), and the origin of the immune response is endogenous. In hemolytic anemia due to α-methyl dopa the antigen is endogenous and the origin of the immune response is endogenous. *Cephalosporins* alter the red cell membrane in a way that allows nonspecific protein absorption. Thus, patients on cephalosporins may have a positive Coombs test without hemolytic anemia.

Leukocytes (Agranulocytosis)

Antibody effects similar to those described above for erythrocytes may also occur with polymorphonuclear leukocytes, resulting in loss of neutrophils (*agranulocytosis*). However, most

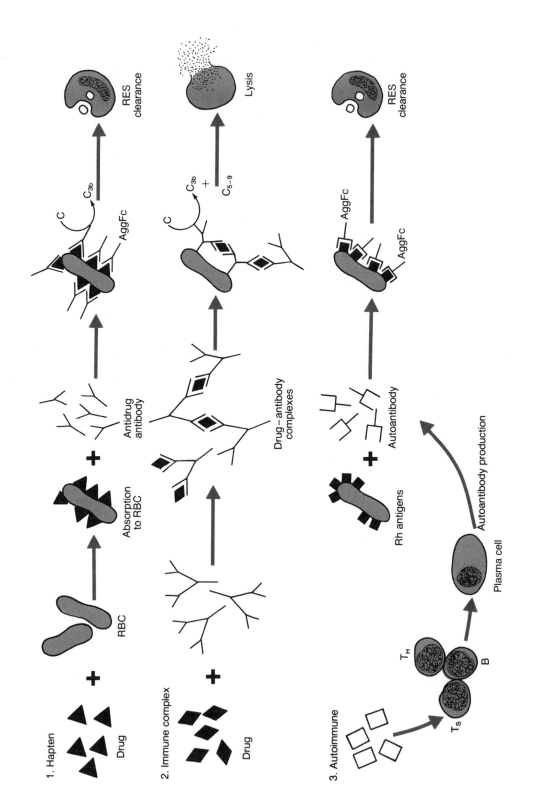

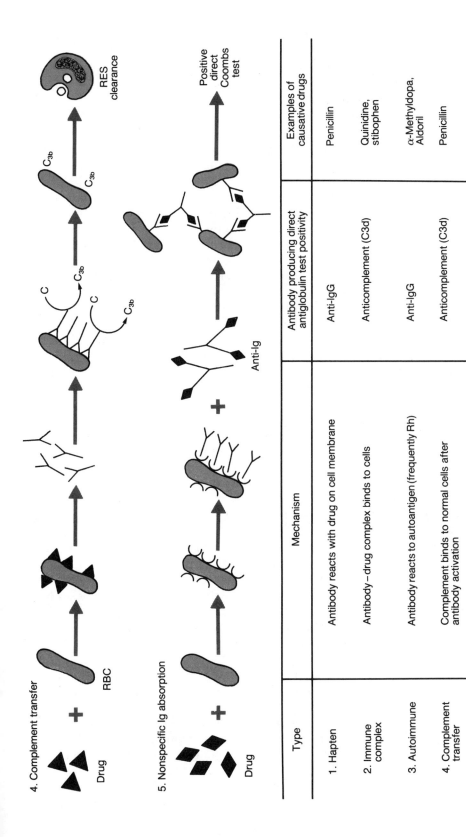

Figure 15-7. Mechanisms of drug-induced hemolytic drug reactions (see text).

cases of agranulocytosis are secondary to a lack of proliferation of granulocytes in the bone marrow on a metabolic basis. Many drugs are known to inhibit granulocyte production. The consequence of leukocyte destruction is a decreased ability to defend against infection.

Neonatal Leukopenia

Destruction of fetal white blood cells may be accomplished by antibodies formed by maternal immunization to fetal leukocyte antigens that cross the placenta.

Drug-Induced Agranulocytosis

Destruction of a patient's own white blood cells may be caused by autoantibodies or by antibodies to certain drugs that adhere to white blood cells and function as haptens. Sulfapyridine and aminopurine are two of the drugs that have been implicated.

In some situations drugs may have a direct nonimmune cytotoxic effect (idiosyncrasy), and some cases of agranulocytosis are caused by a congenital metabolic defect. In nonimmune agranulocytosis, more than one line of leukocyte is usually involved; for instance, in some cases all leukocytes containing granules are destroyed or fail to develop. Antibodies to lymphocytes are found in a variety of human diseases, particularly in acquired immune deficiency syndromes (see Chapters 26 and 28), and may be associated with lymphocyte deficiencies.

Platelets (Bleeding Diathesis or Purpura)

Immune reactions to platelets may cause destruction of platelets with resulting purpura and other hemorrhagic manifestations. The word *purpura* (purple) describes hemorrhage into the skin, easily recognized by the red or purple discoloration produced by the presence of extravasated red cells. The color is first red but becomes darker (purple) and fades to a brownish yellow as the red cells are destroyed or cleared from the site of hemorrhage by macrophages. Since platelets function to prevent such hemorrhages, a loss of platelets permits purpuric lesions to develop. An antiplatelet antibody can be demonstrated in about 60% of the affected individuals. Recent studies reveal that, in some diseases, antigen–antibody complexes cause thrombocytopenia. Currently, sensitive immunoassays are being developed that should increase the sensitivity of antiplatelet antibody tests. Thrombocytopenia may also occur congenitally or secondarily because of increased splenic function (hypersplenism) or other nonimmune consumptive disorders.

Post-transfusion Thrombocytopenic Purpura

This occurs as a result of the production of alloantibody following transfusions of blood products containing allogeneic platelets. The cause of autologous platelet destruction is unclear. This reaction is very rare. It presents as an acute, severe thrombocytopenia occurring about 1 week after a transfusion. Antibodies to the platelet antigen PI^{A1} are invariably found; rarely, other platelet antibody specificities have been implicated. Treatment consists of plasma exchange. This reaction is essentially seen only in women who have been pregnant, suggesting that sensitization may originally occur to platelet antigens from a fetus.

Neonatal Thrombocytopenic Purpura

Neonatal thrombocytopenic purpura occurs as a result of maternal immunization of fetal platelet antigens, with thrombocytopenia occurring in the fetus when this antibody crosses the placenta. Most cases are due to antibodies to PI^{A1} and affect platelets in a way analogous to the effect of anti-Rh on red blood cells in hemolytic disease of the newborn. This can be distinguished from autoimmune neonatal thrombocytopenia by detection of normal levels of platelet bound IgG on maternal platelets.

Idiopathic Thrombocytopenic Purpura

Acute idiopathic thrombocytopenic purpura (ITP) is more common in children than in adults. Most affected individuals have a history of infection (e.g., rubella) occurring 1 to 2 weeks previously. The destruction of platelets may be due to antibodies to antigens of infectious agents adherent to platelets, to antibody–antigen complexes adsorbed to platelets (innocent bystander), or to antibodies to platelets altered by the infectious process. Platelets are destroyed rapidly when transfused into an affected individual. Chronic idiopathic thrombocytopenic purpura is caused by the production of autoantibodies against altered or naturally occurring platelet antigens and is more common in adults. The chronic form is frequently associated with systemic lupus erythematosus or a lymphoproliferative disorder (leukemia, myeloma).

Quinine (Sedormid) Purpura

Quinine purpura is an example of a reaction to a drug acting as a hapten on the platelet surface.

Immune Suppression of Blood Cell Production

Antibody to blood cell precursors may injure proliferating cells in the bone marrow, producing an aplastic anemia or agranulocytosis. Hematopoietic stem cells may have a variety of cell surface antigens, and cells in the erythrocyte, granulocyte, or lymphocyte line may carry differentiation antigens unique for the line. Thus immune suppression may affect all cell lines, or one cell line. Antibodies to stem cells have rarely been found spontaneously in man. Such antibodies to red or white cell precursors have been found associated with aplastic anemia, red cell aplasia, profound panleukopenia, and systemic lupus erythematosus. Thus, although rare, antibodies to blood cell precursors may produce a clinical picture similar to a metabolic defect in blood cell maturation (see also Erythropoietin, Chapter 14).

Vascular Purpura

Hemorrhagic phenomena may occur due to destruction of vascular endothelium. A loss of integrity of small blood vessels permits blood cells to escape, causing purpura and other hemorrhagic manifestations. The syndrome of anaphylactoid purpura may be in this category. Clinically urticarial and hemorrhagic lesions are the most prominent features and tend to occur around joints. Variations in the clinical syndrome include abdominal involvement with edema and hemorrhage into the gastrointestinal tract (Henoch's syndrome); joint involvement with effusion, swelling of the soft tissues, redness, and pain (Schonlein's syndrome); or renal lesions of focal proliferative glomerulonephritis. Vascular purpura may be induced in experimental animals by the injection of heterologous antisera to endothelial antigens.

The immunopathogenic mechanism of vascular purpura is not necessarily direct cytolysis. In fact, most instances of vascular purpura are believed to be caused by focal deposition of antibody–antigen complexes (see Chapter 16), and activation of complement leading to cell lysis or inflammation with polymorphonuclear leukocytes. Henoch–Schonlein purpura is frequently found in association with an IgA immune complex nephritis. Thus vascular purpura may be caused by antibody to vascular endothelium or by a particular form of immune complex reaction. In either case, the clinical manifestation is focal bleeding due to a loss of the integrity of small vessels.

Other Cytotoxic Reactions

Sperm

Autoimmune Diseases

Autologous or allogenic sperm is antigenic when injected into adults, and such immunization may decrease fertility in both females and males. This effect is correlated with serum agglutinating antibodies to sperm after decomplementing the sera by heating. Antibodies to sperm may occur in men who have had a vasectomy, because of extravasation of immunogenic sperm, but no disease manifestations have been documented because of this. Antisperm antibodies are found more frequently in prostitutes than in normal age-matched control women. Intentional sperm immunization of women as a method for controlling pregnancy is possible, but has not been considered practical because of possible deleterious effects of producing autoimmune reactions.

Autoimmune Diseases

Cytotoxic antibody may produce damage in allergic thyroiditis, allergic aspermatogenesis, and other autoallergic diseases, although it is generally believed that the primary mechanism of these diseases is delayed hypersensitivity.

Homograft Rejection

Chandler Stetson in the 1950s showed that specific antisera injected into a graft site may cause an acute "white" graft rejection. Although homograft rejection is usually mediated by sensitized cells (delayed sensitivity), antibody-mediated acute rejection is now well recognized (see Chapter 19).

Forssman Antigen

Forssman antigen is a generic term for a family of carbohydrate antigens with overlapping specificities found in some plants (corn, spinach), some microorganisms (pneumococcus, *Shigella dysenteriae, Bacillus anthracis*), and some fish and animal tissues (carp, toad, chicken, horse, guinea pig, sheep, hamster, dog, cat, human). The injection of anti-Forssman serum into guinea pigs or chick embryos causes vascular damage and hemorrhage. The possibility of such a reaction occurring in humans is uncertain.

Nephritis and Endocarditis

The acute nephritis or acute endocarditis following streptococcal infection may be caused by the production of cytotoxic antibodies to antigens produced by the attachment of bacterial products to normal tissue components, by the production of antibodies to streptococcal antigens that cross-react with normal tissue antigens, or by the formation of antibody–streptococcal antigen complexes in vivo. However, such reactions are most likely mediated through the immune complex reaction (see Chapter 16).

Skin

The role of cytotoxic antibodies in the destruction of epithelial cells producing "bullous" lesions is discussed in Chapter 16.

Demonstration of Cytotoxic Antibodies

The effect of the antibody may be produced by passive transfer of serum-containing antibody into a normal recipient (see Fig. 15-2). If this antibody is associated with cellular injury, for example, platelet destruction in ITP, a specific cytopenia may develop.

In Vitro (Coombs Test)

The addition of the patient's serum to the target cells in a test tube, or the addition of the patient's serum to normal cells in the presence of the antigen, produces agglutination or lysis (complement present). In some cases, antibody does not result in agglutination unless a second antibody is added. Such non-agglutinating antibodies are termed incomplete and may be detected by the Coombs test. In the *direct Coombs test*, target cells are already coated with incomplete antibody and/or complement. The addition of an antiserum containing antibodies directed against Ig or complement components then causes agglutination of the target cells. Thus, human Rh^+ erythrocytes coated with incomplete anti-Rh antibody agglutinate when sheep anti-human gamma-globulin serum is added. In the *indirect Coombs test*, the target cells are not coated with antibody but are mixed with a serum containing incomplete antibody to the target cells. The treated cells are then agglutinated by the addition of anti-gamma-globulin serum. Human Rh$^+$ cells are added to human serum containing incomplete anti-Rh antibodies. These sensitized cells are agglutinated by sheep anti-human gamma globulin serum (Fig. 15-8). In suspected Rh hemolytic

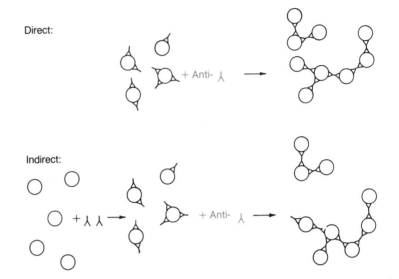

Figure 15-8. Coombs antiglobulin tests. The Coombs test for antibody to erythrocytes is carried out in two forms: direct and indirect. Direct: cells taken from the patient are coated with antibody in vivo and are agglutinated by the addition of anti-Ig, which reacts with the antibodies coating the cells. Indirect: the patient's serum contains free antibody that binds to but does not agglutinate erythrocytes added in vitro. Agglutination is accomplished by addition of a second antibody, which reacts with the first antibody (anti-Ig).

disease, both the direct and the indirect Coombs tests must be done to rule out the presence of incomplete Rh antibodies. The direct test is usually positive for fetal erythrocytes coated with maternal anti-Rh, when free antibody is not present in the fetal serum. On the other hand, the mother's serum will contain anti-Rh antibody detectable by the indirect test; maternal serum added to fetal cells results in coating of the fetal Rh$^+$ cells, which are then agglutinable by antibody to human IgG. Coombs' test may also be used to reveal agglutination of a patient's own cells in acquired hemolytic anemia, thus demonstrating an incomplete autoantibody.

Summary

Cytotoxic or cytolytic reactions are caused by circulating antibody to cell surface structures or by antigen–antibody complexes with subsequent complement fixation. The cell surface antigens may be an integral part of the cell membrane or may be acquired by passive absorption. Reaction of antibody of the IgM or IgG class with the cell surface antigens results in activation of complement and destruction of the cell by complement-mediated lysis or by phagocytosis by macrophages with receptors for activated complement components or aggregated immunoglobulin. Cells in contact with the circulating blood are most often the target cells; these include red blood cells, white blood cells, platelets, and vascular endothelium. The disease states are the result of a loss of the function of the affected cells. Examples of such diseases are hemolytic anemia, agranulocytosis, thrombocytopenia, and vascular purpura.

References

General

Atkinson JP, Frank MM: Studies on the in vivo effects of antibody: interaction of IgM antibody and complement in the immune clearance and destruction of erythrocytes in man. J Clin Invest 54:339, 1974.

Beck WS: Hematology, 4th ed. Cambridge, Mass, MIT Press, 1985.

Boyle MDP, Borsos T: The terminal stages of immune hemolysis: a brief review. Mol Immunol 17:425, 1980.

Schreiber AD, Frank MM: Role of antibody and complement in the immune clearance and destruction of erythrocytes. II. Molecular nature of IgG and IgM complement-fixing sites and effects of their interaction with serum. J Clin Invest 51:583, 1972.

Swisher SN: Immune hemolysis. Am Rev Med 15:1, 1964.

Wintrobe MM: Clinical Hematology, 7th ed. Philadelphia, Lea & Febiger, 1974.

Zmijewski CM: Immunohematology. New York, Appleton–Century–Crofts, 1968.

Transfusion Reaction

Salmon C, Carton JP, Rouger P: The Human Blood Groups. New York, Masson, 1984.

Schmidt PJ: Transfusion reaction: status in 1982. Clin Lab Med 2:221, 1982.

Solanki D, McCurdy PR: Delayed hemolytic transfusion reactions: an often missed entity. JAMA 239:729, 1978.

Springer GF: Blood group and Forssman antigenic determinants shared between microbes and mammalian cells. Prog Allergy 15:9, 1971.

Race RR, Sanger R: Blood Groups in Man. Philadelphia, Davis, 1962.

Watkins WM: Blood group substances. Science 152:172, 1966.

Watkins WM: Genetics and biochemistry of some human blood groups. Proc R Soc Lond [Biol] 202:31, 1978.

Erythroblastosis Fetalis

Bowman JM: The management of Rh isoimmunization. Obstet Gynecol 52:1, 1978.

Bowman JM: Fetomaternal ABO incompatibility and erythroblastosis fetalis. Vox Sang 50:104, 1986.

Freda VJ, Gorman JG, Pollack W: Suppression of the primary Rh immune response with passive Rh IgG immunoglobulin. N Engl J Med 277:1022, 1967.

Freda VJ, Pollack W, Gorman JG: Rh disease: How near the end? Hosp Pract 13:61, 1978.

Gorman JG, Freda VJ, Pollack W. Prevention of rhesus isoimmunization. Clin Immunol Allergy 4:473, 1984.

Hamilton EG: Intrauterine transfusion for Rh disease: a status report. Hosp Pract 13:113, 1978.

Levine P: Influence of ABO system in Rh hemolytic disease. Hum Biol 30:14, 1958.

Levine P: The discovery of Rh hemolytic disease. Vox Sang 47:187, 1984.

Levine P, Stetson R: An unusual case of intragroup agglutination. JAMA 113:126, 1939.

Szulman AE: The histologic distribution of the blood group substances in man as determined by immunofluorescence. III. The A, B, and H antigens in embryos and fetuses from 18 mm in length. J Exp Med 119:503, 1964.

Taylor JF: Sensitization of Rh-negative daughters by their Rh-positive mothers. N Engl J Med 276:547, 1967.

Voak D: The pathogenesis of ABO hemolytic disease of the newborn. Vox Sang 17:481, 1969.

Walker RH: Hemolytic Disease of the Newborn. Chicago, Ill, Am Soc Clin Pathol, 1971.

Zawadnik SA, Bonnard GD, Gautier E, MacDonald HR: Antibody dependent cell-mediated destruction of human erythrocytes in ABO and rhesus fetal–maternal incompatibilities. Pediat Res 10:791, 1976.

Autoimmune Hemolytic Anemia

Adams J, Moore VK, Issitt DD: Autoimmune hemolytic anemia caused by anti-D. Transfusion 13:214, 1973.

Bell CA, Zwicker H, Sacks HJ: Autoimmune hemolytic anemia: routine serologic evaluation in a general hospital population. Am J Clin Pathol 60:902, 1973.

Cline MJ, Golde DW: Immune suppression of hematopoiesis. Am J Med 64:301, 1978.

Dacie JV, Wolledge SM: Autoimmune hemolytic anemia. Prog Hematol 6:1, 1969.

Donath J, Landsteiner K: Über paroxysmale Hämoglobinurie. Munch Med Wochenschr 51:1590, 1904.

Frank M, Schreiber AD, Atkinson JP, Jaffe CJ: Pathophysiology of immune hemolytic anemia. Ann Intern Med 87:210, 1977.

Hinz CG Jr, Picken ME, Lepow IH: Studies on immune human hemolysis. II. The Donath–Landsteiner reaction as a model system for studying the mechanism of action of complement and the role of C′1 and C′1 esterases. J Exp Med 113:193, 1961.

Petz LD, Garraty G: Acquired Immune Hemolytic Anemias. New York, Churchill Livingstone, 1980.

Pirofsky B: Clinical aspects of autoimmune hemolytic anemia. Semin Hematol 13:251, 1976.

Poschmann A, Fisher K: Autoimmune hemolytic anemia: recent advances in pathogenesis, diagnosis and treatment. Eur J Pediat 143:258, 1985.

Pruzanski W, Shumar KH: Biologic activity of cold-reacting autoantibodies. N Engl J Med 297:538, 583, 1977.

Roelcke D: Cold agglutination: antibodies and antigens. Clin Immunol Immunopathol 2:266, 1974.

Shohet SB: Hemolysis and changes in erythrocyte membrane lipids. N Engl J Med 286:577, 1972.

Worlledge SM, Rousso C: Studies of the serology of paroxysmal cold haemoglobinuria (P.C.H.) with special reference to relationship with P blood group system. Vox Sang 10:293, 1965.

Drug-Associated Hemolytic Reactions

Ackroyd JF: Sedormid purpura, an immunologic study of a form of drug hypersensitivity. Prog Allergy 3:531, 1952.

Sedormid

Dausset J, Coutu L: Drug induced hemolysis. Annu Rev Med 18:55, 1967.

Kerr R-O, Cardamone J, Dalmasso AP, Kaplan ME: Two mechanisms of erythrocyte destruction in penicillin-induced hemolytic anemia. N Engl J Med 287:1322, 1972.

Lo Buglio AF, Jandl JH: The reaction of the alpha-methyldopa red cell antibody. N Engl J Med 276:658, 1967.

Molthan L, Reidenberg MM, Elchman MF: Positive direct Coombs test due to cephalothin. N Engl J Med 277:123, 1967.

Petz LD, Fudenberg HH: Coombs-positive hemolytic anemia caused by penicillin administration. N Engl J Med 274:171, 1966.

Weiss RB, Bluno S: Hypersensitivity reactions to cancer chemotherapeutic agents. Ann Intern Med 941:66, 1981.

Wolledge SM: Immune drug-induced hemolytic anemias. Semin Hematol 10:327, 1973.

White Blood Cell Reactions

Bagby GC, Lawrence HJ, Neerhout RC: T-lymphocyte-mediated granulopoietic failure. N Engl J Med 309:1073, 1983.

Cannon DC: Clinical aspects of the leukocyte autibody reaction. Postgrad Med 47:51, 1970.

Cline MJ, et al: Autoimmune panleukopenia. N Engl J Med 295:1489, 1976.

Dehoratius RJ: Lymphocytotoxic antibodies. Clin Immunol 4:151, 1980.

Gilliand BC, Evans RS: The immune cytopenias. Postgrad Med 54:195, 1973.

Jacob HJ, et al: Complement induced granulocyte aggregation. N Engl J Med 302:789, 1980.

McCullough J, et al.: A comparison of methods for detecting leukocyte antibodies in autoimmune neutropenia. Transfusion 21:483, 1981.

Pisciotta AV: Immune and toxic mechanisms in drug induced agranulocytosis. Semin Hematol 10:279, 1973.

Platelets

Ackroyd JF: Sedormid purpura: an immunologic study of a form of drug hypersensitivity. Prog Allergy 3:531, 1952.

Aster RH: Post-transfusion purpura. Immunologic aspects and therapy. N Engl J Med 291:1163, 1974.

Aster RH: Immune thrombocytopenias. Hosp Pract 18:187, 1983.

Baldini M: Idiopathic thrombocytopenic purpura. N Engl J Med 274:1245, 1302, 1360, 1966.

Cines DB, et al: Immune thrombocytopenic purpura and pregnancy. N Engl J Med 306:826, 1982.

Delfraissy JF, et al: Suppressor cell functions after intravenous gammaglobulin treatment in adult chronic idiopathic thrombocytopenic purpura. Br J Haematol 60:315, 1985.

Fehr J, Hofmann V, Kappelar U: Transient reversal of thrombocytopenia in idiopathic thrombocytopenic purpura by high-dose intravenous gamma globulin. N Engl J Med 306:1254, 1982.

Hoffman R, et al: An antibody cytotoxic to megakaryocyte progenitor cells in a patient with immune thrombocytopenic purpura. N Engl J Med 312:1170, 1985.

Imbach PA: Multicenter European trial of intravenous immune globulin in immune thrombocytopenic purpura in childhood. Vox Sang 49(Suppl):25, 1985.

Karpatkin S: Autoimmune thrombocytopenic purpura. Blood 56:329, 1980.

Kollar CA: Immune thrombocytopenic purpura. Med Clin North Amer 64:761, 1980.

McCarthy LJ, Menitove JE: Immunologic Aspects of Platelet Transfusion. Arlington, Va., Am Assoc Blood Banks, 1985.

Peterson OH, Larson P: Thrombocytopenic purpura in pregnancy. Obstet Gynecol 4:454, 1954.

Shulman NR, Aster RH, Leitner A, Hiller MC: Immunoreactions involving platelets. V. Post-transfusion purpura due to a complement-fixing antibody against a genetically controlled platelet antigen. A proposed mechanism for thrombocytopenia and its relevance in autoimmunity. J Clin Invest 40:1597, 1961.

Walsh CM, Nardi MA, Karpatkin S: On the mechanism of thrombocytopenic purpura in sexually active homosexual men. N Engl J Med 331:635, 1984.

Other Cytolytic Diseases

Iwai J, Mei-Sai N: Etiology of Raynaud's disease. Jap Med World 5:119, 1925.

Jones WR: Immunologic infertility: fact or fiction. Fert Steril 33:577, 1980.

Li TX: Sperm immunology, infertility and fertility control. Obstet Gynecol 44:607, 1974.

Samuel T, Rose NR: The lessons of vasectomy—a review. J Clin Lab Immunol 3:77, 1980.

Stetson CA: The role of humoral antibody in the hemograft rejection. Adv Immunol 3:97, 1963.

Taichman NS, Tsai C-C: Heterophile antibodies and tissue injury. II. Ultrastructure of dermal vascular lesions produced by Forssman antiserum in guinea pigs. Int Arch Allergy 42:78, 1972.

Waksman BH: Cell lysis and related phenomena in hypersensitivity reactions, including immunohematologic diseases. Prog Allergy 5:340, 1958.

Assays (Laboratory Diagnosis)

Bohnen RF, et al: The direct Coombs test: Its clinical significance: study in a large university hospital. Ann Intern Med 68:19, 1968.

Coombs RRA, Mourant AE, Race RR: A new test for the detection of weak and "incomplete" Rh agglutinins. Br J Exp Pathol 26:255, 1945.

Coombs RRA, Roberts F: Antiglobulin reaction. Br Med Bull 15:113, 1959.

Gilliand BC, Leedy JP, Vaughn JH: The detection of cell-bound antibody on complement coated human red cells. J Clin Invest 49:898, 1970.

Henry JB: Clinical Diagnosis and Management. Philadelphia, Saunders, 1984.

Koepke JA ed: Laboratory Hematology. New York, Churchill Livingstone, 1984.

McPherson AJ: Antibody detection and identification in a hospital blood bank. Pathology 8:299, 1976.

Immune Complex Reactions

Immune complex reactions are caused by immunoglobulin antibody reacting directly with antigens in tissue or by antibody reacting with soluble antigen in the blood to form soluble antigen–antibody complexes that deposit in tissues. Although these initiating events are clearly different, the subsequent inflammatory reaction, mediated by complement, is essentially the same (Fig. 16-1). IgG antibody reacting with antigen in tis-

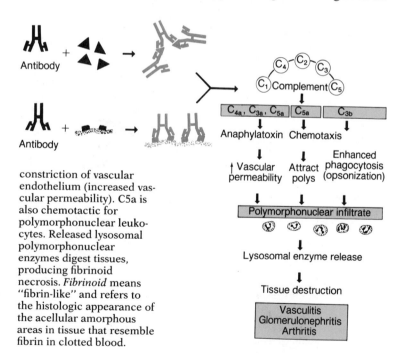

Figure 16-1. Antibody (usually IgG) reacts with soluble antigens to produce soluble circulating immune complexes, or with basement membranes (such as renal glomerular basement membrane). Antibody–antigen complexes cause activation of complement with formation of inflammatory (phlogistic) complement fragments. Fragments C3a, C4a, and C5a (anaphylatoxin) cause constriction of vascular endothelium (increased vascular permeability). C5a is also chemotactic for polymorphonuclear leukocytes. Released lysosomal polymorphonuclear enzymes digest tissues, producing fibrinoid necrosis. *Fibrinoid* means "fibrin-like" and refers to the histologic appearance of the acellular amorphous areas in tissue that resemble fibrin in clotted blood.

sue forms aggregated IgG Fc's, which fix complement. Soluble complexes, formed in the circulation by a single IgG molecule reacting with a soluble antigen, form aggregates of IgG when two or more complexes from the blood deposit closely in tissue.

373

These antigen–antibody complexes fix complement with activation of the anaphylatoxic and chemotactic activities of C4a, C3a, and C5a. This results in the accumulation of neutrophilic polymorphonuclear leukocytes, which release lysosomal enzymes and reactive oxygen metabolites that cause destruction of the elastic lamina of arteries (serum sickness), basement membrane of the kidney glomerulus (glomerulonephritis), walls of small vessels (Arthus reaction), or articular cartilage of joints (rheumatoid arthritis).

The alternate pathway for complement activation, entered by activation of C3 (the C3 shunt; see Complement System, Chapter 12) is active in the pathogenesis of some types of lesions that are similar to immune complex–mediated lesions. Activation of this pathway also results in formation of C3a and C5a, production of complement chemotactic factor (C5a), accumulation of polymorphonuclear cells, and destruction of tissue. Complement mediators such as anaphylatoxin may induce endothelial cell contraction and open cell junctions so that soluble complexes can deposit in basement membranes or inflammatory cells can enter into tissue spaces.

Arthus Reaction

The Arthus reaction is a dermal inflammatory response caused by the reaction of precipitating antibody with antigen placed in the skin (Fig. 16-2). The reaction is characterized grossly by

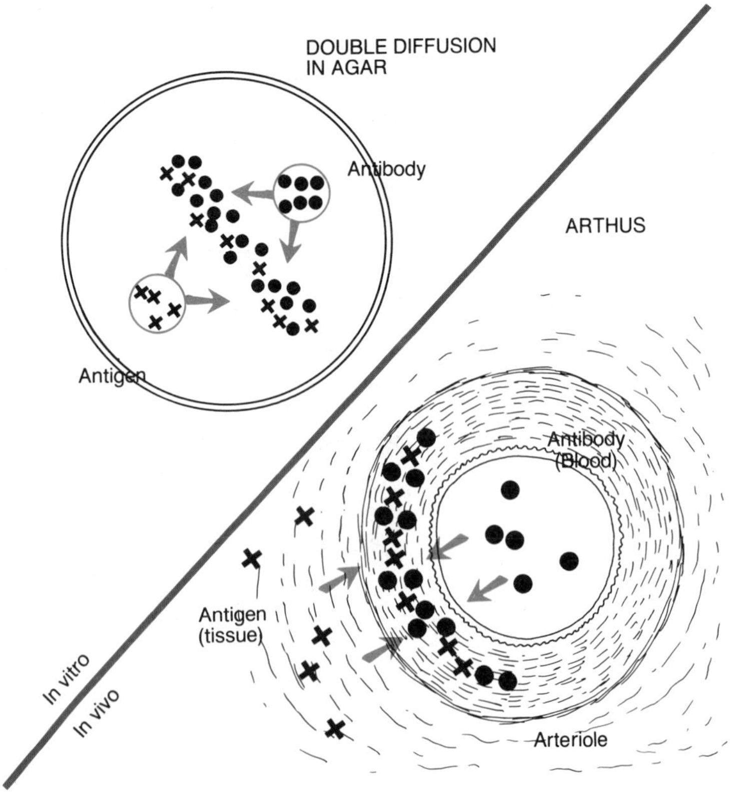

Figure 16-2. Comparison of double-diffusion-in-agar precipitin reaction and Arthus reaction. When antibody and antigen are allowed to diffuse toward each other in agar a precipitation band forms when the antigen and antibody concentrations in the agar are in equivalence. Similarly if antigen is injected into the skin it will diffuse toward the vessels. The major precipitin reaction occurs in the walls of small vessels, usually arterioles, where antibody in the circulation diffuses out to meet antigen diffusing in.

edema, erythema, and hemorrhage, all of which develop over a few hours, reaching a maximum in 2 to 5 hours or even later if the reaction is severe (Fig. 16-3). Histologically hemorrhage,

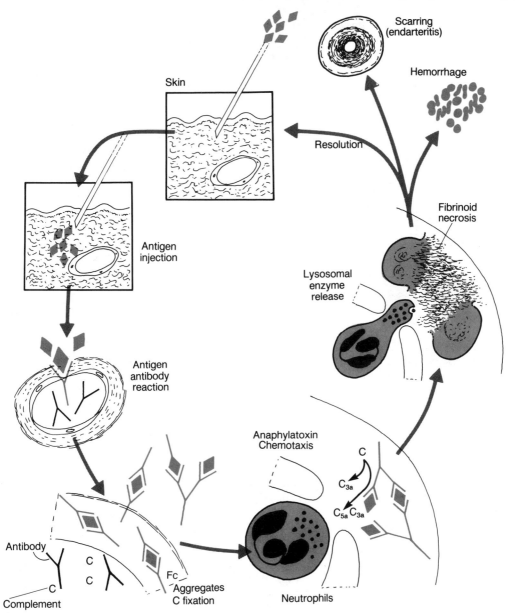

Figure 16-3. Steps in Arthus reaction. (1) Injection of antigen into the dermis. (2) Diffusion of antigen in tissue to vessels. (3) Reaction of antigen with circulating antibody in wall of small arterioles. (4) Formation of antibody–antigen complexes, aggregation of Fc of antibody, and activation of complement. (5) Contraction and separation of endothelial cells by C3a and C5a (anaphylatoxin), and attraction of neutrophils by C5a and C5a des-Arg chemotactic factor. (6) Activation of neutrophils in vessel wall with release of lysosomal enzymes. (7) Digestion of vascular wall, producing fibrinoid necrosis. (8) Resolution or scarring depending on severity of reaction.

vascular fibrinoid necrosis, and emigration of neutrophils and eosinophils are seen. If the reaction is severe, there is thrombosis, with resulting ischemic necrosis. This lesion is caused by the reaction of antigen with antibody, forming microprecipitates in vessel walls or in adjacent tissue spaces, and activation of complement. Polymorphonuclear-cell infiltrate and lysosomal enzymes released secondarily to phagocytosis of immune complexes damage vascular endothelium. Clumping of cells and activation of the clotting system may result in occlusion of small vessels and ischemic necrosis. The presence of antigen and antibody may be demonstrated in vascular wall deposits by the fluorescent antibody technique. In this reaction complexes in different ratios of antibody to antigen (antibody excess, equivalence, or antigen excess) are present and are active in fixing complement if the Fc's of two antibody molecules are juxtaposed.

Serum Sickness

The syndrome of serum sickness was first recognized by von Pirquet and Schick in 1905. It consists of arthritis, glomerulonephritis, and vasculitis appearing 10 days to 2 weeks following passive immunization with horse serum (i.e., horse antitetanus toxin). The disease is the result of the production by the treated individual of circulating precipitating antibody to the injected horse serum (Fig. 16-4). Arnold Rich produced the disease by injections of large amounts of bovine serum albumin (BSA) into rabbits. Frank Dixon and his colleagues, by following the fate of radiolabeled BSA, demonstrated that the lesions appeared at the time of immune elimination of the labeled antigen when soluble complexes in antigen excess could be demonstrated in the serum (Fig. 16-5). By a continuous infusion of BSA, they were able to identify three types of immune responses in rabbits: (1) the production of no antibody to BSA (high dose tolerance) or the production of antibody in such small amounts that it was overwhelmed by the massive doses of antigen so that serum sickness did not develop; (2) the production of large amounts of antibody, which formed complexes with antigen in antibody excess that did not induce lesions; or (3) the production of a moderate amount of antibody. In the latter instance, soluble antigen–antibody complexes were formed in antigen excess and lesions typical of serum sickness developed. Complexes formed in vitro and injected into animals may also produce lesions, but only if the complexes are formed in antigen excess. Immune complexes in antibody excess or equivalence are cleared by the reticuloendothelial system (RES) due to the presence of aggregated Fc's or C3b. The phagocytic cells of the RES have receptors for aggregated Fc's and C3b. However, soluble complexes in antigen excess (toxic

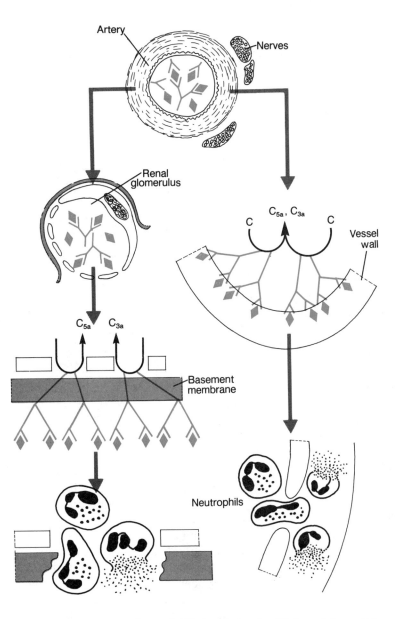

Figure 16-4. Steps in serum sickness. (1) Formation of soluble antibody–antigen complexes in circulation. Such complexes do not fix complement, because Fc's are not aggregated. (2) Soluble complexes pass through open endothelial spaces in glomeruli and deposit on epithelial side of basement membrane or deposit in walls of small arteries. Accumulation of complexes results in formation of aggregates of Ig, activating complement. (3) Neutrophils are attracted, pass into basement membrane or vessel wall, and release lysosomal enzymes causing destruction of basement membrane.

complexes) are not cleared efficiently by the RES and deposit in vessels and glomeruli, where accumulation of complexes results in aggregation of Fc and complement activation.

Horse serum contains at least 30 different, separate antigens, so that complexes of one or more of these antigens may be present in the circulation even though excess antibody or other free antigens may be present at the same time. Therefore, demonstration of circulating antibody to some components does not rule out the presence of complexes from another antigen–antibody system. In addition, some individuals may produce

Figure 16-5. Comparison of antigen elimination, precipitin reaction, and serum complement levels during experimental serum sickness. Immune elimination of antigen follows production of antibody that binds to antigen in the circulation. When antibody first appears there is an excess of antigen, so that soluble immune complexes in antigen excess are formed. These complexes lodge in arteries and, in particular, in glomeruli where aggregates of immunoglobulin fix complement. This results in lesions of serum sickness and a fall in serum complement. As more antibody is produced complexes in equivalence and then antibody excess are found. Since these complexes contain aggregated Fc pieces of Ig they will be cleared from the circulation by the reticuloendothelial system, because of receptors on macrophages for aggregated Fc and C3b.

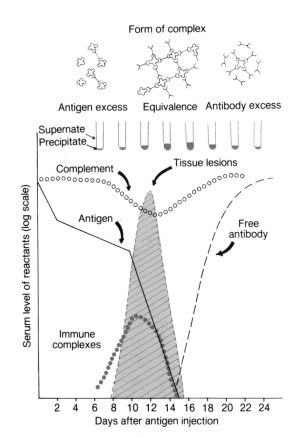

reaginic (IgE) antibodies or a state of delayed hypersensitivity to some of the antigens in horse serum, resulting in a very complicated clinical picture.

Immune Complexes in Infectious Diseases

Transient serum sickness–like episodes are frequently associated with infections. In many instances, antibody–antigen complexes may be demonstrated, and in some cases the antigen has been identified as a component of the infectious agent. Immune complexes have been documented in glomerular or vascular deposits in animals infected with lymphocytic choriomeningitis virus, *Schistosoma mansoni*, leprosy bacilli, *Treponema pallidum*, and a number of other agents. In humans, vasculitis, glomerulonephritis, arthritis, and skin lesions may be associated with deposition of hepatitis antigen (HBsAg)–antibody complexes. Circulating immune complexes may also be found in high frequency in patients with recurrent infections in the absence of serum sickness–like lesions. The presence of immune complexes in the circulation does not necessarily correlate with lesions. The form of the complexes, the class of the antibody, and the properties of the antigen are all important factors, as is the integrity of the RES.

Glomerulo-nephritis

Inflammation of the glomeruli of the kidney is known as *glomerulonephritis*. The kidney is probably the organ most frequently affected by immune complex deposits. Immune complexes may produce lesions in various ways. Lesions are caused either by deposition of antibody–antigen complexes formed elsewhere and deposited in the glomeruli or by direct reaction of antibody with glomerular basement membrane or other antigens. To appreciate the nature of antibody-mediated glomerulonephritis, an understanding of the normal structure of the glomerulus and the form of deposition of antibody or immune complexes is necessary (Fig. 16-6). The nephron is the unit of the kidney that filters metabolites and electrolytes from the blood and produces urine. It is made up of glomerulus and tubule. The glomerulus is that portion of the nephron responsible for producing an ultrafiltrate of blood. The tubule collects the filtrate and resorbs electrolytes as urine passes into the collecting system. The glomerulus is made up of four principal cell types, each of which has a specific function: endothelial cells, which line the glomerular capillary network, mesangial cells, which form a stalk that supports the capillaries, and two types of epithelial cells, visceral and parietal. The mesangium is made up of cells of the reticuloendothelial system and frequently may contain immune complexes. The visceral epithelial cells cover the external surface of the capillary basement membrane, and the parietal epithelial cells line the internal surface of the external capsule of the glomerulus. The critical feature of the glomerulus is that the capillary basement membrane is not completely covered by endothelial cells. This permits antibody to basement membrane or immune complexes to filter into the basement membrane. Complement activation (anaphylatoxin) or mast cell mediators may produce further separation by causing contraction of endothelial cells. Lesions are produced by alteration of the basement membrane by two mechanisms: (1) directly by the deposition of complexes or antibody that cause changes in the electrostatic properties of the basement membrane and consequent leakage of serum proteins, or (2) indirectly by complement-mediated attraction of polymorphonuclear leukocytes, which in turn release enzymes that digest the basement membrane. The lesions may resolve or progress into a chronic stage of inflammation with infiltration by mononucler cells. Mononuclear cell infiltration represents a stage of progression to chronic glomerulonephritis. In addition, chronic deposition of complexes may cause thickening of the basement membrane and fusion of the foot processes of the epithelial cells. Dissolution of the basement membrane is associated with leakage of blood components into the urine (proteinuria, hematuria, the nephrotic syndrome), whereas thickening of the basement membrane causes a loss in filtration capacity and uremia (the uremic syndrome).

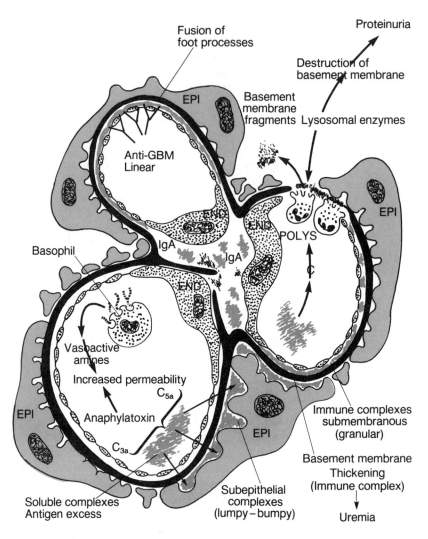

Figure 16-6. Pathogenesis of glomerulonephritis. Depicted is a glomerular tuft. The mesangial cells are located in the center and support the endothelial cells (END), which line the inside of the basement membrane. There are gaps in the cytoplasm of the endothelial cells, which expose the basement membrane to blood components. The upper right illustrates deposition of antiglomerular basement membrane antibody (anti-GBM) as a linear deposit of immunoglobulin on the endothelial side of the basement membrane. The upper left depicts deposition of soluble immune complexes on exposed basement membrane after contraction of endothelial cells by vasoactive amines or activation of anaphylatoxin. The lower left illustrates that the complexes may deposit as large clumps, distorting the foot processes of the endothelial cells. Dissolution of the basement membrane by release of lysosomal enzymes from polymorphonuclear leukocytes activated by complement or alteration in the electrostatic properties of the basement membrane by anti-GBM or immune complex deposition leads to leakage of proteins into the urine (proteinuria) (lower right). If more extensive destruction of the basement membranes occurs, cellular elements of the blood as well as basement membrane fragments may be detected in the urine. Prolonged accumulation of immune reactants leads to thickening of the basement membrane and fusion of the foot processes of epithelial cells. Clinically, this is expressed as a loss of the filtering capacity of the kidney and retention of toxic metabolites (uremia).

The charge of the immune complex in the glomerular basement membrane may also determine the extent and location of the lesions. The basement membrane is strongly negatively charged. In experimental disease models highly cationic antigens, in the form of soluble antigen or soluble immune complexes, tend to localize within or pass through the basement membrane, whereas anionic antigens may be prevented from localizing in the membrane and deposit on the endothelial side (Fig. 16-7). "Neutralization" of the cationic basement membrane by anionic depositions may result in increased permeability to smaller serum proteins, such as serum albumin. In this way proteinuria may occur without neutrophil-mediated basement membrane damage.

Immune Complex Glomerulonephritis

One of the features of experimental serum sickness produced using foreign albumin as antigen is acute glomerulonephritis. There is accumulation of large amounts of soluble antibody–antigen complexes (antigen excess) that become lodged on the epithelial side of the glomerular basement membrane and appear as lumpy deposits of antigen–antibody complex when examined by immunofluorescence. Granular deposits of immune complexes may also be seen on the endothelial side of the glomerular basement membrane when other antigens are used. Presumably the overall charge of an albumin–antialbumin soluble complex is determined more by the charge of the antibody than of the albumin. Thus the complex is overall positively charged and deposits on the epithelial side of the basement membrane. Following localization, there may be changes in the electrostatic properties of the membrane or fixation of complement components, resulting in the production of the complement chemotactic factors, attraction of polymorphonuclear leukocytes, and release of lysosomal enzymes leading to destruction of glomerular basement membrane. Chronic repeated deposition leads to proliferation of endothelial cells and thickening of the basement membrane. Experimentally, this process may be produced by an appropriate host antibody response to an exogenous antigen (serum sickness), passive transfer of exogenous antigen and exogenous antibody, or injection of preformed soluble antigen–antibody complexes.

A chronic form of immune complex glomerulonephritis may be produced by repeated injections of small amounts of antigen into an appropriately immunized animal or by repeated injections of soluble complexes. The resulting lesion produced is a chronic membranous glomerulonephritis with a variable amount of polymorphonuclear leukocyte infiltration and endothelial proliferation that leads to scarring and destruction of the

A. Soluble complexes — cationic antigen (subepithelial)

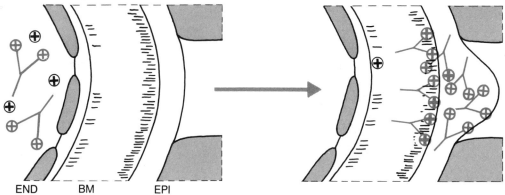

END   BM   EPI

B. Soluble cationic antigen (subepithelial & intramembranous)

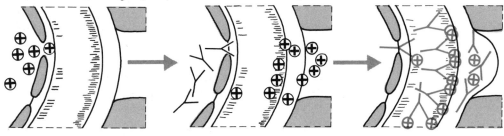

C. Anionic antigens or complexes (subendothelial)

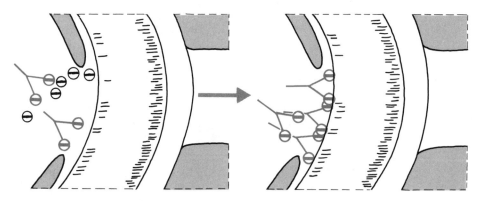

D. Soluble anionic antigen (mesangial)

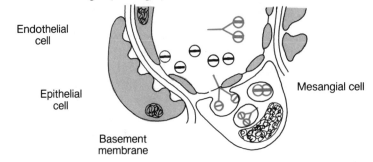

Endothelial
cell

Mesangial cell

Epithelial
cell

Basement
membrane

◀ **Figure 16-7.** Postulated effect of antigen charge on localization in glomeruli. Cationic antigens (positively charged) preferentially localize in the glomerular basement membrane either in the form of soluble immune complexes (A) or as free antigen (B). Subepithelial localization may be explained by the higher density of anions (negative charge) on the epithelial side of the basement membrane (A). Anionic complexes tend to be taken up by the mesangial cells (D) and are less pathogenic but may localize on the endothelial side of the basement membrane (C). Accumulation of complexes may result in functional aggregation of immunoglobulin and complement activation. In the case of free antigen deposition in the glomerulus, subsequent formation of antibody may result in reaction of circulating antibodies with antigen localized in the basement membrane, formation of immunoglobulin aggregates, complement fixation, and glomerulonephritis.

glomerulus. This type of mechanism is responsible for the glomerulonephritis associated with various human diseases, such as lupus erythematosus (DNA–anti-DNA), diabetes mellitus (insulin–anti-insulin), and thyroiditis (thyroglobulin–antithyroglobulin). In addition, the deposition of toxic complexes of antibody and viral antigens is responsible for some cases of human glomerulonephritis. Deposits of the tumor antigen *carcinoembryonic antigen* (CEA; see Chapter 29) and antibody to CEA have been identified as being responsible for renal damage in some patients with colonic carcinoma. Rare instances of glomerulonephritis from the deposition of IgE antibody–antigen complexes may occur in atopic individuals.

Experimental Autoallergic Glomerulonephritis

Experimental glomerulonephritis may be induced by injection of animals with glomerular basement membrane extract in complete Freund's adjuvant, which stimulates the production of antibody to glomerular basement membrane. This antibody then localizes on the capillary side of the basement membrane and may be observed by immunofluorescence as a continuous thin layer along the membrane, in contrast to the location and form of the soluble complex deposition described above. The reaction of antibody with the basement membrane results in the binding of complement, polymorphonuclear leukocyte infiltration, and basement membrane destruction. A transient form of the experimental disease may be transferred with serum from an affected sheep injected into a normal sheep if the affected sheep is nephrectomized several days prior to transfer. Nephrectomy is necessary because the nephritogenic antibody is absorbed in vivo by the glomerular tissue of the serum donor.

Nephrotoxic Serum (Masugi) Nephritis

Experimental glomerulonephritis may also be produced in animals by the passive transfer of heterologous antisera to glomeruli. For example, the passive transfer of rabbit anti-rat glomerulus serum to rats causes nephrotoxic serum nephritis. The nephritis consists of a biphasic response: (1) an acute transient proteinuria is observed as a result of the formation of complexes of rabbit antibodies and antigens present in rat glomerulus; (2) after 10 days to 2 weeks, a potentially fatal chronic proliferative glomerulonephritis may develop. This second lesion is caused by the production of host (rat) antibodies to donor (rabbit) immunoglobulin. These rat antibodies react with the rabbit antiglomerular antibodies localized on the rat glomeruli, causing the second-phase lesions.

Poststreptococcal Glomerulonephritis

The occurrence of acute glomerulonephritis in humans is associated with exposure to some strains of group A β-hemolytic streptococci. Such streptococcal strains have been termed *nephritogenic*. The acute infection usually presents as a sore throat and fever. There is a characteristic latent period following the onset of infection, during which no significant renal symptoms are observed. Acute poststreptococcal glomerulonephritis is characterized by the onset of proteinuria and hematuria. This corresponds in time with the appearance of host antibodies to streptococcal antigens. Immunofluorescence examination of affected kidneys reveals a morphologic alteration typical of immune complex glomerulonephritis (described above); complement, immunoglobulins, and streptococcal antigens are found in glomeruli. Although several immune mechanisms have been invoked to explain the pathogenesis of acute glomerulonephritis, the findings are most consistent with an immune complex–mediated inflammatory reaction. It is not clear why only certain strains of streptococci are nephritogenic. Poststreptococcal glomerulonephritis, as the name implies, may occur after all other clinical evidence of infection is gone. It was once thought that certain streptococcal antigens, namely, streptococcal M protein, might have an unusual affinity for the glomerulus. If an appropriate antibody–antigen complex between streptococcal M protein and host antibody could be produced, this complex would be selectively bound to the glomerulus. The fixation to the glomerulus of this complex could be followed by the binding of complement and the attraction of polymorphonuclear leukocytes, leading to glomerular inflammation. However, existence of such a glomerular-binding antigen has not been demonstrated. It is also possible that these nephritogenic streptococci have antigenic specificities that cross-react with some human tissue antigens, and that circulating antibody produced to these streptococcal antigens reacts with glomerular antigens. If this were the case, immunofluorescence examination should reveal linear lesions such as are seen in experimental allergic glomerulonephritis, rather than the lumpy–bumpy deposits that are usually found. In addition, convincing demonstration of such cross-reacting antigens is lacking.

Anti-Basement Membrane Glomerulonephritis

There is evidence that direct anti-basement membrane antibodies are responsible for some cases of human glomerulonephritis. Immunofluorescence examination of such kidneys reveals immunoglobulin deposits in a linear pattern on the basement membrane. It has been postulated that the reaction to an infectious agent (streptococcus, virus) has caused destruction and dissolution of the host basement membrane and that the host produces an antibody to this material that reacts with the remaining basement membrane. Potential basement membrane antigens are present in the circulation of normal individuals and it is possible that streptococcal or viral infections may provide an adjuvant function for such antigens. However, only 5% to 10% of patients with glomerulonephritis appear to develop such an autoantibody. The basement membrane of the glomerulus shares some cross-reacting antigens with the basement membrane of the pulmonary alveoli. A disease caused by antibody that reacts with these antigens is called *Goodpasture's disease* (see below).

Hypocomplementemic Glomerulonephritis

A chronic form of glomerulonephritis without evidence of Ig in the glomerulus but associated with low levels of serum complement has been termed *hypocomplementemic glomerulonephritis*. The etiologic mechanism has not been clearly established. Nonimmune activation of complement via the alternate pathway may lead to deposition of complement in renal glomeruli and produce glomerulonephritis. There may be a so-called C3 nephritic factor, which acts like an autoantibody to altered C3, resulting in chronic deposition of C3 in the glomerulus and lowered serum levels of C3. It is also possible that immune complexes may initiate the deposition of complement but be undetectable when the complement components are still active. C3 receptors may be present on glomerular endothelial cells and serve to activate C3 in some circumstances. In any case, glomerulonephritis associated with deposits of complement components without detectable immunoglobulin and lowering of the serum complement is termed hypocomplementemic glomerulonephritis.

IgA Nephritis

A usually, but not always, mild proliferative form of glomerulonephritis is associated with mesangial deposition of IgA. The reason for this remains undefined, but the more limited nature of the disease may be because IgA does not activate the classical complement pathway. It is likely that IgA antibody–antigen complexes are formed in the circulation and are cleared by the glomerular mesangial cells (IgA is less cationic than IgG). The disease is usually a mild acute glomerulonephritis, with only a small proportion of patients progressing to renal failure. No specific antigens have yet been identified, and no epidemiologic clues support an infectious agent. Mesangial IgA deposits have been found in patients with Henoch–Schönlein purpura, systemic lupus erythematosus, and viral hepatitis. The etiologic implications of such associations are not clear, although the presence of shared antigens between mesangium and cutaneous capillaries might account for the IgA deposits seen in Henoch–Schönlein purpura.

Henoch–Schönlein Nephritis

Henoch–Schönlein purpura is a unique form of immune complex-mediated systemic vasculitis that involves the skin (purpura), kidneys (hematuria), and gastrointestinal tract (abdominal pain). Granular deposits of IgA and C3 are found in the walls of small vessels in intestine and skin, and in the glomerular mesangium. This syndrome usually occurs in children below age 15. There is evidence that polyanionic (negatively charged) immune complexes tend to localize in the mesangium, whereas polycationic complexes lodge in the basement membrane. It is possible that an abnormal mucosal immune response to negatively charged antigens may result in IgA complexes that preferentially lodge in the mesangium. Complement is then activated via the alternate pathway, leading to glomerular damage. This disease is self-limiting and does not lead to chronic renal disease.

Heymann Nephritis

Experimental immunization of rats with renal cortex extract may result in production of autoantibodies to the brush border of the proximal renal tubular cells, immune complex deposition on the epithelial side of the basement membrane, and vacuolization of the proximal tubular cells. The tubular cell damage may be caused by a cytotoxic effect of the antibody. The role of this mechanism in human disease is not clear at this time.

Experimental Allergic Interstitial Nephritis

Immune injury to renal tubules may be induced by immunization of experimental animals with whole kidney or an antigen from the basement membrane of the renal tubule. The lesion begins as a polymorphonuclear infiltrate but progresses to a chronic mononuclear infiltrate with atrophy and degeneration of the tubules. Linear deposits of IgG may be detected along the basement membrane of the proximal tubules. Immune-mediated interstitial nephritis may occur in association with collagen diseases or renal graft rejection in humans.

Clinical–Immunopathological Correlations in Glomerulonephritis

Glomerulonephritis may be caused by deposition of immune complexes formed elsewhere, by reaction of antibody directly with glomerular basement membrane antigens, or by the activation of complement by the alternate pathway. Each of these mechanisms may produce an identical clinical picture or pathologic lesion (Fig. 16-8). Clinically, glomerulonephritis is a syn-

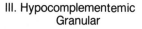

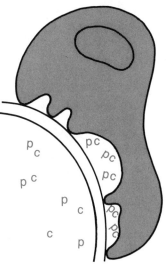

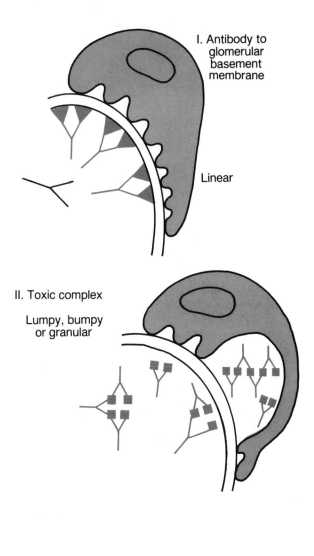

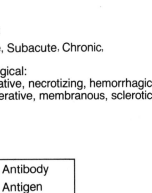

I. Antibody to
glomerular
basement
membrane

Linear

III. Hypocomplementemic
Granular

II. Toxic complex

Lumpy, bumpy
or granular

Clinical:

  Acute, Subacute, Chronic,

Pathological:
  infiltrative, necrotizing, hemorrhagic,
  proliferative, membranous, sclerotic

⋎—	Antibody
■	Antigen
P	Properdin
C	Complement

Figure 16-8. Glomerulonephritis: clinical–pathological correlations. The three pathological mechanisms of glomerulonephritis illustrated may produce a varied clinical and pathological picture. No single mechanism produces a particular type of clinical picture or pathological lesion, although hypocomplementemic glomerulonephritis is usually of the chronic variety. A capillary lumen, basement membrane endothelial cell foot plates, and an epithelial cell are illustrated. (I) Antiglomerular basement membrane antibody reacts with antigens on the lumenal side of the glomerular basement membrane and produces a linear deposition when examined by immunofluorescence. (II) Soluble immune complexes formed elsewhere pass through the glomerular basement membrane and lodge on the epithelial side, producing lumpy–bumpy subepithelial complexes, or lodge within or on the endothelial side of the basement membrane as granular deposits. (III) Complement in the absence of immunoglobulin may be detected as a granular deposit. Hypocomplementemic glomerulonephritis may be caused by a preceding immunoglobin deposit or by the action of properdin, both of which may activate complement. (Modified from illustration of C. Wilson, Scripps Clinic and Research Foundation, La Jolla, Calif.)

drome with markedly variable expression, but the disease can be classified generally into acute, subacute, and chronic. The acute disease may include proteinuria, gross hematuria, oliguria or anuria, edema, azotemia, and rapid death because of renal failure. However, recovery from the acute disease occurs in over 99% of the cases. A more persistent subacute or chronic progression to renal failure may develop. Pathologically, a variety of lesions may be seen in the glomeruli. During the acute stage, the lesions may be minimal (proteinuria associated with fusion of epithelial foot plates), necrotic (death of glomerular cells), infiltrative or exudative (glomeruli full of polymorphonuclear leukocytes), or hemorrhagic (red blood cells in glomeruli). Subacute glomerulonephritis is associated with proliferative (increased number of mononuclear cells or glomerular epithelial cells) or embolic (fibrin thrombi in glomerular capillaries) lesions. Chronic glomerulonephritis features membranous (thickening of glomerular basement membrane) or sclerotic (scarring of glomeruli) changes. Intermediate stages of the disease usually demonstrate an overlap of lesions.

Any of these lesions may be produced by one of the three basic immunopathological mechanisms. The pathological type of lesion depends upon the degree of injury produced in a given period of time, not upon the immunopathological mechanism. Thus, the deposit of large amounts of immune complexes, or antibody to the basement membrane, causing acute complement activation, will lead to infiltration of the glomerulus with a large number of polymorphonuclear leukocytes and extensive dissolution of the basement membrane. The dissolution permits proteins of large molecular weight to pass through the basement membrane. If larger segments of the basement membrane are destroyed, larger blood components such as erythrocytes will pass through the basement membrane, producing hematuria. The loss of protein leads to hypoproteinemia, decreased intravascular osmotic pressure, edema, and heart failure—the clinical picture of acute glomerulonephritis. The deposit of small amounts of immune complexes over long periods of time may produce some disruption of the basement membrane and leakage of serum proteins, but mainly causes a buildup on or in the basement membrane, leading to thickening of the basement membrane and a gradual loss of the filtering capacity of the glomeruli (membranous glomerulonephritis). This results in retention of nitrogen and waste products (azotemia) and gradual renal failure. The pathologist cannot identify the immunopathological mechanism responsible for a given case of glomerulonephritis by defining the histopathological lesion. Identification of the mechanism requires immunofluorescent studies, serologic workup, electron microscopy, and careful clinical documentation of the course of the disease.

Human Glomerulonephritis

Some of the more common forms of glomerulonephritis in humans are listed in Table 16-1. The involvement of immune complex mechanisms in these diseases is proven for some and suspected for others. The different diseases are recognized by the pathologic and clinical findings as indicated in the table.

Other Immune Complex Diseases

In addition to the renal glomerulus, other organs of the body also contain capillary basement membrane exposed to circulating blood: the lung, the synovial capillaries, the choroid plexus of the brain, and the uveal tract of the eye. These organs are susceptible to anti-basement membrane antibody attack and deposition of immune complexes.

Goodpasture's Disease

The combination of pulmonary hemorrhage and glomerulonephritis is known as *Goodpasture's syndrome*. In severe cases there is extensive intraalveolar hemorrhage and marked proliferative glomerulonephritis. The disease is caused by antibody to basement membrane antigens shared by lung and kidney (Fig. 16-9). Immunoglobulin and complement may be identified in the basement membrane of pulmonary alveoli and renal glomeruli. Antibody eluted from the kidneys of such patients binds to lung tissue, and antibody eluted from lung tissue binds to kidney, indicating the presence of cross-reacting antigens in lung and kidney basement membranes. Antibody to lung tissue induces pulmonary hemorrhage and glomerulonephritis when injected into animals. Glomerulonephritis may be induced in animals by immunization with human lung tissue, and antibody eluted from involved kidneys demonstrates strong binding to human lung and kidneys. Experimental Goodpasture's disease has been produced using passively transferred antibody to type IV collagen and/or laminin, both components of the basement membrane.

Cellular Interstitial Pneumonia

Immune-complex deposition and subsequent inflammation may also cause an interstitial inflammation in the lung. These lesions have been identified morphologically as an infiltration of the lung with different cellular elements. Cellular interstitial pneumonia (CIP) is often found associated with various collagen diseases. Immunoglobulin and complement have been identified in the lungs of patients with active interstitial disease in a manner similar to an experimental systemic immune complex–induced pneumonitis in rabbits. In addition, circulating immune complexes have been found in the sera of patients with interstitial pneumonias. A chronic form of interstitial pneumonia (diffuse fibrosis) is not associated with

Table 16-1. Some Forms of Glomerulonephritis of Humans

Type	Mechanism
Post-infectious glomerulonephritis (human counterpart of acute serum sickness)	Immune complex
Membranous nephropathy (human counterpart of chronic serum sickness)	Immune complex
Minimal change disease	Immunological (exact mechanism unknown)
IgA nephropathy (Berger's disease)	Immune complex (IgA)
Goodpasture's disease	Antibasement membrane (kidney, lung)
Membranoproliferative GN (type I)	Immune complex
Dense deposit disease (membranoproliferative GN, type II)	Alternate pathway of complement

Abbreviations: LM, light microscopy; EM, electron microcopy; GN, glomerulonephritis.
Note: These are basic characteristic features; variations occur in pathological and clinical findings.

circulating immune complexes. This may be a later stage of a cellular interstitial pneumonia when complexes are no longer present, or there may be a different pathogenesis. Patients with active stages of the disease (when immune complexes are

Pathologic Findings	Immunofluorescence	Clinical Features	Prognosis
LM: diffuse cellular proliferation, neutrophils EM: subepithelial deposits ("humps")	Coarse granular or lumpy–bumpy pattern in basement membranes (IgG, C3)	Acute nephritis	Good
LM: diffuse basement membrane thickening EM: subepithelial deposits, several, small	Fine granular along basement membranes (IgG, C3)	Nephrotic syndrome	Slowly progressive (renal failure)
LM: normal glomeruli EM: effacement of epithelial cell foot processes	Negative or nonspecific	Nephrotic syndrome	Good
LM: increase in mesangial matrix and cells EM: electron-dense deposits in the mesangium	Positive in the mesangium (IgA, IgG, C3)	Hematuria	Usually good
LM: crescentic glomerulonephritis EM: no evidence of deposits	Linear positivity along basement membranes (IgG, C3)	Acute renal failure, hemoptysis (lung hemorrhage)	Rapidly progressive (renal failure)
LM: mesangial proliferation, basement membrane alteration EM: split basement membranes, subendothelial deposits	Granular irregular pattern in basement membranes (IgG, C3)	Variable (nephrotic syndrome, nephritis)	Progressive (renal failure)
LM: Mesangial proliferation, basement membrane alteration EM: Very dense material of unknown nature deposited in basement membranes	Focal C3 (IgG and early-acting complement components absent)	Variable (nephrotic syndrome, nephritis, hypocomplementemia)	Progressive (renal failure)

Nephrotic syndrome: proteinuria > 3.5 g/24 h.
Nephritis: hematuria, red cell casts, hypertension.
Table contributed by Dr. Regina Varani, University of Texas Medical School, Houston.

present) are responsive to steroid therapy. The spectrum of interstitial pneumonias resembles the stages of glomerulonephritis described above. It is also possible that immune-complex formation is secondary to, and not the cause of, cellular interstitial inflammation.

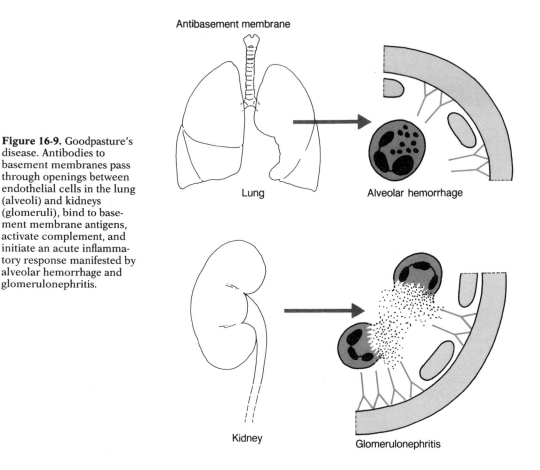

Figure 16-9. Goodpasture's disease. Antibodies to basement membranes pass through openings between endothelial cells in the lung (alveoli) and kidneys (glomeruli), bind to basement membrane antigens, activate complement, and initiate an acute inflammatory response manifested by alveolar hemorrhage and glomerulonephritis.

Arthritis

Subsynovial capillaries are also a site for immune complex deposition. Transient arthritis is seen in many infectious diseases and is also often associated with collagen diseases. A classic example is the arthritis seen during acute attacks of rheumatic fever. It is likely that such transient arthritis episodes are due to immune complex–initiated inflammation.

Choroid Plexus

The choroid plexus is a frequent site of immune-complex deposition in experimental animals injected with immune complexes and with infections associated with circulating immune complexes. In humans, depositions of immune complexes in the choroid plexus are found in some diseases, such as systemic lupus erythematosus (SLE). In the choroid plexus, the endothelial cells are fenestrated so that, in contrast to other parts of the cerebral vasculature, there is not a tight blood–brain barrier. Immune complexes pass through the endothelial cells to lie between the endothelial and epithelial cells. The epithelial cells overlying the basement membrane are tightly joined and prevent increased filtration after complex deposition such as is seen in renal glomeruli. The role of these immune complexes in producing neurological symptoms of SLE remains undefined.

Uveitis

Some forms of uveitis may be caused by deposition of immune complexes in the ocular basement membrane. In rabbits, circulating immune complexes may deposit in ocular tissue and be responsible for inflammation of the uveal tract (iris, ciliary body, and choroid). In humans, uveitis is associated with circulating immune complexes, and immune complexes have been detected in the aqueous humor of the anterior chamber of the eye. Thus, the uveal tract may also be a preferential site for immune-complex deposition and subsequent inflammation. Other forms of uveitis may be caused by cellular autosensitivity to uveal antigens (see Chapter 19).

Vasculitis

Inflammation of vessels is a primary feature of immune complex–mediated diseases. There are definite associations between the size of the vessel and the underlying disease or syndrome. Table 16-2 depicts the distribution of vascular le-

Table 16-2. Human Immune Vasculitides

Disease	Principal Vessels Involved	Cells
Takayasu's arteritis	Aorta, large arteries	Mononuclear
Giant cell arteritis	Cranial arteries	Mononuclear
Polyarteritis nodosa	Medium/small arteries	PMN[a]
Wegener's granulomatosis	Small	PMN/Monos
Hypersensitivity angitis	Small	PMN/Monos
Burger's disease	Veins	Lymphocytes
Behçet's syndrome	Large arteries and veins	PMN

Modified from Penny R: Vasculitis: an approach for physicians. Aust NZ J Med 11:302–308, 1981.

[a] Polymorphonuclear neutrophils.

sions related to vessel size in some human diseases. Each of these vascular lesions has a component of neutrophil infiltrate as well as lesions associated with other immune mechanisms. Often biopsies of the lesions are done at a stage of development when the neutrophils have partially disintegrated. This is referred to as *leukoclastic vasculitis*. The presence of vasculitis in the early stages of the collagen–vascular disease implies an important role for immune complexes in the pathogenesis of these diseases.

Behçet's Syndrome

Behçet's syndrome, described in 1937, includes oral and genital aphthous ulcerations, vascular skin lesions, arthritis, and inflammation of the eye. It is believed to be an immune complex–mediated disease, perhaps related to a virus infection.

Kawasaki's
Syndrome
(Mucocutaneous
Lymph Node
Syndrome)

This is similar to rheumatic fever (see Chapter 17) involving the heart (vasculitis and pancarditis) but with frequent involvement of the coronary arteries leading to thrombosis, infarction, aneurysms, and scarring. The acute disease features fever, conjunctivitis, erythematous skin rash, mucous membrane ulcerations, edema, and lymphadenopathy.

Hypocomplemente-
mic Vasculitic
Urticarial Syndrome

This syndrome includes urticaria, leukoclastic vasculitis, arthritis, and neurologic abnormalities. Laboratory findings are a low C1q, C4, C2, and C3, with normal C1r and C1s, C5–9, and properdin. A 7 S protein which precipitates C1q is found (C1q activating factor) and is believed to be responsible for complement activation.

Post-Cardiac Bypass
Syndrome

Patients who have been on cardiac bypass develop fever, leukocytosis, and edema believed to be secondary to nonimmune activation of C3 to C3a.

Aleutian Mink
Disease

This disease is caused by the immune response to a persistent virus infection and offers an animal model for the relationship of the humoral immune response to the development of lesions found during a viral infection. The disease is characterized by a proliferation of lymphoid tissues, hypergammaglobulinemia, glomerulonephritis, hepatitis, and arteritis. There is overproduction of IgG antibody and formation of immune complexes because the humoral immune response is unable to control viral reproduction. This results in hyperplasia of IgG-forming cells, formation of antibody–virus complexes, and immune complex lesions of vasculitis and glomerulonephritis. The intracellular virus infection could possibly be controlled by the cellular reactivity of delayed hypersensitivity. However, for as yet undefined reasons, the affected mink produce a nonprotective, lesion-producing IgG antibody response. Thus Aleutian mink disease is a prime example of the destructive effects of an immune response when the response is inappropriate (e.g., humoral rather than cellular; see also Leprosy (Chapter 21) and Chronic Mucocutaneous Candidiasis (Chapter 26)). If the mink manifested a cellular rather than a humoral immune response to the virus, the disease in this form would not occur.

**Skin Diseases
Mediated by
Immune Complex
Mechanisms**

Skin reactions are one of the most common manifestations of immune reactions. These may be caused by different immune mechanisms, such as the acute wheal and flare or hive reaction of cutaneous anaphylaxis (Chapter 18) and the delayed skin reaction of cellular hypersensitivity (Chapter 19). Studies using immunolabeling procedures indicate that many different kinds of lesions are the result of the action of antibody and complement. These may be caused by cytotoxic autoantibody to skin antigens or by immune complexes formed elsewhere and deposited in dermal vessels. Some lesions, such as pemphigus or pemphigoid or the skin lesions of SLE, may be the result of the cytotoxic action of antibody directly upon a target cell, whereas others, such as erythema nodosum and erythema multiforme, require the mediation of acute inflammatory cells for full expression. A comparison of these skin diseases is given in Table 16-3 and Figure 16-10. They may be divided into vascular lesions and nonvascular lesions.

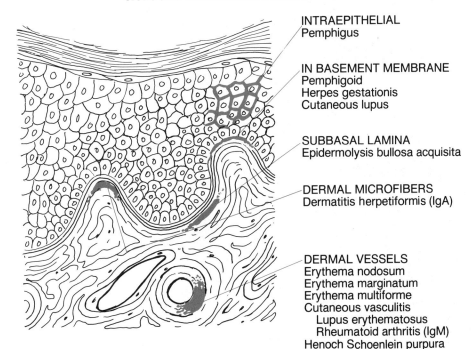

INTRAEPITHELIAL
Pemphigus

IN BASEMENT MEMBRANE
Pemphigoid
Herpes gestationis
Cutaneous lupus

SUBBASAL LAMINA
Epidermolysis bullosa acquisita

DERMAL MICROFIBERS
Dermatitis herpetiformis (IgA)

DERMAL VESSELS
Erythema nodosum
Erythema marginatum
Erythema multiforme
Cutaneous vasculitis
Lupus erythematosus
Rheumatoid arthritis (IgM)
Henoch Schoenlein purpura

Figure 16-10. Diagrammatic representation of lesion location and deposits of immunoglobulin and complement in some skin diseases. Vascular lesions are mediated by immune complex mechanisms, bullous lesions by cytotoxic mechanisms.

Vascular Lesions

Erythema Nodosum

The lesions of erythema nodosum are painful red nodules that appear bilaterally on the shins. The lesions occur predominantly in women in the fall and winter months. Their appearance is usually associated with an infection, a reaction to a drug, or a granulomatous disease such as sarcoidosis. In particular, erythema nodosum is associated with SLE and leprosy (see Chapter 21). The major pathological finding is a subcutaneous vasculitis featuring a polymorphonuclear infiltration of small veins or arterioles. It is generally believed that erythema nodosum is caused by an immune complex allergic reaction. The skin reactions usually fade and do not require treatment.

Erythema Marginatum

An uncommon feature of rheumatic fever, classic erythema marginatum is described as a bright pink, ringlike lesion that

Table 16-3. Immune Findings in Some Skin Diseases

Disease	Lesion	Association	Immune Mechanism
Erythema nodosum	Subcutaneous vasculitis	Infection, SLE	Immune complex
Erythema marginatum	Subcutaneous vasculitis	Rheumatic fever	Immune complex (?anaphylactic)
Erythema multiforme	Subcutaneous vasculitis	Drug reaction	Immune complex
Cutaneous vasculitis	Subcutaneous vasculitis	Infection	Immune complex
Dermatitis herpetiformis	Subepidermal bullae	Gluten enteropathy (sprue)	IgA and complement deposition in dermal microfibers and basement membrane (autoantibody or immune complex)
Herpes gestationis	Subepidermal bullae	Pregnancy	Properdin, C3, and IgG in basement membrane (autoantibody or immune complex)
Pemphigus	Intraepithelial bullae	Autoallergic diseases	Autoantibody to epithelial cells
Pemphigoid	Subepidermal bullae	Neoplasm, autoallergy	Autoantibody to basement membrane
Psoriasis	Corneum parakeratosis, acanthosis	Rheumatoid arthritis	?Autoantibody to keratin
Cutaneous lupus	Basement membrane degeneration, subcutaneous vasculitis	Systemic and discoid lupus	Autoantibody to BM or immune complex deposition
Vitiligo	Melanocytes, depigmentation	Autoallergic diseases, endocrinopathy	??Antibody to melanocytes
Alopecia areata	Loss of hair		Antibody to capillary of endothelium hair bulb

spreads irregularly through pale skin. It is flat and is not pruritic or painful. The center fades as the peripheral pink edge spreads. The lesions change appearance quite rapidly (in hours or even minutes) and may fade and reappear within a few minutes. It is associated with cardiac involvement and may go on intermittently for months, even when all other signs of rheumatic fever are gone. The pathology is not well documented, although a nonspecific perivascular mononuclear infiltrate is sometimes seen. The lesions may be mediated by the inflammatory activity of anaphylatoxin as well as by inflammatory cells. Erythema chronicum migrans, which resembles erythema marginatum, follows a tick bite introducing the *Borellia* organism responsible for Lyme disease.

Erythema Multiforme

Erythema multiforme may vary from a mild skin eruption consisting of erythematous or edematous flat lesions to widespread eruptions with bullous formation and extensive sloughing of the surface of the skin, involvement of the mucous membranes of internal organs, and rapid progression to death (Stevens–Johnson syndrome). The skin lesions consist of large circular macules or papules with a central blue depression and an elevated red periphery. The variety of types of lesions is reflected in the term *erythema multiforme*. Vesicules and bullae may occur and new crops of lesions may appear in the center of fading plaques, resulting in a targetlike appearance. These eruptions usually resolve in a few weeks, but a mortality rate of up to 20% occurs with the more severe form of the disease. Lesions begin in the dermal vessels with an extensive lymphocytic infiltrate; edema fluid accumulates, leading to formation of a cavity of fluid and inflammatory cells lying between the dermis and epidermis — subepidermal bullae. Necrosis of epidermal cells may occur in the absence of inflammatory cell infiltrate. The occurrence of the disease is associated with infections and the use of certain drugs. Evidence of an allergic reaction includes (1) a latency period of 10 to 12 days between initial exposure to a drug and development of the disease, (2) the appearance of lesions in a few hours on second exposure to the drug, (3) recurrence of the disease after subsequent exposure to the offending drug, (4) changes in the small blood vessels consistent with the allergic vasculitis, and (5) skin tests with a suspected antigen that elicit the cutaneous lesion. No circulating autoantibodies to epidermal or dermal antigens have been demonstrated, and Ig and complement are not present in the lesions. It is suspected that erythema multiforme is an immune complex reaction, but the mechanism of production of this disease is still unclear. Severe cases benefit from corticosteroid treatment.

Cutaneous Vasculitis in Infectious Diseases

A variety of skin lesions may be associated with infections such as viral hepatitis, infective endocarditis, infectious mononucleosis, and a number of bacterial infections, in particular streptococcal and pseudomonal infections. In some cases, immunoglobulin and complement have been identified in cutaneous vessels, and circulating immune complexes are present. Often these patients have glomerular or pulmonary lesions as well.

Nonvascular Lesions (Cytotoxic)

Dermatitis Herpetiformis and Gluten-Sensitive Eneropathy (Sprue, Celiac Disease)

Dermatitis herpetiformis is a blistering skin lesion with papillary edema, microabscesses containing polymorphonuclear cells in dermal papillae, and subepidermal blisters. There may be intense burning and itching. Immunoglobulin A and complement are prominent in microfibers in the dermal papillae, and some patients have a bandlike granular deposition of IgA and complement in the dermal papillae along the epidermal basement membrane. IgA activates complement by the alternate pathway, and C3 is regularly found in areas of IgA deposition. Patients with dermatitis herpetiformis usually have sprue, a gluten-sensitive enteropathy (i.e., an inability to absorb nutrients from the gastrointestinal tract), and increased amounts of gastrointestinal IgA. Gluten is a gelatinous protein found in wheat and other grains. Elimination of gluten from the diet frequently results in reversal of the gastrointestinal lesions as well as the skin lesions. Thus it may be that these patients have IgA antibody to gluten protein. It is postulated that the dermal IgA originates in the gastrointestinal lymphoid tissue. When gluten protein is absorbed, IgA gluten protein complexes may circulate and deposit preferentially in the skin because of genetically determined characteristics or properties of the IgA–gluten complex.

Herpes Gestationis

Herpes gestationis is a rare, blistering skin disease associated with pregnancy and the postpartum period. The skin lesions are large subepidermal bullae. Properdin and complement have been identified in the epidermal basement membrane, indicating that the alternate pathway of complement is activated. However, IgG may be identified by more sensitive techniques, and a more recent interpretation is that IgG antibody is involved but may not be identified by the usual immunofluorescent techniques. The antibody specificity of the IgG deposited remains unknown.

Pemphigus and Pemphigoid

Pemphigus and pemphigoid are skin lesions caused by denudation of the epidermis. In pemphigus, the epidermis separates above the basal layer, resulting in either formation of large fluid-filled spaces (pemphigus vulgaris) or stripping of the upper (horny and granular) layer of epidermis (pemphigus foliaceus). In pemphigoid, separation occurs between the basal layer of the epidermis and the dermis, leading to the formation of subepidermal bullae. Antibodies to intracellular substances specific to the stratified epithelium are found in the sera of patients with pemphigus; in contrast, antibodies to the subepidermal basement membrane are found in patients with pemphigoid. Thus, pemphigus antibodies attack the epithelial cells in the stratified layers, leading to their separation from each other, cell death, and formation of bullae, whereas pemphigoid antibodies attack the basement membrane, separating the epidermis from the dermis and producing subepidermal bullae. Evidence that antiepithelial autoantibodies cause the lesions includes the following facts: the patient's own immunoglobulin binds to his skin cells; both IgG and complement are demonstrable to the lesions; and the site of the lesion, either intraepithelial or subepithelial, is directly related to the site of Ig binding in pemphigus and pemphigoid. Although it has been suggested that antibodies in these lesions may activate epithelial proteases, most evidence indicates an antibody-mediated complement-dependent cytotoxicity mechanism. Lesions similar to those of the human may be induced by injection of pemphigus antibodies into monkey mucosa, and antiepidermal cell surface antibody from pemphigus patients detaches viable epidermal cells from tissue culture dishes. The autoantigen is not well characterized, but is a protein of molecular weight of about 20,000. Several clinical courses are recognized, from rapidly fatal to relatively benign. Corticosteroid and immunosuppressive therapy have been highly efficacious in severe cases. Successful therapy not only reverses the skin lesions but also causes a reduction in the titer of autoantibodies. Pemphigoid lesions are frequently associated with other autoallergic diseases and antitissue antibodies.

Epidermolysis Bullosa Acquisita

Epidermolysis bullosa acquisita is a rare skin disease characterized by blisters and extreme fragility of the skin due to subepidermal bullae similar in appearance to bullous pemphigoid. As in bullous pemphigoid, linear depositions of immunoglobulin and complement are seen along the dermal–epidermal junction. However, immune electron microscopy shows that these depositions are localized below the subbasal lamina-anchoring fibril zone of the basement membrane, whereas in bullous pemphigoid the deposits are localized within the lamina lucida, suggesting involvement of a different antigen in these otherwise similar lesions.

Psoriasis

Psoriasis is a chonic, brownish, scaly sharply demarcated skin lesion associated with arthritis. Psoriasis is characterized by an abnormality in keratinization with elongation of dermal papillae, parakeratosis (imperfect keratinization), and intraepithelial collections of polymorphonuclear leukocytes. Immunoglobulin deposition in the epidermal layer has been reported. The immunoglobulin deposition has a characteristic intracellular and diffuse staining pattern in the stratum corneum. The pathogenic role of stratum corneum antibody is implied but not established in psoriasis. Many normal individuals apparently have such autoantibodies, and the antibody may be able to gain access to the stratum corneum only because of an as yet undefined abnormality in psoriatic individuals. Multiple HLA antigens, particularly HLA-CW6, have been associated with psoriasis.

Lupus Erythematosus

The skin lesions associated with lupus erythematosus are quite variable. The term *lupus* refers to the wolflike appearance of individuals with the full-blown facial rash. In chronic discoid lupus there is extensive accumulation of keratin in hair follicles (keratotic plugging). The epidermis is atrophic and there is a patchy mononuclear cell infiltrate near the hair follicles. In SLE the epidermis is atrophic with dissolution of the basal layer (liquefaction degeneration). There is less inflammatory filtrate, usually limited to a perivascular cuffing, and less keratotic plugging than seen in discoid lupus. There may be small vacuoles within, above, and below the basement membrane, and marked thickening of the basement membrane occurs in chronic lesions. Immunoglobulin and complement are found in the walls of blood vessels and at the dermal–epidermal junction. The characteristic lesion is described as a band of immunoglobulin at the dermal–epidermal junction and may be seen prior to development of a positive LE cell test. Granular depositions of immunoglobulin and/or complement may help predict those patients with glomerulonephritis, even those patients where clinically the skin is not involved. It is likely that in lupus, deposition of antinuclear antibody–antigen complexes occurs in epidermal basement membrane as well as in renal glomerular basement membrane, but autoantibodies to basement membrane of the skin are also present.

Vitiligo

Vitiligo is sharply delineated patches of depigmentation of the skin that occur in various sizes and shapes. Histologically, all that can be identified is an absence of melanin pigment although melanocytes are present in normal numbers. The occurrence of vitiligo is associated with autoallergic diseases and a variety of autoantibodies. Autoantibodies to melanin have been reported in some patients with vitiligo, but there has not been uniform confirmation of this observation. In addition, complement deposits have been found. Therefore an autoimmune etiology of vitiligo is unsubstantiated but remains an interesting hypothesis.

Alopecia

Alopecia is a loss of hair either in circumscribed areas (alopecia areata) or in the entire body (alopecia totalis). There is a loosely arranged nonspecific inflammatory infiltrate around the lower third of the hair follicle. Later the hair follicle becomes atrophic and the inflammatory infiltrate disappears. An association between alopecia and endocrine disease has been noted. An antibody that reacts with the capillary endothelium of the hair bulb has been reported to be eluted from lymphocytes in these patients, suggesting an antibody-dependent cell-mediated mechanism (see Chapter 19).

Amyloidosis

Amyloidosis is a disease in which there is an extracellular deposition of a hyaline, microscopically amorphous material that stains with dyes such as Congo red, which usually stains only linear polysaccharides — hence the name *amyloid* (starchlike). Amyloid is now known to be a hydrophobic proteinaceous substance containing numerous fibrils. Its protein content is heterogeneous; both fibril and plasma protein components are present (see below). Although the lesion of amyloidosis is different from those of the collagen diseases listed above, amyloidosis is included here because it may be found rarely associated with collagen–vascular diseases and frequently involves immunoglobulin deposition.

The deposition of amyloid is found in a variety of forms: primary familial, primary sporadic, secondary, localized, senile, and associated with multiple myeloma.

1. Primary familial amyloidosis is characterized by its appearance in families.
2. Primary sporadic amyloidosis is the most common form of amyloidosis. It appears in individuals with no familial tendency. Infiltrations of amyloid are usually located around small blood vessels and are found in the heart, kidney, spleen, liver, tongue, gastrointestinal tract, and other organs.
3. Secondary amyloid occurs in association with a prolonged inflammatory disease (such as tuberculosis or ankylosing spondylitis). Deposits are found in many organs but most often in kidney, liver, and spleen. Separation of primary and secondary on the basis of the organs involved (e.g., primary: heart and tongue; secondary: liver, spleen, and kidney) no longer appears to be valid.
4. Localized amyloid may be seen in tumorlike masses, primarily in the upper respiratory tract and frequently in association with neoplastic masses.
5. Senile amyloid deposits are frequently (approximately 30%) seen in the hearts of individuals over 60 years of age. No apparent clinical manifestations result.
6. Amyloidosis may be found in 10% to 20% of patients with plasma cell neoplasia (multiple myeloma), suggesting a relationship to increased immunoglobulin production.
7. Amyloid deposits resulting from excessive levels of β_2-microglobulin occur in patients on chronic dialysis.

Table 16-4. Characteristics of Amyloid Proteins

Protein	Disease Association
V_L dimer	Primary myeloma
Protein AA	Secondary familial FMF
Protein P	All
β_2-Microglobulin	Chronic dialysis

The symptoms observed in patients with amyloidosis depend upon the organ involved. Enlargement of the spleen and liver is frequent. Cardiac or renal failure may occur and localized neurological symptoms may be found as amyloid deposition impinges upon nerve fibers. Until recently the diagnosis of amyloidosis was infrequently made prior to death, but now the diagnosis may be apparent upon microscopic examination of tissue biopsies.

Amyloid deposition is caused by the overproduction of precursor molecules of plasma proteins, which are incompletely catabolized and accumulate in tissues. The chemical analysis of amyloid was not successful until the 1970s because of difficulties in solubilizing extracts of amyloid. George Glenner found that amyloid proteins are not soluble with mild solvents but will solubilize in 0.1 N NaOH or 6 M guanidine hydrochloride. Using such extraction procedures, at least four chemically distinct classes of amyloid fibrils have been demonstrated (Table 16-4).

One of these classes is a component of the immunoglobulin light chain. It is found in primary amyloidosis and amyloid associated with multiple myeloma. These amyloid depositions contain immunoglobulin when stained by specific fluorescent-labeled antibody, and amino acid sequence analysis indicates a homology between amyloid fibril proteins and immunoglobulin light chains. The immunoglobulin deposits usually consist of dimers of two variable halves of the light chain, of a variable half and a complete light chain, or of two complete light chains. Mixing V_L's from some Bence Jones proteins in vitro results in the formation of β-pleated sheet structures characteristic of amyloid. It is postulated that these structures are difficult to catabolize and may have particular affinity for deposition in certain tissues because of a Fab-like structure produced by the V_L–V_L dimers. The light chain type of the dimer is almost always the same as the amyloid protein.

A second form of amyloid is found in secondary amyloidosis and familial amyloidosis. It is made up of a nonimmunoglobulin protein called protein AA. Protein AA found in tissues has a molecular weight of 8500 and is related to a larger (MW 14,000) serum protein, SAA. A proteolytic enzyme in macrophages clips off 30 to 40 amino acid residues from the carboxy-

Amino Acid Sequence, Antigenicity	MW	Electron Microscopy	Precursor (MW)
Unique	$10,000 \times 2$	Fibril β-Sheet	L-chain (20,000)
Common	8,500	Fibril β-Sheet	SAA (14,000)
Common	$23,000 \times 10$	Doughnut 80 Å	CRP ($23,000 \times 5$)
Common	?	?	β_2-Microglobulin

terminal end of SAA to produce AA protein. AA is extremely sticky and is believed to deposit in tissues, forming typical fibrils. SAA is present in small amounts in the sera of normal patients, but patients with secondary amyloidosis most likely are stimulated to produce increased amounts of SAA that cannot be completely metabolized.

A third component of amyloid deposits is protein P. Protein P is a minor component ($<10\%$) of all amyloid and is related to C reactive protein. C reactive protein is an acute phase serum protein that can react with pneumococcal polysaccharide or various polycations to activate complement through the classical pathway. Protein P is made up of a double pentamer composed of ten MW-23,000 molecular weight subunits. C reactive protein is a single pentamer. C reactive protein most likely serves as the precursor for protein P deposition, perhaps by aggregration rather than catabolism. Protein P is responsible for the 80-Å doughnut-like structures seen in amyloid deposits.

Experimental amyloidosis may be produced in mice by repeated injections of endotoxin, casein, or bacterial products that stimulate the reticuloendothelial system. However, passive infusions of serum from a donor mouse with hypergammaglobulinemia do not cause amyloidosis in the recipient mouse. Therefore, hyperglobulinemia alone is not sufficient for amyloid deposition. On the other hand, the passive transfer of cells, cell products, or serum from mice with experimental amyloidosis may cause amyloid deposition in recipient mice. How this is accomplished in the recipient animal is not known, but the deposition is in the form of protein A. Presumably the amyloidogenic serum proteins SAA are transferred and act as precursors for protein A.

Evaluation of Circulating Immune Complexes

There are a number of laboratory assays for immune complexes (Table 16-5). Since these assays depend upon different properties of immune complexes, different tests may give different results. It is recommended that at least three tests be used: C1q binding, the Raji test, and monoclonal 19 S rheumatoid factor with high reactivity to IgG in complex form. The interpretation of positive tests for circulating immune complexes is compli-

Table 16-5. Some Techniques for Detecting Immune Complexes

ANTIGEN SPECIFIC

Isolation of complex (i.e., anti-Ig precipitation) followed by specific identification of antigen

ANTIGEN NONSPECIFIC

Physical techniques
  Ultracentrifugation
  Sucrose gradient centrifugation
  Gel filtration
  Ultrafiltration
  Electrophoresis
  Polyethyleneglycol precipitation
Biological techniques
  Complement reactivity (C1q binding, PPT)
  C3 precipitation
Antiglobulin (anti-IgG)
  Rheumatoid factors with specificity for IgG in complexes
Cellular
  Platelet aggregation
  Release of enzymes from mast cells
  Rosette inhibition
  Raji cell (Fc receptor)
Other
  Binding to Staph A protein

Modified from Theofilopoulos AN: Evaluation and significance of circulating immune complexes. In Schwartz RS (ed): Progress in Clinical Immunology, Vol 4. Grune & Stratton, 1980, p63.

cated. Many asymptomatic individuals have detectable circulating immune complexes (CIC) with no symptoms or lesions. However, in symptomatic individuals the level of immune complexes often correlates with the severity of disease.

Summary

Immune complex reactions are caused by reaction of immunoglobulin antibody with tissue antigens, by formation of antibody–antigen complexes that deposit in vessel walls or basement membrane of capillaries, or by reaction of antibodies with basement membrane antigens. Tissue destruction is mediated by lysosomal enzymes released from polymorphonuclear leukocytes attracted and activated by complement components (C3a, C5a). Acute lesions result from tissue digestion by enzymes, whereas chronic lesions may be caused by deposition of large amounts of immune complexes or scarring. Typical diseases caused by this mechanism include serum sickness, glomerulonephritis, collagen–vascular diseases (see Chapter 17), and many types of skin eruptions. The antigens involved may be host tissue antigens (autoallergic reaction) or foreign (bacterial, viral) antigens.

References

Arthus Reaction

Arthus M: Injections répétées de sérum de cheval chez le lapin. CR Soc Biol (Paris) 55:817, 1903.

Cochrane CG: Mediators of the Arthus and related reactions. Prog Allergy 11:1, 1967.

Cochrane CG, Weigle WO, Dixon FJ: Factors responsible for decline of inflammation in Arthus hypersensitivity vasculitis. Proc Soc Exp Biol Med 101:695, 1959.

Cochrane CG, Weigle WO, Dixon FJ: The role of polymorphonuclear leukocytes in the initiation and cessation of the Arthus vasculitis. J Exp Med 110:481, 1959.

Crawford JP, Movat H, Ranadive NS, Hay JB: Pathways to inflammation induced by immune complexes: development of the Arthus reaction. Fed Proc 41:2583, 1982.

Gell PGH, Hinde IT: Observations on the histology of the Arthus reaction and its relation to other known types of skin hypersensitivity. Int Arch Allergy 5:23, 1954.

Humphrey JH: The mechanism of Arthus reactions. II. The role of polymorphonuclear leukocytes and platelets in reversal of passive reactions in the guinea pig. Br J Exp Pathol 36:283, 1955.

Margaretten W, McKay DG: The requirement for platelets in the active Arthus reaction. Am J Pathol 64:257, 1971.

Movat HZ, Fernando NVP: Allergic inflammation. The earliest fine structural changes at the blood–tissue barrier during antigen–antibody interaction. Am J Pathol 42:41, 1963.

Opie EL: Pathogenesis of the specific inflammatory reaction of immunized animals (Arthus reaction). J Immunol 9:259, 1924.

Opie EL: The fate of antigen (protein) in an animal immunized against it. J Exp Med 39:659, 1924.

Rich AR, Follis RH: Studies on the site of sensitivity in the Arthus phenomenon. Bull Johns Hopkins Hosp 66:106, 1940.

Serum Sickness

Cochrane CG: The role of immune complexes and complement in tissue injury. J Allergy 42:113, 1968.

Dixon FJ: The role of antigen–antibody complexes in disease. Harvey Lect 58:21, 1962.

Dixon FJ, Vasquez JJ, Weigle WO, Cochrane CG: Pathogenesis of serum sickness. Arch Pathol 65:18, 1958.

Germuth FG: A comparative histologic and immunologic study on rabbits of induced hypersensitivity of serum sickness type. J Exp Med 97:257, 1953.

Griswold WR, Brams M, McNeal R: The rapidly changing nature of acute immune complex disease. J Lab Clin Med 96:57, 1980.

Kniker WT, Cochrane CG: Pathogenic factors in vascular lesions of experimental serum sickness. J Exp Med 122:83, 1965.

von Pirquet CF, Schick B: Serum Sickness, 1905 (Schick B, trans). Baltimore, Williams & Wilkins, 1951.

Immune Complex Injury

Cochrane CG: Immunologic tissue injury mediated by neutrophilic leukocytes. Adv Immunol 9:97, 1968.

Cochrane CG, Koffler D: Immune complex disease in experimental animals and in man. Adv Immunol 16:185, 1973.

Cochrane CG, Ward PA: The role of complement in lesions induced by immunologic reactions. *In* Graber P, Miesher P (eds): Immunology, Vol IV. Basel, Schwabe, 1966.

Dixon FJ: The role of antigen–antibody complexes in disease. Harvey Lect 58:21, 1962.

Gotze O, Muller-Eberhard HJ: The C3 activator system: an alternate pathway of complement activation. J Exp Med 134:905, 1971.

McCluskey RT, Hall CL, Colvin RB: Immune complex mediated diseases. Hum Pathol 9:71, 1978.

Movat HZ: Pathways to allergic inflammation: the sequelae of antibody–antigen complex formation. Fed Proc 35:2435, 1976.

Weigle WO: Fate and biological action of antigen–antibody complexes. Adv Immunol 1:283, 1961.

Glomerulonephritis

Adler S, Baker P, Pritzl P, Couser WG: Effects of alterations in glomerular charge on deposition of cationic and anionic antibodies to fixed glomerular antigens in the rat. J Lab Clin Med 106:1, 1985.

Atkins RC, Holdsworth SR, Hancock WW, et al: Cellular immune mechanisms in glomerulonephritis: the role of mononuclear leukocytes. Springer Semin Immunopathol 5:269, 1985.

Balow JE: Steroids in immunologically mediated renal disease. Hosp Pract 18:85, 1983.

Batsford S, Oite T, Takamiya H, Vogt A: Anionic binding sites in the glomerular basement membrane: possible role in the pathogenesis of immune complex glomerulonephritis. Renal Physiol 3:336, 1980.

Burkholder PM: Atlas of Human Glomerular Pathology. Hagerstown, Harper & Row, 1974.

Camussi G, Noble B, Van Liew J, et al: Pathogenesis of passive Heymann glomerulonephritis: chlorpromazine inhibits antibody-mediated redistribution of cell surface antigens and prevents development of the disease. J Immunol 136:2127, 1986.

Coimbra TM, Gouveia MA, Ebisul L, et al: Influence of antigen changes in the pathogenicity of immune complexes in rats. Br J Exp Pathol 66:595, 1985.

Costanza ME, Pinn V, Schwartz RS, Nathanson L: Carcinoembryonic antigen–antibody complexes in a patient with colonic carcinoma and nephrotic syndrome. N Engl J Med 289:520, 1973.

Couser WG, Salant DJ: In situ immune complex formation and glomerular injury. Kidney Int 17:1, 1980.

D'Amico G: Idiopathic IgA mesangial nephropathy. Nephron 41:1, 1985.

Gauthier VJ, Striker GE, Mannik M: Glomerular localization of preformed immune complexes prepared with anionic antibodies or with cationic antigens. Lab Invest 50:636, 1984.

Kashgarian M, Hayslett JP, Spargo BH: Renal disease. Am J Pathol 89:187, 1977.

Klassen J, Andres GA, Brennan JC, McClusky RT: An immunologic renal tubular lesion in man. Clin Immunol Immunopathol 1:69, 1972.

Klassen J, McClusky RT, Milgrom F: Non-glomerular renal disease produced in rabbits by immunization with homologous kidney. Am J Pathol 63:333, 1971.

Knisser MR, Jenis EH, Lowenthal DT, Bancroft WH, Burus W, Shalhoob R: Pathogenesis of renal disease associated with viral hepatitis. Arch Pathol Lab Med 97:193, 1974.

Lampert PH, Dixon FJ: Pathogenesis of the glomerulonephritis of NZB/W mice. J Exp Med 127:507, 1968.

Lehman DH, Wilson CB, Dixon FJ: Interstitial nephritis in rats immunized with heterologous tubular basement membrane. Kidney Int 5:187, 1974.

Lerner RW, Dixon FJ: Transfer of ovine experimental allergic glomerulonephritis (EAG) with serum. J Exp Med 124:431, 1966.

Lowance DC, Mullins JD, McPhaul JS Jr: IgA associated glomerulonephritis. Int Rev Exp Pathol 17:144–172, 1977.

McPhaul JJ, Dixon FJ: Characterization of human anti-glomerular basement membrane antibodies eluted from glomerulonephritic kidneys. J Clin Invest 49:308, 1970.

Nagai T, Tadao T, Ogino K, Kith T: IgE deposits in glomeruli with membrane nephropathy and marked asthmatic predisposition in humans. Jpn Circ J 37:1227, 1973.

Steblay RW, Rudofsky V: Autoimmune glomerulonephritis induced in sheep by injections of human lung and Freund's adjuvant. Science 160:204, 1968.

Stevenson JA, Leona LA, Cohen AH, Border WA: Henoch–Schönlein purpura. Arch Pathol Lab Med 106:192, 1982.

Tisher CC: Functional anatomy of the kidney. Hosp Pract 13:53, 1978.

Unanue ER, Dixon FJ: Experimental glomerulonephritis: immunological events and pathologic mechanism. Adv Immunol 6:1, 1967.

Van Marck EAE, Peelder AM, Gigase PLJ: Effect of partial portal vein ligation on immune glomerular deposits in Schistosoma mansoni–infected mice. Br J Exp Pathol 58:412, 1977.

Vernier RL: Clinical aspects of glomerulonephritis. In Sampter M (ed): Immunological Diseases, 2nd ed. Boston, Little, Brown, 1971, p1134.

Verroust PJ, Wison CB, Cooper NR, Edgington TS, Dixon FJ: Glomerular complement components in human glomerulonephritis. J Clin Invest 53:77, 1974.

Westberg NG, Naff GB, Boyer JT, Michael AF: Glomerular deposition of properdin in acute and chronic glomerulonephritis with hypocomplementemia. J Clin Invest 50:642, 1971.

Wilson CB, Dixon FJ: Immunologic mechanisms in nephritis. Hosp Pract 14:57, 1979.

Zabriskie JB: The role of streptococci in human glomerulonephritis. J Exp Med 134:180, 1971.

Other Immune Complex Diseases

Benoit FL, Rulon DB, Theil GB, Doolan PD, Watten RH: Goodpasture's syndrome: a clinicopathologic entity. Am J Med 37:424, 1964.

Brentjens JR, O'Connel DW, Pawlowski IB, Hsu KC, Andres CA: Experimental immune complex disease of the lung: the pathogenesis of a laboratory model resembling certain interstitial lung diseases. J Exp Med 140:105, 1974.

Buchmeier MJ, Oldstone MBA: Virus-induced immune complex disease: identification of specific viral antigens and antibodies deposited in complexes during chronic lymphocytic choriomeningitis virus infection. J Immunol 120:1297, 1978.

DeGowin RL, Oda Y, Evans RH: Nephritis and lung hemorrhage: Goodpasture's syndrome. Arch Intern Med 111:62, 1963.

Dreisin RB, Schwartz MI, Theofilopoulis AN, Stanford RE: Circulating immune complexes in the idiopathic interstitial pneumonias. N Engl J Med 298:353, 1978.

Fernandez R, McCarty DJ: The arthritis of viral hepatitis. Ann Intern Med 74:207, 1971.

Grey HM, Kohler PF: Cryoimmunoglobulins. Semin Hematol 10:87, 1973.

Henson JB, Gorham JR: Animal model of human disease: Aleutian disease of mink. Am J Pathol 71:345, 1973.

Ingram DG, Cho HJ: Aleutian disease in mink: virology, immunology and pathogenesis. J Rheumatol 1:1, 1974.

Lampert PW, Garrett R, Lampert A: Ferritin immune complex deposits in the choroid plexus. Acta Neuropathol (Berl) 38:83, 1977.

Lampert PW, Garret RS, Oldstone MBA: Immune complex deposits in the choroid plexus. Birth Defects 14:237, 1978.

Liebow AA: Definition and classification of interstitial pneumonias in human pathology. Hum Pathol 8:1, 1975.

Maumenee AE, Silverstein AM (eds): Immunopathology of Uveitis. Baltimore, Williams & Wilkins, 1964.

Melish M, Hicks RV, Reddy V: Kawasaki Syndrome: an update. Hosp Pract 17:99, 1982.

Penny R: Vasculitis: an approach for physicians. Aust NZ J Med 11:302, 1981.

Porter DD, Larsen AE, Porter HG: The pathogenesis of Aleutian disease of mink. I. Viral replication and the host antigen. J Exp Med 130:575, 1969.

Rotter JI, Henner DC: Are there immunologic forms of duodenal ulcer? J Clin Lab Immunol 7:1, 1982.

Steere AC, Hardin JA, Malawista SE: Lyme arthritis: a new clinical entity. Hosp Pract 13:143, 1978.

Behçet's Syndrome

Behçet H: Über rezidivierende Aphtose durch ein Virus verursachte Geschwure am Mund, am Auge und an den Genitalien. Dermatol Wochenschr 105:1152, 1937.

Cohen L: Etiology, pathogenesis and classification of aphthous stomatitis and Behçet's syndrome. J Oral Pathol 7:347, 1978.

Hooks JJ, Benezra D, Cohen L, et al: Classification, pathogenesis and etiology of recurrent oral ulcerative diseases and Behçet's syndrome. J Oral Pathol 7:436, 1978.

Lakhanpal S, Tani K, Lie JT, et al: Pathologic features of Behçet's syndrome: a review of Japanese autopsy registry data. Hum Pathol 16:790, 1985.

Lehner T, Barnes CG (eds): Behçet's Syndrome: Clinical and Immunological Features. Academic Press, New York, 1980.

Immune Skin Diseases

Bedi TR, Pinkus H: Histopathologic spectrum of erythema multiforme. Br J Dermatol 95:243, 1976.

Beutner EH, Jordon RE, Shorzelski TP: The immunopathology of pemphigus and bullous pemphigoid. J Invest Dermatol 51:63, 1968.

Bor S, Feiwel M, Chanarin I: Vitiligo and its aetiological relationship to organ specific autoimmune disease. Br J Dermatol 81:83, 1969.

Cavenish A: A case of dermatitis from 9-bromofluorene and peculiar reaction to a patch test. Br J Dermatol 52:155, 1940.

Chorzelski TP, Von Weiss JF, Lever WF: Clinical significance of autoantibodies in pemphigus. Arch Dermatol 93:570, 1966.

Clark WH, Reed RJ, Mihm MC: Lupus erythematosus. Histopathology of cutaneous lesions. Hum Pathol 4:157, 1975.

Claxton RC: Review of 31 cases of Stevens–Johnson syndrome. Med J Aust 50:963, 1963.

Cochran REI, Thompson J, MacSween RNM: An autoantibody profile in alopecia totalis and diffuse alopecia. Br J Dermatol 95:61, 1976.

Cormane RH: Diagnostic procedures in immunodermatology. J Invest Dermatol 67:129, 1976.

Cunliff WJ, Hall R, Newell DJ, Sevenson CJ: Vitiligo, thyroid disease and autoimmunity. J Dermatol 80:135, 1968.

Diaz LA, Calvauico NJ, Tomasi TB Jr, Jordon RE: Bullous pemphigoid antigen: isolation from normal human skin. J Immunol 118:455, 1977.

Epstein WL: Erythema nodosum. *In* Sampter M (ed): Immunological Diseases, 2nd ed. Boston, Little, Brown, 1971, p944.

Farb RM, Dykes R, Lazarus GS: Anti-epidermal-cell-surface pemphigus antibody detaches viable epidermal cells from culture plates by activation of proteinases. Proc Nat Acad Sci USA 75:459, 1978.

Fletcher MWC, Harris RC: Erythema exudativum multiforme (Mebra) —bullous type. J Pediatr 27:465, 1945.

Hertz KC, Gazze LA, Kirkpatrick CH, Katz SI: Autoimmune vitiligo. Detection of antibodies to melanin-producing cells. N Engl J Med 297:634, 1977.

Holubar K, Konrad K, Stingl G: Detection by immuno-electron microscopy of immunoglobulin G deposits in skin of patients with herpes gestationis. Br J Dermatol 96:569, 1977.

Jablonska S, Beutner EH, Michel B, et al: Cooperative study: uses for immunofluorescence tests of skin and sera. Arch Dermatol 111:371, 1975.

Jablonska S, Chorzelski TP, Jarzabek-Chorzelska M, Beutner EH: Studies in immunodermatology. VIII. Four-compartment system studies of IgG in stratum corneum and of stratum corneum antigens in biopsies of psoriasis and control dermatosis. Int Arch Allergy 48:324, 1975.

Jordon RE, Heine KG, Tappeiner G, Bushkell LL, Provost TT: The immunopathology of herpes gestationis. Immunofluorescence studies and characterization of "HG Factor." J Clin Invest 57:1426, 1976.

Katz SI, Strober W: The pathogenesis of dermatitis herpetiformis. J Invest Dermatol 70:63, 1978.

Krogh HK, Tonder O: Immunoglobulins and antiimmunoglobulin factors in psoriatic lesions. Clin Exp Immunol 10:623, 1972.

Langhof HV, Feverstein M, Schabinski G: Anti-melanin antibody in vitiligo. Hautarzt 5:209, 1965.

Lever WF: Histopathology of the Skin, 3rd ed. Philadelphia, Lippincott, 1961.

Murphy GF, Guillen FJ, Flynn TC: Cytotoxic T lymphocyte and phenotypically abnormal epithelial dendritic cells in fixed cutaneous eruptions. Hum Pathol 16:1264, 1985.

Pearson RW: Advances in the diagnosis and treatment of blistering disease: a selective review. *In* Malkinson FW, Pearson RW (eds): 1977 Year Book of Dermatology. Chicago, Year Book Med Pub, 1977.

Pedro SD, Dahl MV: Direct immunofluorescence of bullous systemic lupus erythematosus. Arch Dermatol 107:118, 1973.

Person JR, Rogers RS: Bullous and cicatricial pemphigoid. Clinical, histopathologic and immunologic correlations. Mayo Clin Proc 53:54, 1977.

Provost TT, Tomasi TB Jr: Evidence for the activation of complement via the alternate pathway in skin diseases. II. Dermatitis herpetiformis. Clin Immunol Immunopathol 3:178, 1974.

Schultz JR: Pemphigus acantholysis: A unique immunologic injury. J Invest Dermatol 74:359, 1980.

Shelley WB: Herpes simplex virus as a cause of erythema multiforme. JAMA 201:153, 1967.

Starr JC, Brasher CW: Erythema marginatum preceding hereditary angioedema. J Allergy Clin Immunol 53:352, 1974.

Tan EM, Kunkel HG: An immunofluorescent study of the skin lesions in systemic lupus erythematosis. Arthritis Rheum 9:37, 1966.

Thomas BA: The so-called Stevens–Johnson syndrome. Br J Med 1:1393, 1950.

Weiss TD, Tsai CG, Baldassare AR, Zuckner J: Skin lesions in viral hepatitis: histologic and immunofluorescent findings. Am J Med 64:269, 1978.

Woolfson H, Finn OA, Mackie RM, McQueen A, MacSween RNM: Serum anti-tumor antibodies and auto-antibodies in vitiligo. Br J Dermatol 92:395, 1975.

Yaoita H, Briggaman RA, Lawley TJ, et al: Epidermolysis bullosa acquisita: ultrastructural and immunological studies. J Invest Dermatol 76:288, 1981.

Amyloidosis

Anders RF, Natvig TE, Michaelsen TE, Husby G: Isolation and characterization of amyloid serum protein SAA as a low molecular weight protein. Scand J Immunol 4:397, 1975.

Cathcart ES, Skinner M, Cohen AS: Immunogenicity of amyloid. Immunology 20:945, 1971.

Cohen AS: Amyloidosis. N Engl J Med 277:522, 1967.

Cohen AS, Cathcart ES, Skinner M: Amyloidosis—current trends in its investigation. Arthritis Rheum 21:153, 1978.

Glenner GG: Amyloid deposits and amyloidosis: The β-fibrilloses. N Engl J Med 302:1283,1333, 1980.

Glenner GG, Ein D, Eanes ED, Bladen HA, Terry W, Page DL: Creation of "amyloid" fibrils from Bence Jones proteins in vitro. Science 174:712, 1971.

Glenner GG, Terry W, Harada M, Isersky C, Page D: Amyloid fibril proteins: proof of homology with immunoglobulin light chains by sequence analysis. Science 172:1150, 1971.

Glenner GG, Terry WD, Isersky C: Amyloidosis: its nature and pathogenesis. Semin Hermatol 10:65, 1973.

Gorevic PD, Cleveland AB, Franklin EC: The biologic significance of amyloid. Ann NY Acad Sci 77:380, 1982.

Gorevic PD, Franklin EC: Amyloidosis. Annu Rev Med 32:261, 1981.

Howes EL Jr, Incus T, McKay DG, Christian CL: A model for amyloidosis. Arthritis Rheum 6:278, 1963.

Jaffee RH: Amyloidosis produced by injections of proteins. Arch Pathol Lab Med 1:25, 1926.

Janigan DT, Druet RL: Experimental immune amyloidosis in x-irradiated recipients of spleen homogenates or serum from immunized donors. Am J Pathol 52:381, 1968.

Levo Y, Frangione B, Franklin EC: Amino acid sequence similarities between amyloid P, component C1q and CRP. Nature 268:56, 1977.

Linder E, Anders RF, Navig JB: Connective tissue origin of the amyloid-related protein SAA. J Exp Med 144:1336, 1976.

Pras M, Reshef T: The acid soluble fraction of amyloid—a fibril-forming protein. Biochim Biophys Acta 271:193, 1972.

Puchtler H, Sweat F: A review of early concepts of amyloid in context with contemporary chemical literature from 1839 to 1859. J Histochem Cytochem 14:123, 1965.

Rosenthal CJ, Franklin EC, Frangione B, Greenspan J: Isolation and partial characterization of SAA—an amyloid relative protein from human serum. J Immunol 116:1415, 1976.

Vazquez JJ, Dixon FJ: Immunohistochemical analysis of amyloid by fluorescence technique. J Exp Med 104:727, 1956.

Watanabe S, Jaffee E, Pollock S, Sipe S, Glenner G: Amyloid AA protein: cellular distribution and appearance. Am J Clin Pathol 67:540, 1977.

Willerson JT, Asofsky R, Barth WF: Experimental murine amyloid. IV. Amyloidosis and immunoglobulin. J Immunol 103:741, 1969.

Immune Complex Evaluation

Delire M, Masson PL: The detection of circulating immune complexes in children with recurrent infections and their treatment with human immunoglobulins. Clin Exp Immunol 29:385, 1977.

Dernouchamps JP, Vaermau JP, Michaels J, Masson PL: Immune complexes in the aqueous humor and serum. Am J Ophthalmol 84:24, 1977.

Ploth DW, Fitz A, Schnetzler D, Seidenfeld J, Wilson CB: Thyroglobulin–antithyroglobulin immune complex glomerulonephritis complicating radioiodine therapy. Clin Immunol Immunopathol 9:327, 1978.

Ritzmann SE, Daniels JC: Immune complexes: characteristics, clinical correlations and interpretive approaches in the clinical laboratory. Clin Chem 28:1259, 1982.

Theofilopoulos AN: Evaluation and clinical significance of circulating immune complexes. Prog Clin Immunol 4:63, 1980.

Theofilopoulos AN, Dixon FJ: Detection of immune complexes: techniques and implications. Hosp Pract 15:107, 1980.

Theofilopoulos AN, Dixon FJ: Immune complexes in human disease. Am J Pathol 100:531, 1980.

17 | Connective Tissue (Collagen–Vascular, Rheumatoid) Diseases

Klemperer in 1942 coined the term *collagen disease* for a number of disorders that had in common a morphologically similar lesion in connective tissue. The characteristic lesion is fibrinoid necrosis — an increase in ground substance with swollen, fragmented collagen fibers and necrosis, resulting in a structureless eosinophilic area resembling fibrin in appearance. The collagen diseases include polyarteritis nodosa, systemic lupus erythematosus (SLE), dermatomyositis, progressive systemic sclerosis (scleroderma), thrombotic thrombocytopenic purpura, rheumatic fever, rheumatoid arthritis, and Sjögren's syndrome. The concept that one disease could affect the function of many organs was revolutionary at the time. We now think that most of the lesions of the collagen diseases may be explained by immune complex–mediated mechanisms, but other mechanisms, in particular delayed hypersensitivity (see Chapter 19), may also contribute. Since the major lesion of Sjögren's syndrome is mediated by delayed hypersensitivity, this disease will be covered in the next chapter.

The collagen diseases vary markedly in their clinical features, time course, location of lesions, pathological picture, and immune findings. As depicted in Figure 17-1, there is considerable overlap of pathological features within the collagen disease group. The incidence of collagen diseases is increased in association with autoimmune and granulomatous diseases. Many individuals with a collagen disease have angiitis or glomerulonephritis, immunoglobulin abnormalitites, and autoantibodies with varied specificies of reactivity, including falsely positive tests for syphilis. Some of the protean manifestations of syphilis, and other chronic infectious diseases, are not unlike many of the features of the collagen diseases, and may be the result of autoimmune reactions caused by alteration of host tissue or allergic reactions to infecting organisms located in host tissue. Similarly, the lesions seen in the collagen

413

414

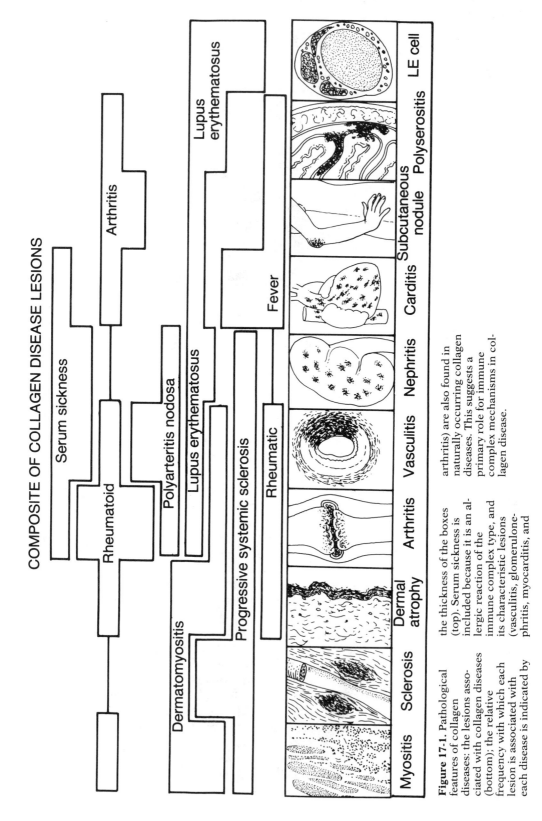

COMPOSITE OF COLLAGEN DISEASE LESIONS

Figure 17-1. Pathological features of collagen diseases: the lesions associated with collagen diseases (bottom); the relative frequency with which each lesion is associated with each disease is indicated by the thickness of the boxes (top). Serum sickness is included because it is an allergic reaction of the immune complex type, and its characteristic lesions (vasculitis, glomerulonephritis, myocarditis, and arthritis) are also found in naturally occurring collagen diseases. This suggests a primary role for immune complex mechanisms in collagen disease.

diseases may result from immune reactions to as yet undetected infectious agents.

The variable clinical and pathological features of the collagen diseases may be the result of the operation of different types of immune reactions with different degrees of severity at different times, directed toward different antigenic specificities with different tissue locations. The interplay of these variables could produce varying clinical pictures during the course of a disease in a given individual. It is within the scope of this text to cover only selected clinical and pathological features of these diseases. For further information, the reader is referred to the standard textbooks of medicine and pathology or to the *Primer on Rheumatic Disease* published by the Arthritis Foundation, Atlanta, Georgia.

Polyarteritis Nodosa

This disease consists of multiple foci of localized infarcts affecting almost any organ or combination of organs in the body. Inflammation of medium-sized arteries results in thrombosis and obstruction of blood flow, leading to many areas of necrosis and scarring. There is characteristically necrosis of a portion of the arterial wall with sparing of the remaining wall. The necrotic segment may become distended due to intraarterial pressure, resulting in the formation of microaneurysms and giving rise to the term *nodosa;* hence *polyarteritis nodosa.*

The arterial lesion is similar to that seen in serum sickness arteritis, and immunoglobulin may be identified in the areas of fibrinoid necrosis. The role of this immunoglobulin in the production of the lesion is unclear. The immunoglobulin may be antibody that is reacting with antigen that is part of the vessel wall; it may be part of an antigen–antibody complex formed in the circulation and deposited in the vessel wall; or the immunoglobulin may be nonspecifically absorbed to an arterial lesion evoked by an unrelated mechanism.

Complexes of viruses and immunoglobulin appear to be responsible for some cases of polyarteritis nodosa (PAN). A substantial number of patients with polyarteritis nodosa have hepatitis B antigenemia, suggesting that polyarteritis occurring naturally may be due to an immune response to viral hepatitis infection with hepatitis B antigen release. The association of polyarteritis with drug administration also suggests that some cases of polyarteritis may be caused by an immune response to drugs administered for therapy of other diseases. Polyarteritis nodosa has been reported rarely in patients undergoing hyposensitization for asthma.

Only about half of the cases of histologically proven polyarteritis nodosa survive over 5 years. Early and vigorous treatment with corticosteroids and cyclophosphamide may significantly improve the prognosis, but this has not been documented in a controlled study.

Systemic Lupus Erythematosus

Systemic lupus erythematosus (SLE) is a complex syndrome caused by autoantibodies produced to a wide variety of the patient's own cellular antigens, particularly nuclear antigens. This disease appears most frequently in women of childbearing age and characteristically involves many different tissues. There is an increased incidence in individuals of HLA-DR2 and HLA-DR3 major histocompatibility complex (MHC) type and in individuals with inherited deficiencies of complement. The fatal form is a rapidly advancing systemic disease featuring high fever, skin rash, nephritis, polyarthritis, polyserositis (pleural, pericardial, and peritoneal effusions), and central nervous system symptoms. With recent diagnostic techniques (mainly tests for antinuclear antibodies), milder forms of SLE have been recognized that may include only a remitting arthralgia, myalgia, and malaise. Degrees of severity between these extremes are common, and the clinical course is usually characterized by spontaneous remissions and exacerbations. Diagnosis and classification of SLE in a given patient are based on the results of a series of clinical findings and laboratory tests (Table 17-1).

Table 17-1. American Rheumatism Association Criteria for the Diagnosis of Systemic Lupus Erythematosus

1. Butterfly rash (facial erythema)
2. Skin rash of discoid lupus (raised keratotic patches)
3. Raynaud's phenomenon (transient ischemia of fingers)
4. Alopecia (rapid loss of hair)
5. Photosensitivity (unusual skin reaction to light)
6. Oral or nasopharyngeal ulceration
7. Arthritis without deformity
8. Positive antinuclear antibody test
9. Chronic false positive serologic tests for syphilis
10. Proteinuria > 3.5 g/day
11. Urinary casts
12. Pleuritis or pericarditis
13. Psychosis and/or convulsions
14. Hemolytic anemia, leukopenia, or thrombocytopenia

Note. Four or more positive criteria are required for diagnosis.

Pathology of SLE

The pathological changes of SLE include proliferative and/or membranous glomerulonephritis that may result in formation of so-called wire loops, hyaline thrombosis, and hematoxylin bodies; periarteriolar fibrosis in the spleen; scattered focal thickening, necrosis, and fibrosis of medium-sized arterioles in many different organs; and patchy atrophy of the epidermis and collagen degeneration of the dermis, both of which occur more frequently in areas of the skin exposed to sunlight.

Antinuclear Antibodies

A major diagnostic advance in SLE was the recognition of the LE cell by Hargraves in 1948. The LE cell is a polymorphonuclear neutrophil that has phagocytosed nuclear material. Its formation depends upon the presence of an antibody capable of reacting with nucleoprotein. When whole anticoagulated peripheral blood from a patient with SLE is incubated in vitro, this antibody reacts with the nuclei of lymphocytes. The swollen nuclear material is then phagocytosed by polymorphonuclear neutrophils in the peripheral blood, and LE cells are formed (Fig. 17-2).

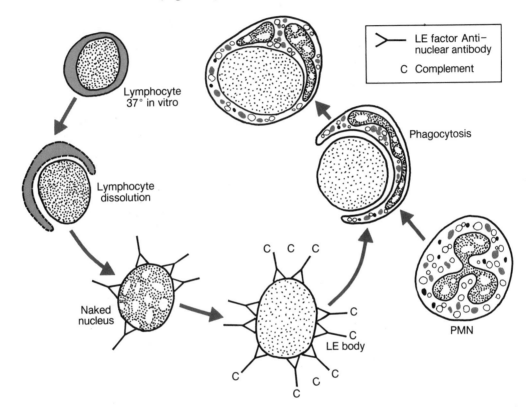

Figure 17-2. Formation of LE cell. LE cells are polymorphonuclear leukocytes that have phagocytosed the nuclei of lymphocytes by coating the nuclei with antibody. This takes place at 37°C upon incubation of the whole blood of a patient with SLE who has antibody to nucleoprotein or other nuclear antigens. Lymphocytes break up, and lymphocyte nuclei become coated with antibody (LE factor), swell, and are phagocytosed by polymorphonuclear leukocytes. LE cells may also be formed by phagocytosis of the nuclei of cells other than lymphocytes.

A variety of antinuclear antibodies have been identified in the sera of patients with SLE, and identification of these has replaced the LE cell test in the clinical laboratory. These include anti-DNA, antinucleoprotein, antihistones, antiacidic nuclear proteins, antinucleolar RNA, and antibodies to fibrous or particulate nucleoprotein (Table 17-2). The immunofluorescent staining pattern observed when serum from a patient with SLE is allowed to bind to tissue nuclei provides some clues to diagnosis. The localization of the bound immunoglobulin is determined by addition of fluorescent-

Table 17-2. Some Reactivities of Antinuclear Antibodies

Type of Antibody	Disease in Which Antibodies Seen
Antibody to DNA	
1. Reacts only with double-stranded DNA	Characteristic of SLE; few cases reported
2. Reacts with both double- and single-stranded DNA	High levels in SLE; lower levels in other rheumatic diseases
3. Reacts only with single-stranded DNA	Rheumatic, nonrheumatic diseases
Deoxynucleoprotein, soluble form	LE cell antibody in SLE, drug-induced LE
Histone	SLE, drug-induced SLE
Sm	Highly diagnostic of SLE
Nuclear RNP (Mo)	High levels in mixed connective tissue disease; lower levels in other rheumatic diseases
Cytoplasmic RNP (Mu)	SLE
Scl-70	Highly diagnostic of scleroderma
SS-A (Ro)	High prevalence in Sjögren's syndrome sicca complex (40%); lower prevalence in other rheumatic diseases (SLE 25%)
SS-B (La) (Ha)	High prevalence in Sjögren's syndrome sicca complex (20%); lower prevalence in other rheumatic diseases (SLE 10%)
Ma	SLE
RANA	Present in RA and Sjögren's syndrome with RA
Pn-Scl	High prevalence in myositis and scleroderma overlaps
PCNA	SLE
Nucleolar	High prevalence in progressive systemic sclerosis; SLE
Centromere	High prevalence in mild scleroderma (CREST syndrome)
Jo-1	Highly specific for polymyositis
Ni-2	Specific for dermatomyositis

Abbreviations: ANA, antinuclear antibodies; DNA, deoxyribonucleic acid; RNA, ribonucleic acid; LE, lupus erythematosus; SLE, systemic lupus erythematosus; RNP, ribonuclear protein; RA, rheumatoid arthritis; Sm, Smith; Scl, scleroderma; SS,

Characteristic of Antigenic Determinants	Nuclear Pattern Observed by Indirect Immunofluorescent Test
Double-strandedness of DNA essential	Rim and/or homogeneous
Related to deoxyribose, purines, and pyrimidines, but not dependent on double helix	Same as No. 1
Related to purines and pyrimidines, with ribose or deoxyribose equally reactive	Not detected on routine screen; special treatment necessary
DNA–histone complex necessary; dissociated components are nonreactive	Rim and/or homogeneous
Different classes of histones may have different determinants	Homogeneous and/or rim
U1-RNP, U2, U4-6	Speckled
U1-RNP (RNA splicing enzymes)	Speckled
Ribosomal fraction	Nucleolar, cytoplasm
Extractable antigen, topoisomerase I	Atypical speckled
Chemical nature unknown	Negative
Extractable antigen, RNA polymerase III transcript	Speckled
Chemical nature unknown	?
Chemical nature unknown, relates to EBNA	Negative
Chemical nature unknown	Nucleolar
Chemical nature unknown	Speckled in proliferating cells
4–6 S RNA	Nucleolar
Centromere antigens	Discrete centromeric staining
Histidyl tRNA synthetase	Cytoplasmic or nuclear
Chemical nature unknown	Homogeneous

Sjögren's syndrome; RANA, rheumatoid arthritis nuclear antigen; EBNA, Epstein–Barr virus nuclear antigen; PCNA, proliferating cell nuclear antigen.
Table contributed by Frank Arnett, University of Texas Medical School, Houston.

labeled antibody to immunoglobulin (indirect fluorescent antibody test). Four major patterns are seen: nuclear rim (anti-DNA or anti-nucleoprotein), speckled (antiacidic nuclear proteins), nucleolar (antinucleolar RNA), and diffuse (not antigenically specific). The association of antibodies of different specificities with certain collagen–vascular diseases is shown in Table 17-3.

Table 17-3. Nuclear Staining Patterns Observed in Patients with Collagen Diseases

Staining Pattern	Major Disease Association	Specificities of Antibody
Rim	SLE	DNA or nucleoprotein
Speckled	SLE, scleroderma, other connective tissue diseases	Ribonucleoprotein
Nucleolar	Scleroderma, Sjögren's syndrome	4–6 S RNA
Diffuse	SLE, Sjögren's syndrome, rheumatoid arthritis	Nucleoprotein, unknown

Patients with SLE may have a number of serologic abnormalities in addition to antinuclear antibodies. These include antibodies to basement membranes of the skin, antibodies to red blood cells (positive Coombs test), antibodies to blood clotting factors (lupus anticoagulant), antibodies to lymphocytes (usually to T suppressor cells), falsely positive serologic reactions for syphilis, and antibodies to cytoplasmic antigenic components. These "autoantibodies" may be responsible for some SLE lesions (Table 17-4). A transient annu-

Table 17-4. Systemic Lupus Erythematosus

Organ Involvement	Associated Autoantibodies	Proposed Mechanism
Glomerulonephritis	Anti-double-stranded DNA Anti-Ro(SS-A) Other (?)	Immune complexes
Cerebritis (psychosis), seizures, infarction	Antineuron Antilymphocyte Anti-DNA, anti-Sm Antiphospholipid	Antibody mediated Immune complex vasculitis Vascular thrombosis
Dermatitis	Anti-Ro(SS-A) Anti-DNA Others (?)	Immune complexes Antibody-dependent cytotoxicity (?)
Red blood cell	Anti-RBC	Antibody mediated
Lymphocyte	Antilymphocyte	Antibody mediated
Platelet	Antiplatelet	Antibody mediated
Arthritis, serositis	None	Immune complexes

From the lecture notes of Dr. Frank Arnett, University of Texas, Houston.

lar erythematous skin rash or permanent heart block that appears in neonates of mothers with antibody to Ro(SSA) antigen has been recognized as due to passive transfer of antibody from mother to fetus. This may occur when the mother is asymptomatic.

The membranous glomerulonephritis of SLE may contain

deposits of immunoglobulin and DNA; both granular and linear deposits of Ig have been observed. Immunoglobulin and complement may also be detected in the vascular lesions of the spleen and other organs, in the basement membrane of skin, and along the dermal–epidermal junction of grossly normal-appearing skin (positive lupus band test). These latter antibodies are associated with a high incidence of renal disease. In addition, antibodies to lymphocyte antigens that cross-react with neurons may be found in LE sera, and immune complexes are frequently found in the basement membrane of the choroid plexus (see above). The relationship of these to the central nervous system (CNS) symptoms associated with lupus erythematosus remains unclear.

The etiology of naturally occurring SLE remains unsolved, but two major theories are offered:

1. SLE is a virus-induced disease. Antibodies to viral antigen and intracellular tubular inclusions consistent with viral particles are frequently found in patients with SLE. However, a specific virus responsible for SLE has not been identified.
2. There is an imbalance of humoral immunity. This leads to abnormal antibody formation to a variety of antigens, including host molecules. Multiple MHC and non-MHC genes appear to predispose to this imbalance.

The most acceptable explanation at the present time is a combination of the above: an abnormal humoral antibody response to a chronic viral-like infection and formation of antibodies that cross-react with a wide variety of human tissues.

Drug-Induced Lupus Erythematosus

In recent years, the features of SLE have been identified in patients receiving certain drugs. The important difference between drug-induced SLE and naturally occurring SLE is that the drug-induced symptoms generally disappear upon discontinuation of the drugs. Drugs associated with SLE include diphenylhydantoin, isoniazid, hydralazine, and procainamide, used for the treatment of epilepsy, tuberculosis, hypertension, and cardiac arrhythmias, respectively. Other drugs produce SLE-like syndromes less frequently. The mechanisms of induction of drug associated SLE-like syndromes are not yet fully understood. Patients with hydralazine-induced SLE may have antibodies to hydralazine as well as antibodies to native DNA. In contrast, procainamide induces antibodies to denatured DNA, presumably because of complexes of the drug and host DNA; antibodies to native DNA or to procainamide alone are not produced. Procainamide acts by stabilization of cell membranes. It may bind to erythrocyte surfaces, alter red cell membranes, and produce immunogenic membrane fragments that lead to autoantibody formation and a Coombs-positive hemolytic anemia. Hydralazine and isoniazid may form reactive intermediate radicals that inactivate and alter DNA, producing immunogenic DNA fragments. Thus the induction of autoantibodies or formation of drug–antibody toxic complexes results in drug-induced SLE-like syndromes; different drugs may act by different mechanisms.

Treatment

Treatment of SLE is generally designed to reduce both the inflammatory reaction of the disease and the amount of pathogenic antibodies (see Chapter 27). Treatment for mild or moderate manifestations of SLE includes avoidance of the sun, rest, and aspirin or other nonsteroidal anti-inflammatory drugs. Two agents are used for life-threatening episodes: corticosteroids and immunosuppressive drugs (azathioprine, cyclophosphamide), and in some cases, a combination of the two. The protocol used for steroid treatment calls for high initial doses (1 mg/kg/day) with tapering off after 7–10 days when fulminant disease manifestations are controlled. Steroid therapy not only prolongs the lives of patients with severe SLE but also significantly changes the character of the syndrome. Prior to steroid therapy, patients frequently died of an acute crisis; now the disease is more protracted, and chronic renal or neurological problems cause death. Lower doses of steroids and anti-inflammatory drugs may control symptoms in patients with less severe disease. Effective therapy reduces the acute symptoms (fever, joint pain, others) and reverses the immunological abnormalities. The intensity of therapy depends upon the severity of the disease and the degree of response, which may vary considerably from patient to patient. Two important prognostic indicators are the severity of renal disease (a creatinine greater than 0.3 mg/ml) and the presence of antibodies to skin basement membrane (lupus band test). These are associated with a poor prognosis. Patients with acute disease that responds to steroids should have steroids withdrawn as soon as possible. The major deleterious effect of steroids is a decrease in immune defensive reactions, resulting in susceptibility to a variety of opportunistic infections (see Secondary Immune Deficiencies, Chapter 26). Although the present therapy considerably improves the prognosis and condition of patients with SLE, it is far from satisfactory. Ninety percent of well-managed SLE patients have at least a 10-year survival, but over 50% of those with renal or neurological involvement die within 10 years of the onset of symptoms. Plasmapheresis may be used as a last resort.

"Lupus Mice"

New Zealand black (NZB) mice and F_1 hybrids of NZB mice and some other inbred mouse strains spontaneously develop lesions similar to human SLE, and serve as animal models of lupus erythematosus. The NZB inbred mouse strain was developed by Marianne Bielchowsky in New Zealand in the 1950s for cancer research. These mice were found to respond immunologically quite differently from other mouse strains. After immunization with a variety of exogenous antigens, NZB mice produce abnormally high humoral antibody responses but less intense delayed (cellular) hypersensitivity than other mice. The "lupus" strains of mice spontaneously develop a number of immunopathological abnormalities, including a Coombs-positive hemolytic anemia, LE- and rheumatoid-like factors, hypergammaglobulinemia, circulating immune complexes, and glomerulonephritis. The thymi of NZB mice develop germinal centers with aging; germinal centers are not normally found in the thymus, but sometimes occur in humans with myasthenia gravis (see Chapter 14). Other lupus mouse strains have atrophy of the thymic cortex. The development of these immunological abnormalities occurs after about 4 to 6 months of age. Female mice develop more severe abnormalities than male mice, and at an earlier age.

The reason for development of "lupus" in these mice is not clearly understood but appears to depend on multiple factors including genetically controlled tendencies to abnormally high antibody responses associated with virus infections. Multiple immune controlling factor abnormalities have been described including polyclonal B cell activation, decreased T suppressor cell activity, increased T helper activity, antilymphocyte antibodies, increased complement activation, and increased T killer cell activity. A constellation of these incompletely understood factors appears to contribute to the lupus erythematosus disease syndrome in these mice.

Dermatomyositis

Symptoms of this disease complex include an erythematous skin rash, mild arthritis, and progressive muscular weakness, each of which may occur with a different degree of severity. The primary lesion is in muscle and consists of a degeneration of muscle fibers associated with infiltration of mononuclear cells (polymyositis). This may occur with or without a skin rash. The cause is unknown. Several clinical subdivisions have been suggested. The characteristic symptom is muscle weakness of insidious onset. The incidence of dermatomyositis is increased in association with malignant tumors, lymphoproliferative syndromes, and certain autoallergic diseases. Females are affected twice as commonly as males. The diagnosis is most often confirmed by electromyography and muscle biopsy, and the activity of the diseases process may be followed by detection of enzymes (especially creatine phosphokinase) released from affected muscle tissue. An experimental disease, experimental allergic myositis, may be produced in animals by immunization with xenogeneic muscle tissue in complete Freund's adjuvant.

This experimental disease is more likely a delayed hypersensitivity reaction than an antibody-mediated inflammation. The inflammatory lesions in the muscles of patients with myositis are also more consistent with a delayed hypersensitivity reaction and/or an antibody-dependent cell-mediated mechanism. This suggests that more than one type of allergic reaction may be responsible for the lesions of dermatomyositis. Newer antinuclear antibodies have been found in myositis patients. Jo-1 antibodies directed against histidyl tRNA synthetase are very specific for polymyositis with lung involvement, while Ni-2 occurs only (3%) in patients with dermatomyositis. Pn-Scl is seen frequently in patients with myositides in the setting of scleroderma (see Table 16-3). The disease frequently has remissions and exacerbations, but the natural course is progressive. Corticosteroid therapy provides effective relief, and death from progressive muscular weakness producing respiratory failure occurs rarely. Immunosuppressive drugs have been reported to induce remissions in some steroid-resistant cases.

Progressive Systemic Sclerosis (Scleroderma)

This disease, primarily involving the skin, is characterized by fibrotic thickening (sclerosis) of connective tissue in association with mild to moderate mononuclear cell infiltration. Scleroderma refers to scarring of the skin, the only lesion in some cases, but systemic involvement of synovia, gastrointestinal tract, kidneys, heart, and lungs may occur and lead to a number of symptoms (Table 17-5). The five major findings that make up

Table 17-5. Symptoms and Lesions of Scleroderma

CLASSIC SCLERODERMA	
Pulmonary	Dyspnea, cough, failure
Gastrointestinal	Dysphagia, dysmobility, constipation, malabsorption
Renal	Proteinuria, azotemia, hypertension, failure
Musculoskeletal	Polyarthralgia, contractures, myositis
Cardiovascular	Arrhythmias, failure
CREST COMPLEX	
Calcinosis	In subcutaneous connective tissue
Raynaud's	Temporary vasospasm of fingers
Esophageal dysmobility	Dysphagia
Sclerodactyly	Thickening of the skin of the fingers
Telangectasia	Hyperplasia of small blood vessels in skin and mucous membranes

the CREST complex designate a more benign form of the disease usually limited to cutaneous manifestations. Females are affected approximately twice as frequently as males. Skin thickening is usually noted first on the fingers, then on the upper extremities and upper torso. The skin loses its flexibility and becomes taut and shiny. The dermis of the skin or the muscular wall of the gastrointestinal tract is replaced with compact bundles of collagen. Inability to move fingers and difficulty in swallowing may be prominent symptoms. Arthralgia is usually present. Joint lesions show focal collections of chronic inflammatory cells; the appearance may essentially be identical to that of early rheumatoid arthritis. The kidneys have concentric intimal thickening of small renal arteries, and sometimes fibrinoid necrosis of the arterial wall. The course of the disease may be rapidly progressive or slowly evolving over a number of years. Progression of the disease occurs in three phases: edematous, indurative, and atrophic. The major feature is the overproduction of connective tissue. The mechanism for this is not known, but there is some evidence that lymphocytes or mast cells from scleroderma patients may produce soluble factors that enhance synthesis of collagen by fibroblasts. A variety of serologic abnormalities occur, including the presence of LE factors, antinuclear antibodies (especially Scl-70, centromere, Pn-Scl, and nucleolar), rheumatoid factors, and other autoantibodies. No satisfactory treatment is known.

Shulman's syndrome (diffuse fasciitis with eosinophilia) is a very rare disease consisting of diffuse fasciitis of rapid onset, hypergammaglobulinemia, and eosinophilia associated with scleroderma-like lesions with firm taut skin and flexion contractures. There is often a dramatic response to prednisone therapy. There is an absence of Raynaud's phenomenon or visceral involvement, but immune-mediated aplastic anemia and/or thrombocytopenia may occur. Immunoglobulin and C3 are localized in the affected fascia.

Thrombotic Thrombocytopenic Purpura

Thrombotic thrombocytopenic purpura (TTP) consists of thrombocytopenia (decreased number of blood platelets), hemolytic anemia, hemorrhagic skin lesions (purpura), and central nervous system signs and symptoms. Autopsy reveals widespread thrombotic occlusion of arterioles and capillaries by hyaline masses that are usually located beneath the endothelium. The central nervous system symptoms are presumably due to microvascular occlusions. The anemia is microangiopathic, secondary to mechanical destruction of erythrocytes by the physical trauma of contact with the altered vascular walls. The etiology of the vascular lesions is unknown, but they may be caused by a form of toxic complex or autoantibody deposits leading to focal fibrinoid necroses and hyaline scarring or by activation of the clotting mechanism by toxic complexes.

Rheumatic Fever

Rheumatic fever is an acute systemic disease that includes inflammation of the heart (carditis), joints (polyarthritis), and skin (erythema marginatum) and development of subcutaneous nodules and involuntary movements of muscles (chorea,

St. Vitus' dance). These findings occur in a variety of combinations that together permit the diagnosis of rheumatic fever.

Rheumatic fever occurs as a sequel to group A streptococcal infections. There are cross-reacting antigenic specificities between certain streptococcal antigens and host tissue. Antibodies with cross-reacting specificity appear in the sera of patients with rheumatic fever and in animals inoculated with group A streptococci. The most important is streptococcal M protein. Antibodies to M proteins cross-react with heart muscle. The antigen is protein in nature, but has been only partially characterized. It is possible that these antibodies react with heart tissue and are responsible for the production of lesions. On the other hand, some of the lesions of rheumatic myocarditis are more consistent with cell-mediated destruction (see Chapter 19), and animals inoculated with group A streptococci have lymphocytes that are cytotoxic for myocardial cells in vitro. Thus, rheumatic myocarditis may be caused by the action of autoantibody, autosensitized cells, or both. The chorea of rheumatic fever is associated with autoantibodies to basal ganglia that can be removed by absorption with streptococcal cell walls. Cross-reacting antibodies to other tissue antigens and immune complexes of antibody and streptococcal antigen most likely account for other manifestations of rheumatic fever (Table 17-6).

Table 17-6. Cross-Reacting Antibodies in Streptococcal Infections

Strep A Antigen	Host Tissue	Lesion
Streptolysin O		
Streptokinase		
Hyaluronidase ———————→	Cartilage ——————→	Arthritis
Group A carbohydrate ———→	Heart valves ——————→	Endocarditis (Valvulitis)
Cell walls —————————	Basal ganglia ——————→	Chorea
M protein ————————	Heart muscle ——————→	Myocarditis
	Immune complexes ————→	Vasculitis
		Erythema marginatum
		Rheumatic nodule
		Glomerulonephritis

The cardiac lesion consists of foci of fibrinoid necrosis, usually in perivascular areas in the myocardium. These areas of fibrinoid necrosis contain variable numbers of mononuclear inflammatory cells and peculiar oval cells with striated nuclei (Anitschkow's myocytes) that appear to arise from the inflamed myocardium. The composite of fibrinoid necrosis and cellular reaction has a characteristic microscopic appearance and is called an *Aschoff body*. The appearance is that of a cluster of cells similar to a granuloma (see Chapter 21). The affected areas evolve into thick fibrous tissue so that old Aschoff bodies appear as focal perivascular scars. The endocarditis may be extensive, with formation of Aschoff bodies in the valve leaflets. This leads to vascularization, fibrosis, fusion, and distortion of the valve leaflets. Loss of function of affected heart valves may lead to chronic cardiac failure; the type of failure, however, depends upon the cardiac valve involved. Variable degrees of polyarthritis, vasculitis, and glomerulonephritis may be associated with rheumatic carditis, and subcutaneous nodules histologically similar, but not identical, to those seen in rheumatoid arthritis may occur. Erythema marginatum, a red, flat-topped lesion with a pale center, is a skin manifestation of the vasculitis associated with rheumatic fever.

The natural course of rheumatic fever is now understood fairly well because of recognition of the relationship between a preceding group A streptococcal infection and development of the disease. Rheumatic fever occurs after bacterial infection, but the lesions of rheumatic fever are sterile. Refinement of the diagnosis of streptococcal infection and prompt introduction of measures to eliminate the infection, usually by intensive therapy with penicillin, significantly reduce the occurrence of cardiac sequelae. The most important prognostic finding is evidence of carditis during an acute attack of rheumatic fever. If carditis is present, subsequent development of significant disease is likely; if carditis is not present, then development of rheumatic heart disease, even if subsequent attacks of rheumatic fever occur, is unlikely. The decreased incidence of rheumatic fever over the last 20 years appears to correlate with the increased use of penicillin. However, very recently the incidence of rheumatic fever appears to be increasing in many areas.

Rheumatoid Arthritis

Rheumatoid arthritis is a systemic syndrome in which inflammation of the joints caused by autoantibodies is the major feature. The autoantibodies are directed to self immunoglobulin determinants (rheumatoid factor). The formation of immune complexes in the joint spaces leads to activation of complement and destructive inflammation (see below). Cytotoxic T cells may contribute to chronic articular damage, and T cells are present in large numbers in rheumatoid synovium.

Diagnosis

The precise diagnosis of mild rheumatoid arthritis is difficult, as evidenced by the arbitrary criteria for classic, definite, and possible rheumatoid arthritis established by a committee of the American Rheumatism Association. The most common symptoms include a symmetric arthritis usually involving the knee joints or the small joints of the hands. The arthritis is the result of an inflammatory synovitis that begins as a chronic inflammatory infiltration but usually proceeds to destructive inflammation and proliferation (pannus) eroding the articular surface. The synovia become hyperplastic and filled with lymphocytes and plasma cells. Muscle wasting and the formation of subcutaneous nodules are found in about 20% of patients. The subcutaneous nodules consist of a stellate center of fibrinoid necrosis surrounded by a palisade of mononuclear cells and a variable amount of fibrous tissue. Nodules are believed to arise from vasculitis leading to fibrinoid necrosis and resultant tissue reaction. Serositis, myocarditis, vasculitis, and peripheral neuropathy may also be found.

Rheumatoid Factor

One of the diagnostic features of rheumatoid arthritis is rheumatoid factor, a circulating autoantibody with reactivity to immunoglobulins. Three general reactive specificities are recognized: (1) to xenogeneic immunoglobulins (rabbit, horse), (2) to allogeneic immunoglobulins (denatured human IgG), and (3) to autologous immunoglobulins (the patient's own IgG). Rheumatoid factor usually is an IgM (19 S) antibody that reacts with one or more of the above antigens, although 7 S rheumatoid factors are also found in some cases. The formation of rheumatoid factor is the result of an immune reaction by the host to one or more specific antigenic determinants present in his/her own immunoglobulins. Rheumatoid factor is usually detected by agglutination of particles (erythrocytes, latex) coated with IgG; it also reacts with antigen–antibody complexes. Rheumatoid factors often react with antigenic groupings of IgG that are buried in the native molecule. These antigenic specificities may be revealed by unfolding of the IgG molecule due to various denaturing processes or to the reaction of IgG antibody with antigen. Reaction of rheumatoid factor with IgG occurs in vivo and may be responsible for some of the lesions associated with rheumatoid arthritis. Necrotizing arteritis is especially likely to evolve in patients with high titers of rheumatoid factor.

In most cases rheumatoid factor (anti-IgG) forms large complexes with IgG in vivo. These complexes appear to be cleared from the circulation by the reticuloendothelial system with no further tissue damage. In rare cases the rheumatoid factor–immunoglobulin complexes are soluble at body temperature but can be precipitated from the patient's serum by cooling (cryoglobulins). Patients with cryoglobulins are more apt to develop secondary vascular lesions. Some cryoimmunoglobulins are not immune complexes but abnormal immunoglobulins found in the sera of patients with collagen diseases and patients with lymphoproliferative disorders. These "monoclonal" cryoimmunoglobulins do not cause the significant vascular and glomerular lesions found with the immune complex (mixed) cryoimmunoglobulins.

The relation of rheumatoid factor in serum to arthritis remains obscure. Pertinent findings are that rheumatoid factor is found in some normal individuals, rheumatoid arthritis may occur in agammaglobulinemic individuals, and infusion (transfer) of large amounts of rheumatoid factor into a normal individual causes no noticeable lesions. However, the serum levels of rheumatoid factor do correlate well with the appearance of subcutaneous nodules, the presence of deforming arthritis, and the incidence of systemic disease. It is possible that rheumatoid factor represents antibodies to antigen–antibody complexes formed in vivo during the course of the disease. Rheumatoid factor may also react with genetically controlled isoantigens (allotypes) located on immunoglobulins.

Pathogenesis

Although most of the serologic findings do not support an etiologic role for serum rheumatoid factor in the pathogenesis of rheumatoid arthritis, observations on synovial fluid (the fluid of the articular cavity) support an immune complex autoimmune mechanism for the early inflammation of rheumatoid arthritis. The synovial fluid aspirated from patients with active rheumatoid arthritis may contain demonstrable immune complexes, and the polymorphonuclear leukocytes in such fluids have complexes of rheumatoid factor and IgG in their cytoplasm. There is also a selective lowering of complement components in the synovial fluid during active rheumatoid arthritis. The possible role of antibody and cellular immune mechanisms in rheumatoid arthritis is depicted in Figure 17-3. The synthesis of complement components by synovial inflammatory tissue may also contribute to the severity of the arthritis.

A search for an infectious agent initiating rheumatoid arthritis has yielded a number of possibilities, but as yet there is no clear identification of an etiologic agent. There has been some evidence that the Epstein–Barr (EB) virus may be associated with rheumatoid arthritis. EB virus is believed to be the causative agent for infectious mononucleosis and lymphoid tumors in humans (Burkitt's lymphoma; see Chapter 28). The sera of patients with rheumatoid arthritis contain antibody activity to a nuclear antigen found only in B cell lymphoid cell lines that have been transformed (immortalized) by EB virus. This antigen is not the same as the EB virus antigen found in Burkitt's lymphoma and has been termed *rheumatoid arthritis–associated nuclear antigen* (RANA). An etiologic relationship between EB virus infection and rheumatoid arthritis has not been demonstrated, but further studies on this possibility are under way.

Clinical Course

The clinical course of rheumatoid arthritis is quite variable; in some cases, there is rapid progression to severe disability, and in others, a prolonged benign course with little or no joint deformity. Spontaneous remissions and exacerbations occur frequently and make evaluation of therapy difficult. Rheuma-

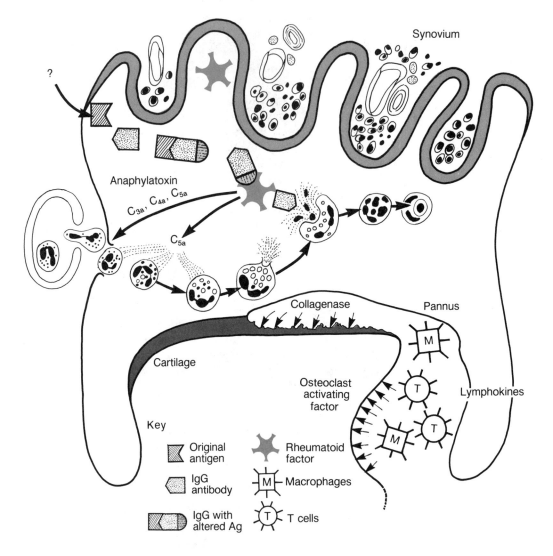

Figure 17-3. Current concepts of the pathogenesis of rheumatoid arthritis postulate that an as yet unidentified antigen (infectious agent, host autoantigen) present in the joint cavity stimulates the production of an antibody. Antigen–antibody complexes are formed that produce an alteration in the tertiary structure of the antibody, revealing new or buried antigenic determinants. These determinants in turn stimulate the production of another antibody, rheumatoid factor (IgM or IgG), which can react with IgG. Complexes form in the synovial fluid and activate complement components that attract polymorphonuclear leukocytes. A proliferation of lymphocytes and plasma cells in the synovial lining tissue converts the synovium into a lymphoid organ, which produces rheumatoid factor that is released locally into the synovial fluid. T lymphocytes in the synovium are activated to produce lymphokines that attract and activate macrophages. Macrophages produce osteoclast-activating factor that leads to destruction of adjacent bone. Hyperplasia of granulation tissue and inflammatory cells occurs and extends as a mass (pannus) over the articular cartilage. The pannus produces collagenase and elastase that destroys the joint cartilage. This pannus may progress to form a scar in the joint that leads to immobilization.

toid arthritis does not usually shorten life, but can lead to total disability in about 10% of the cases. Inflammation of the heart, small or medium vessels, and lung (diffuse interstitial pulmonary fibrosis) is infrequent but may occur and is believed to be part of the rheumatoid process. Rheumatoid nodules may form in any tissue of the body. In the lung, rheumatoid nodules are worsened or exacerbated by tissue injury, such as that produced by silica exposure in hard-coal miners (Caplan's syndrome).

Therapy

Therapy is directed toward controlling pain, reducing inflammation, and preventing severe deformities by active physical therapy or orthopedic surgery. Salicylates and other nonsteroidal anti-inflammatory agents have a beneficial effect and, along with low doses of steroids, are the drugs of choice in most cases. The synovium of rheumatoid arthritics contains mast cells and macrophages. Mast cells release arachidonic acids, and macrophages process arachidonic acids to prostaglandins. Prostaglandins are present in high concentrations in rheumatoid synovium and are believed to contribute to the disease. Salicylates or other cyclooxygenase inhibitors may function to reduce prostaglandin synthesis in synovial tissues. Corticosteroids may provide temporary relief of pain but do not effectively control the disease. Other antirheumatic agents include gold salts and antimalarial drugs. Immunosuppressive therapy and plasmapheresis have also been applied in severe cases.

Mixed Connective Tissue Disease

In 1972 G. C. Sharp described a syndrome characterized by features of different rheumatic diseases that has been designated *mixed connective tissue disease*. These patients have a variety of the clinical features of collagen diseases, which overlap with SLE, dermatomyositis, rheumatoid arthritis, and scleroderma, including arthritis and arthralgia, Raynaud's phenomenon, myositis, serositis, splenomegaly, anemia, leukopenia, hyperglobulinemia, and glomerulonephritis. These patients usually have high titers of antibody to ribonucleoprotein. The impression is that this disease eventually progresses to systemic sclerosis.

Summary

Connective tissue (collagen – vascular) diseases include a number of diseases believed to be caused primarily by immune complex mechanisms. These diseases are polyarteritis nodosa, systemic lupus erythematosus, dermatomyositis, progressive systemic sclerosis (scleroderma), thrombocytopenic purpura, rheumatic fever, and rheumatoid arthritis. The shared lesions include fibrinoid necrosis, glomerulonephritis, and vasculitis. Other immune effector mechanisms (neutralization, cytotoxic, delayed, and granulomatous reactions) play a pathogenic role in some lesions seen in these diseases, but the major manifestations may be attributed to immune complex reactions. The causes of these diseases are quite variable. Fulminant manifestations may be controlled by anti-inflammatory drugs or steroids, but chronic progression is usual.

References

General

Comroe BI, Hollander JL: Arthritis and Allied Conditions, 4th ed. Philadelphia, Lea & Febiger, 1949.

Fauci AS: Corticosteroids in autoimmune disease. Hosp Pract 18:99, 1983.

Klemperer P: The concept of collagen diseases in medicine. Am Rev Resp Dis 83:331, 1961.

Klemperer P, Pollack AD, Baehr G: Diffuse collagen disease: acute disseminated lupus erythematosus and diffuse scleroderma. JAMA 119:331, 1942.

Kunkel HG, Tan EM: Autoantibodies and disease. Adv Immunol 4:352, 1964.

Lasser A: Serum antibodies in connective tissue diseases. Hum Pathol 12:1, 1981.

Rodnan GH, Schumacher HR, Zvaifler NJ (eds): Primer on Rheumatic Disease, 8th ed. Atlanta, Ga., Arthritis Foundation, 1983.

Symposium on immunologic aspects of rheumatoid arthritis and systemic lupus erythematosus. Arthritis Rheum 6:402, 1963.

Tan EM, Northway JD, Pinnas JL: The clinical significance of antinuclear antibodies. Postgrad Med 54:143, 1973.

Vaughan JH: Rheumatologic disorders due to immune complexes. Postgrad Med 54:129, 1973.

Polyarteritis Nodosa

Alarcon-Segovia D, Brown AL: Classification and etiologic aspects of necrotizing angiitides: an analytical approach to a confused subject with a critical review of the evidence for hypersensitivity in polyarteritis nodosa. Mayo Clin Proc 39:205, 1964.

Fronhert PP, Sheps SG: Long-term follow-up study of periarteritis nodosa. Am J Med 43:8, 1967.

Gocke DJ, Hsu K, Morgan C, Bombardieri S, Lockshin M, Christian CL: Association between polyarteritis and Australia antigen. Lancet 2:1149, 1970.

Kauffmann RH, et al: Circulating and tissue bound immune complexes in allergic vasculitis: relationship between immunoglobulin class and clinical features. Clin Exp Immunol 41:459, 1980.

Kussmaul A, Maier R: Über eine bisher nicht beschriebene eigenthumliche Arterienerkrankung (Periarteritis nodosa), die mit Morbus Brightii und rapid fortschreitender allgemeiner Muskellahmung einhergeht. Dtsch Arch Klin Med 1:484, 1866.

Mackel SE: Treatment of vasculitis. Med Clin North Am 66:941, 1982.

McCombs RP: Systemic "allergic" vasculitis: clinical and pathological relationships. JAMA 194:1059, 1965.

Moskowitz RW, Baggenstoss AH, Slocumb CH: Histopathologic classification of periarteritis nodosa: a study of 56 cases confirmed at autopsy. Proc Mayo Clin 38:345, 1963.

Phanuphak P, Kohler PF: Onset of polyarteritis nodosa during allergic hypersensitization treatment. Am J Med 68:479, 1980.

Rich AR, Gregory JE: The experimental demonstration that polyarteritis nodosa is a manifestation of hypersensitivity. Johns Hopkins Med J 72:63, 1943.

Rose GA, Spencer H: Polyarteritis nodosa. Q J Med 26:43, 1957.

Trepo CG, Thivolet J, Prince AM: Australia antigen and polyarteritis nodosa. Am J Dis Child 123:390, 1972.

Systemic Lupus Erythematosus

Arnet FC: HLA and genetic predisposition to lupus erythematosus and other dermatologic disorders. J Am Acad Dermatol 13:472, 1985.

Blomgren SE: Drug-induced lupus erythematosus. Semin Hematol 10:345, 1973.

Blomgren SE, Condemi JJ, Vaughan JH: Procainamide-induced lupus erythematosus. Am J Med 52:388, 1972.

Bluestein HG, Zvaifler NJ: Brain-reactive lymphocytotoxic antibodies in the serum of patients with systemic lupus erythematosus. J Clin Invest 57:509, 1976.

Burnham TK, Fine G: The immunofluorescent band test for lupus erythematosus. III. Employing clinically normal skin. Arch Dermatol 103:24, 1971.

Burnham TK, Neblett TR, Fine G: The application of the fluorescent antibody technique to the investigation of lupus erythematosus and various dermatoses. J Invest Dermatol 4:451, 1963.

Cheatum DE, Hurd ER, Strunk SW, Ziff M: Renal histology and clinical course of systemic lupus erythematosus. A prospective study. Arthritis Rheum 16:670, 1973.

Cohen AS, Canoso JJ: Criteria for the classification of systemic erythematosus. Arthritis Rheum 15:540, 1972.

Donadio JV, Holley KE, Wagoner RD, Ferguson RH, McDuffie FC: Treatment of lupus nephritis with prednisone and combined prednisone and azathioprine. Ann Intern Med 77:829, 1972.

Freese E, Sklarow S, Freeze EB: DNA damage caused by anti-depressive hydrazines and related drugs. Mutat Res 5:343, 1968.

Gilliam JN, Cheatum DE, Hurd ER, Stastny P, Ziff M: Immunoglobulin in clinically uninvolved skin in systemic lupus erythematosus. Association with renal disease. J Clin Invest 53:1434, 1974.

Hahn BH, Sharp GC, Irwin WS, Kantor OS, Gardner CA, Bagby MK, Perry HM, Osterland CK: Immune responses to hydralazine and nuclear antigens in hydralazine-induced lupus erythematosus. Ann Intern Med 76:365, 1972.

Hargraves MM, Richmond H, Morton R: Presentation of 2 bone marrow elements: the "tart" cell and the "LE" cell. Mayo Clin Proc 23:25, 1948.

Harvey AM, Shulman LE, Tumulty PA, Conley CL, Schoenrich EH:

Systemic lupus erythematosus: review of the literature and clinical analysis of 138 cases. Medicine 33:191, 1954.

Holman HR: Systemic lupus erythematosus. *In* Sampter M (ed), Immunological Diseases, Vol 2. New York, Little, Brown, 1971, p995.

Koffler D, Schur PH, Kunkel HG: Immunological studies concerning the nephritis of systemic lupus erythematosus. J Exp Med 126:607, 1967.

Lampert PW, Oldstone MBA: Host immunoglobulin G and complement deposits in the choroid plexus during spontaneous immune complex disease. Science 180:408, 1973.

Lief PD, Barland P, Bank N: Diagnosis of lupus nephritis by skin immunofluorescence, in the absence of extrarenal manifestations of systemic lupus erythematosus. Am J Med 63:441, 1977.

Luciano A, Rothfield NF: Patterns of nuclear fluorescence and DNA-binding activity. Ann Rheum Dis 32:337, 1973.

Nakamura RM, Tan EM: Recent progress in the study of autoantibodies to nuclear antigens. Hum Pathol 9:85, 1978.

Phillips PE, Christian CL: Virus antibodies in systemic lupus erythematosus and other connective tissue diseases. Ann Rheum Dis 32:450, 1973.

Siegel M, Lee SL, Peress NS: The epidemiology of drug-induced systemic lupus erythematosus. Arthritis Rheum 10:407, 1967.

Steinberg AD, et al: Systemic lupus erythematosus: insights from animal models. Ann Intern Med 100:714, 1984.

Tan EM, et al: The 1982 revised criteria for classification of systemic lupus erythematosus. Arthritis Rheum 25:1271, 1982.

Wierzchowiecki MO, Quismoro FP, Friou GJ: Immunoglobulin deposits in skin in systemic lupus erythematosus. Arthritis Rheum 18:77, 1975.

Zurier RB: Systemic lupus erythematosus. Hosp Pract 14:45, 1979.

Progressive Systemic Sclerosis (Scleroderma)

Cathcart MK, Krakauer RS: Immunologic enhancement of collagen accumulation in progressive systemic sclerosis. Clin Immunol Immunopathol 21:128, 1981.

Claman HN: Mast cell, T cells and abnormal fibrosis. Immunol Today 6:192, 1985.

Claman HN, Jafee BD, Huff JC, Clark RAF: Chronic graft vs host disease as a model for scleroderma. Cell Immunol 94:73, 1985.

Fennel RH Jr, Reddy CRRM, Vasquez JJ: Progressive systemic sclerosis and malignant hypertension. Arch Pathol 72:209, 1961.

Fu TS, et al: Eosinophilic fasciitis. JAMA 240:451, 1978.

Hochberg MC: The spectrum of systemic sclerosis: Current concepts. Hosp Pract 16:61, 1981.

Huffstutter JE, Delustro FA, Leroy EC: Cellular immunity to collagen and laminin in scleroderma. Arthritis Rheum 28:775, 1985.

McCoy RC, et al: The kidney in progressive systemic sclerosis: immunological histochemical and antibody selection studies. Lab Invest 35:124, 1976.

Rodnan GP: Progressive systemic sclerosis (diffuse scleroderma). *In* Sampter M (ed): Immunological Diseases, 2nd ed. Boston, Little, Brown, 1971.

Rothfield MF, Rodman GP: Serum anti-nuclear antibodies in progressive systemic sclerosis (scleroderma). Arthritis Rheum 11:607, 1968.

Tuffanelli DL, Winkelman RK: Systemic scleroderma: a clinical study of 727 cases. Arch Dermatol 84:359, 1961.

Winkelman RK (ed): Symposium on scleroderma. Mayo Clin Proc 46:83, 1971.

Dermatomyositis

Adams RD, Denny-Brown D, Pearson CM: Diseases of the Muscle: A Study of Pathology, 3rd ed. New York, Harper & Row, 1975.

Crowe WE, et al: Clinical and pathogenetic implications of histopathology in childhood polydermatomyositis. Arthritis Rheum 25:126, 1982.

Dawkins RL: Experimental myositis associated with hypersensitivity to muscle. J Pathol Bacteriol 90:619, 1965.

Haas DC: Treatment of polymyositis with immunosuppressive drugs. Neurology (Minneap) 23:55, 1973.

Kissel JT, Mendell JR, Rammohan KW: Microvascular deposition of complement membrane attack complex in dermatomyositis. N Engl J Med 314:331, 1986.

Mastaglia FL, Ojeda VJ: Inflammatory myopathies. Ann Neurol 17:215,317, 1985.

Reichlin M et al: Antibodies to a nuclear/nucleolar antigen in patients with polymyositis overlap syndromes. J Clin Immunol 4:40, 1984.

Salmeron G, Greenberg D, Lidsky MD: Polymyositis and diffuse interstitial lung disease: a review of the pulmonary histopathologic findings. Arch Intern Med 141:1005, 1981.

Thrombotic Thrombocytopenic Purpura

Antes EH: Thrombotic thrombocytopenic purpura: a review of the literature with a report of a case. Ann Intern Med 48:512, 1958.

Breckenridge RT, Moore RD, Ratnoff OD: A study of thrombocytopenia—new histologic criteria for the differentiation of idiopathic thrombocytopenia and thrombocytopenia associated with disseminated lupus erythematosus. Blood 30:39, 1967.

Rheumatic Fever

Feinstein AR: A new look at rheumatic fever. Hosp Pract 2:71, 1968.

Gillum RF: Trends in acute rheumatic fever and chronic rheumatic heart disease: a national perspective. Am Heart J 111:430, 1986.

Gordis L: Effectiveness of comprehensive-care programs in preventing rheumatic fever. N Engl J Med 289:331, 1973.

Gross L, Ehrlich JC: Studies on the myocardial Aschoff body. I. Descriptive classification of the lesions. Am J Pathol 10:467, 1934.

Husby G, van de Rijn I, Zabriskie JB, et al: Antibodies reacting with cytoplasm of subthalamic and caudate nuclei neurons in chorea and acute rheumatic fever. J Exp Med 144:1094, 1976.

Leirisalo M: Rheumatic fever: clinical picture, differential diagnosis and sequelae. Ann Clin Res 9(suppl 20):1, 1977.

Marboe CC, et al: Monoclonal antibody identification of mononuclear cells in endomyocardial biopsy specimens from a patient with rheumatic carditis. Hum Pathol 16:332, 1985.

Markowitz M: The decline of rheumatic fever: role of clinical intervention. J Pediatr 106:545, 1985.

Martin DR, Kick KJ: M-associated antibodies in patients with rheumatic fever. J Med Microbiol 17:189, 1984.

McCarty M: Lewis W Waunamaker in the campaign against rheumatic fever. Zentralbl Bakteriol Hyg A260:151, 1985.

Rijn I, Zabriske JB, McCarty M: Group A streptococcal antigens cross-reactive with myocardium. Purification of heart reactive antibody and isolation and characterization of the streptococcal antigen. J Exp Med 146:579, 1977.

Stollerman GH: Rheumatic Fever and Streptococcal Infection. New York, Grune & Stratton, 1975.

Williams RC: Host factors in rheumatic fever and heart disease. Hosp Pract 17:125, 1982.

Williams RC, et al: Studies of streptococcal membrane antigen-binding cells in acute rheumatic fever. J Lab Clin Med 105:531, 1985.

Yang LC, Soprey PR, Wittner MK, Cox EN: Streptococcal-induced cell-mediated-immune destruction of cardiac myofibrils in vitro. J Exp Med 146:344, 1977.

Zabriskie JB: Mimetic relationships between group A streptococci and mammalian tissues. Adv Immunol 7:147, 1967.

Rheumatoid Arthritis

Alspaugh MA, Jensen FC, Rabin H, Tan E: Lymphocytes transformed by Epstein–Barr virus. Induction of nuclear antigen reaction with antibody in rheumatoid arthritis. J Exp Med 147:1018, 1978.

American Rheumatism Association: On criteria for rheumatoid arthritis: review of the rheumatic diseases. JAMA 171:1213, 1959.

Bartfeld H, Epstein WV: Rheumatoid factors and their biologic significance. Ann NY Acad Sci 168:1, 1969.

Dayer JM, Graham R, Russel G, Krane M: Collagenase production by rheumatoid synovial cells: stimulation by a human lymphocyte factor. Science 195:181, 1977.

Freemont-Smith K, Bayles TB: Salicylate therapy in rheumatoid arthritis. JAMA 192:1123, 1965.

Harris ED: Pathogenesis of rheumatoid arthritis. Clin Orthoped 182:14, 1984.

Jasin HE: Autoantibody specificities of immune complexes sequestriated in articular cartilage of patients with rheumatoid arthritis and osteoarthritis. Arth Rheum 28:241, 1985.

Konttinen YT, et al: Cellular immunohistopathology of acute, subacute and chronic synovitis in rheumatoid arthritis. Ann Rheum Dis 44:549, 1985.

Krakauer T, Oppenheim JJ, Jasin HE: Human interleukin 1 mediates cartilage matrix degranulation. Cell Immunol 91:92, 1985.

Kurosaka M, Ziff M: Immunoelectron microscopic study of the distribution of T cell subsets in rheumatoid synovium. J Exp Med 158:1191, 1983.

Mizel S, Dayer JM, Krane SM, Mergenhagen SE: Stimulation of rheumatoid synovial cell collagenase and prostaglandin production by partially purified lymphocyte-activating factor (interleukin 1). Proc Nat Acad Sci USA 78:2474, 1981.

Novri AME, Panayi GS, Goodman SM: Cytokines and chronic inflammation of rheumatic disease. I. The presence of interleukin 1 in synovial fluids. Clin Exp Immunol 55:259, 1984.

Perper RJ (ed): Mechanism of Tissue Injury with Reference to Rheumatoid Arthritis. NY Acad Sci 256, 1975.

Ruddy S, Colten HR: Rheumatoid arthritis. Biosynthesis of complement components by synovial tissue. N Engl J Med 290:1284, 1974.

Short CL, Bauer W, Reynolds WE: Rheumatoid Arthritis. Cambridge, Harvard University Press, 1957.

Williams RC: Immunopathology of rheumatoid arthritis. Hosp Pract 13:53, 1978.

Young CL, Adamson TC, Vaughn JH, Fox RI: Immunohistologic characterization of synovial membrane lymphocytes in rheumatoid arthritis. Arthritis Rheum 27:32, 1984.

Zvaifler NJ: Further speculation on the pathogenesis of joint inflammation in rheumatoid arthritis. Arthritis Rheum 13:895, 1970.

Zvaifler NJ: Immunoreactants in rheumatoid synovial fluid. J Exp Med 134:2765, 1971.

Zvaifler NJ: Rheumatoid synovitis. An extravascular immune complex disease. Arthritis Rheum 17:297, 1974.

Zvaifler NJ: Rheumatoid arthritis: a dissertation on its pathogenesis and future directions for research. Aust NZ J Med 8 (Suppl):44, 1978.

Mixed Connective Tissue Disease

Alarcón-Segovia D: Mixed connective tissue disease—a decade of growing pains. J Rheumatol 8:535, 1981.

Sharp GC, Irvin WS, Tan EM, Gould RG, Holman HR: Mixed connective tissue disease: an apparently distinct rheumatic disease syndrome associated with a specific antibody to an extractable nuclear antigen. Am J Med 52:148, 1972.

18 | Atopic or Anaphylactic Reactions (Allergy)

The term *anaphylaxis* was coined by Porter and Richet in 1902 to indicate adverse reactions to horse serum injected for passive therapy of infections. The term implies a damaging reaction that is the opposite of prophylaxis or protective reaction. Coca applied the term *atopy* in the 1920s for a variety of strange reactions in humans not then believed to occur in lower animals, from the Greek word *atopia,* meaning strangeness. These are now identified as allergies. The term *allergy* was introduced by von Pirquet in 1906 to designate "altered reactivity" as a result of previous exposure. The term *allergy* is now mostly used for atopic or anaphylactic reactions.

The effects produced by atopic or anaphylactic reactions are the result of a two-phase inflammatory reaction initiated by mediators that are released by the reaction of antigen with effector cells passively sensitized by IgE antibody (Fig. 18-1). The mast cell (tissue) or basophil (peripheral blood) is the cell responsible (see Chapter 12). Following reaction with antigen these cells release a number of biologically active substances including histamine, heparin, and serotonin (early phase), as well as arachidonic acid, which is converted by other cells into prostaglandins and leukotrienes responsible for the later-phase inflammatory reaction. The acute phase is characterized by immediate smooth muscle constriction or dilation. On the one hand, the smooth muscle of arterioles is stimulated to dilate by reaction of histamine with H-2 receptors (blocked by cimetidine). On the other hand, the smooth muscle of pulmonary bronchi, the gastrointestinal tract, and the genitourinary system, in addition to endothelial cells, is stimulated to contract by the action of histamine on H-1 receptors (blocked by antihistamines) (see Table 18-1). The role of the later-acting prostaglandins and leukotrienes is discussed in detail in Chapter 12.

Prostaglandin E is a potent dilator of bronchial smooth muscle, whereas prostaglandin F is a potent constrictor. Leu-

439

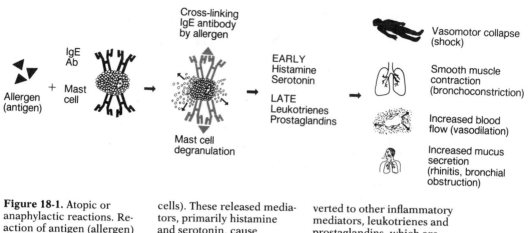

Figure 18-1. Atopic or anaphylactic reactions. Reaction of antigen (allergen) with reaginic antibody (IgE) fixed to effector (mast) cells causes release of pharmacologically active agents stored in cytoplasmic granules (degranulation of mast cells). These released mediators, primarily histamine and serotonin, cause contraction of endothelial cells and bronchial smooth cells and produce edema and bronchoconstriction. Other products released from mast cells are converted to other inflammatory mediators, leukotrienes and prostaglandins, which are responsible for later stages of the reactions. The acute effects are termed *anaphylactic*, the more chronic effects *atopic*.

Table 18-1. Allergic Symptoms: Five Organ Systems

Histamine Receptor	Reactive Tissue	Constriction	Dilation	Symptom
H$_2$	Vascular		X	Shock
H$_1$	Lung	X		Asthma
	Gastrointestinal tract	X		Vomiting and diarrhea
	Genitourinary system	X		Involuntary urination
	Endothelium	X		Edema

kotriene E4 (slow reacting substance of anaphylaxis) causes later vasoreactions, whereas leukotriene B4 is chemotactic for acute inflammatory cells. The late phase occurs 6 to 12 hours after antigen exposure and is characterized by a more prolonged reaction involving infiltration by neutrophilic, eosinophilic, and basophilic polymorphonuclear cells, as well as lymphocytes and macrophages. This late phase causes an indurated, erythematous, painful reaction in the skin, or, in the lung, a more prolonged deterioration in air flow as compared with the rapidly appearing wheal and flare skin reaction or with asthma characterized by rapidly reversible bronchoconstriction in the immediate or early phase. A better understanding of the production, release, and effects of these mediators may lead to improved therapeutic approaches.

The effects of these agents include contraction of smooth

muscle, increased vascular permeability, early increase in vascular resistance followed by collapse (shock), and increased gastric, nasal, and lacrimal secretion. The type of lesion observed depends upon the dose of antigen, the route of contact with antigen, the frequency of contact with antigen, the tendency for a given organ system to react (shock organ), and the degree of sensitivity of the involved individual. This final factor may be genetically controlled or may be altered by environmental conditions (temperature), unrelated inflammation (presence of a viral upper respiratory infection), or the emotional state of the individual. Some of the reactions seen clinically are urticaria (wheal and flare, hives), hay fever, asthma, eczema, angioedema, and anaphylaxis.

Acute reactions (wheal and flare and systemic shock) are generally referred to as *anaphylactic;* chronic recurring reactions (hay fever) are referred to as *atopic.* However, this distinction is not always made, and there is considerable overlap in the use of the terms. An atopic individual is one who is prone to develop this type of allergic reaction. The antigen responsible for elicitation of an anaphylactic or atopic reaction is referred to as an *allergen.* The antibody involved is termed *reagin.*

Reaginic Antibody

Reaginic antibody has a special ability to bind to skin or other tissues. The term *atopic reagin* was adopted to refer to the particular tissue-fixing antibody found in the serum of patients with hay fever and asthma. The original use of the word *reagin* was to designate the reacting serum component responsible for the Wassermann reaction, the serologic test for syphilis. The Wassermann reagin is a particular serum reactant found in individuals infected with syphilis. The Wassermann reagin is demonstrable by its ability to combine with an antigen extracted from ungulate heart muscle and has no relation to anaphylactic or atopic reactions. It has been reported that atopic reaginic antibody may be found in all the major immunoglobulin groups (IgA, IgG, IgM). However, in most cases reagin is found in a separate immunoglobulin class, IgE. In humans it may be assumed that atopic or anaphylactic reactions are essentially always due to IgE antibody.

IgE Antibody

IgE antibody is termed *skin fixing* because it binds to mast cells in skin or basophils in the blood and sensitizes these cells to react to allergen. IgE anaphylactic antibodies have structures on the Fc piece of the molecule that fits receptors of the basophils (mast cells). The average number of IgE molecules on a basophil is 10,000–40,000. The number of cell-bound IgE antibody molecules determines the sensitivity of basophils to an allergen. However, the amount of mediators released from a given cell depends on enzyme systems that regulate the biochemical mechanisms of mediator release. Antigen binding two adjacent IgE molecules on the cell surface initiates events leading to mediator release (see Fig. 12-5). Mediator release may also be initiated by reaction of anti-IgE with IgE on the cell surface.

Passive Anaphylaxis

The reaginic activity of an immunoglobulin is determined by its ability to fix to skin of the same species. If serum from a sensitive individual is passively transferred to the skin of a normal recipient, the classic wheal and flare reaction can be elicited at this site upon application of the antigen (Prausnitz–Kustner test). In 1921 Carl Prausnitz and Heinz Kustner reported the passive transfer of anaphylactic reactions both systemically and cutaneously, by serum from a patient sensitive to fish, to a normal individual. Because the antibody fixes to the skin, the transfer site may be tested up to 45 days later and still elicit a positive reaction. In contrast, with local passive transfer of nonreaginic antibody (passive Arthus), the skin site must be tested within a few hours in order to obtain a positive reaction before the non-skin-fixing antibody diffuses away (Table 18-2).

Table 18-2. Passive Transfer of Antibody-Mediated Skin Reactions

	Passive Cutaneous Anaphylaxis (Prausnitz–Kustner)	Passive Cutaneous Arthus
Time after antibody transfer	Up to 90 days	1–2 days
Time after antigen challenge	15 min	5–6 hr
Reaction	Wheal and flare	Induration and erythema
Histology	Edema and congestion Spongiosis[a]	Vasculitis

[a]Spongiosis—intercellular epidermal edema.

The passive transfer of atopic or anaphylactic reactions may be accomplished by a variety of methods, all of which depend upon the ability of reagins or IgE antibodies to fix the tissue (mast) cells.

1. For the local passive cutaneous anaphylaxis transfer (Prausnitz–Kustner) test, antibody-containing serum is injected into the skin and after an appropriate period of time (usually several days) the same skin site is challenged with antigen.
2. For systemic passive cutaneous anaphylaxis, either the antibody is injected intravenously and the antigen intradermally or the antibody is injected intradermally and the antigen intravenously (methods used only in experimental animals).
3. Transfer of a systemic reaction (passive systemic anaphylaxis) is best elicited by injection of the antibody intravenously, followed by injection of the antigen intravenously 24 hours later.

4. Reverse passive cutaneous anaphylaxis may be elicited if the antigen fixes to skin; in this instance the antibody does not require tissue-fixing capacities. For reverse reactions, the antigen is injected into the skin, and after a suitable period, the antibody is injected intravenously or at the same site. Reverse tests are useful for determining the skin-fixing properties of the immunoglobulins of one species for the skin of another species.

In most species studied the antibody that fixes to the skin of the same species (e.g., human reagin fixing to human skin) belongs to a special class of immunoglobulin with properties similar to human IgE. If a given antibody in a species fixes to the skin of individuals of the same species, it is termed *homocytophilic*. In some instances the immunoglobulins that fit tissue receptors of another species belong to a class other than IgE. For instance, human IgG antibodies may fix to guinea pig skin, but IgA, IgM, or IgE does not fix to guinea pig skin. Immunoglobulins that fix to the skin of a species different from their source are termed *heterocytophilic*.

IgE (reaginic) antibody has other properties different from usual antibody: it does not fix complement in the usual manner and is heat labile (56°C for 30 min). IgE antibody precipitates with antigen if sufficient amounts of antibody can be obtained. However, the amount of IgE antibody present in the serum of a sensitive individual is usually too small to be detected by precipitation, but can be detected by more sensitive techniques involving the anaphylactic response.

Skin Tests

Because of the unusual properties noted above, there is no simple test for reagin. The most commonly used clinical test is a skin test. Suspected allergens are injected into the skin of an individual to test for cutaneous anaphylaxis. In this way, allergenic antigens may be identified. Skin testing must be done under careful supervision because systemic anaphylactic shock may be induced. Antianaphylactic drugs (e.g., epinephrine) must be kept on hand for rapid use, if necessary. The local transfer of skin-fixing antibody may be used to demonstrate reaginic activity in serum (passive) cutaneous anaphylaxis. This is the basis of the Prausnitz–Kustner test. Another in vivo test that is extremely sensitive is bronchoprovocation. Inhalation of small amounts of the allergen elicits acute bronchospasm (asthma). This test is rarely done except in well-controlled settings because of the obvious danger of inducing fatal anaphylaxis.

In Vitro Tests

The Schultz–Dale test, histamine release by mast cells (degranulation), and the radioallergosorbent test (RAST) are included in this group.

Schultz–Dale Test

This test utilizes organs containing smooth muscle (guinea pig intestine or rat uterus) in an organ bath. When the organ is taken from a sensitized animal or incubated with serum from a sensitized individual, contraction occurs when the specific antigen is added. Contraction may also be induced by the addition of mediators (histamine, leukotrienes).

Histamine Release

Histamine release from mast cells in vitro may be induced by contact of sensitized mast cells with antigen. The amount of histamine release may be determined spectrophotometrically or by morphologic observation of mast cell degranulation. Nonsensitized mast cells may be passively sensitized by incubation with reagin-containing serum. The passive leukocyte-sensitizing (PLS) activity of a given serum is determined by incubating a reaginic serum with blood leukocytes from nonallergic donors for about 2 hours. The cells are then washed and treated with antigen for 1 hour. The amount of histamine present in the supernate is then determined photometrically. The extent of histamine release is used as an index of the serum reagin content. The PLS activity of ragweed-sensitive individuals is highest in the early fall (during the pollen season) and lowest in summer just prior to the pollen season.

RAST Test

The radioallergosorbent test depends upon the binding of IgE antibody to specific antigen and the subsequent binding of radiolabeled anti-IgE to the IgE antibody–antigen complex. Fluorescent and enzyme-labeled antibodies are also being used. The suspected antigen is first covalently bound to insoluble particles. The insoluble antigen is then added to samples of serum. Those sera containing antibodies to the antigen will have antibody immunoglobulin that binds to the insoluble antigen. The particles are washed and treated with a labeled antibody to IgE. The labeled anti-IgE will bind to the IgE antibody, which is bound to the insoluble antigen. By determining the amount of labeled anti-IgE bound, an estimation of the IgE antibody to the specific antigen may be made. At present the indiscriminate use of these tests to diagnose allergy has resulted in an unfortunately high incidence of the misdiagnosis of allergy. Many false positive results occur that do not correlate with in vivo testing. Reliable allergists conduct careful history taking and skin testing before attempting therapy.

Mediator Release from Mast Cells

Two types of mechanisms may operate for release of mediators from mast cells or basophils: *nonlytic*, in which mast cell lysosomal membranes fuse with each other and with the cell surface membrane, resulting in release of lysosomal contents (degranulation), and *lytic*, in which antibody–antigen complexes on the surface of mast cells bind complement components with subsequent cytolysis of the mast cell. Nonlytic release is the usual mechanism active in anaphylactic reactions involving reaginic antibody. The mast cell is not destroyed and granules re-form. Lytic release provides a mechanism whereby cytolytic allergic reactions mediated by IgG or IgM may produce anaphylactic symptoms. The mechanism by which reaction of antigen with reaginic antibody on mast cells or basophils causes the release of mediators is described in Chapter 12 (see Fig. 12-5).

Anaphylaxis

Cutaneous Anaphylaxis

Cutaneous anaphylaxis (urticaria, wheal and flare, hive) is elicited in a sensitive individual by skin test (scratch or intradermal injection of antigen). Grossly visible manifestations are erythema; itching; a pale, soft, raised wheal; pseudopods, and a spreading flare, reaching a maximum in 15 to 20 minutes and fading in a few hours. Early there is edema, with essentially no cellular infiltration until 12–18 hours. The mechanism is the same as in systemic anaphylaxis, but the reaction is localized because of the antibody fixation in the skin and release of histamine or histamine-like substances into the skin with local changes in vascular permeability. Cutaneous anaphylaxis should be differentiated from the Arthus reaction in terms of both time of appearance and morphology of the reaction (see Table 18-2).

Systemic Anaphylaxis

Anaphylaxis or anaphylactic shock is a generalized reaction elicited in a sensitized animal by the intravenous injection of antigen. However, in highly sensitive individuals, a severe systemic reaction to small doses of the allergen placed on the skin (scratch or patch test) may occur. For this reason, the clinical allergist must be prepared to administer epinephrine to any patient during skin testing. This counteracts the systemic effects of the anaphylactic reaction. The nature of the systemic reaction is species dependent. In all species, smooth muscle contraction is prominent, with increased permeability of small vessels, leukopenia, fall in temperature, hypotension, slowing of the heart rate, and decreased serum complement levels.

Guinea Pig. Death occurs in 2 to 5 minutes, with prostration, convulsions, respiratory embarrassment, involuntary urination, defecation, itching, sneezing, and coughing. At autopsy the lungs are inflated because of bronchial constriction with air trapping.

Rabbit. Death occurs in minutes; the course is similar in other respects to that in the guinea pig, except for the absence of respiratory difficulty. Autopsy shows right heart failure attributed to obstruction of the pulmonary circulation.

Dog. Death occurs after 1 to 2 hours. There is a profound prostration with vomiting and bloody diarrhea. Liver engorgement from hepatic vein obstruction is revealed at postmortem examination.

Rat. Death occurs in 30 minutes to 5 hours. There is congestion of the small intestine and midzonal and periportal necrosis of the liver.

Humans. Humans exhibit a combination of the above reactions. For instance, the description by Prausnitz and Kustner of a positive reaction after skin injection of fish muscle extract into a patient with a fish allergy in 1921 follows:

> After half an hour: itching of the scalp, neck, lower abdomen, dry sensation in the throat; soon afterwards swelling and congestion of the conjunctivae, severe congestion and secretion of the respiratory mucous membranes, intense fits of sneezing, irritating cough, hoarseness merging into aphonia, and marked inspiratory dyspnoea. The skin of the entire body, especially the face, becomes highly hyperaemic, and all over the skin of the body there appear numerous very itching wheals, 1–2 cm large, which show a marked tendency to confluence. Increased perspiration has not been noted. After about 2 hours heavy salivation starts and is followed by vomiting, after which the symptoms very gradually fade away. Temperature, cardiac and renal function have always been normal. After 10 or 12 hours all the symptoms have disappeared; only a feeling of debility persists for a day or so. After each attack there is a period of oliguria and constipation; this may be due to dehydration and vomiting.

Circulatory shock with dizziness and faintness may be the only manifestation, but collapse, unconsciousness, and death can occur within 16 to 120 minutes. There is obstruction and edema of the upper respiratory tract, laryngeal edema, and increased eosinophils in sinusoids of spleen and liver. Acute systemic anaphylaxis in man is often iatrogenic, that is, produced by injection of drugs (penicillin), but can occur naturally following insect (bee, wasp) stings.

Angioedema

Angioedema is an hereditary condition involving nonimmune mechanisms that produce lesions resembling those seen in anaphylaxis. Edema and swelling are more extensive than the localized hive. The lesion may involve the eyelids, lips, tongue, and areas of the trunk. Involvement of the gastrointestinal tract may produce symptoms of acute abdominal distress, but the symptoms almost always disappear in a few days without surgical intervention. The most significant life-threatening complication is severe pharyngeal involvement, which may lead to asphyxia. The pathological alteration is firm, nonpitting edema of the dermis and subcutaneous tissue, which can be differentiated from a wheal and flare reaction by the absence of erythema. In addition, antihistamines have no effect upon angioedema, and the lesions cause a burning or stinging sensation rather than itching.

Angioedema is inherited as a autosomal dominant trait. Biochemically, there is a deficiency of C1 esterase inhibitor (C1-INH) or C1 esterase inhibitor is present in an inactive form. C1 esterase is the active form of the first component of complement. If normal serum is incubated at 37°C there is a gradual "spontaneous" loss of complement activity. In patients with angioedema this spontaneous decrease may not occur because of a lack of C1-INH. During attacks the C4 and C2 levels in the serum are decreased, indicating that activation of the complement system is important in this phenomenon. The injection of C1 esterase into the skin of normal individuals produces a wheal and flare reaction, but the injection of C1 esterase into the skin of patients with angioedema produces a firm, nonpitting induration with no flare (localized angioedema). Production of the lesions of angioedema may involve factors other than failure to inactivate C1 esterase. C1-INH is an α_2-neuroaminoglycoprotein that is a serine esterase inhibitor. It is effective not only on activated C1 but also on plasmin, activated Hageman factor (XIIa), and kallikrein. Thus, interactions of different inflammatory systems due to C1-INH deficiency may be responsible for the clinical picture observed.

It has been claimed that attacks of angioedema may be terminated by the injection of fresh frozen plasma from normal individuals, presumably because of the presence of C1 esterase inhibitors in such preparations. However, this observation has not been generally reproducible. Episodes of local angioedema may follow surgical procedures such as dental extractions. It thus becomes important to prevent such attacks. Short-term administration of tranexamic acid does prevent these attacks. It is believed that tranexamic acid may inhibit plasmin-dependent conversion of the product of C1, C4, and C2 interaction to a pathologically active peptide.

Urticaria

Giant urticaria is manifested by the widespread development of firm, raised wheal-like lesions over large areas of the skin. They are superficial, erythematous, and intensely pruritic, with raised serpiginous edges and blanched centers. Individual lesions last about 48 hours, but new eruptions may appear for an indefinite period. Although allergic mechanisms may be operative, identification of an eliciting allergen is not possible in most instances and nonimmunologic stimuli such as heat, cold, or sunlight frequently initiate urticarial lesions. However, in some instances, the lesions of cold urticaria can be transferred with serum factors: either IgM, suggesting the involvement of a cryoimmunoglobulin, or IgE, indicating that an IgE-mediated reaction can cause giant urticaria.

Atopic Allergy

Atopic allergy is a term applied to a group of chronic human allergies to natural antigens, including asthma, hay fever, allergic rhinitis, urticaria (hives), eczema, serous otitis media, conjunctivitis, and food allergy. The mechanisms are essentially the same as those involved in systemic and cutaneous anaphylaxis. Anaphylaxis is included by many under the general term *atopy*.

The clinical features of atopic allergy are itching and whealing, sneezing, and respiratory embarrassment. The pathological features include edema, smooth muscle contraction, and leukopenia. The pharmacological characteristics are reported episodes of histamine release and partial protection by antihistamines as well as involvement of leukotrienes and prostaglandins. The type of reaction seen clinically depends upon four factors.

Route of Access of Antigen

If contact occurs via the skin, hives (wheal and flare) predominate; if contact is via respiratory mucous membranes, asthma and rhinitis occur; if contact occurs via the eyes, conjunctivitis predominates, or if through the ears, serous otitis; if contact occurs via the gastrointestinal tract, food allergy, with cramps, nausea, vomiting, and diarrhea, results.

Dose of Antigen

The rarity of death from atopic allergy, in contrast to anaphylaxis, is most likely because of the dose and route of access of the antigen. In systemic anaphylaxis, large doses of antigen are given intravenously; in atopic allergy, the doses are low and contact is across mucous membranes. Such a conclusion is justified by the observation that anaphylactically sensitized guinea pigs exposed to small amounts of antigen by inhalation develop typical asthmatic symptoms. However, in highly sensitive individuals minute doses of allergen may elicit a fatal reaction.

"The Shock Organ"

Individual differences in reactivity depend upon individual idiosyncrasies, pharmacological abnormalities of the target tissue (increased histamine content), or increased susceptibility of a given organ because of nonspecific irritation or inflammation. Many affected individuals commonly have an atopic reaction involving one organ system (asthma) without involvement of other organs.

Familial Susceptibility

Members of an atopic family have an increased incidence of atopic-type reactions. This may be because of a tendency to form a particular type of antibody (IgE). Individuals of HLA type DW2 tend to form IgE antibodies to ragweed pollen extract. The serum IgE concentrations of pairs of monozygotic twins are significantly more similar to each other than are the levels of otherwise comparable pairs of dizygotic twins. In addition, the concept of genetic control of basal IgE levels in man is supported by statistical analysis of serum IgE levels in normal adults. It is possible, although not yet established, that genetic control of the immune responses by immune response genes (see Chapter 10) may extend to the IgE immunoglobulin class; certain individuals inherit genes that select an IgE antibody response to a given antigen rather than a response with another immunoglobulin class. Elevated serum IgE levels during the first year of life frequently occur in infants who develop atopic disease later, suggesting the early expression of a genetically controlled propensity of atopic individuals to produce IgE immunoglobulin.

Asthma

Allergic and Nonallergic

The characteristic symptoms of asthma have been known since as early as the first century AD. Asthma presents clinically as reversible acute respiratory distress from airway obstruction, presumably caused mainly by constriction of the smooth muscles of the small bronchi. A number of factors predispose to development of allergic asthma, the most important being repeated exposure to the allergen. Other correlations with an allergic proclivity are listed in Table 18-3. There are at least two

Table 18-3. Factors Predisposing to Development of Allergic Disease

1. Heredity — Positive family history (HLA-DW2)
2. Prenatal effects (high cord blood IgE levels, prenatal exposure to allergens)
3. High postnatal IgE serum level
4. Birth during pollen season
5. Birth in urban environment
6. Stressful perinatal period
7. Early diet: early exposure to eggs, wheat, and bovine products (cow's milk vs breast feeding)
8. Low serum IgA levels at 3 months of age
9. Low levels of T lymphocytes at 3 months of age
10. Early surgery or hospitalization
11. Exposure to animals, molds, tobacco smoke, and pollen
12. Frequent infections

Modified from Johnston DE: Some aspects of the natural history of asthma. Ann Allergy 49:257, 1982.

forms of asthma: one clearly mediated by the anaphylactic mechanism and one that is not mediated by known allergic reactions. The allergically mediated form is caused by the activation of effector cells (mast cells) sensitized by IgE antibody. Allergic asthma is termed *extrinsic* because of the clear identification of an exogenous eliciting antigen in most cases. The mechanism of activation of the nonallergic form of asthma is not well understood but is probably due to an imbalance of the physiological control of smooth muscle tone (see below). Immune mechanisms are not believed to be involved and a specific eliciting antigen cannot be identified. Drugs that block β-adrenergic effects used for treatment of angina pectoris, cardiac arrhythmias, hypertension, glaucoma, migraine headache, and other diseases are contraindicated in patients with bronchial asthma.

Constriction of bronchial smooth muscle may be triggered by a variety of nonimmune mechanisms, including chemical irritation, change in temperature, physical activity, and emotional stress, as well as by a variety of respiratory infections. The nonimmune form of asthma is termed intrinsic because no exogenous eliciting antigen can be identified. One possible explanation is that intrinsic asthma is caused by sensitivity to a chronic infecting organism, but proof of this hypothesis is lacking. Allergic asthma is usually seasonal, although it is year-round in parts of the world where pollen allergens are present for most of the year (e.g., Bermuda grass pollen in Southern California), or if nonpollen allergens such as animal dander are responsible. Intrinsic asthma occurs throughout the year without seasonal exception. A condition of intrinsic asthma may evolve from a background of seasonal asthma or from a nonatopic background of chronic bronchitis.

Pathological Changes

A number of pathological changes have been found in the lungs of patients with either type of asthma. In the acute attack, which may be fatal because of acute asphyxiation, there is marked constriction of the bronchi and occlusion of the bronchi with a particularly thick mucous secretion (mucous plugs). In chronic asthma the pulmonary changes are (1) marked thickening of the basement membrane of the bronchial mucosa, (2) hypertrophy of the bronchial smooth muscle, (3) hypertrophy of the bronchial mucous glands, (4) eosinophils and chronic inflammatory cells in the bronchial wall, with a substantial increase over normal in the number of mast cells, and (5) the presence of mucus in the bronchi, containing large numbers of eosinophilic leukocytes. The thickened basement membrane may contain deposits of IgG or IgM, but IgE has not been detected often. Other stigmata of chronic inflammation and airway obstruction not specific for asthma, including focal fibrosis and scarring, emphysema, and atelectasis, may be found in the periphery of the lung. Since repeated asthma attacks are also associated with increased susceptibility to pulmonary infections, some of the pathological changes may be because of repeated bronchopneumonia.

Therapy

Therapy for asthma depends on whether or not a specific eliciting antigen can be identified. If it can, the best treatment is avoidance of the antigen. Immunotherapy by injection of the antigen in a manner that will change the reactivity of the patient may also be successful. Drugs that produce bronchodilation or that alter the state of activation of effector mast cells may be effective in both extrinsic and intrinsic allergy, and prompt administration by aerosol or injection may be required to prevent death in an acute attack. Psychotherapy may be effective in some cases because the extent of a given attack may be increased by anxiety; the frequency of asthma is higher for individuals in emotional distress. Breathing exercises may reduce symptoms, especially in growing children. Steroid therapy is of limited value because of undesirable side effects but does produce dramatic relief of asthmatic symptoms (see below).

Allergic Aspergillosis

An acute form of infective asthma may occur in persons with *Aspergillus* infection. *Aspergillus* is a genus of mold that may cause a pulmonary infection. A small number of individuals with pulmonary aspergillosis develop allergy to the infecting agent; this causes obstruction of the involved bronchi with mucous plugs (bronchopulmonary impaction).

Hay Fever (Seasonal Allergic Rhinitis)

Seasonal upper respiratory reactions to pollen are commonly referred to as *hay fever*. The eliciting antigens represent a variety of airborne plant pollens that cause a reaction in the nasal passages and eyes of affected individuals. Symptoms include sneezing, nasal congestion, watery discharge from the eye, conjunctival itching, and cough with mild bronchoconstriction. Pathological changes are not extensive. Usually there is edema of the submucosal tissue with an infiltration of eosinophils that is reversible. The degree of reaction and severity of symptoms are directly related to the amount of exposure to the allergen responsible. Treatment consists of avoidance, antihistamines, or specific immunotherapy. Psychological factors may determine the degree of discomfort considerably. Hay fever may progress to asthma, but usually the severity of symptoms gradually diminishes with aging.

Nasal Polyps

Nasal polyps are tumorlike masses that form in the nasal air passages, causing chronic airway obstruction and rendering nasal breathing very difficult or impossible. These masses can be removed surgically but usually recur promptly. The relationship between nasal polyps and allergic rhinitis (inflammation of the nasal mucous membranes as a result of atopic reactivity) is uncertain, although some observers feel that sinusitis and polyps may be caused by bacterial allergy. Nasal polyps characteristically show marked edema, swelling of hydrophilic ground substance, and scattered eosinophilic infiltration. Eosinophilic polymorphonuclear leukocytes are associated with severe persistent allergic rhinitis, and it has been suggested that persistent contact with small amounts of antigen leads to the characteristic picture. The prolonged nature of the swelling may be explained by continued production of hydrophilic ground substance by tissue fibroblasts.

Food Allergy

Ingestion of allergens may lead to remarkable gastrointestinal reactions known collectively as *food allergy*. The relationship of the GI reaction to atopic sensitivity is not clear. Many individuals with positive skin reactions to an allergen do not react to ingestion of the allergen, whereas individuals with repeated episodes of vomiting or diarrhea that occur on eating a given food may not produce a skin reaction to the food. Allergy to cow's milk is the most frequently suspected GI reaction to food. Milk contains over 16 proteins that might be allergenic, and skin reactions to a number of these proteins occur in some sensitive children. In addition, unsuspected food additives such as penicillin may be present in milk and elicit allergic reactions. Food allergy may lead to hypoproteinemia from the loss of protein in the GI tract and persistent diarrhea. Other manifestations of food allergy are extensive skin eruptions (urticaria or eczema) or systemic shock. Avoidance of the allergen is the primary therapy, and artificial diets are sometimes required to prevent food allergy reactions.

Atopic Allergens

Atopic reactions may occur to very unusual antigens. Systemic anaphylactic reactions have been unleashed by ingestion of beans, rice, shrimp, fish, milk, cereal mixes, potatoes, Brazil nuts, and tangerines. Men have complained about being allergic to their wives, but usually they are reacting to some component of makeup, hair spray, or other cosmetic agent. Rarely, women have developed systemic anaphylactic symptoms shortly after intercourse, and appropriate tests demonstrate anaphylactic sensitivity to seminal fluid. Several such cases have been reported in which the allergy is an IgE-mediated reaction to a seminal plasma protein. About 10% of individuals who work with laboratory animals develop anaphylactic reactions to the dander from these animals that are severe enough to prevent them from further work with the animals. The incidence of such sensitivity increases with the amount of contact with the animals. During the days of cavalry many officers and troops had to be discharged or moved to different tasks because of an allergic reaction to horse dander. As many as 20% of the cavaliers were involved. Documentation of allergic reactions of horses to humans has not been found. Several laundry detergents contain enzymes derived from *Bacillus subtilis*. These may cause severe reactions to laundry detergent involving occasional unsuspecting users. Since the use of such enzyme additives is not necessary, one must question why they are allowed to be added at all.

Aspirin Intolerance

Aspirin, one of the world's most widely used drugs, was once generally thought to be almost completely devoid of undesirable effects when used within a therapeutic dose range. However, it is now known to be responsible for a variety of atopic and anaphylactic-like reactions, including asthma, rhinitis, nasal polyps, and even anaphylactic shock. A strong plea has been made to reevaluate the uncontrolled use of aspirin.

Aspirin is a chemically active molecule that acetylates serum proteins, including human serum albumin, so that it is possible that chronic aspirin intolerance may be caused by alteration in the antigenicity of albumin or by aspirin acting as a hapten. On the other hand, an idiosyncratic effect of aspirin in disruption of the physiologic control of smooth muscle and mucus secretion has also been proposed as responsible for aspirin intolerance. Aspirin intolerance may develop in children or appear in adults with no previous history of atopy. Aspirin intolerance manifested by asthma represents a minority of asthmatic children; the onset is usually later than for asthma not related to aspirin.

In adults the symptoms of aspirin intolerance appear suddenly with a watery rhinorrhea followed by development of nasal polyps, chronic asthma, and in some cases even shock reactions to ingestion of aspirin. The chronic asthma related to aspirin intolerance responds well to drug therapy, but, of course, avoidance of aspirin is the obvious treatment. This is easier said than done, because aspirin is included in many drug mixtures, where it is unsuspected, and other cross-reacting haptens may elicit reactions in aspirin-sensitive individuals. Yellow food color number 5 contains such a related hapten.

Insect Allergy

Atopic or anaphylactic reactions to insects may be divided into three groups: inhalant or contact reactions to insect body parts or products, skin reactions (wheal and flare) to biting insects, and systemic shock reactions to stinging insects. Asthmatic or hay fever–like reactions may occur following airborne exposure of a sensitive individual to large numbers of insects or their body parts. This happens outdoors with insects that periodically appear in large numbers, such as locusts or grasshoppers, and indoors, more chronically, with beetles, flies, and spiders.

Bites

Biting insects may produce delayed hypersensitivity or acute wheal and flare skin reactions. A delayed reaction to insect bite may convert to an anaphylactic one with aging of the individual. The common reaction to a mosquito or flea bite is a localized cutaneous anaphylactic reaction. There is a very limited toxic effect of the saliva introduced by the insect bite; the reaction is an allergic one. An individual who has little or no reaction to a mosquito bite may not have developed an allergic response or may be tolerant to the allergen. Among the author's children, one has essentially no reaction to mosquito bites; one produces large, delayed hypersensitivity skin reactions; a third has large wheal and flare reactions, and the fourth produces a small, limited wheal with no flare. Serious effects of a reaction to insect bites may occur in parts of the world where large numbers of mosquitos appear in waves; multiple mosquito bites to a sensitive individual may produce systemic effects. Immunotherapy is warranted in a highly sensitive individual who risks extensive exposure.

Stings

Fatalities occur more frequently from stinging insects, such as bees and wasps. More people die each year as a result of being stung by an insect than from being bitten by a snake. Deaths from stinging insects are caused by systemic anaphylaxis and usually occur within 1 hour of being stung. Therefore, immediate therapy is required. This may be provided by injection of epinephrine (see below). Immunotherapy may prevent subsequent severe reactions. People who raise bees may permit a bee to sting them and limit the amount of venom injected; if the amount is increased on subsequent stings, the degree of reaction to a larger dose becomes less.

It is not clear what survival advantage these acute allergic reactions to insect bites and stings provide. It has been postulated that the reaction induces immediate avoidance behavior and may limit the exposure of a bitten individual to a dose of a toxic venom that could be even more damaging, or to insects that might be causes of diseases such as malaria. On the other hand, a systemic anaphylactic reaction to an insect sting may be interpreted as an immune mechanism that should be protective but is instead deleterious and potentially fatal.

Atopic Eczema – Atopic Dermatitis

In 1892 Besnier described a familial, pruritic skin disease beginning in infancy and often occurring in association with hay fever and asthma. The term *atopic dermatitis* was coined by Wise and Sulzberger in 1933. *Eczema* refers to the weeping phase of early lesions, and *dermatitis* the more chronic dry, hyperkeratotic lesions. Atopic dermatitis is a chronic skin eruption of varied etiology that usually occurs in young individuals who develop atopic reactions (hay fever) at a later age. The pathological changes in the skin are consistent with those of a severe contact dermatitis (see Chapter 19). Erythema, papules, and vesicles are accompanied by intense pruritus. There is perivascular accumulation of mononuclear cells followed by infiltration into the epidermis with epidermal spongiosis. As the affected child becomes older, thickening of the skin of the affected areas occurs (lichenification). Atopic dermatitis features thickened patches with frequent, acute, itching episodes. Identification of an antigen that elicits the eczema is very difficult, but in some cases there is evidence that the antigens are those that also elicit other allergic reactions (pollen, house dust, animal dander). Atopic eczema is morphologically more like a reaction of cellular or delayed hypersensitivity, but is discussed here because of its association with atopic conditions.

The pathogenic mechanism of atopic dermatitis remains unclear. Patients with atopic dermatitis will produce wheal and flare reactions when challenged with allergen, and this reactivity is IgE mediated. On the other hand, cutaneous antigen exposure does not elicit the skin lesion characteristic of atopic dermatitis. Atopic dermatitis patients frequently have increased delayed hypersensitivity skin reactivity and decreased in vitro blast transformation responses to various test antigens; thus atopic dermatitis may be caused by increased anaphylactic activity due to a lack of T suppressor cells.

An allergic etiology of all eczema must be questioned because typical eczema may occur in children with severe combined immune deficiency. Therefore, although proven eczema of atopic allergic origin exists, eczema-like (eczematoid) skin lesions may be produced in other ways. An abnormality in the activation, production, or inactivation of arachidonic acid metabolites has been considered as a possibility.

Immunotherapeutic Modification of Atopic Allergy

Atopic or anaphylactic conditions may be treated by injecting small amounts of the offending allergen and increasing the amount of antigen over a protracted period of time. "Desensitization" therapy for hay fever was introduced in England in 1911 by L. Noon. He was following the lead of Pasteur who had had success in "vaccination" against infectious disease. Many farmers in England at that time developed severe reactions to hay during the harvest season and were unable to continue farming. Noon prepared aqueous extracts of hay, "immunized" the affected farmers, and obtained significant beneficial effects. Although his reasoning was incorrect, the result was favorable. Injection immunotherapy may result in a significant decrease in allergic symptoms. The major factors contributing to successful immunotherapy are selection of the proper antigen and adequate doses of the antigen. Frequently in the present application of inoculation therapy in office practice, not enough of the allergen is given to be effective, but the placebo effect (estimated to be up to 30%) deludes the physician and patient into believing that the low doses of allergen are effective. Controlled clinical trials demonstrate up to 70% effective use with high dose immunotherapy for required allergy, but only 10–20% with low doses (the placebo effect). Effective immunotherapy has been accomplished using various preparations of plant antigens, insect venoms, cat dander, and more recently fire ant toxin, but the proper antigens for immunotherapy of insect or animal dander reactions remain controversial. Purified allergen preparations must be used; "whole body" insect extracts are not effective.

The mechanism of the beneficial effect of immunotherapy of allergies is not always clear. Possible mechanisms include hyposensitization (blocking), desensitization, tolerance, and suppression (Fig. 18-2).

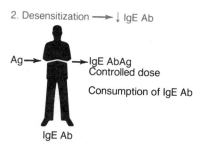
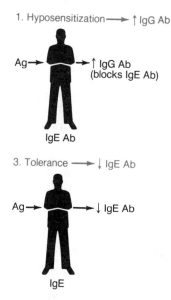
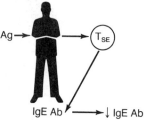
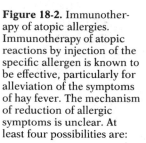

Figure 18-2. Immunotherapy of atopic allergies. Immunotherapy of atopic reactions by injection of the specific allergen is known to be effective, particularly for alleviation of the symptoms of hay fever. The mechanism of reduction of allergic symptoms is unclear. At least four possibilities are: (1) hyposensitization, production of IgG blocking antibody; (2) desensitization, consumption of IgE antibody by repeated small doses of allergen; (3) tolerance, a loss or significant decrease in IgE antibody production to the allergen; and (4) production of suppressor T cells specific for IgE/B cells. Another possible mechanism not yet identified as resulting from specific immunotherapy is the production of nonspecific IgE that might block the effector cell receptors for IgE allergen-specific antibody.

Hyposensitization

The production of blocking antibody is referred to as *hyposensitization*. By careful immunization with the offending allergen, it may be possible to induce the formation of nonreaginic, precipitating IgG antibody. Since the precipitation antibody reacts with the same antigen as the reaginic antibody, the precipitating antibody will compete with the reaginic antibody in the reaction with antigen and help prevent atopic symptoms. The formation of precipitating antigen–antibody complexes may also produce tissue changes, but many more molecules of precipitating antibody reacting with antibody are needed to produce a reaction of clinical significance than molecules of reaginic antibody. Such blocking antibody may be demonstrated in vitro by its ability to inhibit the release of anaphylactic mediators from sensitized mast cells upon exposure to antigen, and passive transfer of IgG antibody under controlled conditions reduces anaphylactic responses to bee venom. However, in some individuals who have had a beneficial response to injection therapy, no blocking antibody is demonstrable. Another possibility is that IgA antibodies in nasal or bronchial secretions may block IgE-mediated reactions, but the small changes in mucosal IgA levels measured do not account for the marked beneficial effect seen. Thus, the decrease in sensitization of many individuals must be due to some other mechanism.

Desensitization

Desensitization may be produced by providing enough antigen in small doses to combine with the IgE antibody so that IgE antibody is not available for reactive tissue sites. Desensitization may occur with injection therapy for hay fever. Frequently a series of injections of allergen binds the available antibody as it is produced without producing significant symptoms. With cessation of injections, continued IgE antibody production is able to overcome the antigen and become available for tissue sensitization.

Tolerance

Tolerance may be defined as the specific failure of responding T or B cells for a given antigen (see Chapter 11). Specific deletion of responding cells has been difficult to demonstrate. However, it is possible that specific immunotherapy might produce a temporary loss of responsiveness by specific deletion. More recent experimental studies suggest that such lack of responsiveness is due to the action of T suppressor cells.

Suppressor T Cells

Suppressor T cells specific for IgE production have been found by several investigators using mouse model systems. Suppressor T cells for IgE may be preferentially induced by controlled immunization. Factors selecting for IgE suppressor activity as opposed to IgE production include high doses (1 mg versus 1 ng) of allergen, use of particulate antigens such as alum precipitates, conjugation of antigens with polyethylene glycol, intramuscular or intraperitoneal injection of antigens rather than aerosol exposure via mucous membranes, and the use of large carrier antigens such as bacterial or parasitic extracts. Suppressor activity may be demonstrated by passive transfer of T cells from suppressed donors to primed B cells in culture or to syngeneic recipient animals (Fig. 18-3). Suppressor cells may actually turn off ongoing IgE antibody responses. There is evidence that there are separate populations of T helper cells for different Ig classes of B cells. IgE-specific T suppressor cells may act on T helper cells for IgE, IgE B cells, or T cell–B cell interactions, perhaps by production of a specific suppressor factor. There is evidence that IgE B cells may be more susceptible to T cell suppression than are IgG B cells. IgE suppressor T cells appear to control the degree of responsiveness of high and low IgE responder strains of mice, thus providing an explanation for the observation of the role of heredity in determining the class of immunoglobulin response to a given antigen. It is not clear that the same phenomenon is being studied in these experimental systems, because some investigators find that the T suppressor cells for IgE are antigen specific, whereas others do not. T cells of humans have type 1 and type 2 histamine

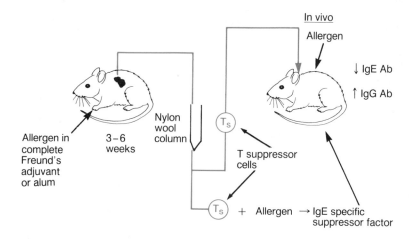

Figure 18-3. Demonstration of IgE-specific suppressor cells. In a mouse model, antigen-specific T suppressor cells that act to inhibit production only of IgE and not other Ig classes have been identified. After immunization with allergen in complete Freund's adjuvant, a population of T cells (nylon wool passed, killed by anti-T cell serum and complement) will inhibit the production of IgE antibody by primed B cells in vitro and depress IgE production in vivo after passive transfer. IgG antibody production to the same antigen is not affected. Suppression is also accomplished using a soluble factor (SF_E) derived from the T suppressor cells exposed to the specific antigens. This suppressor factor contains an Ia marker (I-E) (see Chapter 11) and acts only on B cells of the IgE response when passively transferred in vivo.

receptors. T cells bearing histamine type 2 receptors are activated by reaction with histamine to express suppressor function. This subclass of T cells appears to be lower than normal in allergic individuals, and allergic individuals are less able to generate histamine-induced suppressor activity. The role of this activity in controlling allergy is not known.

Hyperimmuno-globulin E

The presence of high concentrations of an IgE that does not bind a particular antigen (nonantibody IgE) could saturate mast cell binding sites and prevent the functional sensitization of mast cells by IgE with specific antibody activity. This would be an IgE "blocking" effect, that is, nonantibody IgE blocking IgE antibody. Support for this concept comes from the observations that experimental animals with helminth infections who have high IgE serum concentrations have a decreased incidence of "allergic" reactions. On the other hand, in endemic areas of intestinal helminthiasis in Venezuela, there is a decreased incidence of allergies in rural populations as compared with urban populations, even though both have elevated IgE serum concentrations as compared with other populations. A final possibility that must be considered is a decrease in the threshold for activation of mast cells or decreased numbers of mast cells in effector organs, such as the bronchial and nasal submucosa, but the evidence for such changes is not consistent.

Pharmacological Control of Atopic Reactions

The severity of reaction by an anaphylactically sensitized individual upon exposure to the specific allergen depends not only on the amount of allergen and reaginic antibody, but also on the reactivity of mast cells, the excitability of the end organ (smooth muscle), and the effect of the autonomic nervous system (Fig. 18-4). Imbalance of these homeostatic control mechanisms ex-

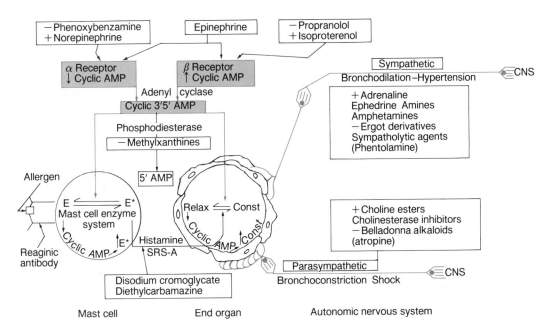

Figure 18-4. Pharmacological control of atopic–anaphylactic reactions. Effects of atopic or anaphylactic reactions are mediated by biologically active mediators released by mast cells that affect end organ smooth muscle. Amount of mediators released and reactivity of end organ to mediators are controlled by cellular messenger systems. Mast cell sensitivity depends on amount of reaginic antibody sensitizing the cell and on relative intracellular levels of cyclic and cyclic GMP. Cyclic AMP and cyclic GMP levels are controlled by adrenergic receptors. Stimulation of α-receptors causes decrease of cyclic AMP, increase of cyclic GMP, and increased reactivity; stimulation of β-receptors activates adenyl cyclase and produces increased cyclic AMP, decreased cyclic GMP, and decreased reactivity. A similar mechanism is operative for end organ smooth muscle. Degree of mast cell and end organ excitability may be modified by pharmacological agents that operate through adrenergic or autonomic systems. Cyclic AMP is broken down to 5′-AMP by phosphodiesterase, so that inhibition of phosphodiesterase activity by methylxanthines increases cyclic AMP and decreases sensitivity of mast cell and end organs. Epinephrine stimulates both α- and β-receptors but generally has pronounced ability to reverse acute allergic reactions at the usual therapeutic dose. Disodium chromoglycate and diethylcarbamazine inhibit histamine release from mast cells. Excitation of end organs is controlled by a balance of the autonomic nervous system. Parasympathetic effects are similar to anaphylactic effects (bronchial constriction, endothelial contraction, increased peristalsis, dilatation of bladder sphincter, and so on), whereas sympathetic effects are the opposite. Certain situations may result in a temporary imbalance of these systems and increase the severity of reaction, as in patients with chronic asthma.

plains how exposure to nonimmunological stimuli, such as heat, cold, physical exercise, and light, may, in some individuals, serve to excite physiological reactions that mimic allergic reactions (anaphylactoid reactions).

In fact, over 80% of asthma in adults is caused not by extrinsic antigen exposure but by physiological imbalance of the responsive smooth muscle end organs. The concept of cyclic nucleotides as "second messengers" in controlling cellular responses has led to a theoretical appreciation of the mechanisms controlling anaphylactic reactions (β-adrenergic blockade theory of asthma).

Mast Cells

Control or sensitivity of mast cells to allergen (the amount of mediators released by sensitized mast cells following contact with allergen) is accomplished by balanced adrenergic receptors (α- and β-receptors) that control the cellular level of enzyme systems, such as methyltransferase phosphorylating enzymes and phospholipases, the activation of which leads to mediator release. Contact of the sensitized mast cell with antigen causes activation of the enzyme system and release of mediators (see Fig. 12-5). The amount of enzymes available is determined by the cellular level of cyclic AMP, which in turn is controlled by stimulation of α- and β-receptors. Stimulation of β-receptor activates adenyl cyclase, causes an increase in cyclic AMP, and decreased reactivity, whereas activation of α-receptor results in decreased cyclic AMP and increased reactivity. Cyclic AMP is normally broken down to 5'-AMP by phosphodiesterase, so that inhibition of phosphodiesterase leads to increased cyclic AMP and decreased reactivity. The extent of reaction of mast cells to antigen may be controlled by stimulating or blocking the controlling receptors. Norepinephrine stimulates α-receptors, which results in a decrease in cellular cyclic AMP (increased enzymes and increased sensitivity to allergen), whereas isoproterenol stimulates β-receptors (decreased sensitivity to allergen). Phenoxybenzamine blocks α- and β-receptors, but selective stimulation may be achieved by the use of epinephrine combined with one of the blocking drugs. Methylxanthines (theophylline) inhibit phosphodiesterase and thus prevent cyclic AMP breakdown (decreased sensitivity to antigen). Two drugs block the release of mediators after contact of sensitized mast cells with allergen. The way in which these drugs, diethylcarbamazine and disodium chromoglycate, inhibit histamine release is not known. Specific desensitization of sensitized cells occurs as patients treated with sodium chromolyn and challenged with antigen remain refractory to subsequent challenge with the same antigen but not a different antigen when retested after 5 hours.

End Organ Sensitivity

The unleashing of severe atopic reactions not only is controlled at the mast cell level but also depends upon the balance between homeostatic α- and β-adrenergic end organ (smooth muscle) receptors. The cyclic AMP levels of the end organ cells may be controlled in a similar manner to that described above for mast cells. Thus, stimulation of α-receptors leads to a decrease in cyclic AMP and increased anaphylactic effects; stimulation of β-receptors leads to increased cyclic AMP and decreased end organ effects. The β-adrenergic theory states that atopic individuals do not have the normal adrenergic end organ homeostatic mechanism. Activation of α-receptors in normal nonatopic individuals does not produce significant anaphylactic symptoms because such activation is counterbalanced by activation of the β-adrenergic system. Thus, in the terms of this theory, bronchial asthma is not primarily an immunologic disease but is due to an abnormality in the β-adrenergic end organ system. The marked beneficial effect of epinephrine upon anaphylactic symptoms is due to its apparent stimulation of end organ β-receptors and not because of its effect on mast cells.

Autonomic Nervous System

The excitability of the end organ smooth muscle (bronchial muscles, arteries, gastrointestinal muscles) is also controlled by the autonomic nervous system and is maintained by a balance of sympathetic (adrenergic) and parasympathetic (cholinergic) effects. In general, parasympathetic effects are similar to anaphylactic effects (bronchial constriction, increased gastrointestinal peristalsis, dilatation of bladder sphincter, dilatation of arteries, pupil constriction), whereas sympathetic effects are the opposite (bronchial and pupil dilatation, arterial and sphincter constriction). In a normal individual the effects of the two components of the autonomic system are usually in balance, with a tendency to sympathetic dominance. It is known that certain situations may result in a temporary imbalance of these systems. Thus, stimulation of the parasympathetic system by injection of mecholyl or acetylcholine in a normal individual results in a temporary drop in blood pressure. Immediately after this effect the individual may be hyperresponsive to sympathetic stimulation; this phenomenon is called *sympathetic tuning*. A permanent imbalance may be produced in experimental animals by producing lesions in the pituitary. Ablation of areas of the anterior pituitary that reduces parasympathetic discharge protects against the lethal effects of anaphylaxis. Anaphylactically sensitized individuals may have a permanent imbalance of autonomic control that predisposes them to increased reactivity to mediator release. The shock organ effect (i.e., selective reactivity of certain organs) may be explained by a local imbalance of autonomic effects. Anaphylactoid reactions may be overreactions of this balancing system induced by physiological change. Because the autonomic nervous system is indirectly connected through neuronal synapses to higher areas of the brain, it is possible for emotional conditioning to affect the autonomic balance. Thus, emotional states may lead to parasympathetic tuning with resultant atopic or anaphylactic symptoms (cholinergic urticaria).

An imbalance of any or all of three levels — mast cells, end organ, or autonomic nervous system — may explain the increased sensitivity of atopic individuals to anaphylactic mediators. Atopic individuals injected with small doses of histamine have a much greater reaction than nonatopic individuals. It has been shown that the lymphocytes of atopic individuals have a decreased ability to respond to certain stimuli by increased cyclic AMP levels. Thus, atopic individuals may be unable to balance the effects of α-stimulation or allergen contact.

Autoantibodies to β-Adrenergic Receptors

Some individuals at high risk for development for asthma have autoantibodies for β_2-adrenergic receptors. Since such antibodies might block β_2-adrenergic receptors, it is possible that this blockade could increase mast cell sensitivity to IgE-mediated degranulation (β_2-adrenergic receptor stimulation decreases mast cell sensitivity). Autoanti-β_2-adrenergic receptors might also affect end organ responsiveness. Presently, only clinical correlations have been made; that is, such antibodies are found in 10% of severe asthmatics, but not in sera of nonasthmatic individuals. Questions regarding the role that these antibodies play in the pathogenesis of asthma, how they arise (for instance, are they stimulated by therapy with synthetic β-adrenergic ligand?), and whether or not they have any prognostic value remain to be answered (see also Chapter 14).

Anaphylactoid Reactions

Any event causing histamine release may cause atopic symptoms that may be confused with a true allergic reaction. Anaphylactoid shock is produced in normal (nonimmune) animals by injection of a variety of agents capable of releasing histamine without the mediation of an antigen–antibody reaction. The resulting clinical, physiological, and pathological picture is virtually indistinguishable from true anaphylaxis, but is not produced by immune reaction. Physical agents (heat, cold), trauma (dermatographia), emotional disturbances, or exercise may evoke pharmacological mechanisms that mimic allergic reactions. Dermatographia is most likely caused by the release of anaphylactic mediators from mast cells by a degree of physical trauma that does not induce a reaction in normal individuals. Such a reaction may confuse the results of skin testing, because a wheal may result from insertion of a needle alone. In some patients, a reaction to a physical agent may actually have an immune basis. A physical agent may cause release or production of altered tissue antigens to which a patient is sensitive. The reaction of idiopathic cold urticaria may be transferred with IgE and it is possible that this reaction is caused by reaction of an IgE autoantibody to a cold-dependent skin antigen. Reactions to light (photoallergy) may be caused by agents activated by sunlight that are applied to the skin to form haptens. Such reactions are usually contact dermatitis reactions (see Chapter 19). Cholinergic urticaria is believed to be produced by an abnormal response to acetylcholine released from efferent nerves after emotional stress, physical activity, or trauma. Cholinesterase levels of the skin may be reduced in cholinergic urticaria, leading to prolonged survival of acetylcholine that may act to release histamine from tissue mast cells.

The clinical findings in an atopic reaction are often confused by associated nonimmune factors. Thus, asthma is frequently complicated by infection or bronchiectasis that may overshadow the allergic condition. The severity and duration of asthmatic attacks may be greatly influenced by psychological conditions, and typical attacks may occur because of emotional stress, with no known contact with an allergen. These anaphylactoid reactions may be mediated by nonimmunologic mediator release, an imbalance of the sympathetic nervous system, or hyperreactivity of end organ smooth muscles (see below).

Treatment of Atopic Allergy

Therapeutic procedures to prevent or decrease atopic reactions may be applied at the various levels of the reaction: contact with antigen, IgE receptor, sensitivity of the mast cell to stimulation, degranulation of mast cell, mast cell mediator activity, sensitivity of end organ cell, autonomic nervous system balance, and emotional state of the reactive individual (Fig. 18-5).

Protective Role of IgE

The protective role of atopic or anaphylactic reactions has been the subject of considerable speculation. The most popular hypothesis is that anaphylactic reactions serve to open small blood vessels via endothelial cell contraction and thus permit the exudation of other immunoglobulin classes of antibodies and inflammatory cells into the tissue containing the offending antigen. Experimental support for this concept has been obtained. In immunized animals containing IgG antidiphtheria toxin antibodies, the simultaneous injection of ragweed antigen and diphtheria toxin into the skin results in an increase in toxin neutralization if the skin site is prepared by previous sensitization with reaginic antibody for the ragweed antigen. It is concluded that the increased toxin neutralizing capacity of the local skin sites in passively immunized animals is due to increased transudation of serum IgG antibody into the skin test sites ("gatekeeper effect").

Anaphylactic reactions may also serve to protect the individual against intestinal parasites. Parasitic worm infestations

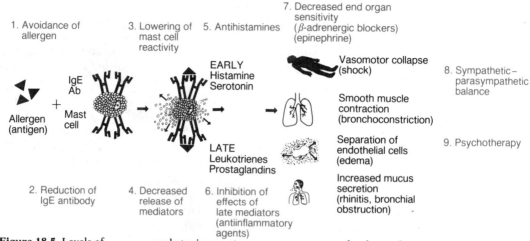

Figure 18-5. Levels of possible therapeutic or preventive intervention in allergy. 1. Avoidance of contact with the allergen is the most effective means of preventing atopic allergic reactions, thus removing antigen activation of IgE receptors. Avoidance is not always feasible and other methods must be used. 2. The availability of the IgE receptor may be reduced by hyposensitization, desensitization, or tolerance as the result of injection therapy (see above). 3. The sensitivity of the mast cell upon reaction of IgE receptors with allergen may be controlled by the amount of cyclic AMP available. This level may be affected by drugs as indicated in Figure 18-4. If mast cell cyclic AMP can be increased by the methods indicated above, the extent of mast cell mediator release upon reaction of sensitized cells with allergen may be decreased and atopic symptoms controlled. 4. Two drugs, diethylcarbamazine and disodium chromoglycate, significantly decrease the release of mediators from mast cells upon contact with allergen. 5. The effect of mast cell mediators may be partially controlled by drugs that interfere with histamine activity (antihistamines). The fact that antihistamines are only partially effective in decreasing atopic symptoms indicates that other mediators play an important role. 6. The rapidly increasing understanding of the role of arachidonic acid metabolites in allergic reactions could well lead to more effective therapy. In particular, nonsteroidal anti-inflammatory agents or agents that could control the balance of effects of prostaglandin E (bronchodilation) and prostaglandin F (bronchoconstriction) could have great potential beneficial effects. Steroids are used only as a last resort. 7. The sensitivity of the end organ (smooth muscle) to atopic mediators also depends on β-adrenergic control of cellular cyclic AMP levels. If end organ cyclic AMP can be increased, then atopic symptoms should be decreased. 8. Sympathetic stimulation or parasympathetic blockade may also have a significant beneficial effect upon atopic reactions through the effect of the autonomic nervous system on end organ excitability (Fig. 18-4). 9. It is well known that severity of atopic reactions (particularly asthma) depends upon the emotional state of the individual. Anxious or insecure patients have more severe symptoms than more secure or stable patients. Thus, the emotional state of the reactive individual should be evaluated and treated with psychotherapy, if necessary.

are frequently associated with IgE antibody response. Gastrointestinal anaphylactic reactions may help expel intestinal parasites by acute severe diarrhea. It is also possible that the sneezing associated with acute asthma dislodges potential infectious agents from the lungs.

Finally, acute anaphylactic reactions may force the sensitized individual to avoid further exposure to the offending allergen. By avoiding exposure to the antigens, more prolonged extensive immune-mediated damage may be prevented. Avoidancé may prevent formation of immune complex disease or delayed hypersensitivity to the same antigen, since anaphylactic reactions may be elicited by extremely small doses of an antigen.

Summary

Anaphylactic (acute) or atopic (chronic) reactions are caused by activation of mast cells via reaction of reaginic antibody fixed to the mast cell surface. Reaginic antibody belongs to a unique class of immunoglobulin, IgE, which has the capacity to bind to receptors on mast cells — to "fix." Mast cells are stimulated by reaction with allergen to release pharmacologically agents stored in cytoplasmic granules (degranulation), such as histamine and serotonin, which produce acute reactions. In addition, arachidonic acid from membrane phospholipids is converted to leukotrienes and prostaglandins, which produce or cause later inflammatory lesions. These released mediators act on smooth muscle cells and endothelial cells, causing constriction. This in turn produces clinical symptoms because of bronchoconstriction (asthma), loss of intravascular fluid (edema, cutaneous anaphylaxis, shock), or chronic accumulation of mucus (hay fever, nasal polyps). The degree of reactivity of the system is controlled by a balance between adrenergic and cholinergic receptors, and the extent of these reactions may be controlled by drugs that affect this physiological balance. Many allergic symptoms are believed to result from an imbalance of this controlling system rather than from exposure to allergen. The extent of production of reaginic (IgE) antibody may be influenced by specific immunization (immunotherapy). The mechanism of action of immunotherapy remains poorly defined.

Anaphylactic reactions may serve a protective role in providing rapid egress of other antibodies or cells into sites of antigen deposition by inducing endothelial cell separation. However, allergic reactions cause problems for a large number of people and constitute the basis for the practice of a major clinical specialist — the allergist.

References

See also Basophils and Mast Cells, Chapter 12.

IgE, Reaginic Antibody, and Receptors

Adkinson NF: The radioallergosorbent test in 1981 — limitations and refinements. J Allergy Clin Immunol 67:87, 1981.

Bazaral M, Orgel HA, Hamburger RN: The influence of serum IgE levels of selected recipients, including patients with allergy, helminthiasis and tuberculosis, on the apparent P-K titer of a reaginic serum. Clin Exp Immunol 4:117, 1973.

Bazaral M, Orgel HA, Hamburger RN: Genetics of IgE and allergy: serum IgE levels in twins. J Allergy Clin Immunol 52:211–244, 1974.

Block KS: The anaphylactic antibodies of mammals including man. Prog Allergy 10:84, 1967.

Coca AF, Grove EF: Studies on hypersensitiveness. XIII. A study of the atopic reagins. J Immunol 10:445, 1925.

Conrad DH, Froese A: Characterization of the target cell receptor for IgE. III. Properties of the receptor isolated from rat basophilic leukemia cells by affinity chromatography. J Immunol 120:429, 1978.

Hamburger RN, Fernandez-Cruz E, Arnaiz A, Perex B, Bootello A: The relationship of the P-K titer to the serum IgE level in patients with leprosy. Clin Exp Immunol 17:253, 1974.

Ishizaka K, Ishizaka T, Hornbrook MH: Physico-chemical properties of human reaginic antibody. IV. Presence of a unique immunoglobulin as a carrier of reaginic activity. J Immunol 97:75, 1966.

Metzger H, Rivnay B, Henkart M, et al: Analysis of the structure and function of the receptor for IgE. Mol Immunol 21:1167, 1984.

Moller G (ed): Immunoglobulin E. Immunol Rev 41:1, 1978.

Mota I: Biological characterization of mouse "early" antibodies. Immunology 12:343, 1967.

Orgel HA, Hamburger RN: Development of IgE and allergy in infancy. J Allergy Clin Immunol 56:296, 1975.

Osler AG, Lichtenstein LM, Levy DA: In vitro studies of human reaginic allergy. Adv Immunol 8:183, 1968.

Perelmutter L: IgG$_4$: non-IgE-mediated atopic disease. Ann Allergy 52:64, 1984.

Prausnitz C, Kustner H: Studies on sensitivity. Zentralbl Bakteriol (Orig) 86:160, 1921. English trans *in* Gell PGH, Coombs RRA: Clinical Aspects of Immunology. Philadelphia, Davis, 1963, p808.

Stanworth DR: Reaginic antibodies. Adv Immunol 3:181, 1963.

Anaphylaxis

Austen KF, Humphrey JH: In vitro studies of the mechanism of anaphylaxis. Adv Immunol 3:1, 1963.

Halpern BN, Ky T, Robert B: Clinical and immunological study of an exceptional case of reaginic type sensitization to human seminal fluid. Immunology 12:247, 1967.

James LP, Austen KF: Fatal systemic anaphylaxis in man. N Engl J Med 270:597, 1964.

Reunala T, Koskimies AI, Bjorksten F, Janne J, Lassus A: Immunoglobulin E–mediated severe allergy to human seminal plasma. Fert Steril 28:832, 1977.

Wicher K, Reisman RE, Arbesman CE: Allergic reaction to penicillin present in milk. JAMA 208:143, 1969.

Atopic Allergy

Cochrane CG: Immunologic tissue injury mediated by neutrophilic leukocytes. Adv Immunol 9:97, 1968.

Ellis EF: Immunologic basis of atopic disease. Adv Pediatr 16:65, 1969.

Frier S, Kletter B: Clinical and immunological aspects of milk protein intolerance. Aust Paediatr J 8:140, 1972.

Goldman AS, Sellars WA, Halpern SR, Anderson DW, Furlow TE, Johnson CH: Milk allergy. II. Skin testing of allergic and normal children with purified milk proteins. Pediatrics 32:572, 1963.

Golert TM, Patterson R, Pruzansky JJ: Systemic allergic reactions to ingested antigens. J Allergy 44:96, 1969.

Levine BB: Genetic controls of reagin production in mice and man: role of Ir genes in ragweed hayfever. *In* Goodfriend L, Sehon AH, Orange RP (eds): Monographs in Allergy, Vol 4. Basel, Karger, 1969.

Rowe AH, Rowe A Jr: Food Allergy. Springfield, Ill., Thomas, 1972.

Savilahti E: Cow's milk allergy. Allergy 36:73, 1981.

Slavin RG, Lewis CR: Sensitivity to enzyme activities in laundry detergent workers. J Allergy Clin Immunol 48:262, 1971.

Waldmann TA, Wochner RD, Laster L, Gordon RS Jr: Allergic gastroenteropathy: a cause of excessive gastrointestinal protein loss. N Engl J Med 276:761, 1967.

Asthma

Aas K: Heterogeneity of bronchial asthma: Subpopulation or different stages of the disease. Allergy 36:3, 1981.

Austen KF, Lichtenstein LM (eds): Asthma: Physiology, Immunopharmacology and Treatment. New York, Academic Press, 1973.

Austen KF, Orange RP: Bronchial asthma: the possible role of the chemical mediators of immediate hypersensitivity in the pathogenesis of subacute chronic disease. Am Rev Resp Dis 112:432, 1975.

Farr RS: Asthma in adults: the ambulatory patient. Hosp Pract 13:113, 1978.

Hinson RFW, Moon AJ, Plummer NS: Bronchopulmonary aspergillosis. Thorax 7:317, 1952.

Johnstone DE: Some aspects of the natural history of asthma. Ann Allerg 49:257, 1982.

Lichtenstein LM, Austen KF: Asthma: Physiology, Immunopharmacology, and Treatment. New York, Academic Press, 1977.

Lichtenstein LM, Osler AG: Studies on the mechanism of hypersensitivity phenomena. IX. Histamine release from human leukocytes by ragweed pollen antigen. J Exp Med 120:507, 1964.

Aspirin

Abrishami MA, Thomas J: Aspirin intolerance — a review. Ann Allergy 39:28, 1977.

Falliers CJ: Aspirin and subtypes of asthma: risk factor analysis. J Allergy Clin Immunol 52:141, 1973.

Farr RS: Presidential message. J Allergy 45:321, 1970.

Fein BT: Aspirin shock associated with asthma and nasal polyps. Ann Allergy 29:589, 1971.

Hawkins D, Pinckard RN, Crawford IP, Farr RS: Structural changes in human serum albumin induced by ingestion of acetylsalicylic acid. J Clin Invest 48:536, 1969.

Sampter M: Intolerance to aspirin. Hosp Pract 8:85, 1973.

Sampter M, Beers RF Jr: Intolerance to aspirin. Ann Intern Med 68:975, 1968.

Van Dellen RG, Peters GA: Acute anaphylactic reactions and aspirin allergy. Postgrad Med 49:197, 1971.

Insect Allergy

Barr SE: Allergy to hymenoptera stings—review of the world literature: 1953–1970. Ann Allergy 29:49, 1971.

Feinberg AR, Feinberg SM, Benaim-Pinto C: Asthma and rhinitis from insect allergies. J Allergy 27:437, 1956.

Feingold BF, Benjamini E, Michaeli D: The allergic responses to insect bites. Annu Rev Entomol 13:137, 1968.

Frazier CA: Insect Allergy. St. Louis, Green, 1969.

Frazier CA: Biting insect survey: a statistical report. Ann Allergy 32:200, 1974.

Killby VA, Silverman PH: Hypersensitive reactions in man to specific mosquito bites. Am J Trop Med Hyg 16:374, 1967.

Perlman F: Stinging insect allergy—a historical sketch and confused state. Ann Allergy 39:285, 1977.

Shulman S: Insect allergy: biochemical and immunochemical analyses of the allergens. Prog Allergy 12:246, 1968.

Atopic Dermatitis

Blaylock WK: Atopic dermatitis. Diagnosis and pathology. J Allergy Clin Immunol 57:62, 1976.

Hanifin JM: Atopic dermatitis. J Allergy Clin Immunol 73:211, 1984.

Kay JW: Atopic dermatitis: an immunologic disease complex and its therapy. Ann Allergy 38:345, 1977.

McGready SJ, Buckley RH: Depression of cell-indicated immunity in atopic eczema. J Allergy Clin Immunol 56:393, 1975.

Rajka G: Atopic Dermatitis. London, Saunders, 1975.

Wise F, Sulzberger MB: Year Book of Dermatology and Syphilology. Year Book Med Pub, Chicago, 1933, p59.

Immunotherapy

Chiorazzi N, Fox DA, Katz DH: Hapten-specific IgE antibody responses in mice. VII. Conversion of IgE "non-responder" strains to IgE "responders" by elimination of suppressor T cell activity. J Immunol 118:48, 1977.

Ishizaka K: Cellular events in the IgE antibody response. Adv Immunol 23:1, 1976.

Ishizaka K: Regulation of IgE synthesis. Annu Rev Immunol 2:159, 1984.

Lee WY, Sehon AH: Suppression of reaginic antibodies with modified allergens. II. Abrogation of reaginic antibodies with allergens conjugated to polyethylene glycol. Int Arch Allergy 56:193, 1978.

Lichtenstein LM, Levy DA. Is "desensitization" for ragweed hay fever immunology specific? Int Arch Allergy 42:615, 1972.

Noon L: Prophylactic inoculation against hay fever. Lancet 1:1572, 1911.

Norman PS: Specific therapy in allergy. Med Clin North Am 58:111, 1974.

Norman PS: Immunotherapy. Prog Allergy 32:318, 1982.

Platts-Mills TAE: Desensitization treatment for hay fever. Immunol Today 1:35, 1981.

Tada T: Regulation of reaginic antibody formation in animals. Prog Allergy 19;122, 1975.

Tamura S-I, Ishizaki K: Reaginic antibody formation in the mouse. X. Possible role of suppressor T cells in transient IgE antibody response. J Immunol 120:837, 1978.

Watanabe N, Kojima S, Ovary Z: Suppression of IgE antibody producton in SJL mice: non-specific suppressor T cells. J Exp Med 143:833, 1976.

Pharmacology of Atopic Reactions

Beer DJ, Osband ME, McCaffery RP, et al: Abnormal histamine-induced suppressor cell function in atopic subjects. N Engl J Med 306:454, 1982.

Fraser CM, Venter JC: Autobodies to beta-adrenergic receptors and asthma. J Allerg Clin Immunol 74:227, 1984.

Gellhorn E: Autonomic Imbalance and the Hypothalamus. Minneapolis, University of Minnesota Press, 1957.

Goodfriend L, Sehon AH, Orange RP (eds): Mechanisms in Allergy: Reagin-Mediated Hypersensitivity. New York, Dekker, 1973.

Ishizaka T, Ishizaka K: IgE molecules and their receptor sites on human basophil granulocytes. *In* Goodfriend L, Sehon AH, Orange RP (eds): Mechanisms in Allergy. New York, Dekker, 1973, p221.

Ishizaka T, Ishizaka K, Johansson SGO, Bennich H: Histamine release from human leukocytes by anti-E antibodies. J Immunol 102:884, 1969.

Levy DA, Carlton JA: Influence of temperature on the inhibition by colchicine of allergic histamine release. Proc Soc Exp Biol Med 130:1333, 1969.

Luparello JJ, Stein M, Park CD: Effect of hypothalamic lesions on rat anaphylaxis. Am J Physiol 207:911, 1964.

Morley J (ed): Beta-Adrenergic Receptors in Asthma. New York, Academic Press, 1984.

Orange RP, Austen KF: Chemical mediators of immediate hypersensitivity. Hosp Pract 6:79, 1971.

Parker CW: Autoantibodies and beta-adrenergic receptors. N Engl J Med 305:1212, 1981.

Robinson GA, Butcher RW, Sutherland EW: Cyclic AMP. New York, Academic Press, 1971.

Sibley DR, Lefkowitz RJ. Molecular mechanisms of receptor desensitization using the β-adrenergic receptor coupled adenylate cyclase system as a model. Nature 317:124, 1985.

Sutherland EW, Robinson GA, Butcher CW: Cyclic AMP. Circulation 37:279, 1968.

Szentivanyi A: The beta adrenergic theory of the atopic abnormality in bronchial asthma. J Allergy 42:203, 1968.

Wasserman SI, Center DM: The relevance of neutrophil chemotactic factors to allergic disease. J Allergy Clin Immunol 64:231, 1979.

Willis T: Pharmaceutic Rationales on the Operations of Mechanics in Humane Bodies. London, Dring, 1684, Sect 1, Pt 2, pp78–85.

Anaphylactoid
Reactions

Cohen G, Peterson A: Treatment of hereditary angioedema with frozen plasma. Ann Allergy 30:690, 1972.

Donaldson VH, Ratnoff OD, DaSilva WD, Rosen FS: Permeability-increasing activity in hereditary angioneurotic edema plasma. J Clin Invest 48:642, 1969.

Ebken RK, Bauschard FA, Levin MI: Dermatographism: its definition, demonstration, and prevalence. J Allergy 41:338, 1968.

Epstein JH: Photoallergy, a review. Arch Dermatol 106:741, 1972.

Grolnick M: An investigative and clinical evaluation of dermatographism. Ann Allergy 28:395, 1970.

Sheffer AL, Austen KF, Gigli I: Urticaria and angioedema. Postgrad Med 54:81, 1973.

Sheffer AL, Fearon DT, Austin KF, Rosen FS: Tranexamic acid. Preoperative prophylactic therapy for patients with hereditary angioneurotic edema. J Allergy Clin Immunol 60:38, 1977.

Wanderer AA, Maselli R, Ellis DF, Ishizaka K: Immunologic characterization of serum factors responsible for cold urticaria. J Allergy Clin Immunol 48:13, 1971.

Treatment of Atopic
Allergy

Berglund E, Svedmyr N: Asthma — evaluation of drug therapy. Scand J Resp Dis (Suppl) 1011:1, 1978.

Church MK, Warner JO: Sodium cromoglycate and related drugs. Clin Allergy 15:311, 1985.

Craps L, Greenwood C, Radielovich P: Clinical investigation of agents with prophylactic auto-allergic effects in bronchial asthma. Clin Allergy 8:373, 1978.

Kay AB, Austen KF, Lichtenstein LM (eds): Asthma: Physiology, Immunopharmacology and Treatment. New York, Academic Press, 1984.

Kolotkin BM, Lee CK, Townley RG: Duration and specificity of sodium chromolyn on allergen inhalation challenges in asthmatics. J Allergy Clin Immunol 53:288, 1974.

Orr TSC, Pollard MC, Gwilliam J, Cox JSG: Mode of action of disodium chromoglycate: studies on immediate type hypersensitivity reactions using "double sensitization" with two antigenically distinct rat reagins. Clin Exp Immunol 7:745, 1970.

Protective Role of
Atopic Reaction

Buckle DR, Smith H (eds): Development of Anti-asthma Drugs. London, Butterworths, 1984.

Soulsby EJL: The mechanism of immunity to gastro-intestinal nematodes. In Biology of Parasites. New York, Academic Press, 1966.

Stebbings JH Jr: Immediate hypersensitivity: a defense against arthropods. Perspect Biol Med 17:233, 1974.

Steinberg P, Ishizaka K, Norman PS: Possible role of IgE-mediated reaction in immunity. J Allergy Clin Immunol 54:359, 1974.

19 | Delayed Hypersensitivity Reactions (Cell-Mediated Immunity)

The term *delayed hypersensitivity* is applied to an immune-mediated tissue inflammatory reaction initiated by specifically sensitized T lymphocytes (Fig. 19-1). The reaction is manifested

Figure 19-1. Delayed hypersensitivity (cellular) reactions. Specifically modified T lymphocytes with receptors capable of recognizing antigen initiate the reaction. T_K cells (CTL) may kill target cells directly, whereas T_D cells release mediators that in turn act to influence nonsensitized cells to participate in the reaction.

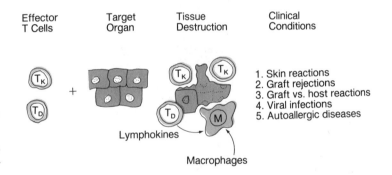

by the infiltration of cells, beginning with a perivascular accumulation of lymphocytes and monocytes at the site where antigen is located. Evidence obtained using labeled, specifically sensitized cells transferred to normal donors indicates that only a few of the infiltrating cells are specifically sensitized. The reaction of these few sensitized cells with the antigen in the tissue causes large numbers of unlabeled cells to infiltrate the area, with subsequent tissue destruction (see below). The inflammatory response is induced and maintained by mediators derived by T lymphocytes (lymphokines) or by macrophages (monokines). Activated macrophages secrete interleukin 1 (see Fig. 12-13) as well as a variety of other inflammatory mediators and enzymes (see Table 12-13). These mediators may stimulate proliferation of fibroblasts, digest tissue components, or activate other inflammatory mechanisms that contribute to later stages of immune-mediated inflammation as well as resolution and healing (see Chapter 12). Destruction of tissue may be due

471

to specific T cytotoxic lymphocytes or to lymphokine-activated macrophages.

The term *delayed* is applied because the time course of the skin reaction is measured in days or even weeks, in contrast to the cutaneous anaphylactic reactions, which reach their peak in a few minutes, and the Arthus reaction, which occurs in hours. The term *tuberculin-type hypersensitivity* is used because for many years the study of delayed hypersensitivity was essentially the study of the immune response to tuberculin and infection with tubercle bacilli. It is now known that delayed hypersensitivity is also the major effector mechanism in many other infectious diseases, as well as in homograft rejections and autoallergic diseases. It differs from the allergic reactions mentioned previously in this text in that no humoral antibody is involved and reactivity cannot be transferred by serum, but only by cells, and the gross appearance and microscopic appearance are different.

Delayed hypersensitivity reactions are initiated by subpopulations of T cells, T_K (cytotoxic T cells or CTL) and T_D cells (Fig. 19-2). Upon reaction with antigen in vivo, these cells be-

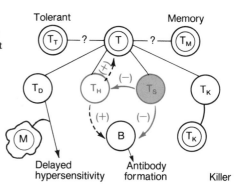

Figure 19-2. Functional T cell populations: Immature T cells may mature into different functional immune competent effector populations, including T_D (delayed hypersensitivity effectors), T_H (helper), T_S (suppressor), and T_K (killer or cytotoxic) cells. T_D cells release lymphokines, which act through macrophages to effect delayed hypersensitivity reactions. T_H and T_S cells act to control the extent of immune reactions, with T_H cells providing them with a positive signal, and T_S cells with negative signals. T_K cells specifically kill (lyse) tissue target cells. In addition, T cells may become tolerant (T_T) or memory (T_M) cells.

come activated and initiate a series of events leading to the delayed inflammatory reactions recognized by infiltration of tissues with mononuclear cells. T_K (killer) cells act by directly reacting with antigens on tissue cells, resulting in their destruction. T_D cells release lymphocyte mediators upon reaction with tissue or soluble antigens. These mediators or "lymphokines" activate inflammatory processes, in particular the attraction and activation of macrophages. The tissue reaction observed is the result of the activity of a number of lymphocyte mediators and the accessory function of macrophages.

A number of in vitro assays have been devised to measure cell-mediated immunity but none of these accurately quantitate the in vivo state of delayed hypersensitivity. Although in vitro tests for T lymphocyte activities have contributed greatly to our understanding of how T cells recognize and react to antigens it is not possible to duplicate in vitro the sequence of events that occurs in vivo during a delayed hypersensitivity reaction. The in vitro correlates of delayed hypersensitivity are presented in detail in Chapter 8. If the reader is not familiar with these phenomena, it is recommended that Chapter 8 be read before proceeding further with this chapter.

Delayed Skin Reactions

Two examples of skin reactions mediated by sensitized cells are presented as examples of the two major effector mechanisms of delayed hypersensitivity. The first, contact dermatitis, is mediated mainly by T killer cells that cross into the epidermis and cause death of epithelial cells. The second, the classic delayed hypersensitivity skin (tuberculin) test, is initiated by T_D cells, which release lymphokines that attract and activate macrophages. Although these represent examples of the different effector arms of cell-mediated immunity, both effector arms may be active in different degrees in other reactions.

Contact Dermatitis

Contact allergy (contact eczema, dermatitis venenata) is exemplified by the common allergic reaction to poison ivy. It also occurs as an allergic response to a wide variety of simple chemicals in such things as ointments, clothing, cosmetics, dyes, and adhesive tape, in any adequately exposed individual. The antigens are usually highly reactive chemical compounds capable of combining with proteins; they are also lipid soluble and can penetrate the epidermis. The antigen often is an incomplete antigen (hapten) that combines with some constituent of the epidermis to form a complete antigen. Sensitization occurs by exposure of the skin once or repeatedly to sufficiently high concentrations of antigen. Langerhans cells within the epidermis (see Chapter 2) are believed to play an important role in antigen processing. All individuals are susceptible if exposed to the antigen in sufficient amounts. A greater amount of antigen is needed for sensitization than for elicitation of skin reaction in an already sensitive individual. When United States soldiers moved into Japan after World War II, the military medical dispensaries noticed the widespread occurrence of a skin rash with the appearance of contact dermatitis. It was the distribution of the rash that was most unusual: it occurred on the elbows and buttocks. After diligent sleuthing, it was discovered that the bars and toilet seats of certain Japanese public establishments were coated with a lacquer made from the sap of a tree that contained small amounts of a substance closely related to the poison ivy antigen. The amounts of this related antigen were not great enough to sensitize the native Japanese, but were sufficient to elicit the characteristic dermatitis in previously sensitized individuals. The American soldiers were sensitive because of previous exposure to poison ivy. Also related are the oleoresins of the cashew nut shell, the rind of the mango, the ginkgo tree fruit pulp, and Indian-marking nut resin. All of these plants belong to the Avacardiaceae family and produce an oleoresin called *urushiol* that cross-reacts in skin tests of sensitive patients.

The characteristic skin reaction is elicited in sensitized individuals by exposing the skin to the antigen (natural exposure, patch tests). Again the classic reaction is that to poison ivy or poison oak. The reaction is a sharply delineated, superficial skin inflammation, beginning as early as 24 hours after exposure and reaching a maximum at 48 to 96 hours (Fig. 19-3). It is characterized by redness, induration, and vesiculation. The reaction may take longer to reach a maximum than the tuberculin skin test because of the longer time required for the antigen to penetrate the epidermis. Histologically the dermis shows perivenous accumulation of lymphocytes and histiocytes and some edema. The epidermis is invaded by these cells and shows intraepidermal edema (spongiosis), which progresses to vesiculation and death of epidermal cells. It was once assumed that the lesion was the result of sensitization of the epidermal cells themselves. However, no reaction occurs when the local vascular supply is interrupted, and careful histologic study shows that infiltration of the epidermis with lymphocytes precedes the epidermal cell damage. Since antibody is not involved, it is clear that hematogenous cells are the carriers of sensitivity, and epidermal death is comparable to the destruction of parenchyma (i.e., of the cells bearing the antigen) in homograft rejection and the autoallergies (see below and Chapter 20). Sensitivity can be passively transferred with lymphocytes. In addition, suppression of the circulating lymphocytes, by radiation or by specific antiserum to lymphocytes, depresses contact reactivity. Because the antigen is present mainly in the epidermis, it takes about 2 days for the reacting mononuclear cells (mainly lymphocytes but also macrophages) to invade and react with the antigen. As a result of this invasion and reaction, epidermal cells are destroyed and small foci (sterile microabscesses) are formed, eventually leading to vesicle formation that can be seen on the skin as small, fluid-filled blebs. Since all of the hapten may not be degraded in the vesicles, rupture of the vesicles by scratching may spread the antigen to uninvolved areas of the skin and provoke new reactions. However, there is not general agreement on this point. Proliferation of the basal epidermal cells results in eventual sloughing of the affected epidermal cells. This process may take up to a week to 10 days, depending on the amount of antigen present and the degree of sensitization of the individual. Poison ivy or poison oak oleoresin may remain stable in the dry state for long periods of time so that indirect exposure may occur from touching clothes, tools, or animals that are contaminated with dried plant resins.

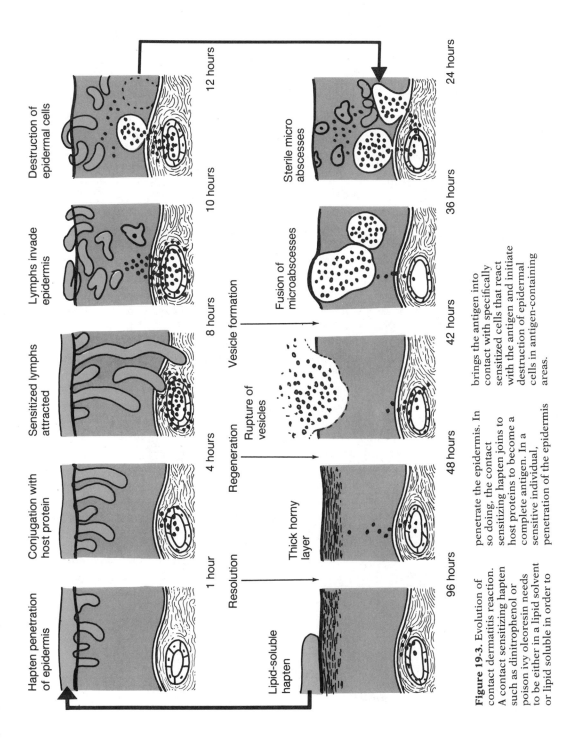

Figure 19-3. Evolution of contact dermatitis reaction. A contact sensitizing hapten such as dinitrophenol or poison ivy oleoresin needs to be either in a lipid solvent or lipid soluble in order to penetrate the epidermis. In so doing, the contact sensitizing hapten joins to host proteins to become a complete antigen. In a sensitive individual, penetration of the epidermis brings the antigen into contact with specifically sensitized cells that react with the antigen and initiate destruction of epidermal cells in antigen-containing areas.

Tuberculin Test

The classic delayed type tuberculin skin reaction is elicited in sensitive individuals by intradermal injection of tuberculoprotein antigens (purified protein derivative, old tuberculin). A delayed skin reaction to tubercle bacilli was noted in 1890 by Koch who injected live tubercle bacilli into guinea pigs previously infected. Redness and swelling were noted 24 hours after injection. The lesion progressed to local tissue necrosis. This reaction was not observed in uninfected animals and could be demonstrated in infected animals using killed bacilli or extracts of the bacilli. The extract originally used was called old tuberculin (OT), a crude extract of cultures of tubercle bacilli. This was replaced by a more purified protein derivative (PPD) of cultures. Because the reaction occurred in hypersensitive animals, not in nonsensitized animals, and occurred much later after testing than the Arthus reaction, the phenomenon was called "delayed hypersensitivity." Following injection of antigen into the skin of an individual sensitive in a delayed manner, there is little or no reaction until after 4 to 6 hours. The grossly visible induration and swelling usually reach a maximum at 24 to 48 hours. Histologically there is accumulation of mononuclear cells around small veins. Later, mononuclear cells may be seen throughout the area of the reaction with massive infiltration in the dermis. Polymorphonuclear cells constitute fewer than one-third of the cells at any time, and usually few are present at 24 hours or later unless the reaction is severe enough to cause necrosis. There may also be infiltration and degranulation of basophils, perhaps contributing to the increased vascular permeability and edema observed.

The role of lymphocyte mediators in delayed hypersensitivity reactions may be delineated as follows: Upon contact with antigen, lymphocytes release migration-inhibitory, skin-reactive, macrophage-specific, chemotactic, and macrophage-activation factors (Chapter 12), all of which serve to attract and hold macrophages in the reaction site. The number of specifically sensitized cells may be increased by lymphocyte-stimulating factor, which induces proliferation of lymphocytes. Cytotoxic factors may cause death of tissue cells in the reactive area; proliferation-inhibitory factor may inhibit nonlymphoid cell

Figure 19-4. Evolution of the delayed skin reaction. In normal skin, lymphocytes pass from venules through the dermis to lymphatics, which return these cells to the circulation. Production of delayed skin reaction involves recognition of antigen by sensitized lymphocytes (T cells), immobilization of lymphocytes at the site, production and release of lymphocyte mediators, and accumulation of macrophages with eventual destruction of antigen and resolution of the reaction. This results in an accumulation of cells seen at 24 to 48 hours after antigen injection. Macrophages degrade the antigen. When the antigen is destroyed, the reactive cells either are disintegrated or return via the lymphatic to the bloodstream or draining lymph nodes. In this way, specifically sensitized lymphocytes may be distributed throughout the lymphoid system following local stimulation with antigen. ▶

growth, and lymphocyte-permeability factor may increase the magnitude of the inflammatory reaction by causing more cells to accumulate.

The evolution of the delayed skin reaction is presented in Figure 19-4. This description incorporates the function of the

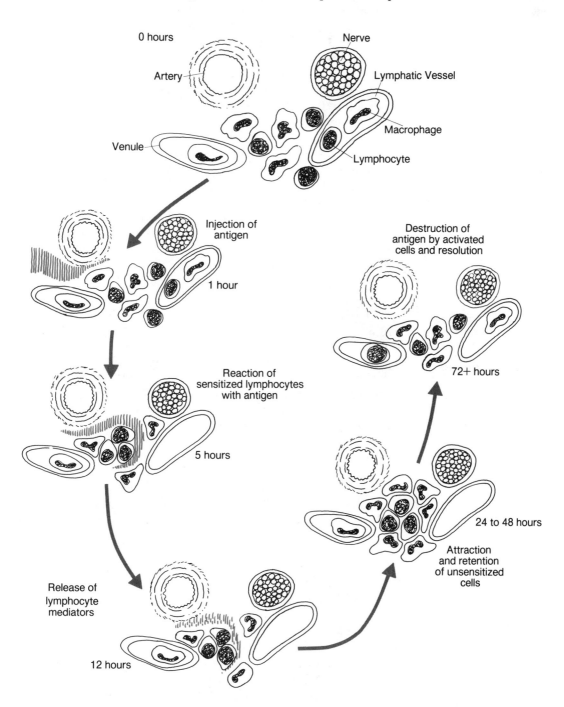

lymphocyte mediators and macrophages. A simplified concept is that the lymphocyte initiates the reaction and the macrophage cleans it up.

Cutaneous Basophil Hypersensitivity

The term *cutaneous basophil hypersensitivity* (CBH) is used to denote a group of lymphocyte-mediated, basophilic reactions that differ histologically from classic delayed type (DH) reactions. Basophils are infrequent or rare in DH, but are numerous in the 24- to 48-hour delayed skin reaction to soluble protein antigens after immunization with the protein in complete Freund's adjuvant, which appears transiently prior to antibody formation. Basophils make up almost half of the inflammatory cells present in these reactions. Basophils may also be found in other situations involving expression of cellular immunity, including skin graft rejection, tumor rejection, reactions to viral infections, and contact allergy. CBH reactions require specifically sensitized lymphocytes. In contact dermatitis infiltration of lymphocytes precedes basophils by at least 12 hours. The lymphocytes probably release a lymphokine responsible for attracting basophils. The function of the basophilic infiltrate is not known, but it might serve as a phagocytic cell that supplements the macrophage.

The term *Jones–Mote reaction* originally referred to the reappearance of a delayed type of sensitivity to serum proteins after the development and regression of an Arthus reaction, noted in humans by Jones and Mote in 1934. This term was extended to cover the transient form of delayed skin reaction to protein antigens occurring prior to antibody production in experimental animals, a finding also previously observed in humans. With a better appreciation of the basophilic nature of these reactions, the term *cutaneous basophil hypersensitivity* has been applied. As an immunological reaction, the significance of CBH-type reactions remains unclear. Since the presence of basophils in varying numbers has been described in human tuberculin as well as in Jones–Mote reactions, it may be that basophils are not really a distinguishing feature but are a variable constituent of delayed hypersensitivity reactions. Some experimental evidence suggests that tissue mast cells must be present in the dermis in order for antigens to elicit a DTH reaction. The mast cells may function to permit vasodilation and increased vascular permeability. However, typical DTH cutaneous reactions have been elicited in strains of mice lacking tissue mast cells.

Graft Rejection

The genetics of graft rejection and methods for matching recipient and donor tissues are presented in Chapter 9. At this point, the pathology and immune mechanism of graft rejection are described. Again both direct killing of target cells by lymphocytes and release of lymphokines that attract and activate macrophages are involved. The mechanism of delivery of immunogenic tissue antigens that sensitize recipients to graft antigens remains incompletely understood. Immunogens for skin, as well as other solid organ grafts, may be provided by "passenger lymphocytes." Passenger lymphocytes are lymphocytes in the grafted tissue that migrate to draining lymph nodes where they provide a strong immunogenic signal.

Morphology

The rejection reaction is perhaps best illustrated by the behavior of two skin grafts from the same donor to the same recipient, with the second graft placed about 1 month after the first graft (Fig. 19-5). During the second or third day following the first grafting procedure, revascularization begins and is complete by the sixth or seventh day. A similar response is observed for autografts, synografts, allografts, or xenografts, in that each type of graft becomes vascularized. However, at about 1 week, the first signs of rejection appear in the deep layers of the allograft or xenograft. A perivascular (perivenular) accumulation of mononuclear cells occurs similar to that seen in the early stages of a tuberculin skin reaction. The infiltration steadily intensifies and edema is grossly visible. At about 9 to 10 days, thrombosis of the involved vessels occurs, with necrosis and sloughing of the graft. This entire process usually requires 11 to 14 days and is called a *first-set rejection*. The synograft or autograft does not undergo this process, but remains viable with little or no inflammatory reaction. When a second graft is transplanted from the same genetically unrelated donor who provided the rejected first graft, a more rapid and more vigorous rejection occurs (*second-set rejection*). For the first 3 days after transplant, the second-set graft looks essentially the same as the first graft. However, vascularization is abruptly halted at 4 to 5 days, with a sudden onset of ischemic necrosis. Because the graft never becomes vascularized and the blood supply is cut off by the second-set rejection, there is little chance for cellular infiltration to occur. The primary target for the second-set rejection appears to be the capillaries taking part in revascularization. Essentially the same events follow grafting of other solid organs, such as kidney or heart.

Rejection of solid tissue grafts is mediated mainly by cellular reactivity. This evidence can be summarized as follows: (1) the ability to reject a solid graft with a second-set reaction may be transferred from a sensitized individual to an unsensitized individual with cells, but not with serum, except in unusual circumstances (see below); (2) extracts of donor tissue injected into the skin of a sensitive recipient induce a delayed skin reaction; (3) individuals with depressed cellular reactivity but apparently normal ability to produce antibody (e.g., Hodgkin's disease) have prolonged homograft survival; (4) antilym-

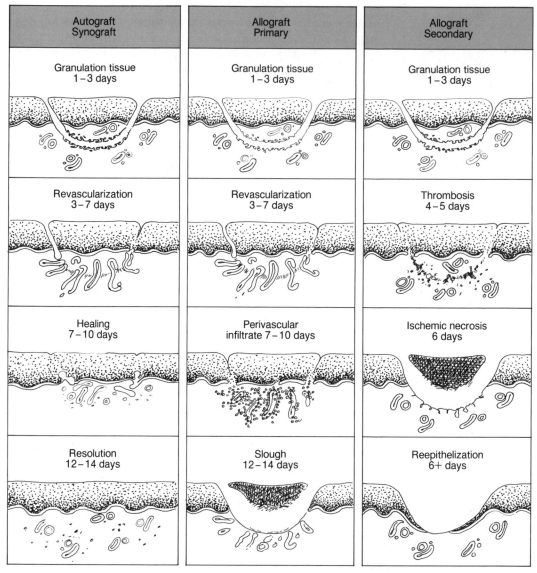

Autograft Synograft	Allograft Primary	Allograft Secondary
Granulation tissue 1–3 days	Granulation tissue 1–3 days	Granulation tissue 1–3 days
Revascularization 3–7 days	Revascularization 3–7 days	Thrombosis 4–5 days
Healing 7–10 days	Perivascular infiltrate 7–10 days	Ischemic necrosis 6 days
Resolution 12–14 days	Slough 12–14 days	Reepithelization 6+ days

Figure 19-5. Stages of skin graft rejection. The type of rejection of an allogeneic skin graft depends upon immune reactivity. An autograft or synograft will "take," that is, survive and heal in the grafted site. An allograft to an unsensitized individual will be rejected after a stage of vascularization by a mononuclear cell infiltrate. An allograft to a sensitized recipient will not become vascularized and will be rejected by ischemic necrosis within a few days after transplantation. (For details see the text.)

phocyte serum and other agents that affect delayed sensitivity more than humoral antibody are effective in prolonging the survival of homografts; (5) xenogeneic tissue grafts survive for long periods of time in nude mice that lack T cell–mediated reactivity. Humoral antibody may contribute to rejection of a tissue allograft, or it may interfere with (block) the action of sensitized cells in rejection. Perhaps the first evidence that circulating antibody does play a role in graft rejection was provided by Chandler Stetson, who demonstrated an acute necrotic rejection of skin allograft when specific antiserum to the graft was injected directly into the site of the skin graft. The failure of any circulation to be established resulted in complete ischemic necrosis—the white graft reaction. The interplay of antibody-mediated and cellular reactions in graft rejection is illustrated by the stages of rejection observed in human renal allografts (see below).

Graft Facilitation

Humoral antibody may also prolong graft survival. This paradoxical situation was first recognized in the 1930s, when it was noted that prior immunization to tumor tissue might increase the incidence and growth of tumors in allogeneic recipients that otherwise would regard the tumor as a foreign graft. This phenomenon was termed *tumor enhancement* (see Chapter 29). Later it was noted that grafts of normal tissues would survive longer if the animal was preimmunized in such a way as to produce circulating humoral antibody to allograft antigens rather than delayed hypersensitivity, or if humoral antibody was passively transferred to the recipient. This effect was termed graft facilitation. The enhancement–facilitation effect may suppress other effects of delayed hypersensitivity, such as graft versus host reactions, rejection of fetal tissues by the mother, autoallergic diseases, and tumor immunity (see below).

The enhancement–facilitation effect of antibody interferes with a potential rejection reaction mediated by sensitized cells. The rejection reaction may be divided into three phases: afferent, central, and efferent. *Afferent* refers to the delivery of antigen to the cells recognizing it; *central* refers to events following recognition, culminating in production of specifically sensitized cells; and *efferent* refers to the delivery of the sensitized cells to the target tissue, the reaction of those cells with target cell antigens, and destruction of the target cell by the sensitized killer cells. The theoretic sites of action of blocking (enhancing–facilitating) antibody are illustrated in Figure 19-6. At present it is impossible to select one mechanism as the most important; it is likely that more than one mechanism is operative in a given situation. In particular, blocking antibodies may mask antigenic sites so that they are not available to recognition cells (afferent effect) or to effector cells (efferent effect). Interference with effector cells by masking of target cell antigens is supported by the finding that humoral antibody to a target cell may block immune attack by T killer cells (CTL) in vitro. In addition, blocking antibodies, or complexes of blocking antibodies and antigen, may react directly with reacting or

482

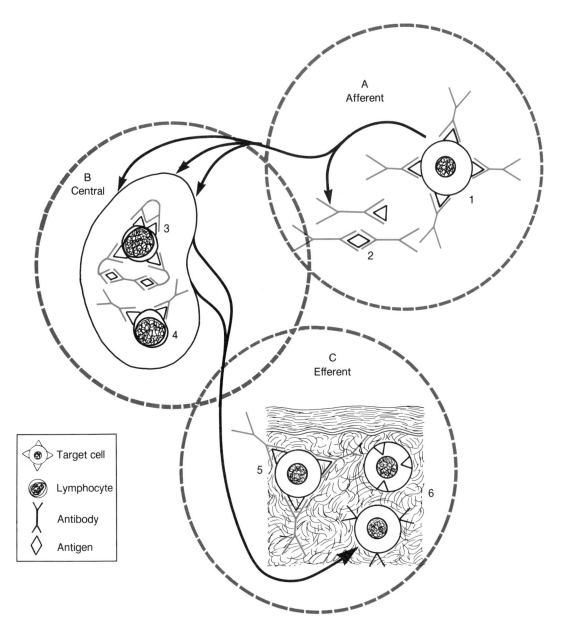

Figure 19-6. Possible mechanisms of immune facilitation of tissue grafts. Blocking antibody may interfere with cellular reactions at one of the three stages of induction and expression of delayed hypersensitivity. (A) Afferent: delivery of antigen to potentially responsive immunocompetent cells may be blocked by reaction of humoral antibody with antigen so that (1) the sites are masked and/or recognizable or (2) the antigen is catabolized in such a manner as to avoid contact with potentially reactive cells. (B) Central: antibody or antibody–antigen complexes may directly block surface receptors of reactive cells and prevent (3) antigen recognition or (4) cellular interactions required for the induction of delayed hypersensitivity. (C) Efferent: (5) antibody-coated target cells may be protected from attack by sensitized killer cells, or (6) antibody may induce disappearance of target cell surface antigens (modulation).

sensitized cells to block either the induction or expression of delayed hypersensitivity.

Stages of Renal Graft Rejection in Man

First-Set Rejection

The morphology of first-set renal allograft rejections in untreated recipients is entirely consistent with cellular mechanisms. The main feature is the accumulation of a mononuclear cell infiltrate. Within a few hours small lymphocytes collect around small venules; later many more mononuclear cells appear in the stroma. After a few days these mononuclear cells are much more varied in structure, with many small and large lymphocytes, immature blast cells, and typical mature plasma cells. Most likely, both T_K and T_D cells are active but many non-T cells are also present. Invasion of the renal tubular cells occurs, with isolation, separation, and death of these cells occurring in a way very similar, if not identical, to that described for tissue culture monolayers and thyroid follicular cells (see Chapter 8). The interstitial tissue of the rejecting kidney accumulates large quantities of fluid (edema). Finally the afferent arterioles and small arteries become swollen and occluded by fibrin and white cell thrombi. Occasionally these vessels show fibrinoid necrosis and contain immunoglobulins and complement consistent with deposition of antibody–antigen complexes. Therefore the first-set renal allograft rejection by an untreated recipient appears to occur primarily via cellular mechanisms, although there is evidence that humoral antibody may contribute.

Second-Set Rejection

A second renal allotransplant from the same donor who provided the first graft is rejected much more rapidly (within 1–3 days). There is little mononuclear cell infiltrate, presumably because adequate circulation necessary for the accumulation of blood mononuclear cells is never established. Morphologically the main features are destruction of peritubular capillaries and fibrinoid necrosis of the walls of the small arteries and arterioles. The glomeruli may contain intercapillary deposition of fibrin clots similar to those observed in the systemic Shwartzman reaction (see Chapter 12). By 24 hours there is widespread tubular necrosis, and the kidney never assumes functional activity. Perfusion of a renal homotransplant with plasma from an animal hyperimmunized against the donor of the kidney produces a similar reaction. Therefore, the acute second-set rejection of renal allograft appears to be mediated by preformed circulating antibodies. This type of acute rejection of a renal allograft has been observed in humans when grafting was attempted across ABO blood group types. A renal allograft from a B or A to an O recipient may lead to complete failure of circulation in the graft. There is distension and thrombosis of afferent arterioles and glomerular capillaries with sludged red cells, presumably owing to the action of cytotoxic anti-blood-group antibodies on blood group antigens located in the vasculature of the grafted kidney.

Late Rejection

Immunosuppressive therapy (see Chapter 27) is widely used to postpone allograft rejection, and the use of immunosuppressive agents has resulted in prolonged survival of human renal allografts. Such therapy appears to be effective in suppressing the development of rapid rejection but does not eliminate later rejection. Some patients with renal allografts survive for many years before rejection results in loss of function of the transplant. Morphologically the major finding in such late-rejected kidneys is a marked intimal proliferation and scarring of the walls of medium-sized arteries. The appearance is much like that of healed or late-stage polyarteritis nodosa. Thus, these late rejections are most likely the result of an antibody-mediated immune complex reaction. The possible fates of renal allografts are depicted in Figure 19-7.

Present Status of Solid Organ Transplantation in Man

Kidney

The initial success of solid tissue grafts indicates that the surgical techniques required for such procedures are well in hand. Most experience in human allografting has involved the kidney, and allografting is the treatment of choice for many types of renal failure. The use of sibling or parent donors is far superior for graft survival. However, most kidneys come from cadaver donors. Although the survival rate for recipients of unrelated cadaver donors is not as good as that of related donors, cadaver donors are much easier to obtain. Fortunately for the recipient, a willing and related living donor is often available.

An important factor in the survival of a renal transplant is the original disease that caused renal failure. The most frequent diseases for which renal transplantation is done include diabetic renal disease, pyelonephritis, and glomerulonephritis. Of these, patients with diabetes (usually males) generally have less success following transplantation than do patients without diabetes. Patients with pyelonephritis will have recurrence of pyelonephritis if the factors predisposing to pyelonephritis are still present. Those recipients whose renal failure resulted from glomerulonephritis may develop glomerulonephritis in the transplanted kidney, but in practice this rarely occurs, indicating that the original situation producing glomerulonephritis is no longer present. In diabetes and other diseases associated with chronic deposition of immune complexes, recurrent glomerulonephritis will occur if production of the complexes is not controlled.

A number of investigators have attempted to identify when a rejection episode may occur. Increased immunosuppressive therapy can usually reduce the effects of such an episode, but the effectiveness of this therapy is directly related to how long the rejection reaction has been going on. It is important to be able to monitor transplant patients for possible rejection reac-

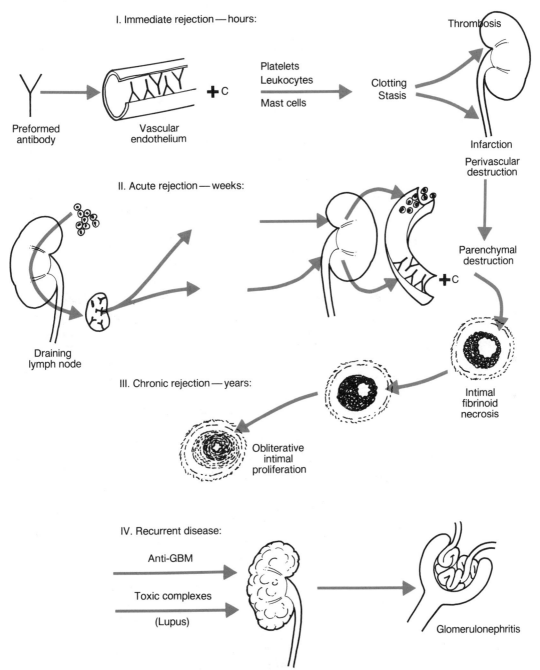

I. Immediate rejection — hours:

Preformed antibody

Vascular endothelium

+ C

Platelets
Leukocytes
Mast cells

Clotting
Stasis

Thrombosis

Infarction
Perivascular destruction

II. Acute rejection — weeks:

Draining lymph node

+ C

Parenchymal destruction

Intimal fibrinoid necrosis

III. Chronic rejection — years:

Obliterative intimal proliferation

IV. Recurrent disease:

Anti-GBM

Toxic complexes

(Lupus)

Glomerulonephritis

Figure 19-7. Some fates of human renal allografts. Renal allografts are subject to immune rejection as well as to recurrence of the original disease. Long-term uncomplicated survival essentially only occurs with completely matched donor and recipient, such as with identical twins. Immune rejection may be caused by either antibody or cell-mediated reactions. Immediate rejection is caused by reaction of preformed antibody with vascular endothelium and activation of the clotting system. Acute rejection is caused mainly by mononuclear cell infiltration (delayed hypersensitivity). Chronic rejection occurs as a result of continuing low-grade endarteritis because of deposition of antibody or immune complexes. Recurrence of the original disease may occur if the predisposing cause is not controlled.

tions. The most important test is that of decreasing renal function as measured by serum creatinine levels.

Presensitization to HLA antigens will affect survival of transplants. Clearly if a recipient has antibody to HLA antigen prior to transplantation, acute antibody-mediated rejection may occur. Recipients with antibody to donor antigens (presensitized) have lower (47%) graft survival rates than patients without antibody to donor antigens (57%). For this reason, blood transfusions to potential recipients have been generally avoided. However, more recent evidence indicates better graft survival in recipients who have had multiple exposures to donor HLA antigens (but are cross-match negative). Thus 44% 1-year graft survival is found in patients who have received no blood transfusions, and 58%, 60%, and 64%, respectively, in patients who have received 1 to 4, 5 to 9, and 10 or more units of blood before the transplantation procedures.

Other Organs

Transplantation of other solid organs, such as heart, lung, liver, and pancreas, has not yet resulted in long-term results as encouraging as with renal transplants. Earlier poor survival rates limited cardiac transplantation to a few experimental centers. However, survival rates have increased significantly. From 1974 to 1981 the survival rates for transplants done at the Stanford Center were 63%, 55%, 51%, 44%, and 39% at 1, 2, 3, 4, and 5 years after transplantation. This corresponds to 44%, 35%, 27%, 21%, and 18% for the period 1968–1973. The improved survival largely reflects better patient management, in particular more careful immunosuppressive therapy, reducing death due to infection. Development of artificial hearts has increased the possibility of eventually finding a donor by prolonging the life of potential recipients. Acute cardiac rejection reactions may be diagnosed by endocardial biopsy, particularly of the right ventricle. The procedure may increase the chances of treating patients by intensive immunosuppression before rejection is advanced. The effectiveness of liver transplantation has also increased substantially as a result of better patient selection and management procedures. Rejection actually accounts for less than 10% of liver transplant failures.

Systematic experimental studies of transplantation of pancreatic islets for treatment of experimental diabetics in animals have provided data indicating that the approaches worked out should be successfully applied to man. The following factors have proved important.

1. Preparation of a suspension of isolated islet cells from pancreatic tissue.
2. Transplantation into an accessible site such as a peritoneal envelope on the omentum.
3. Removal of passenger lymphocytes by cultivation in vitro or treatment of islet cell preparations with anti-class II major

histocompatibility complex (MHC) antibody (islet cells do not express class II (Ia) antigens, whereas passenger lymphocytes do).

4. Matching of donor and recipient for class II MHC antigens.

Prior to 1985 pancreatic islet transplantation in human clinical trials was found to be safe, but unfortunately not successful. The major problem appears to be the ability to obtain sufficient numbers of isolated islet cells. Transplantation of the pancreas as a solid organ is now being attempted, but the results as of the time of this writing are too preliminary to evaluate.

Autotransplantation of parathyroid glands into the forearm musculature has been used following parathyroidectomy for parathyroid hyperplasia. This permits replacement of portions of the gland into easily accessible areas, where their function can be monitored and controlled.

Neural Transplantation

The possibility of brain transplantation has titillated the imagination of science fiction writers for many years, and mammalian neural transplantation has recently been demonstrated to be feasible. The brain is an immunologically privileged site so that the usual graft rejection mechanisms may not be active in neural transplantation. In experimental models it has been possible to transplant neuronal cells to reinnervate damaged zones of the host brain. In these studies small grafts of fetal brain cells can be placed in zones of damage induced in the brain. Small groups of only a few thousand cells are able to restore some neuroendocrine deficits, cognitive disorders, and motor dysfunctions in young adult rodents, and neuroendocrine cells can integrate into brains of aged rodents and improve behavioral performance. It is postulated that it might be possible to alleviate neurotransmitted defects in Parkinson's disease and Alzheimer's disease by neuronal transplantation.

Factors Affecting Graft Survival

Because of the nature of the data and the presence of multiple uncontrolled variables, many of the results reported on human organ transplantation are difficult to evaluate. The survival of the recipient is dependent upon multiple factors, including the original disease, tissue matching, organ source, choice of immunosuppressive treatment, and surgical skill. However, from a pragmatic standpoint, the most important factors for successful renal grafting are careful pretransplant workup and conditioning, and thorough and painstaking post-transplant follow-up of the patient by his physicians, including psychiatric counseling.

Graft versus Host Reactions

Transfer of cell populations such as bone marrow that contain immune competent lymphocytes may lead to a reaction of the transferred cells to antigens of the recipient. This is called a *graft versus host* reaction. Graft versus host (GVH) reactions occur when immune competent cells from an allogenic or xenogenic donor are transferred to a recipient whose own immune responsiveness has been impaired by immune suppression or neoplastic disease, or because of immature development. The transferred cells will colonize in the recipient, recognize host tissue antigens as foreign, and react to them. When the lymphoid tissue of the recipient is not completely destroyed, regeneration of the host immune system in the presence of donor cells may result in a state of mutual tolerance of grafted and recipient cells (lymphoid chimera). In lymphoid cell chimeras, the recipient maintains both its own and the donor lymphoid components.

The reaction of grafted immune cells to host antigens and vice versa produces a wasting syndrome known as graft versus host or secondary disease. This consists of two pathologic processes: infiltration of tissues, especially the skin, intestine, spleen, and liver, with proliferating lymphocytes, resulting in hepatosplenomegaly, diarrhea, and a scaly contact dermatitis skin lesion; as well as loss of immune reactivity to other antigens and increased susceptibility to infections. The hyperplasia of spleen and other lymphoid organs is followed by atrophy, presumably because the grafted cells have attacked and destroyed the host's lymphoid tissue. Chronic GVH disease may lead to scleroderma-like lesions. Proliferating host cells make the major contribution to the lymphoid hyperplasia, and it is the recipient's lymphopoietic tissue that bears the brunt of the attack by the transferred cells. The success of bone marrow transplantation depends largely on controlling the extent of the GVH reaction.

Bone Marrow Transplantation

Bone marrow grafts have been used to treat patients with aplastic anemia (failure of blood cell production), patients with severe combined immune deficiencies (see Chapter 26), or patients with leukemia treated with irradiation or ablative chemotherapy for cancer. With careful follow-up, good results are obtained in most of the cases of aplastic anemia if an HLA-identical sibling donor is used. The use of bone marrow in immune deficiency diseases is discussed in Chapter 26. Irradiation leads to failure of blood cell production and reduction in immune function. The degree and type of immune deficiency depend on the dose of radiation given. Irradiation doses sufficient to cause significant reduction in leukemic cell mass frequently result in death by infection. This can be circumvented by transfer of bone marrow from a healthy donor. Unless an identical twin is available, some degree of graft versus host reactivity seems inevitable. In some situations a fatal outcome can be avoided; the graft can survive, with the recipient eventually having both donor and host lymphoid cells (radiation chimera).

Clinically, bone marrow transplantation following radiation treatment of leukemia and aplastic anemia has had increasing success. Efforts in improving bone marrow transplantation have centered on ways to reduce the severity of the graft versus host reaction, yet provide sufficient bone marrow stem cells to reconstitute the irradiated recipient. Techniques have included HLA matching, particularly using HLA-matched siblings; the use of mixtures of cells from a number of related donors with the hope that the most compatible donor cells will survive; administration of immunosuppressive agents such as cyclophosphamide or antilymphocyte serum to control the GVH reaction, and fractionation of cells in an attempt to eliminate the immunologically reactive cells that would produce the GVH reaction. Recently treatment of cells with "cytotoxic" monoclonal antibodies to donor T cells in an attempt to remove potentially reactive cells or the use of preserved autologous bone marrow obtained during a remission is being attempted. None of these procedures can be considered satisfactory as yet, although many long-term remissions have been obtained. In most remissions a transient GVH reaction occurs and the treated individual demonstrates both host and donor cells after the reaction (chimerism). A particularly interesting and perplexing observation has been that in a few cases of leukemia treated by whole body irradiation and bone marrow from an HLA-matched sibling of the opposite sex, the donor's blood cells became established but developed leukemia. This could be because of excessive antigenic stimulation of donor cells in a foreign environment, an abnormal homeostatic mechanism in the recipient that also applies to donor cells, fusion of donor and recipient cells resulting in transfer of donor chromosome markers to recipient leukemic cells, or transmission of an agent (oncogenic virus) from host to donor cells. Clearly, use of bone marrow transplantation clinically has moved from an experimental procedure to a clinically applicable method and if carefully done may result in a satisfactory therapy for leukemia, lymphoma, aplastic anemia, or immune deficiency diseases.

Graft–Host Relationships in Pregnancy

The effect of the maternal immune response in pregnancy to fetal antigens has been the subject of extensive investigation and speculation. Except for matings within inbred strains of animals, a fetus in utero is a graft of tissue containing transplantation antigens to which the mother can react. Since half of the fetal genetic endowment is contributed by the father, the fetus is a hemiallogeneic graft. Paternal histocompatibility antigens are present on spermatozoa and are represented in fetal tissue. In spite of this potential for immune rejection as an allograft, the fetus is rarely affected. The fetus survives a longer time in the uterus than do other foreign tissue grafts, and gestation is terminated by nonimmune events. The means by which the fetus avoids immune rejection are not fully understood. The following mechanisms have been proposed.

1. Paternal antigens are not present on embryonal or fetal tissues. This is certainly not true. Although histocompatibility antigens are present on postnatal cells in higher amounts than on fetal cells, tissue antigens have been demonstrated on embryonal and fetal cells at essentially all stages of development and are present in sufficient amounts to be killed by sensitized lymphocytes in vitro and in vivo.

2. The fetus is not rejected because half of its histocompatibility antigens are common with those of the mother. This is also an untrue statement, because a mother will reject skin grafts of fetal skin and surrogate mothers will support ova from unrelated parents when transplanted in utero.

3. The mother does not become immunized to fetal tissues during pregnancy. This is unlikely because mothers will develop antibodies to fetal antigens; one of the common sources of HLA typing sera is multiparous women. In addition, a significant hypertrophy of the draining lymph nodes occurs during pregnancy. Furthermore, protection is afforded to the fetus even if the mother is preimmunized to fetal tissues by injection of paternal antigens or rejection of paternal skin graft prior to pregnancy.

4. The uterus is an immunologically privileged site. Skin grafts from F_1 or paternal strains will be rejected if placed in the uterus of a histoincompatible female even if the recipient is hormonally prepared and the uterus has undergone a decidual reaction (i.e., the uterus is hormonally prepared for acceptance of a fertilized ovum). In addition, delayed hypersensitivity reactions can be elicited in the uterus by injection of antigen into the uterus of a sensitized animal.

5. The production of blocking antibody prevents cellular reactivity to fetal antigens. It is well known that mothers will produce antibody to fetal antigens during pregnancy. Whereas in general it has been impossible to induce a graft versus host reaction by immunization of the mother to fetal antigens, such runting can be observed in special circumstances. Female rats of one strain who rejected skin grafts from another produced runted (GVH disease) offspring if mating to fathers of the other strain took place at the time of rejection of the graft. If rejection of the graft took place 2 weeks prior to mating, runting was not observed. Runting is believed to be due to the presence of large numbers of lymphoid cells sensitized to fetal antigens at a time when no humoral antibody is present and the fetus is particularly susceptible to a GVH reaction; rejection of a graft 2 weeks

prior to mating permits cellular sensitivity to decline and blocking antibody to rise so that the fetus is protected. However, this explanation does not appear to hold for other effects seen in pregnancy and may be unique to this experimental system.

6. A factor (soluble serum protein) may be produced during pregnancy that interferes with immune effector mechanisms. Such proposed immunosuppressive factors include α-fetoprotein, pregnancy-associated protein, and α regulatory globulin. The support for immunosuppression is based on the effects of addition of these proteins to in vitro cultures. However, conflicting results have been obtained and a suppressive role in vivo has not been convincingly demonstrated. A suppressive effect on immune induction is not likely, because pregnant animals are not immunosuppressed. However, it is possible that a suppressive factor might function locally at the fetal–maternal interface to block effector mechanisms.

7. The early development of immune competence by the fetus in utero may provide a protective response for the immune elimination of the small number of maternal lymphocytes that get across the placenta. Under carefully defined conditions the passive transfer of cells from unrelated strains of mice immunized against the parental strains will produce runting of the offspring while no GVH reaction occurs in the mother. It is suggested that the passively transferred cells crossed the placenta and produced a GVH reaction in the fetuses that were not yet sufficiently immunologically competent to reject the specifically sensitized transferred cells; but the mother, who was immunologically mature, did reject the transferred cells. In the human, most instances of neonatal GVH disease are associated with an immune deficiency of the fetus. In fact there is speculation that lymphomas in children may be related to production of subclinical runt disease caused by maternal lymphocytes that infiltrated the fetus during pregnancy and were not eliminated by an immune response of the fetus. The high incidence of "autoallergic" reactions found in patients with lymphomas and leukemias suggests that the individual's lymphoid system may be responding to self antigens; perhaps this represents stimulation of maternally derived sequestered lymphocytes and is a GVH reaction.

8. The placenta serves as a barrier to immunization and to maternal immune cells. The fetus is contained in a fluid-filled cyst of fetal origin, the amniotic sac, which separates the mother from the fetus except at the point of attachment of the placenta. At this point, fetal tissue, the trophoblast, actually invades the endometrial wall of the uterus and comes into direct contact with the maternal circulation.

Trophoblastic tissue, although containing histocompatibility antigens in small amounts, is not rejected if transplanted into sites outside the uterus. In fact, the developing fetus may actually be maintained in the abdominal cavity outside of the uterus until nonimmune complications develop (ectopic pregnancy). Trophoblastic cells do not contain H, A, or B blood group antigens; the endothelium of the vessels of the placenta and umbilical cord has only the basic H structure. In contrast, the endothelial cells of the fetus have a large amount of these antigens. The lack of ABH antigens in trophoblasts prevents attack by maternal AB isoantibodies. The trophoblastic cells contain a large amount of glycocalyx, a cell coating of carbohydrate that masks transplantation antigens and repels lymphocytes. However, small numbers of maternal lymphocytes do cross the placenta, but evidently not in sufficient numbers to cause rejection of the fetus. That the placenta may contain lymphocytes that might attack the fetus is supported by the finding that placental size is increased in proportion to the degree of immunity of the mother to the fetus. It is possible that the placental tissue may contain histocompatibility antigens distributed in such a way that specifically sensitized lymphocytes react with placental tissue with minimal effect on placental function, but are prevented from passing into the fetal circulation. Maternal lymphocytes that do cross the placenta may not be reactive to fetal tissue antigens. Passively transferred antibody to fetal tissues is rapidly absorbed from the maternal circulation, most likely by the placenta. Thus the placenta may act not only to provide a simple barrier, but also as a sink to remove and inactivate immune reactants.

Graft Facilitation in Pregnancy

The production of humoral antibody by the mother against paternal antigens on the fetus may actually enhance fetal viability. The placentas of F_1 mice are larger than those of inbred mice. Maternal preimmunization against paternal antigens enhances this effect. In humans the incidence of spontaneous abortions is high in couples that share MHC markers as compared to those who do not, and antibodies to paternal class II MHC are absent in sera of spontaneous aborters. By these mechanisms maternal immunostimulation may result in protection against T cell–mediated graft rejection of the fetus and actually stimulate growth of the fetus and placenta.

Viral Infections

Delayed hypersensitivity reactions to viral antigens may be either protective, by limiting viral infections, or destructive, by destroying functioning host cells that are expressing viral antigens.

Viral Exanthems

It is now generally accepted that delayed hypersensitivity to viral antigens is responsible for the lesions of the viral exanthems. An exanthem is a disease or fever associated with eruptive skin lesions. Von Pirquet in 1907 observed that the local lesion following smallpox vaccination (vaccinia) consisted of a two-stage reaction (see also Chapter 24). Early (first 8 days), there is a papular vesicular lesion because of the growth of the inoculated virus; later (8–14 days) an indurated erythematous reaction (take) follows. The take reaction corresponds to the development of delayed hypersensitivity and is interpreted as evidence that protective immunity has been established. Similar lesions appear at the same time on different parts of the body, even though the different areas are inoculated with the virus at different times. Animal experiments have shown that protection against the virus is associated with delayed hypersensitivity, and that the infective virus disappears from the local lesion when the delayed reaction is maximal. The same concept was considered valid by von Pirquet for other viral exanthems (measles, varicella) in which multiple, disseminated lesions occur as a result of delayed reaction to viruses located at the sites of lesions. There is a suggestion that some of the lesions of the viral exanthems may be modified by humoral antibody reacting with viral antigens to produce an Arthus-like reaction in the skin; however, delayed hypersensitivity is the major mechanism.

Viral Encephalitides of Animals

Several animal models of virus-induced encephalomyelitis illustrate important differences in pathogenesis involving immune mechanisms (Table 19-1).

Table 19-1. Pathogenesis of Some Virus-Related Encephalitides of Animals

Disease	Species	Suspected Mechanism
Lymphocytic choriomeningitis	Mouse	Cellular reaction to virus antigens on neurons
Mouse hepatitis virus encephalitis	Mouse	Viral destruction of myelin
Canine distemper	Dog	Postinfectious autoallergy to myelin or slowly progressing virus demyelination
Theiler's virus myelitis	Mouse	Postinfectious autoallergy to myelin
Marek's disease	Chicken	Postinfectious autoallergy to myelin

Lymphocytic Choriomeningitis

The role of delayed hypersensitivity in producing the lesions of some infectious diseases is exemplified by a viral disease of mice and men, lymphocytic choriomeningitis (LCM). The introduction of the specific virus in mice uniformly results in a fatal brain infection. Certain features of the experimental disease suggest that the brain lesions are due not just to the presence of the virus itself but to a delayed hypersensitivity reaction to the viral antigens located in the brain. Intracranial injection of the virus results in much more severe disease than does intracutaneous injection. If a sublethal intracutaneous injection is followed by a lethal intracranial injection, the eventual outcome depends on the interval between the cutaneous and cranial injections. If the cranial injection follows the cutaneous injection by fewer than 4 days, the outcome is invariably fatal, and the course of the disease is more rapid than when the virus is given only intracranially. If 7 days intervene between the cranial and cutaneous injections, the animals survive. The interpretation is that the sublethal cutaneous injection produces an immune response to the virus. If immunity is developed (7-day interval) when the cranial injection is administered, a specific delayed type reaction prevents dissemination and growth of virus. However, if the virus is already distributed before the delayed reaction develops, the reaction of the specifically sensitized cells with the localized virus produces the lesions. In the 4-day interval situation, the cutaneous injection initiates the development of delayed sensitivity so that it is partially developed but not active (i.e., is in the induction period) when the cranial injection is given. Since the induction of the delayed reactivity is already partially developed, the onset of symptoms occurs earlier than when the induction of the delayed reaction and the cranial injection of the virus occur at the same time. Further evidence that hypersensitivity is the mechanism responsible for the actual production of lesions is that procedures that suppress delayed hypersensitivity (administration of immunosuppressive drugs, irradiation, thymectomy at birth, or antilymphocyte serum) markedly suppress the development of the symptoms of lymphocytic choriomeningitis. Some of the mice so treated may remain completely asymptomatic, even though viable virus can be isolated from brain tissue. However, these mice may develop immune complex–mediated disease because of the production of humoral antibody to LCM virus and the formation of circulating antibody–antigen complexes.

The role of histocompatibility (MHC) restriction in killing of virus-infected target cells was worked out using the LCM model. As described in more detail in Chapter 9, specifically sensitized T killer cells will not lyse LCM virus-infected target cells unless the T_K cells also recognize histocompatibility antigens on the target cells. Adoptive immunization (passive transfer) of T_K cells sensitized to LCM or to immunosuppressed LCM-infected mice causes a fatal reaction within 2 to 4 days. The fatal disease occurs only when the T_K cells can recognize both viral antigens and MHC antigens on the target cells.

Mouse Hepatitis Virus Encephalitis

Virus-induced demyelination that does not depend upon an immune response is exemplified by mouse hepatitis virus.

Mouse hepatitis virus infects oligodendrocytes and produces plaques of demyelination. Viral antigens are detectable in glial cells, which are intimately associated with myelin. Demyelination is believed to be caused by virus infection. In contrast to LCM, immunosuppressive treatment increases the rate of mortality in infected mice. Demyelination occurs randomly with no relation to blood vessels, as is observed in experimental allergic encephalomyelitis (see below). Lymphocyte infiltration is scanty and rarely detected prior to demyelination. Thus some virus infections may cause demyelination directly without the action of immune cells.

Canine Distemper

The relationship of an inadequate or inappropriate immune response to a virus-induced disease is seen in a naturally occurring infectious disease of dogs, canine distemper. The canine distemper paramyxovirus is closely related to human measles virus and produces a disease in dogs similar to human measles and the related neurological diseases—acute encephalitis, postinfectious encephalitis, and subacute sclerosing panencephalitis (SSPE) (see below). Canine distemper produces an acute systemic disease from which most animals recover. Following this disease, however, a certain proportion of the affected animals go on to develop a demyelinating postinfectious encephalomyelitis, the pathology of which is similar to that of experimental allergic encephalomyelitis. The chronic phase of distemper is called "old dog encephalitis" and bears similarities to human SSPE. The distemper virus enters the brain during the acute systemic viremia, and viral inclusions can be found in glial cells. The postinfectious disease develops suddenly after a latent period of several weeks, even though it can be assumed that the virus particles are in the brain throughout the latent period. Although the role of immunopathological mechanisms in the disease remains unclear, antibodies to viral antigens and to myelin appear in high titers in the sera of affected dogs. Since the virus does not appear to cause tissue destruction, it is likely that the demyelination is due to sensitized lymphocytes reacting either to viral antigens present in myelinated tissue or to myelin antigens rendered immunogenic from the viral infection. Humoral antibody may play a role in initiating vascular reactions or may actually be protective (e.g., blocking antibody).

Theiler's Myelitis

This is an inflammatory demyelination of the spinal cord of mice occurring 1 to 3 months following infection with Theiler's mouse encephalitis virus. After initial involvement of the gray matter, patchy demyelination occurs. The pathological picture is similar to that in experimental allergic encephalomyelitis (EAE) (see below). Immunosuppression increases the virus particles that are not present in the areas of demyelination. This demyelination is believed to be caused by a postinfectious auto-sensitization to myelin.

Marek's Disease

Marek's disease is a herpesvirus-induced lymphoproliferative disease of chickens that also induces paralysis associated with perivascular infiltration of mononuclear cells and demyelination. It is postulated that there is an autosensitization to myelin, and a number of observations indicate that the demyelination is T cell dependent. The mechanism of autosensitization in this disease is not known but the lesions are similar to those of EAE of animals and the Guillain–Barré syndrome of humans.

Viral Encephalitides of Man

The viral encephalitides of man occur in a variety of forms, depending on the nature of the infecting agent and the type and intensity of the immune response. The disorders are classified as acute, postinfectious, latent, chronic, and slow (Table 19-2).

Table 19-2. Viral Encephalitides of Man

Acute	Polio, rabies, herpes	Virus destruction of cells, immune response protective
Postinfectious	Postvaccinial	Lymphocyte-mediated destruction (?autoallergic)
	Postvirus infection (mumps, measles, ?multiple sclerosis)	
Latent	Progressive multifocal leukoencephalopathy	Inadequate protective immunity because of secondary immune deficiency (leukemia, lymphoma)
Chronic or slow	Subacute sclerosing panencephalitis Kuru, Creutzfeldt–Jakob syndrome (?amyotrophic lateral sclerosis)	Persistent infection because of lack of protective response, alteration of specialized function of infected cells

In the acute encephalitides (poliomyelitis, rabies, herpes simplex), the virus destroys nerve cells directly in a predictable fashion. The immune response is protective in the sense that it blocks the destructive aspects of the disease by elimination of the virus.

Postinfectious encephalomyelitis follows a mild virus infection and is caused by an autoallergic reaction of sensitized cells with myelin, presumably due to the presence of altered host antigen or virus antigen–host myelin combinations (see Autoallergic Diseases, Chapter 20). The virus alone does not produce significant destruction. Such reactions may follow infections such as mumps, measles, distemper, or vaccination with rabies or vaccinia virus.

Latent viral infections are caused by a change in the relation of the host's immune response to a virus infection that has not produced clinical manifestations, so that clinical symptoms become manifest. This may occur because of an increase or a decrease in the host's immune state. Progressive multifocal leukoencephalopathy occurs in patients whose immune state is lowered (leukemia, lymphoma). Destruction of brain cells occurs in the absence of significant inflammation. Cytomegalic inclusion disease, a systemic virus infection, also occurs in patients with depressed ability to mount an immune response (e.g., kidney transplant recipients undergoing immunosuppression with drugs). On the other hand, symptoms related to lymphocytic choriomeningitis may be produced in experimental animals with latent infections by increasing the immune response to lymphocytic choriomeningitis. The lesions contain a significant inflammatory reaction. Because of an immune response to the virus, infected cells are also destroyed (innocent bystander reaction).

Chronic encephalomyelitis features an irregular protracted course with variation in immune reactivity and brain cell destruction by virus. The condition of subacute sclerosing panencephalitis is believed to be a later manifestation in adults following measles infection in childhood. Affected patients have brain cell inclusions and high antibody titers to measles virus. Some change in the relation between protective immunity and virus infection is believed to occur, but it is not clear whether the allergic reaction or the virus itself is the cause of the destruction. Multiple sclerosis (MS) is a chronic remitting disease with the occurrence of repeated attacks, wheras subacute sclerosing panencephalitis (SSPE) is an unremitting progressive disease caused by the dissemination of a defective yet replicating virus. SSPE is probably caused by an inadequate protective immune response to the virus, whereas MS may be caused by a delayed hypersensitivity response to myelin.

Slow virus infections, represented by kuru and Creutzfeldt–Jakob disease, have a regular protracted fatal course following a long latent period. These diseases are characterized by abnormal membrane accumulations. The responsible agents have not been characterized, but appear to consist of membrane material with no RNA or DNA component. No inflammatory response or immune reactivity of the host can be demonstrated; the course of the disease is determined by characteristics of the agent. Kuru occurs in certain native tribes of New Guinea. Its incidence has decreased sharply since the ritual cannibalism involving removal of the brain, and widespread contamination of those preparing the brain for consumption with tissue containing millions of infective doses of kuru, has been discontinued. Kuru is caused by the progressive proliferation and dissemination of an agent that provokes no immune response and is normally not infective but becomes so if large amounts of the agent are introduced through the skin, as occurs during preparation of brains for ritual eating.

Amyotrophic lateral sclerosis is a disease of unknown origin associated with destruction or injury of anterior cells in the spinal cord and pyramidal cells in the cerebral cortex. It has been shown that persistent infection with virus such as LCM virus can alter luxury functions of certain cells without affecting vital functions. Viral infections of neural cells may not actually destroy the cells but can alter their neurotransmitter function. Thus although the function of these cells is lost, the infected cells are not destroyed by either virus or immune response to the virus. Patients with amyotrophic lateral sclerosis often have circulating immune complexes. Identification of the antigen in these complexes may give an important clue to the etiologic agent.

Viral Hepatitis

Viral hepatitis (inflammation of the liver) is caused by at least three viruses: hepatitis A virus (infectious hepatitis), hepatitis B virus (serum hepatitis), and non-A, non-B hepatitis. The association of a specific virus with hepatitis was made possible by the study of Australia antigen, now known as hepatitis B surface antigen (HBsAg). HBsAg is the coat or surface antigen of hepatitis B virus. Another antigen, the core antigen, HBcAg, contains double-stranded circular DNA with DNA polymerase activity, and is antigenically distinct from HBsAg. The core virus infects and replicates within the hepatocyte nucleus. It then migrates to the cytoplasm, where it is ensheathed in a coat made by the liver cell under the direction of the viral genome.

The viral surface antigen, HBsAg, is detected in the serum of hepatitis patients or antigen carriers by reaction with anti-HBsAg. The association with hepatitis was first made when a patient previously found to be lacking the HBsAg antigen was found to possess the antigen at the time of development of hepatitis. A systemic survey then demonstrated a high incidence of HBsAg antigen among patients with acute viral hepatitis and disappearance of the antigen upon their clinical recovery. Viral antigen may be identified within the liver cells of infected individuals using immunofluorescence, and viral particles may be obtained from the blood of some patients during active stages of the disease. The bloodborne particles consist mainly of viral coat particles, whereas whole viral particles (coat and nucleoprotein core) are rarely found. The detection of HBsAg antigen is now used to confirm the clinical diagnosis of hepatitis. A third antigen, the e antigen, which is distinct from HBsAg and HBcAg, may be present in long-term carriers. The presence of the e antigen is associated with chronic active hepatitis, with cirrhosis, and with an infectious carrier state.

Delayed hypersensitivity reactions to viral antigens expressed on the surface of infected liver cells or to liver cell antigens rendered immunogenic by association with viral particles may be one of the mechanisms of liver cell destruction leading to elimination of virus-infected cells. The acute lesion is destruction of hepatocytes (liver cell necrosis) most likely directly produced by virus infection; later lesions are associated with a marked infiltration of mononuclear cells and may be due to cytotoxic effects of sensitized lymphocytes. Chronic hepatitis may evolve from acute hepatitis or may arise without an obvious acute phase and is most likely due to immune lymphocytes (cytotoxic T cells) attacking virus-infected liver cells.

Antibodies to core antigens (anti-HB$_c$) appear earlier in the disease than anti-surface (anti-HB$_s$) antibodies. Humoral antibody and HBsAg–antibody complexes are present in the sera of patients during disease or recovery. Whereas humoral antibody may act to neutralize the virus, the presence of HBsAg–Ab complexes may lead to systemic immune complex disease; polyarteritis has been found in patients with HBsAg–Ab complexes in their sera (see Chapter 17). The passive transfer of antibody to HBsAg has been suggested as a possible therapy for patients with viral hepatitis, and a successful result in a pregnant patient with fulminant HBsAg-positive hepatitis treated with plasmapheresis and anti-HBsAg plasma has been reported.

The passage of viral hepatitis by transfusion (serum hepatitis) may be significantly reduced by screening blood donors for HBsAg. The possibility of laboratory workers acquiring hepatitis from infected blood or tissues and of the general population becoming infected from contaminated food (shellfish) must be considered and appropriate precautions taken.

In summary, the acute destructive lesions of viral hepatitis are most likely due to direct destruction of liver cells by the virus; chronic destruction is at least partially caused by a cellular reaction to the virus. Protection may be effected by humoral antibody, which probably acts to prevent spread of the infection from cell to cell. However, circulating HBsAg–Ab complexes may cause systemic immune complex disease.

Warts

Warts in humans are caused by a human papilloma virus that, like animal papilloma virus, more commonly causes lesions in young individuals. Spontaneous regression frequently occurs and is associated with the appearance of IgG serum antibodies, or specific cellular immunity. Patients with recurring warts are characterized by a weak or nonexistent specific immune response. Thus a wart is a virus infestation that is effectively controlled by an immune response and occurs persistently only in individuals with an inadequate immune response to the virus.

Summary

Delayed hypersensitivity reactions are initiated by reaction of specifically sensitized lymphocytes with antigen in tissue. Two major T lymphocyte populations are involved: T_D and T_K (killer or cytotoxic) cells. T_D cells release lymphocytic mediators when activated by antigen that produce tissue inflammation mainly by attracting and activating macrophages. Most of the tissue damage seen in vivo is mediated by macrophages. T_K cells react directly with antigens on tissue cells, causing the destruction of the tissue cell. Delayed hypersensitivity reactions include skin test reactions, contact dermatitis, immune rejection of solid organ grafts, reactions to virus infections, and many autoimmune diseases.

References

See also Chapter 8.

Delayed Hypersensitivity

General

Ahmed AR, Blox DA: Delayed-type hypersensitivity skin testing. A review. Arch Dermatol 119:934, 1983.

Askenase PW, Van Loveren H: Delayed type hypersensitivity: activation of mast cells by antigen specific T-cell factors initiates the cascade of cellular interactions. Immunol Today 4:259, 1983.

Bloom BR, Glade PR (eds): In Vitro Methods in Cell Mediated Immunity. New York, Academic Press, 1971.

Bonavida B: Studies on the induction and expression of T cell-mediated immunity. II. Antiserum blocking of cell-mediated cytolysis. J Immunol 112:1308, 1974.

Chase MC: Developments in delayed type hypersensitivity, 1950–1975. J Invest Dermatol 67:136, 1976.

Cohen S: The role of cell-mediated immunity in the induction of inflammatory responses. Am J Pathol 88:502, 1977.

Cohen S: Symposium on cell mediated immunity in human disease. Hum Pathol 17:111, 1986.

Dvorak HF, Galli SJ, Dvorak A: Cellular and vascular manifestations of cell mediated immunity. Hum Pathol 17:112, 1986.

Dvorak HF, Mihm M Jr, Dvorak A, et al: Morphology of delayed type hypersensitivity reaction in man. I. Quantitative description of the inflammatory response. Lab Invest 31:111, 1974.

Frazer IH, et al: Assessment of delayed-type hypersensitivity in man: a comparison of the "multitest" and conventional intradermal injection of six antigens. Clin Immunol Pathol 35:182, 1985.

Galli SJ, Dvorak A: What do mast cells have to do with delayed hypersensitivity? Lab Invest 50:365, 1984.

Gell PGH, Benacerraf B: Delayed hypersensitivity to simple protein antigens. Adv Immunol 1:319, 1961.

Kinker WT, et al.: Cell mediated immunity assessed by multitest CMI skin testing in infants and preschool children. Am J Dis Child 139:840, 1985.

Lawrence HS: The delayed type of allergic inflammatory response. Am J Med 20:428, 1956.

Lawrence HS, Landy M (eds): Mediators of Cellular Immunity. New York, Academic Press, 1969.

Raffel J, Newel JM: The "delayed hypersensitivity" induced by antigen–antibody complexes. J Exp Med 108:823, 1958.

Sell S, Weigle WO: The relationship between delayed hypersensitivity and circulating antibody induced by protein antigens in guinea pigs. J Immunol 83:257, 1959.

Simon FA, Rackeman FF: The development of hypersensitiveness in man. I. Following intradermal injection of the antigen. J Allergy 5:439, 1934.

Turk JL: Delayed Hypersensitivity. New York, Wiley, 1967.

Uhr JW: Delayed hypersensitivity. Physiol Rev 46:359, 1966.

Waksman BH, Namba Y: On soluble mediators of immunologic regulation. Cell Immunol 21:161, 1976.

Waksman BH: A comparative histopathological study of delayed hypersensitivity reactions. *In* Wolstenholme GEW, Connor CE (eds): Cellular Aspects of Immunity. Boston, Little, Brown, 1960.

Waksman BH: Delayed hypersensitivity: a growing class of immunological phenomena. J Allergy 31:468, 1960.

Contact Dermatitis

Arnason BG, Waksman BH: Tuberculin sensitivity: immunologic considerations. Adv Tuberc Res 13:1, 1964.

Auerbuck R, Baer H: Comparison of potency of poison ivy extracts with synthetic pentadecylcatechols in sensitive humans. J Allergy 35:3, 1964.

Epstein E, Clairborne ER: Racial and environmental factors in susceptibility to Rhus. Excerpta Med 12:357, 1958.

Flax MH, Caulfield JB: Cellular and vascular components of allergic contact dermatitis. Am J Pathol 43:1031, 1963.

Foussereau J, Benezra C, Maibach HH: Occupational Contact Dermatitis: Clinical and Chemical Aspects. Philadelphia, Saunders, 1982.

Johnson RA, et al: Comparison of the contact allergenicity of the four pentadecylcatechols derived from poison ivy urushiol human subjects. J Allergy Clin Immunol 49:27, 1972.

Kligman AM: Poison ivy (Rhus) dermatitis: experimental study. Arch Dermatol 77:149, 1958.

Sontheimer RD, Gilliam JN: Immunologically mediated epidermal cell injury. Springer Semin Immunopathol 4:1, 1981.

Spain WC, Newell JM, Meeker MG: The percentage of persons susceptible to poison ivy and poison oak. J Allergy 5:365, 1967.

Stingl G, Katz SI, Green I, Shevach E: The functional role of Langerhans cells. J Invest Dermatol 74:315, 1980.

Thorbecke GJ, et al: The Langerhans cell as a representative accessory cell system, in health and disease. Immunobiology 168:313, 1984.

Tuberculin Test

Fine MH, et al: Tuberculin skin test reactions: effects of revised classification on comparative evaluations. Am Rev Resp Dis 106:752, 1972.

Katz J, Kunofsky S, Krasnitz A: Variation in sensitivity to tuberculin. Am Rev Resp Dis 106:202, 1972.

Koch R: Weitere Mittheilungen über ein Heilmittel gegen Tuberculose. Dtsch Med Wochenschr 16:1029, 1890.

Pietshch JB, Meakins JL: The delayed hypersensitivity response: clinical application in surgery. Can J Surg 20:15, 1977.

Youmans GP: Relation between delayed hypersensitivity and immunity in tuberculosis. Am Rev Resp Dis 111:109, 1975.

Zinsser H, Mueller JH: On nature of bacterial allergies. J Exp Med 41:159, 1925.

Cutaneous Basophil Hypersensitivity

Askanase PW, Atwood JE: Basophils in tuberculin and "Jones–Mote" delayed reactions of humans. J Clin Invest 58:1145, 1976.

Dvorak HF, Dvorak AM: Basophilic leukocytes in delayed-typed hypersensitivity reactions in animals and man. *In* Jankovic BD, Isakovic K (eds): Microenvironmental Aspects of Immunity. New York, Plenum, 1973, p573.

Dvorak HF, Mihm MC Jr: Basophilic leukocytes in allergic contact dermatitis. J Exp Med 135:235, 1972.

Jones TD, Mote JR: The phases of foreign sensitization in human beings. N Engl J Med 210:120, 1934.

Mote JR, Jones TD: The development of foreign protein sensitization in human beings. J Immunol 30:149, 1936.

Richerson HB, Dvorak HF, Leskowitz S: Cutaneous basophil hypersensitivity: a new interpretation of the Jones–Mote reaction. J Immunol 103:1431, 1969.

Graft Rejection

General

Amos DB, Cooper T, Debakey ME, Grondin P, Groth CC, Hanlon CR, Kayhoe DE, Murray JE, Najairian JS, Santos GW, Starzl TE: ACS/NIH Organ Transplant Registry. Third Scientific Report. JAMA 226:1211, 1973.

Billingham RE: Tissue transplantation: scope and prospects. Science 153:266, 1966.

Carpenter CB, Strom TB: Transplantation: immunogenic and clinical aspects. Hosp Pract 17:125, 1982, 18:135, 1983.

Groth C, Ringden O: Transplantation in relation to the treatment of inherited disease. Transplantation 38:319, 1984.

Hellstrom KE, Hellstrom I, Brawn J: Abrogation of cellular immunity to antigenically foreign mouse cells by a serum factor. Nature 224:914, 1969.

Lafferty KJ, Prowse SJ, Simeonovic CJ, Warren HS: Immunology of tissue transplantation. Return to the passenger leukocyte concept. Annu Rev Immunol 1:143, 1983.

Manning DD, Reed ND, Shaffer CF: Maintenance of skin xenografts of widely divergent phylogenetic origin on congenitally athymic (nude) mice. J Exp Med 138:488, 1973.

Mason DW, Morris PJ: Effector mechanisms in allograft rejection. Annu Rev Immunol 4:119, 1986.

Moller G (ed): Intragraft rejection mechanism. Immunol Rev 77, 1984.

Page D, Posen G, Stewart T, Harris J: Immunological detection of allograft rejections. Transplantation 12:341, 1971.

Rappaport FT: The immunobiology of transplantation: investigative trends and clinical implications. Surg Clin North Am 58:221, 1978.

Rappaport FT, Converse JM, Billingham RE: Recent advances in clinical and experimental transplantation. JAMA 237:2835, 1977.

Roberts PS, Hayry P: Effector mechanisms in allograft rejections. II. Density, electrophoresis and size fractionation of allograft-infiltrating cells demonstrating several classes of killer cells. Cell Immunol 30:236, 1976.

Salvatierra O, Perkins HA, Amend W, Feduska NJ, Duca RM, Potter DE, Cochrum KC: The influence of presensitization on graft survival rate. Surgery 81:146, 1977.

Stetson CA: The role of humoral antibody in the homograft rejection. Adv Immunol 3:97, 1963.

Stiller CR, Dossetor JB, Sinclair NR: First international symposium on immunologic monitoring of the transplant patient. Transplant Proc 10:309, 1978.

Stiller CR, Sinclair NR, Abrahams S, McGirr D, Singh H, Howson WT, Ulan RA: Antidonor immune responses in production of transplant rejection. N Engl J Med 294:978, 1976.

Zinkernagel RM: Major transplantation antigens in host response to infection. Hosp Pract 13:83, 1978.

Graft Facilitation

Billingham RE, Sparrow EM: The effect of prior intravenous injections of dissociated epidermal cells and blood on the survival of skin homografts in rabbits. J Embryol Exp Morphol 3:265, 1955.

Casey AE: Experimental enhancement of malignancy in the Brown–Pearce rabbit tumor. Proc Soc Exp Biol Med 29:816, 1932.

Feldman JD: Immunological enhancement: A study of blocking antibodies. Adv Immunol 15:167, 1972.

Hellstrom KE, Hellstrom I: Immunological enhancement as studied by cell culture techniques. Annu Rev Microbiol 24:213, 1970.

Kaliss N: Immunological enhancement of tumor homografts in mice. A review. Cancer Res 18:992, 1958.

Moller G (ed): Regulation of the immune response by antibodies against the immunogen. Immunol Rev 49, 1980.

Nelson DS: Immunological enhancement of skin homografts in guinea pigs. Br J Exp Pathol 43:1, 1962.

Stuart FP, Fitch FW, McKern TJ: Enhancement of rat renal allografts with idiotype and antiidiotype monoclonal antibodies. Transplant Proc 14:313, 1982.

Voisin GA: Immunological facilitation, a broadening concept of the enhancement phenomenon. Prog Allergy 15:328, 1971.

Kidneys

Balch CM, Diethelm AG: The pathophysiology of renal allograft rejections: a collective overview. J Surg Res 12:350, 1972.

Barnes BA, Bergan JJ, Raun WE, Fraumeni JF, Kountz SL, Mickey MR, Rubin AL, Simmons RL, Stevens LE, Wilson RE: The 11th report of the human renal transplant registry. JAMA 226:1197, 1973.

Cameron JS: Glomerulonephritis in renal transplants. Transplantation 34:237, 1982.

Corson JM: The pathologist and the kidney transplant. *In* Sommers SC (ed): Pathology Annual. New York, Appleton–Century–Crofts, 1972, p251.

Ettenger RB, Terasaki PI, Ting A, Malezadeh MH, Pennisi AJ, Vittenbogaart C, Garrison, R, Fine RN: Anti-B lymphocytotoxins in renal allograft rejection. N Engl J Med 295:305, 1976.

Kahan BD: Cyclosporine — Biological Activity and Clinical Applications. Orlando, Fla., Grune & Stratton, 1984.

Kerman RH, Kahan BD: Immunological evaluation of transplant rejections: Pre and postoperative indices detecting immune responsiveness. Ann Clin Res 13:244, 1981.

Monaco AP: Clinical kidney transplantation in 1984. Transplant Proc 17:5, 1985.

Opelz G, et al: Effect of HLA matching, blood transfusion and presensitization in cyclosporine-treated kidney transplant recipients. Transplant Proc 17:2179, 1985.

Porter KA: Morphologic aspects of renal homograft rejection. Brit Med Bull 21:171, 1965.

Porter KA, et al: Human renal transplants. Lab Invest 16:153, 1967.

Rapaport FT, Cortesni R: The past, present, and future of organ transplantation with special reference to current needs in kidney procurement and donation. Transplant Proc 17(Suppl 2):3, 1985.

Rosenau W, Najarian JS: A light, fluorescence, and electron microscopic study of functioning human renal transplants. Surg Gynecol Obstet 128:62, 1969.

Simmons RL, Van Hook J, Yunis EJ, Noreen H, Kjellstraud CM, Condie RM, Mauer SM, Busselmeire TJ, Najarian JS: 100 sibling kidney translants followed 2 to 7½ years: a multifactorial analysis. Am Surg 185:196, 1977.

Waltzer WC, et al: Etiology and pathogenesis of hypertension following renal transplantation. Nephron 42:102, 1986.

Williams G, et al: Current results and expectations of renal transplantation. JAMA 246:1330, 1981.

Williams GM, Lee HM, Weymonth RF, Harlan WR Jr, Holden KR, Stanley CM, Millington GA, Hume DM: Studies in hyperacute and chronic renal homograft rejection in man. Surgery 62:204, 1967.

Zoller K, et al: Cessation of immunosuppressive therapy after successful transplantation: a national survey. Kidney Int 18:110, 1980.

Heart

Baldwin JC, Shumway NE: Cardiac transplantation. Z Kardiol 74:39, 1985.

Carrel A, Guthrie C: The transplantation of veins and organs. Am Med 10:1101, 1905.

Copeland J: Facts to be considered prior to undertaking a heart transplantation program. Heart Transplant 3:275, 1984.

Criepp RB, Stinson EB, Bieber CP, Reitz BA, Copeland JG, Oyer PE, Shumway NE: Human heart transplantation: current status. Ann Thorac Surg 22:171–175, 1976.

Goldstein JP, Wechsler AS: Heart transplantation. Invest Radiol 20:446, 1985.

Haller JD, Cerruti MM: Heart transplantation in man: compilation of cases, II. Am J Cardiol 24:554, 1969.

Pomerance A, Stovin P: Heart transplant pathology: the British experience. J Clin Pathol 38:146, 1985.

Pennock JL: Cardiac transplantation in perspective for the future. J Thorac Cardiovasc Surg 83:168, 1982.

Shumway NE: Recent advances in cardiac transplantation. Transplant Proc 75:1223, 1983.

Pancreas

Baker CF, Frangipane LG, Silvers WK: Islet transplantation in genetically determined diabetes. Am Surg 186:401, 1977.

Lacy PE, Davie JM: Transplantation of pancreatic islets. Annu Rev Immunol 21:183, 1984.

Sutherland DER: Pancreas and islet transplantation. I. Experimental studies. II. Clinical traits. Diabetologia 20:161, 435, 1981.

Liver

Bowers BA, et al: Liver transplantation. Invest Radiol 20:790, 1985.

Eggink HF, et al: Histopathology of serial graft biopsies from liver transplant recipients. Am J Pathol 114:18, 1984.

Fennell RH, Shikes RH, Vierling JM: Relationship of pretransplant hepatobiliary disease to bile duct damage occurring in the liver allograft. Hepatogastroenterology 3:84, 1984.

Kamada N: The immunology of experimental liver transplantation in the rat. Immunology 55:369, 1985.

Scharschmidt BF: Human liver transplantation analysis of data on 540 patients from four centers. Hepatology 4:955, 1984.

Starzl TE, et al: Fifteen years of clinical liver transplantation. Gastroenterology 77:375, 1979.

Vierling JM, Fennell RH: Histopathology of early and late human hepatic allograft rejection: evidence of progressive destruction of interlobular bile ducts. Hepatogastroenterology 5:1076, 1985.

Brain

Freed WJ: Functional brain tissue transplantation: reversal of lesion-induced rotation by intraventricular substantia nigra and adrenal medulla grafts, with a note on intracranial retinal grafts. Biol Psychiatry 18:1205, 1983.

Gash DM, Collier TJ, Slader JR: Neural transplantation: A review of recent developments and potential applications to the aged brain. Neurobiol Aging 6:131, 1985.

Sladek JR, Gash DM: Neural Transplants. New York, Plenum, 1984.

Cornea

Elliot JH: Immune factors in corneal graft rejection. Invest Ophthalmol 10:216, 1971.

Khodadoust AA, Silverstein AM: The survival and rejection of epithelium in experimental corneal transplants. Invest Ophthalmol 8:169, 1969.

Young E, Stark WJ, Prendergast RA: Immunology of corneal allograft rejection: HLA-DR antigens on human corneal cells. Invest Ophthalmol 26:571, 1985.

Graft versus Host Reactions

Deeg HJ, Storb R: Graft-versus-host disease: pathophysiological and clinical aspects. Annu Rev Med 35:11, 1984.

Moller G (ed): Graft-versus-host reactions. Immunol Rev 88, 1985.

Simonsen M: Graft-versus-host reactions: their natural history and applicability as tools of research. Prog Allergy 6:349, 1962.

Snover DC: Acute and chronic graft-versus-host disease: histopathologic evidence for two distinct pathogenic mechanisms. Hum Pathol 15:202, 1984.

Wick MR, et al: Immunologic, clinical and pathologic aspects of human graft-versus-host disease. Mayo Clin Proc 58:603, 1983.

Bone Marrow
Transplantation

Bast RC, et al: Elimination of malignant clonogenic cells from human bone marrow using multiple antibodies and complement. Cancer Res 45:499, 1985.

Congdon CC: Radiation injury: bone marrow transplantation. Annu Rev Med 13:203, 1962.

Deeg HJ, Storb R, Thomas ED: Bone marrow transplantation: a review of delayed complications. Br J Hematol 57:185, 1984.

Gale RP, Opelz G: Second International Symposium on Immunobiology of Bone Marrow Transplantation. Transplant Proc 10(1), 1978.

Genogzian M, Edwards CL, Vodopick HA, Hubner KF: Bone marrow transplantation in a leukemic patient following immunosuppression with antithymocyte globulin and total body irradiation. Transplantation 15:446, 1972.

Good RA: Progress toward a cellular engineering. JAMA 214:1289, 1970.

Leonard JE, Taetle R, To D, Rhyneu K: Preclinical studies on the use of selective antibodies – ricin conjugates in autologous bone marrow transplantation. Blood 65:1149, 1985.

Mathe G, Schwarzenberg L, Amiel JL, Schneider M, Cattan A, Schlumberger JR, Tubiana M, Lalanne C: Immunogenetic and immunological problems of allogeneic haematopoietic radio-chimeras in man. Scand J Hematol 4:193, 1967.

McGovern JJ Jr, Rusell PS, Atkins L, Webster EW: Treatment of terminal leukemic relapse by total-body irradiation and intravenous infusion of stored autologous bone marrow obtained during remission. N Engl J Med 260:675, 1959.

Mouchiroud G, et al: Monoclonal antibodies against human hemopoietic cells and the separation of progenitor cells from bone marrow. Exp Hematol 13:566, 1985.

Quinones RR, et al: Anti-T cell monoclonal antibodies conjugated to ricin as potential reagents for human GVHD prophylaxis. Effect on the generation of cytotoxic T cells in both peripheral blood and bone marrow. J Immunol 132:678, 1984.

Santos GW: Application of marrow grafts in human disease. Am J Pathol 65:653, 1971.

Shearer WT, et al: Epstein – Barr virus – associated B cell proliferations of diverse clinical origins after bone marrow transplantation in a 12 year old patient with severe combined immune deficiency. N Engl J Med 312:1151, 1985.

Slavin RE, Santos GW: The graft versus host reaction in man after bone marrow transplantation: pathology, pathogenesis, clinical features and implications. Clin Immunol Immunopathol 1:472, 1973.

Storb R, Thomas ED, Buckner CD, Clift RA, Johnson FL, Fefer A, Glucksberg H, Giblett ER, Lerner KG, Nieman P: Allogenic marrow grafting for treatment of aplastic anemia. Blood 43:157, 1974.

Sullivan KM, et al: Late complications after marrow transplantation. Semin Hematol 21:53, 1984.

Taliaferro WH, Taliaferro LG, Jaroslow BN: Radiation and Immune Mechanisms. New York, Academic Press, 1964.

Thomas ED, Bryant JI, Buckner CD, Clift RA, Fefer A, Nieman P, Ramberg RE, Strob R: Leukemic transformation of engrafted bone marrow. Transplant Proc 4:567, 1972.

Thomas ED, et al: Bone marrow transplantation. N Engl J Med 292:832,895, 1975.

Van Bekkum DW: Use and abuse of hemopoietic cell grafts in immune deficiency diseases. In Moller G (ed): Lymphoid Cell Replacement. Transplant Rev 9:3, 1972.

Zwaan FE, Heremans J, Barrett AJ, Speck B: Bone marrow transplantation for acute lymphoblastic leukemia: a survey of the European Group for Bone Marrow Transplantation (E.G.B.M.T.). Br J Haematol 58:33, 1984.

Fetal–Maternal Relationship

Beer AE, Billingham RE: Immunobiology of mammalian reproduction. Adv Immunol 14:1, 1971.

Beer AE, Billingham RE: The embryo as a transplant. Sci Am 230:36, 1974.

Billingham RE, Beer AE: Reproductive immunology: past, present and future. Perspect Biol Med 27:259, 1984.

Chaouat G: Forum d'immunologie. The riddle of the fetal allograft. Ann Inst Pasteur 135:301, 1984.

Edidin M: Histocompatibility genes, transplantation antigens and pregnancy. *In* Kahan BD, Reisfeld R (eds): Transplantation Antigens. New York, Academic Press, 1972, p75.

Gill TJ: Immunity and pregnancy. CRC Crit Rev Immunol 5:201, 1985.

Hunziker RD, Wegmann TG: Placental immunoregulation. CRC Crit Rev Immunol, in press.

Moller G (ed): Immunology of Feto-maternal Relationship. Immunol Rev 75, 1983.

Szulman AE: The A, B and H blood group antigens in the human placenta. N Engl J Med 286:1028, 1972.

Wegmann TG, Carlson GA: Allogenic pregnancy as immunoabsorbent. J Immunol 119:1659, 1977.

Viral Infections

See also Chapter 24.

General

Hale JH: Duration of immunity in virus diseases. Adv Immunol 1:263, 1961.

Huppert J, Wild TF: Virus disease without virus. Ann Virol 135E:22, 1984.

Kantor GL, Golberg LS, Johnson L, Derechin MM, Barnett EV: Immunologic abnormalities induced by postperfusion cytomegalovirus infection. Ann Intern Med 73:553, 1970.

Kaarianen L, Ranki M: Inhibition of cell functions by RNA virus infections. Annu Rev Microbiol 38:91, 1984.

Mims CA: Immunopathology in virus disease. Philos Trans R Soc Lond [Biol] 303:189, 1983.

Oldstone MB, et al: Virus-reduced alterations in homeostasis: alterations in differentiated functions of infected cells in vivo. Science 218:1125, 1982.

Oldstone MBA: Immunopathology of persistent viral infections. Hosp Pract 17:61, 1982.

Russell WO: Viruses and autoimmune disease. Fifth Annual ASCP Research Symposium. Am J Clin Pathol 56:259, 1971.

von Pirquet CF: Klinische Studien uber Vakzination und vakzinale Allergie. Leipzig, Deutickie, 1907.

Viral Encephalitides of Animals

Appel MGJ, Gillespie JH: Canine distemper virus. Virology 11:1, 1972.

Daniels JB, Papenheimer AM, Richardson S: Observations on encephalomyelitis of mice (D4 strain). J Exp Med 96:S17, 1952.

Doherty PC, Zinkernagel RM: Capacity of sensitized thymus-derived lymphocytes to induce fatal lymphocyte choriomeningitis is restricted by the H_2 gene complex. J Immunol 114:30, 1975.

Hotchin JE: The biology of lymphocytic choriomeningitis infection: virus-induced immune disease. Cold Spring Harbor Symp Quant Biol 14:479, 1962.

Koestner A, McCullough B, Drakowka GS, Long JF, Olsen RG: Canine distemper: a virus-induced demyelinating encephalomyelitis. *In* Zeman W, Lennette EH (eds): Slow Virus Diseases. Baltimore, Williams & Wilkins, 1974, p86.

Lampert PW, Garrett R, Powell H: Demyelination in allergic and Marek's disease virus induced neuritis, comparative electron microscopic studies. Acta Neuropathol (Berl) 40:103, 1977.

Lampert PW, Sims JK, Kniazeff AJ: Mechanism of demyelination in JHM virus encephalomyelitis. Electron microscopic studies. Acta Neuropathol (Berl) 24:76, 1973.

Oriz-Ortiz L, Weigle WO: Cellular events in the induction of experimental allergic encephalomyelitis in rats. J Exp Med 1244:604, 1976.

Payne LN, Frazier JA, Powell PC: Pathogenesis of Marek's disease. Int Rev Exp Pathol 16:59, 1976.

Stroop WG, Baringer JR: Persistent, slow and latent viral infections. Prog Med Virol 28:1, 1982.

Weiner LP: Pathogenesis of demyelination induced by mouse hepatitis virus (JHM virus). Arch Neurol 28:298, 1973.

Viral Encephalitides of Man

Adams JM: Persistence of measles virus and demyelinating disease. Hosp Pract 87:1970.

Brown P, et al: Potential epidemic of Creutzfeldt–Jakob disease from human growth hormone therapy. N Engl J Med 313:728, 1985.

Budka H, Lassman H, Popow-Krupp T: Measles virus antigen in pan-encephalitis: an immunohistologic study stressing involvement in SSPE. Acta Neuropathol (Berl) 56:52, 1982.

Gajdusek DC: Kuru and Creutzfeldt–Jakob Disease. Experimental models of noninflammatory degenerative slow virus disease of the central nervous system. Ann Clin Res 5:254, 1973.

Gajdusek DC: Unconventional viruses and the origin and disappearance of kuru. Science 197:943–960, 1977.

Lampert PW: Autoimmune and virus-induced demyelinating diseases. Am J Pathol 91:176, 1978.

Manuelidis EE: Creutzfeldt–Jakob disease. J Neuropathol Exp Neurol 44:1, 1985.

Meulen V, Hall WW: Slow virus infections of the nervous system: virological, immunological and pathogenic medications. J Gen Virol 41:1, 1978.

Raine GS: Viral infections of nervous tissue and their relevance to multiple sclerosis. *In* Wolfram F, Ellison GW, Stevens JG, Andrews JM (eds): Multiple Sclerosis. New York, Academic Press, 1972, p91.

Robertson HD, Branch AD, Dahlberg JE: Focusing on the nature of the scrapie agent. Cell 40:725, 1985.

Zeman W, Lennette EN: Slow-Virus Diseases. Baltimore, Williams & Wilkins, 1974.

Viral Hepatitis

Blumberg BS: Australia antigen and the biology of hepatitis B. Science 197:17, 1977.

Burk KH, Oefinger PE, Dreesdian GR: Detection of a non-A non-B hepatitis antigen by immunocytochemical staining. Proc Nat Acad Sci USA 81:3195, 1984.

Deinhardt F: Predictive value of hepatitis virus infection. J Infect Dis 141:299, 1980.

Dienstag JL: Immunopathogenesis of the extrahepatic manifestations of hepatitis infection. Springer Semin Immunopathol 3:461, 1981.

Dmochowski L: Viral type A and type B hepatitis: morphology, biology, immunology and epidemiology. Am J Clin Pathol 65:741–786, 1976.

Edgington TS, Chiasari FV: Immunological aspects of hepatitis B virus infection. Am J Med Sci 270:213, 1975.

Feinstone SM, Purcell RH: Non-A, non-B hepatitis. Annu Rev Med 29:359, 1978.

Hamilton JD: Hepatitis B virus vaccine: An analysis of its potential use in medical workers. JAMA 250:2145, 1983.

Huange S-N, Millman I, O'Connell A, Aronoff A, Gault H, Blumberg GS: Virus-like particles in Australia antigen-associated hepatitis. Am J Pathol 67:453, 1972.

Jones EA, James SP: Circulating immune complexes and the pathogenesis of primary biliary cirrhosis. Gastroenterology 83:709, 1983.

Krugman S, et al: Viral hepatitis, Type B: studies on natural history and prevention re-examined. N Engl J Med 300:101, 1979.

LePore MJ, McKenna PJ, Martinez DB, Stutman LJ, Bonannon CA, Conklin EF, Robilotti JG Jr: Fulminant hepatitis with coma successfully treated by plasmapheresis and hyperimmune Australia-antibody-rich plasma. Am J Gastroenterol 58:381, 1972.

Prier JE, Friedman H: Australia Antigen. Baltimore, University Park Press, 1973.

Prince AM, Szmuness W, Woods KR, Grady GF: Antibody against serum-hepatitis antigen. Prevalence and potential use as immune serum globulin in prevention of serum hepatitis infections. N Engl J Med 285:933, 1971.

Ray MB: Hepatitis B virus antigens in tissues. Baltimore, University Park Press, 1979.

Sabesin SM, Koff RS: Pathogenesis of experimental viral hepatitis. N Engl J Med 290:944.

Senior JR, Sutnick AI, Goeser E, London WT, Danlke MB, Blumbert BS: Reduction of post-transfusion hepatitis by exclusion of Australia antigen from donor blood in an urban public hospital. Am J Med Sci 267:171, 1974.

Shulman NR, Baker LF: Virus-like antigen–antibody and antigen–antibody complexes in hepatitis measured by complement fixation. Science 165:304, 1969.

Sutnick AI, Millman I, London WT, Blumberg BS: The role of Australia antigen in viral hepatitis and other diseases. Annu Rev Med 23:161, 1972.

Szmuness W, et al: Hepatitis B vaccine. Demonstration of efficiency in a controlled trial in a high-risk population in the United States. N Engl J Med 303:833, 1980.

Warts

Howley PM: The molecular biology of papillomavirus transformation. Am J Pathol 113:414, 1983.

Kirchner H: Immunologic surveillance and human papillomavirus. Immunol Today 5:272, 1984.

Lee AKY, Eisinger M: Cell-mediated immunity (CMI) to human wart virus and wart-associated tissue antigens. Clin Exp Immunol 26:419, 1976.

Matthews RS, Shirodaria PV: Study of regressing warts by immunofluorescence. Lancet 1:689, 1973.

Morrison WL: In vitro assay of cell mediated immunity to human wart antigen. Br J Dermatol 90:531, 1974.

Ogilvie MM: Serological studies with human papova (wart) virus. J Hyg (Camb) 68:479, 1970.

Viac J, Thivolet J, Chardonnet Y: Specific immunity in patients suffering from recurring warts before and after repetitive intradermal tests with human papilloma virus. Br J Dermatol 97:365, 1977.

zur Hausen H, et al: Papilloma viruses and squamous-cell carcinoma in man. Perspect Virol 10:93, 1978.

20 | Autoallergic Diseases

Classification of a disease process as autoallergic depends on the demonstration of a damaging effect of an endogenous immune response to an endogenous antigen. The essential mechanism involves loss of tolerance to one's own antigens (see Chapter 11). Acquired hemolytic anemia, idiopathic thrombocytopenic purpura, experimental allergic glomerulonephritis, and lupus erythematosus are examples of autoallergic disease caused by humoral autoantibodies. These have been presented in earlier chapters. However, many other autoallergic diseases are the result of a delayed reaction. Lesions are produced in experimental animals by immunizing an individual with constituents of its own tissues. When the hypersensitive state appears, reactions occur where antigen is situated. Lesions have been produced by immunization with tissues such as lens, uvea, central nervous system myelin, peripheral nervous sytem myelin, thyroid, adrenal, testes, and salivary gland. Antibody has been produced, but no lesions observed, with breast and pancreas. The lesions are irregularly distributed in regions of high antigen concentration (the white matter of the central nervous system in experimental allergic encephalomyelitis). Local inflammatory reactions occur around small veins and consist of lymphocytes, histiocytes, and other mononuclear cells. Necrosis, hemorrhage, and polymorphonuclear leukocyte infiltration occur only in very severe reactions and only in some species. Parenchymal destruction is coexistent with inflammation (i.e., demyelination, destruction of uvea pigment). Byron Waksman has stressed that within the involved tissue the lesion distribution is determined by blood–tissue barriers. There is good experimental correlation between the sites at which lesions appear preferentially and the passage of injection of large colloids, such as trypan blue, from the blood into the tissues. Thus, in the testes, the most severe (though not the only) involvement is in the epididymis and the rete testis, both areas

511

provided with numerous veins that permit passage of trypan blue. The experimental autoallergic diseases are of great interest since they provide good models for the human diseases of unknown etiology listed in Table 20-1. The human diseases in

Table 20-1. Relation of Experimental Autoallergic Diseases to Human Diseases

Experimental Disease	Tissue Involved	Histologically Similar Human Disease	
		Acute Monocyclic	Chronic Relapsing
Allergic encephalomyelitis	Myelin (CNS)	Postinfectious encephalomyelitis	Multiple sclerosis
Allergic neuritis	Myelin (PNS)	Guillain–Barré polyneuritis	
Phacoanaphylactic endophthalmitis	Lens		Phacoanaphylactic endophthalmitis
Allergic uveitis	Uvea	Postinfectious iridocyclitis	Sympathetic ophthalmia
Allergic orchitis	Germinal epithelium	Mumps orchitis	Nonendocrine chronic infertility
Allergic thyroiditis	Thyroglobulin	Mumps thyroiditis	Subacute and chronic thyroiditis
Allergic sialadenitis	Glandular epithelium	Mumps parotitis	Sjögren's syndrome
Allergic adrenalitis	Cortical cells		Cytotoxic contraction of adrenal
Allergic gastritis	Gastric mucosa		Atrophic gastritis
Experimental allergic nephritis	Glomerular membrane	Acute glomerulonephritis	Chronic glomerulonephritis

CNS, central nervous system; PNS, peripheral nervous system.
Modified from Waksman BH: Int Arch Allergy Appl Immunol 14(Suppl), 1959.

general are chronic relapsing processes, since the antigen is consistently present in the tissues and the hypersensitive state may persist or be boosted from time to time by further immunization. The acute monocyclic disease may result from allergic reactions to viruses or to combinations of bacterial products and tissues. The morphologic similarity of these lesions to the experimental autoallergies is indicated by the fact that the same hypersensitivity response is involved in the production of lesions in both instances, even though the antigens may be different.

Encephalomyelitis and Multiple Sclerosis

Experimental allergic encephalomyelitis may be produced by the injection of central nervous system tissue incorporated into complete Freund's adjuvant. In rats, hind leg paralysis occurs after 2 to 3 weeks and is associated with a disseminated focal perivascular accumulation of inflammatory cells involving small veins or venules. The inflammatory cells, which accumulate within the vessel wall and in the perivascular space, are usually mononuclear, but polymorphonuclear leukocytes may be prominent in very acute reactions. Demyelination occurs in intimate association with the focal vasculitis and most likely is a result of the action of specifically sensitized cells; toxic complex activation of polymorphonuclear neutrophils may be responsible for acute lesions. The antigen, encephalitogenic protein, has been studied extensively and the amino acid sequence determined. The major encephalitogenic determinant is a nonapeptide with the amino acid sequence Phe – Ser – Trp – Ala – Glu – Gly – Gln – Lys, the important amino acids being Trp and Gln.

Although the reaction of specifically sensitized cells with myelin antigen is believed to be the major pathological event and T cells are required to transfer the disease in experimental animals, humoral antibody may also play an important part. The venules of the brain do not permit lymphocytes to pass through, as they do in other organs (blood – brain barrier). Humoral antibody may react with myelin antigens released from the brain normally or as the result of a viral infection. The antibody – antigen reaction may activate anaphylactic or complement mediators, causing contraction and separation of endothelial cells, thus permitting extravasation of lymphocytes into brain tissue (Fig. 20-1). The outstanding tissue lesion is perivascular infiltration of the white matter of the brain and spinal cord with lymphocytes. This is followed by migration of macrophages into tissue containing myelinated nerve fibers, and stripping of myelinated fibers by macrophages, culminating in phagocytosis and digestion of the myelin.

The human disease takes three forms: acute hemorrhagic encephalomyelitis, acute disseminated encephalomyelitis, and multiple sclerosis.

Acute Hemorrhagic Encephalomyelitis

This is a rare disease that shows necrosis and fibrin deposits within the walls of venules, hemorrhages through the venule walls with intense polymorphonuclear infiltration, and demyelination in areas of the infiltration. This disease is similar to the acute forms of experimental allergic encephalomyelitis.

Acute Disseminated Encephalomyelitis

This has two variants. The form that occurs following rabies antigen injection appears 4 to 15 days following injection of killed rabies virus and is histologically identical to experimental allergic encephalomyelitis. The lesion is caused by an allergic reaction to the brain tissue used to culture the virus from which the vaccine is prepared. This type of vaccine has been replaced by one prepared from human tissue, and no proven case of post-rabies inoculation encephalomyelitis has been reported after introduction of the new vaccine. The second type of acute disseminated encephalomyelitis occurs after smallpox vaccination or infection with rubella, varicella, or variola (see above). This rare disease is similar to experimental allergic and post-rabies injection encephalomyelitis. Individual cases suggest that acute hemorrhagic encephalomyelitis may progress to

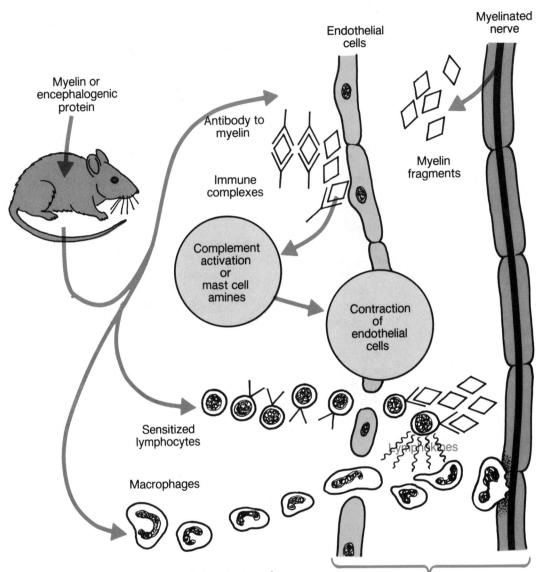

Myelin or
encephalogenic
protein

Endothelial
cells

Myelinated
nerve

Antibody to
myelin

Immune
complexes

Myelin
fragments

Complement
activation
or
mast cell
amines

Contraction
of
endothelial
cells

Sensitized
lymphocytes

Lymphokines

Macrophages

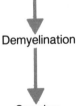

Phagocytosis
and digestion

Demyelination

Scarring

Figure 20-1. Possible pathogenic events in experimental allergic encephalomyelitis. Immunization of experimental animals with myelin or encephalogenic protein results in production of humoral antibody and specifically sensitized cells, which together lead to demyelination by macrophages. Antibody reacting with myelin released into circulation through endothelial venules in white matter (i.e., myelinated area of brain and spinal cord) activates either anaphylatoxin (complement) or mast cell (IgE) degranulation. Contraction of endothelial cells opens up gaps in small venule walls. Sensitized small lymphocytes move into white matter, react with myelin antigen, and release lymphocyte mediators. Macrophages, attracted and activated by these mediators, phagocytose and digest antibody-coated myelin. If zones of demyelination are large, fibrosis occurs and permanent loss of function results.

acute disseminated encephalomyelitis and then to multiple sclerosis.

Multiple Sclerosis

This may be the end stage or chronic form of the encephalitides. There is a pathogenic similarity between multiple sclerosis and chronic experimental allergic encephalomyelitis. However, animals who survive the acute stages of the experimental disease do not go on to develop the chronic scarring lesions typical of multiple sclerosis. It is possible that the chronic lesions of multiple sclerosis are caused by stimulation of glial cell or fibroblast proliferation following abnormal production or response to growth factors. (A "glial cell stimulating factor" produced by lymphocytes has been described.) The lesions are multiple, sharply defined gray plaques, measure up to several centimeters in diameter, and are composed of microglial cells, lymphocytes, and plasma cells usually located around small veins. At later stages, scarring may obscure the small veins and plaques may be found with no vascular component. Complement-fixing antibody capable of causing demyelination of myelin-containing cells in tissue culture has been reported. The titers of this antibody are not related to the titers of complement-fixing antibody in the same serum, and it is possible that the in vitro demyelinating antibody may play a role in demyelination in vivo, but this has not yet been established. Complement-fixing antibody may actually protect against development of the disease. Experimental allergic encephalomyelitis may be consistently transferred with cells, but not with antiserum. The relationship of preceding viral infections to multiple sclerosis and other demyelinating diseases has been discussed above. Viral infections may produce an immunizing event leading to cellular sensitivity to myelin antigens.

Peripheral Neuritis

Experimental allergic neuritis is induced by the injection of peripheral nervous tissue in complete Freund's adjuvant. The lesions are limited to the peripheral nervous tissue; none are found in the central nervous system. The experimental disease is similar to a demyelinating syndrome that follows infection with certain microorganisms — the Guillain–Barré syndrome. An experimental allergic sympathetic neuritis may be induced by immunization with antigens obtained from sympathetic ganglia. The inflammatory lesions are limited to the sympathetic nervous system.

Phacoanaphylactic Endophthalmitis

The lens was probably the first tissue to which an autoallergic reaction was recognized (1903). Experimental lesions have been produced by scratching the lens of rabbits previously sensitized to lens material. The cornea becomes vascularized and infiltrated with mononuclear cells. Because the lens is not vascularized, specifically sensitized cells cannot come into contact with the antigen (lens) unless there is some release of the antigen into the anterior chamber of the eye or other tissue spaces. This is why scratching the lens is necessary to induce the lesion. The disease is not related to circulating antibody, and no lesions are produced by washing the anterior chamber of the eye with large amounts of antibody. An infrequent complication of cataract extraction is an intraocular inflammatory (presumably autoallergic) reaction. In some cases the inflammation may extend to involve the eye not operated on.

Uveitis

Lesions similar to human disease can be produced in experimental animals by injection of uveal tissue in complete Freund's adjuvant (experimental allergic uveitis). A human condition, known as *sympathetic ophthalmia*, is an inflammatory lesion of the uveal tract that appears 2 to 6 weeks after a perforating wound of the eye and affects both the injured and normal eye. Other forms of uveitis are associated with the collagen–vascular diseases. Pain, photophobia, and blurred vision result. The early lesions are focal inflammatory infiltrations of lymphocytes in the choroid, usually related to small veins. As early as 1910, it was proposed that this disease represented an allergic response to uveal antigens. If an individual loses sight in one eye because of injury, the eye is usually removed as soon as possible because the incidence of inflammation occurring in the remaining eye is directly related to the length of time the damaged eye is allowed to remain in situ.

Cogan's Syndrome

Cogan's syndrome is a disease of young adults featuring acute interstitial keratitis (inflammation of the cornea) and disturbances of the ear (vestibulo-auditory dysfunction manifested by nausea, vomiting, ringing in the ear, and vertigo). This syndrome often occurs in association with collagen–vascular diseases. The onset of the syndrome has a clear association with a preceding upper respiratory infection. There is a prompt response to steroid therapy. The etiology of the lesions is not known, but it has been suggested that a local inflammatory reaction mediated by autoantibodies or antibodies to an infectious agent might be responsible.

Orchitis

Focal perivenous accumulations of lymphocytes and macrophages occur 8 to 14 days after sensitization of the animals with testes or spermatozoa in complete Freund's adjuvant. The inflammatory infiltrate is found primarily in the vascular areas of the testes (epididymis) and causes progressive damage of germinal cells, leading to aspermatogenesis. Complement-fixing, sperm-immobilizing, skin-sensitizing antibody may be demonstrated. The destruction of seminiferous tubules is associated with a mononuclear infiltrate, while spermatic ducts have a polymorphonuclear reaction with IgG and C3 present. Therefore antibody and delayed hypersensitivity are both active in allergic aspermatogenesis. Mumps orchitis is a human disease that occurs approximately 14 days after mumps parotitis. The histologic picture is very similar to that of the experimental disease. It has not been possible to demonstrate viruses in the testes of patients with mumps orchitis.

Thyroiditis

This is one of the most extensively studied experimental autoallergic diseases. It occurs 6 to 14 days following immunization of an experimental animal with thyroid extract or thyroglobulin in complete Freund's adjuvant. Evolution of the disease is presented in Figure 20-2. The lesion begins as a perivenous infiltration of lymphocytes, and destruction of the thyroid follicular epithelium is accomplished by the invasion of specifically sensitized cells, in a manner similar to the lesion of contact dermatitis. The experimental disease almost always resolves, although some instances of chronic lesions have been reported. The severity and course of the disease are not related to antibody titer, but do correlate with delayed hypersensitivity skin tests. Experimental thyroiditis may be transferred both with cells and with antiserum in rabbits. Antibody may play a role in initiation of lesions by increasing the permeability of venules to lymphocytes, permitting the passage of sensitized cells that make contact with the target cells. In humans, a disease of unknown etiology, Hashimoto's disease, is characterized by intense lymphocytic infiltration and formation of lymphocytic follicles with prominent germinal centers. There are certain histological similarities between Hashimoto's disease and experimental allergic thyroiditis, and there is a high incidence of antibodies in thyroglobulin and other thyroid antigens in patients with this disease. The role of humoral antibody in the pathogenesis of human thyroiditis remains unclear, but electron-dense deposits have been found in the follicular basement membrane of thyroids from patients with Hashimoto's disease that are similar to the deposits of toxic complex glomerulonephritis.

The role of antithyroid antibodies in the pathogenesis of allergic thyroiditis remains unclear. There is some evidence that circulating antibody may actually suppress the development of experimental allergic thyroiditis. However, circulating thyroglobulin–antithyroglobulin complexes may cause a toxic complex glomerulonephritis. Also, antibody could direct an antibody-dependent cell-mediated cytotoxic effect on follicular cells.

518

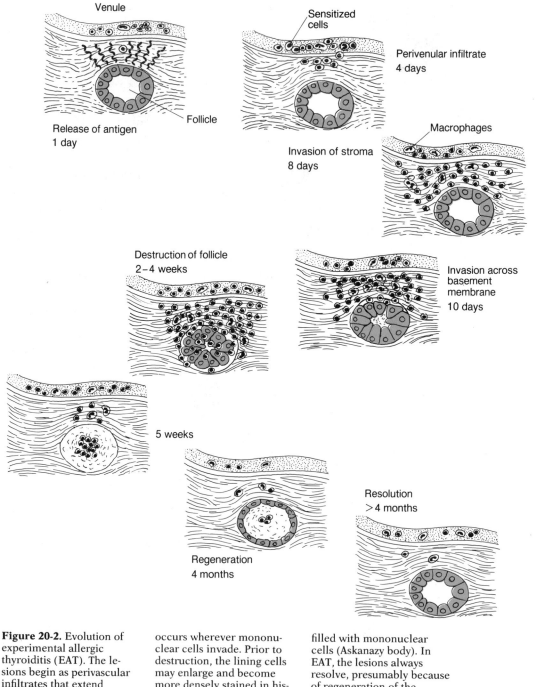

Figure 20-2. Evolution of experimental allergic thyroiditis (EAT). The lesions begin as perivascular infiltrates that extend through the interfollicular stroma to invade the follicular lining cells. Destruction of the lining cells occurs wherever mononuclear cells invade. Prior to destruction, the lining cells may enlarge and become more densely stained in histologic sections (Hurthle or Askanazy cells). After the follicular lining cells are destroyed, the follicles may be filled with mononuclear cells (Askanazy body). In EAT, the lesions always resolve, presumably because of regeneration of the follicular lining cells similar to that of epithelial cells after contact dermatitis.

Sialadenitis (Sjögren's Syndrome; Sicca Complex)

Sialadenitis in an inflammation of the salivary glands. Mononuclear inflammatory lesions have been reported in experimental animals following the injection of salivary gland tissue in complete Freund's adjuvant. However, the validity of these observations is questionable, and the autoallergic nature of such lesions is not well established. It is convenient, however, to consider Sjögren's syndrome as an autoallergic disease. This human disorder, consisting of dryness of the eyes (keratoconjunctivitis sicca) and dryness of the mouth (xerostomia), may occur alone (primary Sjögren's syndrome) or may be associated with connective tissue diseases (rheumatoid arthritis, systemic lupus erythematosus, or scleroderma) and is often included in the list of collagen–vascular diseases. It is associated with HLA-B8 and HLA-DR3 MHC types. Clinically there is swelling of the lacrimal and salivary glands. (If the parotid gland alone is involved, the eponym *Mikulicz's syndrome* has been used). Histologically, lymphocytes and plasma cells infiltrate the salivary and lacrimal glands. Fibrosis, acinar atrophy, and proliferation of the myoepithelial cells of the ducts with obstruction follow. In small lesions B cells predominate; in large lesions T cells are found centrally and B cells peripherally. Similar findings may be observed in the mucosal glands of the pharynx and larynx, and the submucosal glands of the esophagus, trachea, and bronchi. Precipitating and complement-fixing antibody to salivary gland tissue has been found associated with the disease, as have other serologic abnormalities such as antinuclear antibodies (anti-Ro (SS-A), 50%; anti-La (SS-B), 20%), rheumatoid factor, and antibodies to thyroglobulin. The presence of antibodies to salivary ducts is associated with less cellular infiltrate in the salivary glands of patients with Sjögren's syndrome when these lesions are compared with those of patients who lack this antibody. Thus, antibody to salivary gland may block cell-mediated tissue destruction or could contribute to inflammation through an antibody-dependent cell-mediated (ADCC) mechanism.

It is more likely, however, that a major component of Sjögren's syndrome or sialadenitis in humans is caused by an immune complex mechanism (vasculitis is increasingly recognized in lesions). The salivary gland normally may serve as a site for production of secretory antibody responsible for local defense. In experimental autoallergic sialadenitis, as well as in the human disease, there is substantial infiltration of the glandular tissue with plasma cells and local synthesis of large amounts of immunoglobulin with rheumatoid factor activity. Thus it is postulated that Sjögren's syndrome may be caused by a chronic immune complex reaction in the salivary gland similar to that which occurs in the articular (joint) space in rheumatoid arthritis.

Adrenalitis and Multiple Endocrine Deficiency

Immunization of animals with adrenal tissue in complete Freund's adjuvant leads to mononuclear cell infiltration and necrosis of the adrenal cortex. Most cases of adrenal insufficiency in man (Addison's disease) are secondary to endocrine, infectious, or neoplastic processes. However, a type of adrenal insufficiency, primary cytotoxic contraction, is of unknown origin and may be a correlate of experimental autoallergic adrenalitis. Complement-fixing antibody has been found in some patients with Addison's disease. Autoantibodies to endocrine glands are also associated with other endocrine gland deficiencies, including hypothyroidism, hypogonadism, and diabetes, as well as hypoadrenalism. It is not clear in each case what role delayed hypersensitivity and/or antibody inactivation has in these endocrine diseases. Sensitized autoallergic T cells may cause destruction of the glandular cells, and antibody may inactivate the hormonal product.

Ulcerative Colitis

Ulcerative colitis is a chronic disease of the colon. Its cause is unknown, and numerous attempts to isolate an infectious agent have been unsuccessful. Vascular congestion, edema, hemorrhage, and superficial ulceration, with a mixed infiltration of polymorphonuclear leukocytes, lymphocytes, plasma cells, and eosinophils, characterize the lesions. Associated with ulcerative colitis are hypergammaglobulinemia, a prevalence of atopic sensitivities, prominent occurrence of other autoallergic diseases, and antibodies to colonic tissue. Auer's colitis is a hemorrhagic necrotic lesion of the colon with a cellular infiltrate at the base of the crypts and perivascular polymorphonuclear leukocyte accumulation produced experimentally by the injection of antigen (egg albumen) into the colon of sensitized rabbits (Arthus reaction).

Liver Disease

Although direct evidence for the involvement of allergic mechanisms in the initiation or progression of human liver diseases is controversial, considerable circumstantial evidence (presumptive findings) is available to incriminate allergic mechanisms in chronic active hepatitis, primary bilary cirrhosis, and some types of reactions to drugs causing jaundice and viral hepatitis (see above). These presumptive findings include diffuse (polyclonal) hypergammaglobulinemias, tissue lesions containing lymphocytes and plasma cells consistent with a cellular reaction, depression of serum complement at some stages of the disease, demonstration of immunoglobulin and complement in some early lesions, association with other allergic diseases such as lupus erythematosus, Sjögren's syndrome, and scleroderma, beneficial response to drugs that cause depressed immune response, and presence of a variety of autoantibodies. These antibodies can be demonstrated by immunofluorescence to bind to the nuclei, ductular cells, and mitochondria of the liver and to smooth muscle cells. Of particular interest is the antimitochondrial antibody associated with primary biliary cirrhosis.

Chronic active hepatitis may have at least four etiologies: autoimmune, hepatitis B associated, cryptogenic, and drug induced. A classic finding is the destruction of individual liver cells surrounded by mononuclear inflammatory cells, "piecemeal necrosis," at the edge of inflammation of portal areas.

Halothane is an anesthetic agent that has some very desirable properties but produces liver disease similar to viral hepatitis. This reaction rarely, if ever, occurs upon the first exposure to halothane but is induced on subsequent exposures, suggesting that a sensitization event occurs. The destructive lesions are associated with a mononuclear infiltrate similar to that seen in other delayed hypersensitivity reactions. It is possible that halothane acts like a hapten with affinity for a liver protein that leads to a contact dermatitis–like reaction in the liver.

Animal models for autoallergic liver disease (experimental allergic hepatitis), through the induction of liver injury by immunization with liver extract, have not accurately reproduced the human disease, although mild inflammatory lesions may be observed in some immunized animals. An allergic role in alcoholic cirrhosis is unlikely. The lesions of congenital biliary cirrhosis, which occur in very young infants, are similar to those seen in liver transplants that have been rejected. The primary lesion is a mononuclear inflammation of the bile ducts. It has been suggested that congenital biliary cirrhosis may be caused by an "autoallergic" reaction to bile ducts or by a rejection of fetal bile ducts by maternally derived lymphocytes.

Periodontal Disease

Periodontal disease is a chronic inflammatory and proliferative reaction of the gums surrounding the teeth that may be at least partially caused by delayed hypersensitivity reactions. The disease begins as a marginal inflammation of the tissue surrounding the teeth (gingivitis) with a predominant lymphocytic infiltrate. The supporting collagen fibers of the gingiva are destroyed and an extensive reactive proliferation of the epithelial cells occurs. Subepithelial inflammation may extend into the marrow of the bone of the jaw, leading to bony resorption and eventual loss of teeth in the involved zones. The antigens responsible may be oral bacterial products, tissue breakdown products, or dietary material. Periodontal disease is a result of poor dental hygiene, and the best preventive action is keeping the oral cavity clean. The lymphocytic infiltrate in periodontal disease may change from predominantly T cell to predominantly B cell as the form of the disease becomes more aggressive. The lesions of severe periodontal disease regress if the patient is treated with immunosuppressive therapy. This effect on periodontal disease has been noticed in patients with cancer or with a transplanted organ who have received immunosuppressive agents; gingival inflammation subsides while the patient is being treated.

Adjuvant Disease

Following the injection of complete Freund's adjuvant alone into rats, lesions may be found in joint synovia, colon, and skin that resemble human diseases of unknown, but suspected immune, origin. The joint lesions are similar to those of Reiter's syndrome and resemble, but are not identical to, those of rheumatoid arthritis. The lesion of rheumatoid arthritis is a villous or papillary thickening of synovial membrane and a vascular granulation tissue (pannus) that may erode the articular surface of the involved joint. The lesions of rheumatoid arthritis include both immune complex and cellular (delayed hypersensitivity) reaction components (see Chapter 17).

Summary

Autoallergic diseases are caused by an immune reaction to an individual's own tissues. The primary cause is a loss of tolerance to one's own tissue antigens (see Chapter 11). Autoallergic lesions may be caused by each of the six immune effector mechanisms or by mixtures of these mechanisms (see Chapter 22). Those caused by antibody have been presented in Chapters 14–17. Many autoallergic lesions involving solid tissue are mediated by delayed hypersensitivity reactions. These include postinfectious encephalomyelitis, multiple sclerosis, thyroiditis, endocrinopathies, chronic active hepatitis, Sjögren's syndrome (salivary and lacrimal glands), chronic rheumatoid arthritis, and other diseases. These lesions are initiated by reaction of sensitized T cells (T_K or T_D) with antigen and often involve tissue destruction by immune activated macrophages. Humoral immune reactions may play an important role in opening blood vessel barriers to allow sensitized T cells to enter tissues. The effect is destruction of solid organs related to infiltration with mononuclear cells, particularly around vessels (perivascular). Many of these diseases are self limited. This may be because of eventual damping of the autoimmune response by immune control mechanisms.

References

See Chapter 11.

Autoimmune Disease

General

Asherson GL: The role of microorganisms in autoimmune responses. Prog Allergy 12:192, 1968.

Baldini M: Idiopathic thrombocytopenic purpura. N Engl J Med 274:1245, 1302, 1360, 1966.

Baldwin RW, Humphrey JH (eds): Autoimmunity. Philadelphia, Davis, 1965.

Beveridge WIB: Acquired immunity: viral infections. *In* Cruickshank R (ed): Modern Trends in Immunology. London, Whitefriars, 1963.

Burnet FM: A reassessment of the forbidden clone hypothesis of autoimmunity disease. Aust J Exp Biol Med Sci 50:1, 1972.

Dacie JV, Wolledge SM: Autoimmune hemolytic anemia. Prog Hematol 6:1, 1969.

Dameshek W: Chronic lymphocytic leukemia—an accumulative disease of immunologically incompetent lymphocytes. Blood 29:566, 1967.

Dixon FJ: Allergy and immunology: autoimmunity in disease. Annu Rev Med 8:257, 1968.

Ehrlich P: An autoimmunity with special reference to cell life. Proc R Soc Lond [Biol] 66B:424, 1900.

Fairfax AJ: Immunological aspects of chronic heartblock: a review. Proc R Soc Med (Lond) 70:327, 1977.

Isacson EP: Myxoviruses and autoimmunity. Prog Allergy 10:256, 1967.

Kaplan MH: Autoimmunity to heart and its relation to human disease. Prog Allergy 13:408, 1969.

Kunkel HG, Tan EM: Autoantibodies and disease. Adv Immunol 4:231, 1964.

Moller G (ed): Models of autoimmune disease. Immunol Rev 55, 1981.

Pease PE: L-Forms, Episomes, and Autoimmune Diseases. Edinburgh, Livingstone, 1965.

Rose NR, Kong YCM, Sundick RS: The genetic basis of autoimmunity. Clin Exp Immunol 39:545, 1980.

Rose NR, Mackey I: The Autoimmune Diseases. Orlando, Fla., Academic Press, 1985.

Smith HR, Steinberg AD: Autoimmunity—a perspective. Annu Rev Immunol 1:175, 1983.

Talal N: Autoimmunity and the immunologic network. Arthritis Rheum 21:853, 1978.

Unanue ER, Dixon FJ: Experimental glomerulonephritis: immunological events and pathologic mechanisms. Adv Immunol 6:1, 1967.

Waksman BH: Autoimmunization and the lesions of autoimmunity. Medicine 41:93, 1962.

Weigle WO: Analysis of autoimmunity through experimental models of thyroiditis and allergic encephalomyelitis. Adv Immunol 30:159, 1980.

Whittingham S, Mackay IR: Tissue antigens, autoantigens, alloantigens, xenoantigens and neoantigens. NZ J Med 7:172, 1977.

Experimental Allergic Encephalomyelitis and Multiple Sclerosis

Craggs RJ, Webster H de F: Ia antigens in the normal rat nervous systems and in lesions of experimental allergic encephalomyelitis. Acta Neuropathol 68:263, 1985.

Eylar EH: Amino acid sequence of the myelin basic protein. Proc Nat Acad Sci USA 67:1425, 1970.

Kibler RF, Shapira R: Isolation and properties of an encephalitogenic protein from bovine, rabbit and human central nervous system tissue. J Biol Chem 243:281, 1968.

Lampert PW: Mechanism of demyelination in experimental allergic neuritis: electron microscopic studies. Lab Invest 20:127, 1969.

Linthicum DS, Munoz JJ, Blaskett A: Acute experimental autoimmune encephalomyelitis in mice. I. Adjuvant action of Bordatella pertussis is due to vasoactive amino sensitization and increased vascular permeability of the central nervous system. Cell Immunol 73:299, 1982.

Oldstone MBA, Perrin LM, Welsh M Sr: Potential pathologic mechanism of injury in amyotrophic lateral sclerosis. *In* Andrews JM, Johnson RJ, Brazier MAB (eds), Recent Research Trends, Vol 19. New York, Academic Press, 1976, p251.

Paterson PY: The demyelinating diseases: clinical and experimental correlates. *In* Sampter M (ed): Immunological Diseases, 2nd ed. Boston, Little, Brown, 1971, p1269.

Paterson PY, Day ED: Current perspectives of neuroimmunologic disease: multiple sclerosis and experimental allergic encephalomyelitis. Clin Immunol Rev 1:81, 1981–82.

Sobel RA, et al: The immunopathology of experimental allergic encephalomyelitis. I. Quantitative analysis of inflammatory cells in situ. II. Endothelial cell Ia increases prior to inflammatory cell infiltration. J Immunol 132:2393, 2402, 1984.

Waksman BH: Experimental allergic encephalomyelitis and the "autoallergic" diseases. Int Arch Allergy Appl Immunol (Suppl) 14, 1959.

Waksman BH: The distribution of experimental autoallergic lesions: its relationship to the distribution of small veins. Am J Pathol 37:673, 1960.

Webb HE, Gordonsmith CW: Relation of immune response to development of central nervous system lesions in virus infections of man. Br Med J 2:1179, 1966.

Weiner HL, Hauser SL: Neuroimmunology I: immunoregulation in neurologic disease. Ann Neurol 11:437, 1982.

Eye–Ear

Cogan DC: Syndrome of nonsyphilitic interstitial keratitis and vestibuloauditory symptoms. Arch Ophthmol 33:144, 1945.

Easom HA, Zimmerman LE: Sympathetic ophthalmia and bilateral phacoanaphylaxis: a clinicopathologic correlation of the sympathogenic and sympathizing eyes. Arch Ophthalmol 72:9, 1964.

Faure JP: Autoimmunity and the retina. Curr Top Eye Res 2:215, 1980.

Haynes BF, et al: Cogan syndrome: studies in thirteen patients, long term follow up and a review of the literature. Medicine 59:426, 1980.

Leopold IH: Clinical immunology in ophthalmology. Am J Ophthalmol 81:129, 1976.

Meyers-Elliott RH: Autoimmunity and the retina: experimental autoimmune uveitis. *In* Cooper EL, Brazier MAB (eds), Developmental Immunology: Clinical Problems and Aging. New York, Academic Press, 1982.

Silverstein AM, O'Conner GR (eds): Immunology and Immunopathology of the Eye. New York, Masson, 1979.

Wakefield D, Schrieber L, Penny R: Immunological features in uveitis. Med J Aust 1:229, 1982.

Orchitis

Brown PC, Glynn LE: The early lesion of experimental allergic orchitis in guinea pigs: an immunological correlation. J Pathol 98:277–282, 1969.

Fjallbrant B, Obrant O: Clinical and seminal findings in men with sperm antibodies. Acta Obst Gynecol Scand 47:1, 1968.

Teuscher C: Experimental allergic orchitis in mice. II. Association of disease-susceptibility with the locus controlling Bordatella pertussis–induced sensitivity to histamine. Immunogenetics 22:417, 1985.

Tung KSK, Unanue ER, Dixon FJ: The immunopathology of experimental allergic orchitis. Am J Pathol 60:313, 1970.

Waksman BH: A histologic study of the auto-allergic testis lesion in the guinea pig. J Exp Med 109:311, 1959.

Thyroiditis

Askanasy M: Pathologische–anatomische Beiträge zur Kenntnis des Morbus basedowi, insbesondere über die dabei auftretende Muskelerkrankung. Dtsch Arch Klin Med 61:118–186, 1898.

Bech K, et al: Heterogeneity of autoimmune thyroiditis. Allergy 8:39, 1984.

Farid NR, Munro RE, Row VV, Volpe R: Peripheral thymus dependent (T) lymphocytes in Graves' disease and Hashimoto's thyroiditis. N Engl J Med 288:1313, 1973.

Flax MH: Experimental allergic thyroiditis in the guinea pig. II. Morphologic studies on the development of the disease. Lab Invest 12:119, 1963.

Hall R: Immunological aspects of thyroid function. N Engl J Med 266:1204, 1962.

Hashimoto H: Zur Kenntnis der lymphomatosen Veränderung der Schilddruse (Struma lymphomatosa). Arch Klin Chir 97:219, 1912.

Kalderon AE, Bogaars HA, Diamond I: Ultrastructural alterations of follicular basement membrane in Hashimoto's thyroiditis. Am J Med 55:485, 1973.

Nakamura RM, Weigle WO: Transfer of experimental thyroiditis by serum from thyroidectomized donors. J Exp Med 130:263, 1069.

Roitt IM, Doniach D, Campbell PN, Hudson RV: Autoantibodies in Hashimoto's disease (lymphoadenoid goitre). Lancet 2:820, 1956.

Rose NR: The thyroid gland as a source and target of autoimmunity. Lab Invest 52:117, 1985.

Rose NR, Witebsky E: Studies on organ specificity. V. Changes in the thyroid glands of rabbits following active immunization with rabbit thyroid extracts. J Immunol 76:417, 1956.

Strakosch CR, et al: Immunology of autoimmune thyroid disease. N Engl J Med 307:1499, 1982.

Urbaniak SJ, Panhale WJ, Irvine WJ: Circulating lymphocyte subpopulations in Hashimoto's thyroiditis. Clin Exp Immunol 15:345, 1973.

Weigle WO: The induction of autoimmunity in rabbits following injection of heterologous or altered homologous thyroglobulin. J Exp Med 121:289, 1965.

Witebsky E, Rose NR, Terplan K, et al: Chronic thyroiditis and autoimmunization. JAMA 64:1439, 1957.

Sjögren's Syndrome

Adamson TC: Immunologic analysis of lymphoid infiltrates in primary Sjögren's syndrome using monoclonal antibodies. J Immunol 130:203, 1983.

Anderson LG, Cummings NA, Asofsky R, et al: Salivary gland immunoglobulin and rheumatoid factor synthesis in Sjögren's syndrome: natural history and response to treatment. Am J Med 53:456, 1972.

Anderson LG, Talal N: The spectrum of benign to malignant lymphoproliferation in Sjögren's syndrome. Clin Exp Immunol 9:199, 1971.

Anderson LG, Tarpley TM, Talal N, Cummings NA, Wolf RO, Schall GL: Cellular-versus-humoral autoimmune responses to salivary gland in Sjögren's syndrome. Clin Exp Immunol 13:335, 1973.

Bloch KJ, et al: Sjögren's syndrome. A clinical, pathological and serological study of sixty-two cases. Medicine 44:187, 1965.

Boss JH, Sela J, Ulmansky M, Dikton T, Rosenmann E: Experimental immune sialoadenitis. Isr J Med 24:15, 1975.

Cummings NA, et al: Sjögren's syndrome — newer aspects of research, diagnosis and therapy. Ann Intern Med 75:937, 1971.

Hadden WB: On "dry mouth," or suppression of the salivary buccal secretions. Trans Clin Soc London 21:176, 1888.

Manthorpe R, et al: Sjögren's syndrome: a review with emphasis on immunological features. Allergy 36:139, 1981.

Sjögren H: Zur Kenntnis der Keratoconjunctivitis sicca (Keratitis filiformus) bei Hypofunction der Tränendrusen. Acta Ophthalmol (Kbh) 11:1, 1933.

Endocrinopathies

Christy NP, Holub DA, Omasi T: Primary ovarian thyroidal and adrenocortical deficiencies simulating pituitary insufficiency, associated with diabetes mellitus. J Clin Endocrinol 22:155, 1962.

Edmonds M, et al: Autoimmune thyroiditis, adrenalitis and oophoritis. Am J Med 54:782, 1973.

Irvine WJ: Immunologic aspects of premature ovarian failure associated with idiopathic Addison's disease. Lancet 2:883, 1968.

Levine S, Wenk EJ: The production and passive transfer of allergic adrenalitis. Am J Pathol 52:41, 1968.

Richtsmeier AJ, et al: Lymphoid hypophysitis with selective adrenocorticotropic hormone deficiency. Arch Intern Med 140:1243, 1980.

Strickland RG: Pernicious anemia and polyendocrine deficiency. Ann Intern Med 70:1001, 1969.

Van de Casseye M, Gepts W: Primary (autoimmune?) parathyroiditis. Virchows Arch Pathol Anat 361:257, 1973.

Werdelin O, Witebsky E: Experimental allergic rat adrenalitis. A study on its elicitation and lymphokinetics. Lab Invest 23:136, 1970.

Bowel Disease

Broberger O, Perlmann P: Autoantibodies in human ulcerative colitis. J Exp Med 110:657, 1959.

Crohn BB, Ginzburg L, Openheimer GD: Regional ileitis: a pathologic and clinical entity. JAMA 99:1323, 1932.

Deodhar SD, Michener WM, Farmer RG: A study of the immunologic aspects of chronic ulcerative colitis and transmural colitis. Am J Clin Pathol 51:591, 1969.

MacPherson BR, Albertini RS, Beekin WL: Immunologic studies in patients with Crohn's disease. Gut 17:100, 1976.

Nielsen H, et al: Circulating immune complexes in ulcerative colitis. I. Correlation to disease activity. II. Correlations with serum protein concentrations and complement conversion products. Clin Exp Immunol 31:72, 81, 1978.

Rabin BS, Rogers SJ: Cell mediated immune model of inflammatory bowel disease in the rabbit. Gastroenterology 75:29, 1978.

Liver Disease

Doniach D: Autoimmune aspects of liver disease. Br Med Bull 28:145, 1972.

Galbraith RM, Fudenberg HH: Autoimmunity in chronic active hepatitis and diabetes mellitus. Clin Immunol Immunopathol 8:116, 1977.

Kaplan MM: The spectrums of chronic active liver disease. Hosp Pract 18:67, 1983.

Mackay IR: Lupoid hepatitis and primary biliary cirrhosis: autoimmune diseases of the liver. Bull Rheum Dis 18:487, 1968.

Mackay IR: Immunological aspects of chronic active hepatitis. Hepatology 3:724, 1983.

Mackay IR, Popper H; Immunopathogenesis of chronic hepatitis: a review. Aust NZ J Med 1:79, 1973.

Paronetto F: Immunologic aspects of liver disease. Prog Liver Dis 3:299, 1970.

Paronetto F, Sagnelli E: Immunologic observation in chronic active hepatitis: a disease of different etiologies. Pathobiol Ann 10:157, 1980.

Popper H, Paronetto F: Problems in immunology of hepatic diseases. Hepatogastroenterology 31:1, 1984.

Prince AM, Trepo C: Role of immune complexes involving SH antigen in pathogenesis of chronic active hepatitis and polyarteritis nodosa. Lancet 1:7713, 1971.

Stenger RJ: Liver disease. Hum Pathol 8:603, 1977.

Subcommittee on the National Halothane Study: Summary of the National Halothane Study: possible association between halothane anesthesia and post-operative hepatic necrosis. JAMA 197:775, 1966.

Uzunalimoglu B, Yardley JH, Boitnott JK: The liver in mild halothane hapatis. Light and electron microscopic findings with special reference to the mononuclear cell infiltrate. Am J Pathol 61:457, 1970.

Periodontal Disease

Horton JE, Oppenheim JJ, Mergenhagen SE: A role of cell-mediated immunity in the pathogenesis of periodontal disease. J Periodontol 45:351, 1974.

Loe M (ed): Possible role of immune phenomena in periodontal tissue destruction. J Periodontol 45:330, 1974.

Nisengard RJ: The role of immunology in periodontal disease. J Periodontol 48:505, 1977.

Patters MR, et al: Lymphoproliferative responses to oral bacteria in humans with varying severities of periodontal disease. Infect Immunity 28:777, 1980.

Seymour GJ, Cole KL, Powell RN: Analysis of lymphocyte populations extracted from chronically inflamed human periodontal tissue. I. Identification. J Periodont Res 20:47, 1985.

Seymour GJ, et al: Experimental gingivitis in humans. A histochemical and immunochemical characterization of the lymphoid cell population. J Periodont Res 18:375, 1983.

Tollefsen T, Saltvedt E, Koppang HS: The effect of immunosuppressive therapy on periodontal disease in man. J Periodont Res 13:240, 1978.

Adjuvant Disease — Arthritis

Katz H, Piliero SJ: A study of adjuvant-induced polyarthritis in the rat with special reference to associated immunological phenomena. Ann NY Acad Sci 147:515, 1969.

Pearson CM: Development of arthritis, periarthritis and periostitis in rats given adjuvant. Proc Soc Exp Biol Med 91:95, 1956.

Rosenthal ME, Capetola RJ: Adjuvant arthritis: immunological and hyperalgesia features. Fed Proc 41:2577, 1982.

Stuart JM, Townes AS, Kang AH: Collagen autoimmune arthritis. Immunol Rev 2:199, 1984.

Waksman BH, Pearson CM, Sharp JT: Studies of arthritis and other lesions induced in rats by injection of mycobacterial adjuvant. II. Evidence that the disease itself is a disseminated immunological response to exogenous antigen. J Immunol 85:403, 1960.

21 | Granulomatous Reactions

The Nature of Granulomas

Granulomas (Fig. 21-1) are identified by focal collections of mononuclear cells in tissue, including macrophages, histiocytes, epithelioid cells, and giant cells as well as lymphocytes and plasma cells. The characteristic epithelioid cell is derived from a macrophage and has a prominent eosinophilic amorphous cytoplasm and a large, oval, pale-staining nucleus with a sharp, thin nuclear membrane and large nuclei. These cells have been called *epithelioid* because of their resemblance to epithelial cells. Granulomas may progress from highly cellular reactions to fibrous scars or central necrosis surrounded by fibrosis (Fig. 21-2). Although it is not always possible using morphological criteria alone, these reactions should be differentiated from nonspecific chronic inflammatory reactions in which lymphocytes, plasma cells, and eosinophils accumulate.

Granulomatous reactions are cellular responses to irritating, persistent, and poorly soluble substances. These reactions may be initiated by sensitized lymphocytes reacting with antigen and may also occur to antigen–antibody complexes that persist locally. Antibody–antigen complexes may provide a stimulus for granuloma formation inflammation if the complex is insoluble and relatively indigestible. Antigen complexed to insoluble particles will produce granulomas when injected into immunized animals. Not all granulomas have their origin in an immune response. Similar lesions may be induced by foreign bodies. Perhaps the most common granulomatous reaction is that found surrounding insoluble suture material.

The origin of the most characteristic cell of granulomatous hypersensitivity reaction—the epithelioid cell—is most likely from a phagocyte that has ingested foreign material but cannot digest and/or exocytose the material. Multinuclear giant cells are believed to form from fusion of macrophages or epithelioid cells. Granulomatous hypersensitivity reactions

529

530

Figure 21-1. Granulomatous hypersensitivity reactions. Granulomatous reactions may be identified morphologically by the appearance of reticuloendothelial cells, including histiocytes, epithelioid cells, giant cells, and lymphocytes arranged in a characteristic round or oval laminated structure called a *granuloma*. Hypersensitivity granulomas form as a variation of delayed hypersensitivity or antibody reactions. Sensitized lymphocytes react with antigens, releasing lymphokines which attract and activate macrophages. The activated macrophages are unable to "clear" the poorly degradable antigens; they accumulate in the tissues, form epithelioid and giant cells, and organize into granulomas. Granulomas may also form in response to poorly degradable antibody–antigen complexes in tissue.

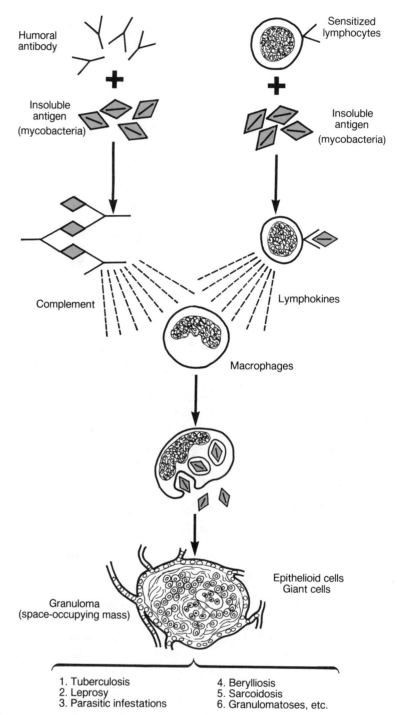

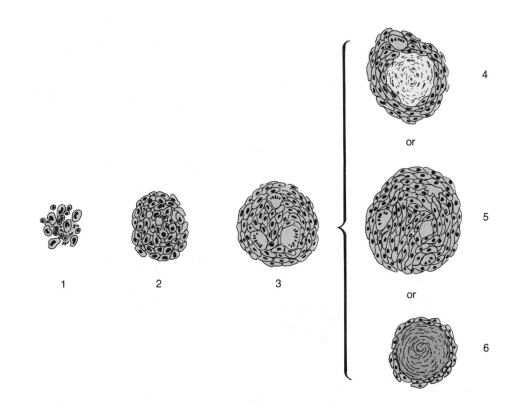

Figure 21-2. Progression of granulomas. (1) Granulomas begin as small collections of lymphocytes and macrophages that form around poorly degradable antigens. (2) Macrophages change to epithelioid cells and become organized into a cluster of cells. (3) Further progression results in ball-like clusters of cells and fusion of macrophages into giant cells. Later progression may include (4) development of necrosis in the center as characteristic of tuberculosis, (5) continued enlargement and replacement of normal tissue (progressive disease), or (6) fibrosis with scar formation, characteristic of "healed" sarcoidosis.

may evolve over weeks or even months because of the persistent nature of the stimulus.

Combinations of immune-mediated lesions in some granulomatous diseases suggest the involvement of different mechanisms in the production of lesions (e.g., immune complex, anaphylactic, and granulomatous). Many diseases demonstrate both granulomatous reactions and vasculitis, varying from essentially pure granulomatous lesions to pure vasculitis (Fig. 21-3). "Allergic granulomatosis" or Churg–Strauss syndrome includes necrotizing vasculitis, extravascular granulomas, and tissue infiltration with eosinophils, which occur in a setting of bronchial asthma.

Granulomatous Diseases

Granulomatous hypersensitivity diseases include infectious diseases (tuberculosis, leprosy, and parasitic infestation), responses to known antigens (zirconium granuloma, berylliosis, and extrinsic alveolitis), and diseases of unknown etiology in

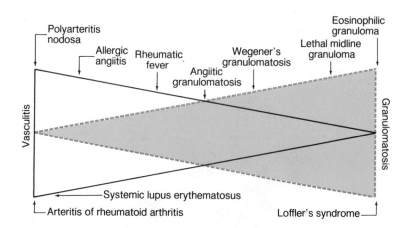

Figure 21-3. Spectrum of association of granulomatous reactions and vasculitis. The lesions of Loffler's syndrome and eosinophilic granuloma are essentially granulomas; those of the vasculitis found with polyarteritis nodosa and collagen diseases are almost pure arteritis. On the other hand, a number of diseases, such as some connective tissue diseases (see Chapter 17) and Wegener's granulomatosis, demonstrate a mixture of granulomatous reactions and vasculitis. In these lesions, which are difficult to classify, it is possible that the granulomatous reactions are secondary to tissue damage initiated by another mechanism.

which epithelioid granulomas are the primary lesions. Epithelioid granulomas occur in such diseases as tertiary syphilis, fungus infections, and some foreign body reactions (e.g., around urate deposits in gout). Granulomas are also a prominent feature of early asbestosis and silicosis.

Infectious Diseases

Tuberculosis

Tuberculosis is the classic example of both immune and nonimmune inflammatory reactions to a single agent. Infection with tubercle bacilli may result in different types of immune responses, including circulating antibody, classic delayed hypersensitivity, increased macrophage activity (immune phagocytosis), and granulomatous inflammation. That protective immunity is successful in limiting the dissemination of the organisms is shown by the finding of a primary (Ghon) complex in many patients at autopsy. The Ghon complex consists of a healed granuloma or scar on the pleural surface of the middle lobes of the lung, and granulomas in the draining hilar lymph nodes. The Ghon complex suggests that the patient resisted a previous tuberculosis infection by a granulomatous reaction. Evidence that the granulomatous reaction is protective is not always definitive. The granulomatous response may not destroy the bacillus, and may even protect it from the other defensive reactions of the host; that is, a few viable organisms evade killing and persist in the granuloma.

Clearly, a granulomatous reaction represents a defensive reaction on the part of an infected individual. T_D cells secrete lymphokines or enable activated macrophages to limit dissemination of the organism. Thus, the immune system can augment the granulomatous inflammatory response to protect the host. The fact that this reaction is not always successful in limiting the infection does not mean that it is not a potentially protective response. If extensive, accumulation of granulomas leads to eventual loss of organ function as the normal tissue is replaced by granulomas. The center of tubercular granulomas frequently becomes necrotic, resulting in a gross appearance similar to that of cheese. This is referred to as *caseous* necrosis. Caseous necrosis may also occur in other granulomatous diseases but is most often seen in tuberculosis. The role of granulomatous reactions in defense against infections is discussed in more detail in Chapter 24.

Leprosy

The clinical features of leprosy depend on the immune reaction of the infected individual. The characteristics of leprosy are presented in Table 21-1. At one pole of the leprosy spectrum

Table 21-1. Immunologic Characteristics of Leprosy[a]

Characteristic	Form of Leprosy		
	Tuberculoid	Borderline	Lepromatous
Mycobacterium leprae in tissues	− or ±	+ or ++	++++
Granuloma formation	++++	+++	−
Lymphocytic infiltration	+++	−	−
Lymph node morphology			
Paracortical lymphocytes	++++	++	−
Paracortical histiocytes	−	++	++++
Germinal center formation	+	++	++++
Plasma cells	±	+	+++
Lepromin test	+++	−	−
Delayed hypersensitivity (%)			
To dinitrochlorobenzene	90	75	50
To hemocyanin	100	100	100
Antimycobacterial antibodies (% patients with precipitins in serum)	11–28	82	95
Autoantibodies in serum (%)	3–11		30–50
Immune complex disease (erythema nodosum leprosum)	−	±	+++

[a] − to ++++ indicates extent of the observation noted.

Modified from Turk JL, Bryceson ADM: Immunological phenomena in leprosy and related disease. Adv Immunol 13:209, 1971.

there are prominent granulomatous lesions with epithelioid cells and many lymphocytes. This is the high-resistance form. Few, if any, *Mycobacterium leprae* organisms can be found in the tissues. Because of a tendency to involve peripheral nerves with loss of sensory function, this is also known as the *anesthetic* form. Affected individuals develop secondary traumatic injury due to loss of pain sensation. There is hyperplasia of the paracortical areas of the lymph nodes, a prominent delayed skin reaction to injection of lepromin, and little or no humoral antibody to mycobacterial antigens.

At the other pole of the clinical spectrum is lepromatous leprosy. This form is the low-resistance type. It is known as the *nodular* form because of a prominence of skin and lymph node involvement and gross nodule formation. There is massive infiltration of tissues with large macrophages filled with numerous mycobacteria. The lymph nodes of lepromatous patients have hyperplastic germinal centers, yet the cell-mediated immune defense against these organisms is diminished. The paracortical areas have a paucity of lymphocytes, and are often filled with large macrophages containing organisms. There are few, if any, lymphocytes in the tissue lesions, the lepromin skin test is negative, and antibodies to mycobacterial antigens are common (see Table 21-1).

The spectrum of leprosy includes many patients who have characteristics that are essentially mixtures of the tuberculoid and lepromatous forms. The manifestations of *M. leprae* infection are therefore quite variable and range from severe tissue destruction to only local depigmented areas of the skin. This latter form is frequently found in the natives of Baja California. Europeans tend to be resistant, South Americans develop little immune response but frequently manifest only depigmented skin, while Southeast Asians usually develop lepromatous leprosy.

The protective function of granulomatous reactivity is exemplified by the spectrum of reactions to *M. leprae* in leprosy. Resistance is associated with granuloma formation and a high degree of delayed hypersensitivity, whereas low resistance is associated with lack of granuloma development and prominence of antibody formation. The position that a given patient occupies on the clinical spectrum frequently changes. A shift from a lepromatous form to a tuberculoid form is associated with a definite clinical improvement.

When the bacterial load diminishes, tissues that contain residual organisms undergo hypersensitivity reactions. There is swelling and erythema of skin lesions associated with fever. The skin lesions show infiltration with lymphocytes. The foamy macrophages lose their content of organisms and became more epithelioid. Although patients with polar tuberculoid or polar lepromatous leprosy usually remain in their part of the spectrum, frequent shifts in the borderline groups occur. Effective chemotherapy frequently precipitates a reversal reaction. Chemotherapy of leprosy with 4,4-diaminodiphenylsulfone may produce a reduction in the antigenic load and permit poorly reactive patients to express a granulomatous reaction.

To produce an effective granulomatous reaction, both macrophages and T cells are required. Cytologic analysis indicates segregation of T_D cells within the aggregate of macrophages and T_{CTL} cells in the mantle of tuberculoid granulomas, whereas T_D and T_{CTL} cells are admixed among the undifferentiated macrophages of lepromatous lesions. The formation of a tuberculoid granuloma appears to require activated T_D cells, which may produce a soluble factor that stimulates giant cell formation. The control of the development of a granuloma may be mediated through the action of T_H and T_S cells on T_D activity. The macrophages of lepromatous patients have a decreased capacity for destroying various target cells as well as the microorganisms (decreased cell-mediated immunity). Treatment of mice with agents that increase the phagocytic and metabolic activity (digestive capacity) of macrophages prevents the development of experimental infection. Leprosy infection is always limited in normal mice but assumes a more virulent course in thymectomized or antilymphocyte serum-treated mice who have depressed cell-mediated immunity. Patients with lepromatous leprosy have a decreased capacity to respond to a variety of cell-mediated reactions, including mitogen activation of lymphocytes, sensitization to contact sensitivity agents, and decreased production of lymphokines.

The lepromin test is a skin reaction to extracts of *M. leprae*. It consists of a two-stage reaction. The first is a typical delayed hypersensitivity reaction that occurs 24 to 48 hours after injection of the antigen (the Fernandez reaction); the second (Mitsuda reaction) appears between 2 and 4 weeks after testing and is an indurated skin nodule caused by the formation of a granuloma. This reaction is over 4 mm in diameter and usually ulcerates. The 24- to 48-hour Fernandez reaction is positive in a large number of persons who have no history of ever contacting leprosy. This is probably because of exposure to cross-reacting antigens of other bacteria. Therefore, the lepromin reaction cannot be used to indicate active or acute infection with *M. leprae*. The clinical importance of the lepromin test in determining the reactivity of infected patients is as a prognostic test. A positive Mitsuda granulomatous reaction is associated with high resistance to the infection, and good prognosis.

Erythema nodosum leprosum is an immune complex–mediated vascular skin reaction (Arthus reaction) found in patients with lepromatous leprosy and antibody to mycobacterial antigens. Crops of red nodules appear in the skin and last for 24 to 48 hours. These may be associated with systemic manifestations, such as arthritis, inflammation of the eye or testes, pain along nerves, fever, and proteinuria. The lesions in the skin show a fibrinoid vasculitis with polymorphonuclear infiltrate. The frequent occurrence of these reactions during chemotherapy suggests that they are related to the release of mycobacterial antigens and deposition of immune complexes in affected tissues. Similar lesions may also be seen in patients with progressive tuberculosis — erythema nodosum tuberculosum. One final feature of lepromatoid leprosy worthy of mention is the high incidence of autoantibodies. These include antinuclear factor, rheumatoid factor, antithyroglobulin antibodies, and false positive serologic tests for syphilis. Most of these autoantibodies do not appear to produce lesions or symptoms in affected patients. The high incidence of autoantibodies in lepromatous leprosy may be because of an adjuvant effect of the organisms, continued tissue destruction releasing potential autoantigens, or altered activity of suppressor cells. (See Chapter 24 for additional information.)

Parasitic Infections

The role of granulomatous reactions in the protective and immunopathological processes in infectious diseases is presented in Chapter 24. Granulomatous reactions occur in response to many parasitic infestations, particularly those from certain helminths. Schistosomiasis and filariasis are mentioned briefly here. In infestations with *Schistosoma mansoni* the eggs are released into the portal bloodstream and lodge in the portal veins of the liver. Here the eggs evoke a severe granulomatous inflammatory reaction that may gradually increase and lead to extensive fibrosis of the portal areas (pipe stem fibrosis). If the liver involvement is severe, collateral circulation of the portal system develops as the portal radicals in the liver become obstructed. The eggs may then pass from the portal system through collateral channels to the pulmonary arteries, resulting in multiple, small granulomatous lesions resembling miliary tuberculosis (pseudotubercles). The eggs of other schistosomes (*S. haematobium* and *S. japonicum*) are deposited in large numbers in the subepithelial connective tissue of the urinary bladder. A severe granulomatous reaction may occur, resulting in obstruction of urinary flow. The extent of granulomatous inflammation may actually decrease in chronic infection, at least in experimental animals. This amelioration of the disease state is termed *modulation*, and may occur because of an active suppressor mechanism mediated by both cellular and humoral systems.

The adult worms of *Wuchereria bancrofti* (filaria) reside in the larger lymphatic channels, particularly those of the extremities. In some persons the presence of these worms evokes an extensive granulomatous inflammatory reaction that causes obstruction of lymphatic flow. This obstruction may lead to massive swelling (lymphedema) of the involved area — elephantiasis. Only a small number of individuals with filaria infestation develop this complication, and it is believed that those persons who do not develop clinical manifestations do not have granulomatous sensitivity to the organism. Therefore, although the granulomatous reaction leads to death and isolation of the offending agent, it is definitely deleterious to the host.

Granulomatous Response to Known Antigens

Some 6 months following the marketing of stick deodorants containing zirconium salts, individuals were observed with axillary granulomas. The injection of zirconium into the skin of

Zirconium Granulomas

such patients resulted in the delayed appearance of a typical epithelioid granuloma. Further studies have clearly implicated zirconium as the causative agent. Some type of hypersensitivity was suspected because only relatively few individuals who used such deodorants actually developed lesions. When the use of zirconium was discontinued, lesions no longer occurred.

Berylliosis

Chronic progressive pulmonary disease featuring multiple small noncaseating granulomas may be caused by the inhalation of beryllium salts. The conclusion that a type of hypersensitivity is involved is based on the observations that only a small number of the exposed individuals actually develop the disease and that there may be a delay of months or years from the time of exposure to the development of berylliosis. Beryllium was once used for the manufacture of fluorescent light bulbs, and many exposed individuals remained symptomless. Beryllium is no longer used for this purpose and the disease is no longer seen; beryllium is still used in the aircraft industry. The chronicity of the disease may also be due to the fact that beryllium tends to remain in the tissue indefinitely. It has been reported that patients with berylliosis give positive patch test reactions with the antigen, but the validity of this observation has been questioned. Further studies have shown that beryllium is an active inducer of contact (delayed type) sensitivity, and a beryllium patch test measures delayed hypersensitivity. A more relevant test is the production of a granuloma upon intradermal application of beryllium in patients with berylliosis. Application of beryllium in a patch test most likely does not stimulate a granulomatous reaction, which requires deposition of the eliciting antigen in tissues. The lymphocytes of patients with berylliosis will transform in vitro upon exposure to beryllium sulfate, further suggesting that cellular sensitization to beryllium occurs. Zirconium as well as beryllium may bind serum proteins and function as a hapten in the production of contact sensitivity. However, the relation of this mechanism to the development of granulomas remains obscure.

Extrinsic Allergic Alveolitis

Allergic reactions to organic dusts, bacteria, or mold products in the lung are believed to be causative in a certain type of interstitial pneumonitis, called by Pepys *extrinsic allergic alveolitis* (Table 21-2). The primary allergic reaction appears to be granulomatous; however, the frequent coexistence of other types of reactions, such as anaphylactic, toxic complex, or delayed hypersensitivity, may produce a complex clinical and pathological picture in a given patient. The pathological reaction is mixed, but inflammation of the alveolar walls is the primary feature, usually consisting of epithelioid cell granulomas. Plasma cell and lymphoid cell infiltration may also be prominent, and granulomas are not always present. In fact, a

Table 21-2. Source and Type of Antigen-Producing Extrinsic Allergic Alveolitis

Disease	Source of Antigen	Antigen against Which Precipitating Antibody Is Present
Farmer's lung	Moldy hay	*Micropolyspora faeni, Thermoactinomyces vulgaris*
Bagassosis	Moldy bagasse[a]	*T. vulgaris*
Mushroom worker's lung	Mushroom compost	*M. faeni, T. vulgaris*
Fog fever in cattle	Moldy hay	*M. faeni*
Suberosis	Moldy oak bark, cork dust	Moldy cork dust
New Guinea lung	Moldy thatch dust	Thatch
Maple bark pneumonitis	Moldy maple bark	*Cryptostroma (Coniosporium)*
Malt worker's lung	Moldy barley, malt dust	*Aspergillus clavatus Aspergillus fumigatus*
Bird fancier's lung	Pigeon/budgerigar/ parrot/hen droppings	Serum protein, droppings
Pituitary snuff taker's lung	Heterologous pituitary powder	Serum protein, pituitary antigens
Wheat-weevil disease	Infested wheat flour	*Sitophilus granarius*
Sequoiosis	Moldy sawdust	*Graphium Aureobasidium pullulans (Pullularia)*
Cheese washer's lung	Moldy cheese	*Penicillium* spp.

[a] Residue of sugar cane after extraction of syrup.

Modified from Pepys J: Hypersensitivity diseases of the lungs due to fungi and organic dusts. In Kallos P, Hasek M, Interbitzen TM, Miescher P, Waksman BH (eds): Monographs in Allergy, Vol 4, Basel/New York, Karger, 1969.

variety of lymphoid cell infiltrates and inflammatory reactions may be found in the lung, suggesting that a mixture of different types of immune reactions may be manifested at any given time. In many cases, precipitating antibodies may be demonstrated to test antigens. However, vasculitis is not a prominent feature, although there are notable exceptions. Patients with these chronic pulmonary diseases often have acute attacks of asthma on exposure to the antigen; these may be caused by the existence of anaphylactic antibodies.

Diseases of Unknown Etiology

Sarcoidosis

Boeck's sarcoidosis is a systemic granulomatous process prominently involving the lymph nodes, lungs, eyes, and skin, with lesions that may be indistinguishable from those of tuberculosis, fungus infections, or other granulomatous hypersensitivity reactions. The clinical presentation of sarcoidosis may masquerade as acute rheumatoid arthritis, lymphadenopathy, erythema nodosum, or Crohn's disease, but usually presents as pulmonary masses and bilateral hilar adenopathy on a chest X ray of a young adult black male with dyspnea. Berylliosis and sarcoidosis may be almost identical in their clinical presentation. About 80% of patients with sarcoidosis resolve spontaneously, 20% progress without treatment, and 5% die from complications of the disease. Corticosteroids are the drugs of choice, but should not be used unless disease progression is noted. The serum levels of angiotensin-converting enzyme are elevated in patients with sarcoidosis, and the serum level of this enzyme may be used to monitor disease activity. Sarcoidosis is noted for its geographic prevalence in the southeastern United States and its relative rarity in the western United States. A cutaneous granulomatous reaction may be elicited 3 to 4 weeks after the subcutaneous injection of crude extracts of sarcoid lymph nodes in patients with sarcoidosis (Kveim reaction). The specificity of this reaction and its use as a diagnostic test are questionable. An infectious agent is suspected, but as yet no specific agent has been identified. Patients with sarcoidosis generally exhibit a depression of delayed type hypersensitivity and increased levels of circulating antibody. The relationship of these findings to the disease process remains unclear, but suggests an imbalance in the immune system, with a relatively incompetent T cell system. This could be due to a redistribution of T cells in the inflammatory process or to an inherent loss of T cell activity (see Chapter 26).

Wegener's Granulomatosis

Wegener's granulomatosis is a triad of granulomatous arteritis, glomerulonephritis, and sinusitis. The glomerulonephritis may or may not be present, and the granulomas may be disseminated but are usually prominent in the lungs, nasal and oral cavities, and spleen. The granulomatous lesions are destructive and contain fibroblastic proliferation, necrosis, and prominent Langhans' giant cells. This disease may be related to polyarteritis nodosa, and some authors have called it polyarteritis of the lungs or a type of hypersensitivity angiitis. However, the lesions of Wegener's granulomatosis are distinctive enough to warrant a separate diagnosis. The relation of Wegener's granulomatosis to other necrotizing granulomatous processes, such as midline lethal granuloma of the face, is not clear. No infectious agent has been consistently isolated from patients with any of these diseases. Circulating immune complexes have been found during the active phase of Wegener's granulomatosis, but disappear with remission. Unfortunately the nature of the antigen in these complexes has not been determined. Thus it appears likely that Wegener's granulomatosis is an immune complex disease caused by the presence of both insoluble and soluble complexes.

Granulomatous Hepatitis

Circumscribed granulomas consisting of epithelioid cells surrounded by plasma cells and lymphocytes may be seen in the liver and are associated with a variety of diseases, including sarcoidosis, histoplasmosis, tuberculosis, cirrhosis, lymphomas, Wegener's granulomatosis, immune deficiency diseases, and malignant tumors. However, in a substantial number of patients, no specific disease association occurs. It is likely that the reaction represents an allergic reaction to a drug or response to an unidentified infectious agent.

Regional Enteritis

Regional enteritis is a chronic inflammatory lesion of unknown etiology. The primary feature is thickening and scarring of the intestinal wall that may occur at any level of the gastrointestinal tract, but usually involves the terminal ileum. Histologically, the inflammatory changes vary from those consistent with a delayed hypersensitivity reaction (dense infiltration of mononuclear lymphoid follicles often containing germinal centers) to those of granulomatous hypersensitivity (typical epithelioid granulomas with prominent giant cells, essentially identical to the pulmonary lesions of sarcoidosis). The mononuclear inflammation of regional enteritis may be the result of the development of delayed hypersensitivity to soluble antigens in the diet, and the granulomatous inflammation may result from the development of granulomatous hypersensitivity to insoluble antigens in the diet, but no causative antigen has yet been identified.

Immune Deficiency Diseases: Granulomatous Disease of Children

Granulomatous disease of children consists of chronic pulmonary disease, recurrent suppurative lymphadenitis, and chronic dermatitis with scattered granulomas in many organs. This disease is due to a defect in nicotinamide adenine dinucleotide phosphate (NADPH) that prevents the phagocytic cell from producing free radicals necessary to kill bacteria following phagocytosis. This results in formation of nonallergic granulomas that consist of collections of large macrophages in affected tissues (see Chapter 26).

Summary

Granulomatous reactions are characterized by the accumulation of oval collections of modified mononuclear cells in tissue. The typical tissue lesion contains large mononuclear cells that look like epithelial cells (epithelioid cells), multinucleated giant cells, lymphocytes, and plasma cells. Granulomatous reactions may be a variant of delayed hypersensitivity reactions to insoluble antigens, but also frequently occur in association with vasculitis or in response to nonantigenic foreign bodies. It is likely that poorly degradable antigens or insoluble antibody–antigen complexes produce granulomas, whereas soluble complexes cause vasculitis or glomerulonephritis. The mechanism of granulomatous reactivity is not clear, but the inability of macrophages to digest antigens is believed to be a major pathogenic feature. Granulomatous tissue reactions serve to isolate infectious agents such as tubercle bacilli, leprosy bacilli, and parasites. Deleterious effects of these reactions occur because of the displacement of normal tissue by granulomas and healing by fibrosis, leading to a loss of normal function.

References

Granulomatous Reactions

General

Adams DO: The granulomatous inflammatory response. Am J Pathol 84:164–192, 1976.

Boros DL: Granulomatous inflammations. Prog Allergy 24:183, 1978.

Boros DL: Basic and Clinical Aspects of Granulomatous Disease. New York, Elsevier/North-Holland, 1981.

Chambers TJ, Spector WG: Inflammatory giant cells. Immunobiology 161:283, 1982.

Epstein WL: Granulomatous hypersensitivity. Prog Allergy 11:36, 1967.

Langhans T: Über Riesenzellen mit mandeständigen Kernen in Tuberkeln und die fibrose Form des Tuberkels. Virchows Arch Pathol Anat Physiol Klin Med 42:382, 1968.

Postlethwait AE, et al: Formation of multinucleated giant cells from human monocyte precursors: mediation by a soluble protein from antigen and mitogen-stimulated lymphocytes. J Exp Med 155:168, 1982.

Spector WG, Heesom N: The production of granulomata by antigen–antibody complexes. J Pathol 98:31, 1969.

Sutton JS, Weiss L: Transformation of monocytes in tissue culture into macrophages, epithelioid cells and multinucleate giant cells. J Cell Biol 28:303, 1966.

Turk JL: The role of delayed hypersensitivity in granuloma formation. Res Monogr Immunol 1:275, 1980.

Infectious Diseases

See also Chapter 24.

Alpert DA, Weissman MH, Kaplan R: The rheumatic manifestations of leprosy (Hansen Disease). Medicine 59:442, 1980.

Baker RD (ed): The Pathologic Anatomy of Mycoses: Human Infection with Fungi, Actinomycetes, and Algae. New York, Springer-Verlag, 1971.

Binford CH: Histoplasmosis: tissue reactions and morphologic variations of the fungus. Am J Clin Pathol 25:25, 1955.

Chaparas SD: Immunity in tuberculosis. Bull WHO 60:447, 1982.

Chaparas SD: The immunology of mycobacterial infections. CRC Crit Rev 139, 1982.

Daniel TM, Janicki B: Mycobacterial antigens: a review of their isolation, chemistry and immunological properties. Microbiol Rev 42:84, 1978.

Dennenburg AM: Cellular hypersensitivity and cellular immunity in the pathogenesis of tuberculosis specificity, systemic and local nature, and associated macrophage enzymes. Bacteriol Rev 32:85, 1968.

Hsu KHK: Thirty years after isoniazid: its impact on tuberculosis in children and adolescents. JAMA 251:1283, 1984.

Kaplan G, et al: An analysis of in vitro T cell responsiveness in lepromatous leprosy. J Exp Med 162:917, 1985.

Marcial-Rojas RA (ed): Pathology of Protozoal and Helminthic Diseases. Baltimore, Williams & Wilkins, 1971.

Rich AR: The Pathogenesis of Tuberculosis. Springfield, Ill., Thomas, 1951.

Skinsness OK: Immunopathology of leprosy: the century in review— pathology, pathogenesis and the development of classification. Int J Leprosy 41:329, 1973.

Turk JL, Bryceson ADM: Immunological phenomena in leprosy and related disease. Adv Immunol 13:209, 1971.

Vanek J, Schwartz J: The gamut of histoplasmosis. Am J Med 50:89, 1971.

Warren KS: Modulation of immunopathology and disease in schistosomiasis. Am J Trop Med Hyg 26:113, 1977.

Response to Known Antigens

Barna BP, et al: Immunologic studies of experimental beryllium lung disease in the guinea pig. Clin Immunol Immunopathol 20:402, 1981.

Denardi JN, Van Ordstrand HS, Curtis GH, Zielinski J: Berylliosis. Arch Indust Hyg 8:1, 1953.

Deodhar SD, Barna B, Van Ordstrand HS: A study of the immunologic aspects of chronic berylliosis. Chest 63:309, 1973.

Kanared DJ, Wainer RA, Chamberlin RI, Weber AL, Kazemi H: Respiratory illness in a population exposed to beryllium. Am Rev Resp Dis 108:1295, 1973.

Keller RH, et al: Immunoregulation in hypersensitivity pneumonitis. I. Differences in T-cell and macrophage suppressor activity in symptomatic and asymptomatic pigeon breeders. J Clin Immunol 2:46, 1982.

Larson G: Hypersensitivity lung disease. Annu Rev Immunol 3:59, 1985.

McCombs RP: Diseases due to immunologic reactions in the lungs. N Engl J Med 286:1186–1245, 1972.

Nicholson DP: Bagasse worker's lung. Annu Rev Resp Dis 97:546, 1968.

Pepys J: Hypersensitivity diseases of the lungs due to fungi and organic dusts. In Kallos P, Hasek M, Interbitzen TM, Miescher P, Waksman BH (eds): Monographs in Allergy, Vol 4. Basel, Karger, 1969.

Richardson HB: Immune complexes in the lung: a skeptical review. Surv Synth Pathol 3:281, 1984.

Solley GO, Hyatt RE: Hypersensitivity pneumonitis induced by penicillin species. J Allergy Clin Immunol 65:65, 1980.

Tepper LB, Hardy HL, Chamberlin RI: Toxicity of Beryllium Compounds. Amsterdam, Elsevier, 1961.

Vacher J: Immunologic responses to guinea pigs to beryllium salts. J Med Microbiol 5:91, 1972.

Diseases of Unknown Etiology

Alarcón-Segovia D, Brown AL: Classification and etiologic aspects of necrotizing angiitis. An analytic approach to a confused subject with a critical review of the evidence for hypersensitivity in polyarteritis nodosa. Mayo Clin Proc 39:205, 1964.

Chumbley LC, Harrison EC Jr, Deremee RA: Allergic granulomatosis and angiitis (Churg–Strauss syndrome). Report and analysis of 30 cases. Mayo Clin Proc 52:477, 1977.

Churg J, Strauss L: Allergic granulomatosis, allergic angiitis, and polyarteritis nodosa. Am J Pathol 27:277–301, 1951.

Churg J: Allergic granulomatosis and granulomatous vascular syndromes. Ann Allergy 21:619, 1963.

Crohn BB, Ginzburg L, Oppenheimer GD: Regional ileitis: a pathologic and clinical entity. JAMA 99:1323, 1932.

Daniele RP: Sarcoidosis diagnosis and management. Hosp Pract 18:116, 1983.

Fahey JL, Leonard E, Churg J: Wegener's granulomatosis. Am J Med 17:168, 1954.

Fauci AS, Wolff SM: Wegener's granulomatosis: studies in eighteen patients and a review of the literature. Medicine 52:535, 1973.

Gugkian JC, Perry JE: Granulomatous hepatitis of unknown etiology: an etiologic and functional evaluation. Am J Med 44:207, 1968.

Howell SB, Epstein WV: Circulating immunoglobulin complexes in Wegener's granulomatosis. Am J Med 60:259, 1976.

Israel HL, Goldstein RA: Relation of Kveim-antigen reaction to lymphadenopathy. Study of sarcoidosis and other diseases. N Engl J Med 284:345, 1971.

Janowitz HD, Sachar DB: New observations in Crohn's disease. Annu Rev Med 27:269, 1976.

Kasdon EJ, Schlossman SF: An experimental model of pulmonary arterial granulomatous inflammation. Am J Pathol 71:365, 1973.

Liebow AA: The J. Burns Amberson Lecture — Pulmonary angiitis and granulomatosis. Am Rev Resp Dis 1081:1, 1973.

Lyons GW, Lindsay WG: Renal transplantation in a patient with Wegener's granulomatosis. Am J Surg 124:104, 1972.

Mir-Madjlessi SH, Farmer RG, Hawk WA: Granulomatous hepatitis: a review of 50 cases.

Oreo GA: Wegener's granulomatosis. Arch Dermatol 81:169, 1960.

Sartor RB, et al: Granulomatous enterocolitis induced in rats by purified cell wall extracts. Gastroenterology 89:587, 1985.

Siltzbach LE: The enigma of sarcoidosis. Hosp Pract 3:80, 1968.

Siltzbach LE (ed): Seventh International Conference on Sarcoidosis and Other Granulomatous Disorders. New York, Academy of Science, 1976.

Simon HB, Wolff SM: Granulomatous hepatitis and prolonged fever of unknown origin: a study of 13 patients. Medicine 52:1, 1973.

Granulomatous
Disease of Children

Berendes H, Bridges RA, Good RA: A fetal granulomatosis of childhood: the clinical study of a new syndrome. Mini Med 40:309, 1957.

Gallin JI, Fauci AS (eds): Advances in Host Defense Mechanisms, Vol 3, Chronic Granulomatous Disease. New York, Raven Press, 1983.

Gallin JI, et al: Recent advances in chronic granulomatous disease. Ann Intern Med 99:657, 1983.

Johnston RB, Baehner RL: Chronic granulomatous disease: correlation between pathogenesis and clinical findings. Pediatrics 48:730, 1971.

Landing BH, Shirkey HS: A syndrome of recurrent infection and infiltration of viscera by pigmented lipid histiocytes. Pediatrics 20:431, 1957.

22 | Interplay of Inflammatory and Immunopathological Mechanisms in Disease

In any inflammatory reaction both immune and nonimmune mechanisms may be activated. In Chapter 12 the interactions of acute inflammatory mechanisms were presented (see Fig. 12-12). In the preceding chapters the distinguishing characteristics of each immune-mediated inflammatory mechanism have been emphasized. In many immune disease processes, more than one immune or nonimmune mechanism may be playing a part sequentially, at the same time, or both. It is important to emphasize again that the clinical manifestations of pathological lesions associated with a given immunopathological reaction are often determined by more than one mechanism.

Nonimmune Inflammation

Inflammation may be activated by nonimmune factors such as tissue necrosis (infarct), release of bacterial products, or physical injury. Such stimuli may activate complement, kinin, coagulation, or mast cell inflammatory mediators that are also activated by immune effector mechanisms. The tissue manifestations may include acute or chronic inflammatory changes that in some cases are indistinguishable from the lesions caused by immune mechanisms. As discussed in the preceding chapter, nonimmune granulomatous reactions to foreign bodies may be very similar, if not identical, to granulomatous hypersensitivity reactions activated by immune mechanisms.

Immune Inflammation

Antibody-Mediated Disease

Neutralization, cytotoxic, atopic, and immune complex reactions result when circulating or humoral antibody combines in vivo with antigen. Considered as immune phenomena, these four types of reactions have the following properties in common:

1. The hypersensitive state is induced by previous exposure to antigen or passive transfer of antibody.
2. There is a definite induction or latent period comparable to that of other immune responses (1 – 2 weeks or longer).
3. The reaction occurs only on exposure to the specific antigen or to closely related chemical substances that cross-react.

545

4. The reaction is determined mainly by the biological properties of the antibody or characteristics of accessory systems (i.e., details of anaphylaxis depend on distribution of smooth muscle). The type of tissue reaction or clinical symptoms also depends on the nature and location of the antigen.
5. The degree of hypersensitivity (titer of antibody) tends to diminish with time.
6. Reexposure to antigen results in reappearance of reactivity more rapidly and in more intense form than primary exposure (secondary or anamnestic response).
7. The hypersensitive state can be passively transferred with serum (antibody).
8. Administration of antigen with proper precautions to avoid death can result in temporary desensitization — loss of the ability to react because of saturation of antibody available at the given time.

Cell-Mediated Disease

Delayed hypersensitivity is characterized by the reaction of specifically sensitized cells (lymphocytes) with antigen. As a result of such reactions, a number of mediators may be released that recruit other mononuclear cells and increase the intensity of the tissue response. The major difference between this type of allergic response and those discussed above is that delayed hypersensitivity reactions cannot be transferred or initiated by circulating immunoglobulin antibody.

Granulomatous reactions feature the formation of organized collections of altered mononuclear cells called *granulomas*. Hypersensitivity granulomas may be a variation of delayed hypersensitivity due to reactivity to poorly degradable antigens, or a chronic response to insoluble antibody–antigen complexes. Granulomas may also form as a nonspecific reaction to foreign material.

Mixed Immunopathologic Mechanisms

The reaction of an antibody with an antigen in vivo may result in activation of more than one effector mechanism. Some possible interactions of allergic mechanisms are illustrated in Figure 22-1. Immune complex reactions may be associated with each of the other immune mechanisms. Antibody reacting with a biologically active antigen not only may cause neutralization, but also may result in the formation of soluble immune complexes and immune complex lesions. In fact neutralization reactions are considered by some to be a particular form of immune complex reaction in which the biological activity of the antigen adds an additional dimension to the effects of an antibody–antigen reaction. The activation of complement or release of enzymes from polymorphonuclear neutrophils as a result of an immune complex reaction may cause mast cell lysis and activation of anaphylactic mechanisms. The release of anaphylactic mediators may, in turn, contribute to the vascular

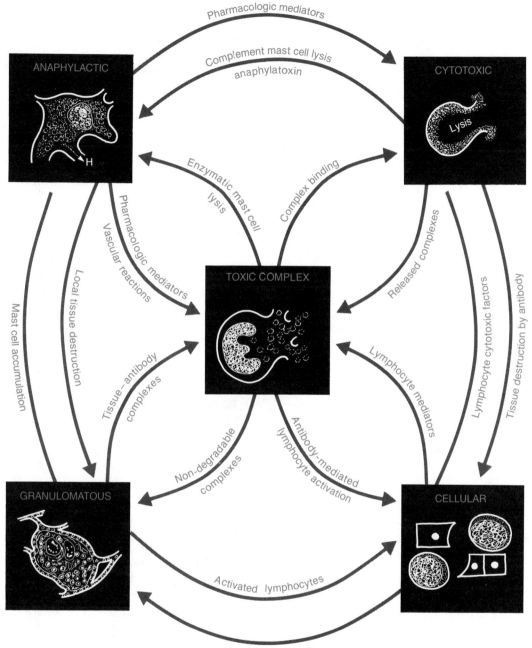

Figure 22-1. Possible interactivation of allergic mechanisms. For a description, see the text.

lesions of immune complex reactions. The reaction of immune complexes with platelets may induce serotonin release, which causes increased vascular permeability, immune complex deposition, polymorphonuclear infiltration, and subsequent tissue damage. Anaphylactic mediators released from mast cells may cause separation of endothelial cells, exposing the basement membrane and thus forming foci where immune complexes can lodge and initiate basement membrane damage by an Arthus mechanism or allow sensitized cells, which initiate delayed hypersensitivity, to pass through the vessels into tissue spaces. Binding of antibody–antigen complexes to red cells may result in their destruction by activation of complement (the innocent bystander reaction), and soluble complexes released by lysed cells may contribute to an immune complex effect. Both immunoglobulin antibody and sensitized cells may play a role in the lesions seen in such autoallergic diseases as thyroiditis, encephalomyelitis, or orchitis. In serum sickness, over 50 serum protein antigens are potentially available to react with different antibodies. Anaphylactic lesions as well as immune complex lesions often coexist in the acute phase of serum sickness. In secondary syphilis, antibody-mediated vasculitis and cell-mediated skin lesions provide a lesion produced by two major mechanisms. Granulomatous lesions frequently occur in association with vasculitis and/or anaphylactic-type reactions. The formation of nondegradable antibody–antigen complexes may initiate granuloma formation, whereas tissue antibody or breakdown products produced by granulomatous reactions may lead to immune complex glomerulonephritis. The role of immune complex reactivity, cell-mediated immunity, macrophage activation, and chronic proliferative response is illustrated by rheumatoid arthritis (see Fig. 17-3).

Other allergic mechanisms may also interreact. Complement-induced mast cell lysis (cytotoxic reaction) may cause anaphylactic symptoms. Cytotoxic antibody may contribute to cell-mediated tissue destruction (e.g., aspermatogenesis); antibody-dependent cell-mediated cytotoxic cells or cytotoxic factors released by activated lymphocytes may produce lysis of cells. Lymphocyte mediators may contribute to the evolution of a granulomatous reaction by attracting and activating macrophages; release of lymphocyte-stimulating factors from granulomatous inflammatory sites may contribute to the cellular component of such reactions. Finally, granulomatous lung diseases (such as farmer's lung) frequently have asthmatic (anaphylactic) components. Granulomatous inflammation may increase the number of mast cells present, and tissue destruction by anaphylactic mechanisms may contribute to granuloma formation. Mixtures of vasculitis, glomerulonephritis, cellular lesions, and granulomas such as seen in Wegener's granulomatosis and some infectious diseases are among the most complex diseases to analyze from the immunopathological standpoint.

Interaction of Immune and Nonimmune Mechanisms

Other systems, such as the blood clotting and the kinin systems, may be activated during the evolution of an inflammatory reaction that also involves allergic reactions. For example, the role that Hageman factor (factor XII of the blood sequence) plays in involvement of other systems is illustrated in Chapter 12. Conversion of plasminogen to plasmin produces activation of complement that may induce lytic or inflammatory reactions. Kinins increase vascular permeability and may expose basement membranes for toxic complex deposition. Complement may be activated by nonimmunological mechanisms (see Alternate Pathway, Chapter 12). Interaction of these "nonimmune" inflammatory mechanisms with allergic (immune) mechanisms may make it very difficult to evaluate the inflammatory processes taking place in a given patient. However, it is important to emphasize that specific inflammatory or immunopathological reactions can be recognized in most patients. In many cases, the nonimmune inflammatory reaction or the clotting system becomes activated secondary to tissue damage caused by immunopathological mechanisms.

References

Cochrane CG: Immunologic tissue injury mediated by neutrophilic leukocytes. Adv Immunol 9:97, 1968.

Johnston MG, Hay JB, Movat HZ: The role of prostaglandins in inflammation. Curr Top Pathol 68:259, 1979.

Lampert PW: Mechanism of demyelination in experimental allergic neuritis: electron microscopic studies. Lab Invest 20:127, 1969.

Marx JL: The leukotrienes in allergy and inflammation. Science 215:1380, 1982.

Movat HZ: The kinin system and its relation to other systems. Curr Top Pathol 68:111, 1979.

Owen CH, Bowie EJW: The Intravascular Coagulation–Fibrinolysis Syndromes in Obstetrics and Gynecology. Kalamazoo, Mich., Upjohn, 1976.

Ratnoff O: The interrelationship of clotting factors and immunologic mechanism. *In* Good RA, Fisher DW (eds): Immunology. Stanford, Sinauer, 1971, p135.

Ryan GB, Majno G: Acute inflammation. A review. Am J Pathol 86:247, 1977.

Scibner DJ, Fahrney D: Neutrophil receptors of IgG and complement: their roles in the attachment and ingestion phases of phagocytosis. J Immunol 116:892, 1976.

Stossel TP: Phagocytosis. N Engl J Med 290:761,774,833, 1974.

Waksman BH: The distribution of experimental autoallergic lesions: its relation to the distribution of small veins. Am J Pathol 37:673, 1960.

Wilkinson PC, Lackie JM: The adhesion, migration and chemotaxis of leucocytes in inflammation. Curr Top Pathol 68:47, 1979.

23 | Drug Allergy

Allergic Mechanisms in Drug Reactions

The untoward or undesirable effects of a drug may be from overdosage, intolerance, idiosyncrasy, side effect, secondary effect, or allergic reaction to the drug (Table 23-1). Drug aller-

Table 23-1. Classification of Drug Reactions

Type	Definition
Overdose	Normal reaction to too much of the drug
Intolerance	Increased sensitivity to normal doses of the drug
Idiosyncrasy	Qualitatively abnormal pharmacological response, not a result of the normal pharmacological effect
Side effect	Normal, but not desired effect of a drug
Secondary effect	Normal, undesired effect of drug as a result of producing the desired effect
Allergic reaction	Reaction mediated by immune response to the drug

gies may be classified, on the basis of the immune mechanism involved, as neutralization or inactivation; cytotoxic; atopic or anaphylactic; immune complex (Arthus); or delayed hypersensitivity or granulomatous reactions. In some instances it is very difficult to differentiate drug allergy from idiosyncrasy. For instance, in patients with glucose-6-dehydrogenase deficiency, phenacetin may induce hemolytic anemia, which closely resembles allergic hemolytic anemia but is not due to antibody. Unless tests for antibody, such as the Coombs test, are positive, it may be impossible to prove an immune pathogenesis. Even if antibody is present, it does not necessarily prove that the patient's symptoms are due to an antibody to the drug.

Allergic reactions to drugs, therefore, include one or more of the immune mechanisms listed in Table 23-2. A given patient may express drug resistance due to neutralization or

551

Table 23-2. Allergic Reactions to Drugs

Mechanism	Manifestations	Examples
Neutralization	Resistance to therapy	Insulin, blood clotting factors, cancer chemotherapeutic agents, penicillin
Cytotoxic	Hemolysis, thrombocytopenia, agranulocytosis, purpura	Penicillin, quinidine, α-methyldopa, quinine
Immune complex	Exanthematous skin rashes, serum sickness, vasculitis, lupus syndrome, nephritis	Penicillin, serum, insulin, hydralazine, isoniazid, sulfa drugs, vaccines
Anaphylactic	Shock, urticaria, asthma, angioedema	Penicillin, antibiotics, cancer chemotherapeutic agents, vaccines
Delayed hypersensitivity	Dermatitis, toxic epidermal necrosis	Penicillin, antibiotics, etc.
Granulomatous	Granulomatous vasculitis, hepatitis	Penicillin, etc.

clearance of antigen–antibody complexes. The capacity of antibodies to drugs to neutralize the therapeutic effect of the drug has not received much attention, yet may be responsible for treatment failure. Clearly, antibodies may cause resistance to antibiotics, insulin, blood clotting factors, or other replacement therapy. In some instances antibody neutralization of a drug may be used to treat an overdose. The passive transfer of $F(ab)_2$ antibody to digitalis is effective in treatment of arrhythmias secondary to digitalis toxicity. Autoantibodies have been shown to inhibit a variety of other effector molecules including steroid hormones, catecholamines, histamine, serotonin, morphine, oxytocin, and vasopressin.

The most striking allergic drug reaction is anaphylactic shock, which occurs within a few seconds or minutes after exposure; less severe anaphylactic symptoms include urticaria and wheezing. Later urticarial reactions may be seen 2 to 48 hours after exposure. Historically, the first conception of an allergic reaction to a ''drug'' was the recognition of serum sickness following administration of horse anti-diphtheria toxin serum to humans with diphtheria. Serum sickness–like symptoms include fever, joint pains, urticaria, and proteinuria (immune complex nephritis). The most common allergic drug reactions are manifested in the skin: exanthematic, erythematous, and maculopapular rashes; urticaria; angioedema; serpiginous lesions; contact dermatitis; erythema multiforme; erythema nodosum; purpura; eczema; and fixed eruptions. Fixed eruptions appear in the same area of the skin each time the responsible drug is administered, and may be macular, eczematous, or bullous. The mechanism involved in fixed eruptions may be delayed hypersensitivity, immune complex, or anaphylactic, but, for as yet unknown reasons, the reaction occurs in the same place. Renal reactions associated with drug reactions include interstitial nephritis, tubular necrosis, membranous nephritis polyarteritis, and acute glomerulonephritis. Hemolytic reactions to drugs are presented in some detail in Chapter 15. Any allergic mechanism, including systemic delayed hypersensitivity and granulomatous reactions, may be found as a reaction to penicillin. Other drug allergies are described in Chapters 14 through 21 in relationship to the immunopathological mechanisms activated.

Sensitization to Drugs

Since drug allergies are manifestations of immunological responses, these reactions have the character of an immune reaction (Table 23-3). Although a clinical reaction is not usually

Table 23-3. Characteristics of Allergic Drug Reactions

1. No response to first exposure; can be reelicited once individual is sensitized.
2. Reaction elicited at doses far below therapeutic dose.
3. Manifestations reflect allergic mechanism and not pharmacological action of drug.
4. Only a small number of treated individuals develop allergic response.
5. Specific antibodies or lymphocytes reactive with drug demonstrable.

seen after the first exposure, often sensitization may occur because of exposure in food or another environmental source not realized by the patient. In addition, if drug therapy is continued over several weeks, or as in the case of serum sickness, if the drug persists in the body for several weeks, sensitization to the drug may occur during the period of first exposure. Reexposure results in a much more rapid and intense reaction and requires much less of the drug. Administration of the drug at low doses, under carefully controlled conditions, in an attempt to induce the suspected reaction is the most clinically reliable test for an allergic reaction. The most common reactions are to antibiotics such as semisynthetic penicillins, sulfa drugs, and erythromycins (Table 23-4). Other common agents are corticotropin and incompatible blood transfusions. The incidence of an allergic reaction to a drug in a patient without a previous history is less than 3% for drugs with the highest rates.

The mechanism of drug sensitization to large polypeptides is similar to that of other complete antigens (immunogens). However, many drugs are molecules that contain fewer than seven amino acids, have molecular weights less than 1000, and are not complete antigens. For the development of drug allergy some mechanism of covalent binding of the drug to an immunogenic carrier must occur. Such reactions are readily accomplished in vitro in the laboratory, but how this occurs in vivo is not clear. It is possible that some drugs may be metabolized in

Table 23-4. Allergic and Toxic Reactions to Some Commonly Used Antibiotics

Drugs	Disease	Contraindications	Untoward and Allergic Reactions
AMEBICIDES			
Chloroquine	Malaria, amebiasis	Psoriasis, pregnancy, G6PD deficiency	Shock, pleomorphic skin reactions, nausea, vomiting (hemolytic anemia)
ANTIBACTERIALS			
Nitrofurantoin	Urinary tract infections, enterococci, S. aureus, E. coli	Impaired renal function, pregnancy	Anaphylaxis, fever, pulmonary edema, exfoliative dermatitis, multiple skin reactions, asthma, hepatitis, anemia, etc.
Penicillin	Many bacterial infections	Hypersensitivity	Multiple skin rashes, serum sickness, anaphylaxis, hemolytic anemia, leukopenia, neuropathy, etc.
Trimethoprim–sulfamethoxazole	Broad spectrum	Hypersensitivity, pregnancy	Skin eruptions, serum sickness, anaphylaxis, arthralgia, myocarditis, anemia, thrombocytopenia, hepatitis diarrhea, polyneuritis, Stevens–Johnson, etc.
Tetracycline	Gram negatives, Rickettsia, mycoplasma, enterococci, etc.	Hypersensitivity, pregnancy, infants	Nausea, vomiting, renal toxicity, enterocolitis, skin eruptions, anaphylaxis, angioedema, pericarditis, SLE, serum sickness, hemolytic anemia, thrombocytopenia, neutropenia, eosinophilia, etc.
Cephalosporin	Broad spectrum, streptococci, S. aureus, H. influenzae, etc.	Hypersensitivity, impaired renal function	Pseudomembranous colitis, urticaria, skin rashes, eosinophilia
Gentamicin, kanamycin (aminoglycoside)	Broad spectrum	Hypersensitivity	Nephrotoxicity, neurotoxicity, various skin rashes, lethargy, anaphylaxis, fever, nausea, vomiting, anemia, alopecia, agranulocytosis
Chloramphenicol	Broad spectrum, used only when others are ineffective	Hypersensitivity, pregnancy, lactation	Bone marrow depression, nausea, vomiting, neurotoxicity, anaphylaxis, vasculitis, skin rashes
Erythromycin	Broad spectrum	Hypersensitivity	Nausea, vomiting, mild skin eruptions, anaphylaxis
Vancomycin	Gram-positive bacteria	Hypersensitivity	Nausea, fever, macular rashes, anaphylaxis, neutropenia, myalgia

Drug	Organism/Use	Contraindications	Adverse effects
ANTIFUNGALS			
Griseofulvin	*Microsporum, Epidermophyton, Trichophyton*	Liver disease, porphyria, hypersensitivity	Multiple skin rashes, urticaria, nausea, granulocytopenia, glomerulonephritis
Myastatin	*Candida*	Hypersensitivity	Relatively nontoxic; diarrhea, vomiting at high doses
MYCOBACTERIALS			
Isoniazid	Tuberculosis	Hypersensitivity	Hepatitis, peripheral neuropathy, neurotoxicity, nausea, vomiting, agranulocytosis, skin eruptions, vasculitis, SLE, rheumatoid arthritis
Rifampicin	Tuberculosis, *Neisseria*	Hypersensitivity, pregnancy	Various skin rashes, hepatitis, hemolytic anemia, thrombocytopenia, renal failure, nausea, vomiting
Streptomycin	Tuberculosis, various bacteria	Hypersensitivity, pregnancy	Vertigo, nausea, vomiting, fever, various skin rashes, hemolytic anemia, anaphylaxis, thrombocytopenia, agranulocytosis
Dapsone	Leprosy	Anemia, G6PD deficiency, hypersensitivity	Multiple cutaneous reactions, hemolytic anemia, neuropathy, nausea, vomiting, vertigo, SLE, glomerulonephritis
ANTIVIRAL			
Adenine arabinoside	Herpes simplex, herpes zoster	Hypersensitivity	Nausea, vomiting, anorexia, encephalopathy, mild skin rashes
Acyclovir	Herpes	Hypersensitivity	None (ointment), inflammation of injection site (IM)
HELMINTHS			
Piperazine	*Ascaris*, pinworm	Impaired liver or renal function, hypersensitivity	Neurotoxicity, nausea, vomiting, fever, skin rashes, arthralgia
Thiabendazole	*Strongyloides, Ascaris*	Hepatic or renal dysfunction, hypersensitivity	Neurotoxicity, nausea, vomiting, leukopenia, various skin rashes, Stevens–Johnson, mild abdominal discomfort, nausea, rare skin rash
Praziquantel	Schistosomiasis	Hypersensitivity, eye lesions	Mild malaise, rare urticaria

G6PD, glucose-6-phosphate dehydrogenase; SLE, systematic lupus erythematosus.
Data extracted from Physician's Desk Reference, Oradell, N.J., Medical Economics Company, 1985.

vivo to active intermediates that combine with host proteins, but this has not yet been clearly established as being chemically important. The best example of sensitization to drugs is penicillin.

Penicillin Allergy: The Epitome

Antibiotics are the drugs that most frequently cause allergic reactions (see Table 23-4). Allergy to penicillin is presented to exemplify antibiotic hypersensitivity. Penicillin is probably the most thoroughly studied drug responsible for producing allergic reactions, not only because it is so widely used but also because it produces a relatively high rate of sensitization. The reported frequency of anaphylactic reactions to penicillin ranges from 1 to 10 per 100,000 injections. The penicillin molecule contains a number of structures that can combine with amino, hydroxy, mercapto, disulfide, or histidine groups on macromolecules due to generation of a number of metabolites (Fig. 23-1). Most studies indicate that sensitization is due to the presence of preformed polymers, high molecular weight aggregates, or impurities present in manufactured penicillin preparations. In addition, presensitization to penicillin may occur from contamination of penicillin in food, particularly milk, or milk products, from cattle who have been fed grain containing penicillin. Penicillin is also present in a number of vaccines and could be responsible for sensitization via this vector.

Experimental studies have shown that a high epitope density (over 30 determinants per carrier molecule) is needed to induce an IgE antibody response to substituted serum albumin in rabbits, and similar densities are needed to induce delayed hypersensitivity to haptens on autologous carriers in guinea pigs. Thus it is unlikely that such immunogenic molecules could be manufactured from small drug haptens and that sensitization to drugs occurs in vivo in this manner. In fact, tolerance to free haptens may be more easily induced than an immune reaction. Penicillin itself may be immunogenic in animals when administered in adjuvants such as complete Freund's adjuvant or together with *Bordatella pertussis*. Complete immunogens may be produced by conjugation of penicillin with host proteins as a result of an adjuvant-induced granuloma or by penicilloylation of adjuvant components. However, high molecular weight contaminants or homopolymers are much more immunogenic than purified penicillin in any circumstances and are more likely to provide the immunogenic stimulus.

The route of application of penicillin is also important as a factor in sensitization. Intravascular and intramuscular exposure produces a low incidence of sensitization. However, topical application, particularly over an inflamed area, or nasal inhalation is associated with a much higher incidence of sensi-

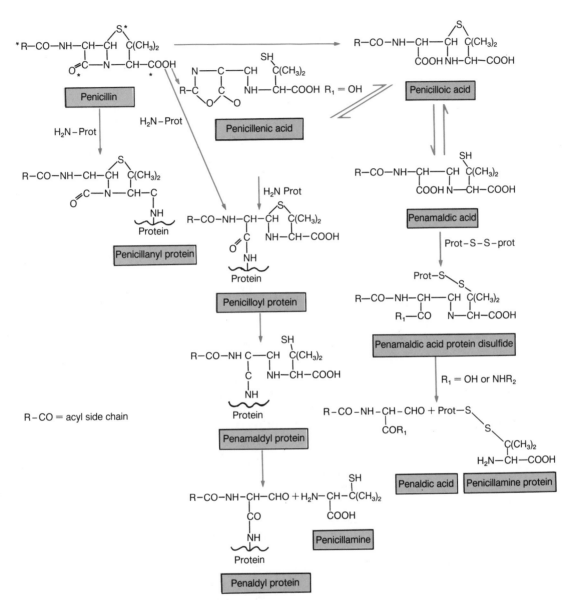

Figure 23-1. Reactive sites of the penicillin molecule and penicillin-derived antigens. Asterisks indicate the reactive sites of the parent penicillin compound. Major metabolic derivatives include penicilloyl compounds (formed by reaction of the β-lactam carbonyl). Homopolymers may be formed by reaction of penicilloyl with aminopenicillin; aminopenicillins contain an amino group that can react with the β-lactam carbonyl of penicilloyl. The penamaldyl and penaldyl determinants are formed from penicilloyl and may bind to proteins, but are of limited importance clinically. S-Penamaldate conjugates are formed from penicilloic and penillic acids, which are included in minor determinants in penicillin preparations. The use of ester prodrugs of penicillin allows the formation of penicilloyl derivatives. The penicilloyl determinant is considered to make the major contribution to penicillin allergy. Once sensitization has occurred to one haptenic form, cross-reactivity allows elicitation of an allergic reaction with other penicillin derivatives.

tization. This may be due to an adjuvant effect of the inflammation, to formation of immunogenic conjugates by bacterial metabolism of penicillin, or to action of inflammatory mediators.

The allergic manifestations of penicillin include each of the immunopathological mechanisms. Neutralization is not usually recognized as it is not usually discriminated from simple treatment failure, and granulomatous reactions are rare, but can occur. The incidence of other reactions to penicillin is given in Table 23-5. Pseudoallergic reactions due to release of

Table 23-5. Frequency of Allergic Reactions to Penicillin

Mechanism	Percentage of Penicillin Allergies
Hemolytic (lysis)	0.5
Immune complex (fever, vasculitis)	20
Anaphylactic (shock, urticaria)	10
Cellular (dermatitis, toxic epidermal necrosis)	0.5
Skin eruptions (?etiology): exanthems, erythema multiforme, purpura	69

bacterial toxins as the result of lysis of bacteria after penicillin treatment or secondary to inflammatory mediators may be responsible for a large number of penicillin reactions. The Jarisch–Herxheimer phenomenon, in which fever, chills, skin rash, edema, lymphadenopathy, and headache appear during the treatment of syphilis, is most likely due to the release of microbial "toxins" or antigens and will subside even if penicillin treatment is continued. This is not caused by an allergic reaction to penicillin but is due to the effects of release of microbial substances secondary to penicillin therapy.

One of the most striking reactions to penicillin is toxic epidermal necrosis. This reaction is characterized by erythema and detachment of skin resembling extensive scalding. It is an acute, life-threatening reaction. There is separation of the epidermis at the basal layer in the detached areas and necrosis and dyskeratosis of cells in the erythematous areas. Such patients demonstrate a positive delayed skin test or lymphocyte transformation to penicillin or to other drugs (phenobarbital, phenylbutazone) associated with this lesion. This is believed to represent an intense delayed reaction to the responsible drug.

Cases of suspected penicillin sensitivity are best detected by skin testing. However, many patients who react positively to skin testing with penicilloyl–lysine, the most frequently used test antigen, do not manifest systemic reactions when injected under controlled conditions with large (over 1,600,000 units) doses of penicillin. In addition, a negative skin test does not always rule out a positive systemic reaction to a larger dose. Even when symptoms consistent with an allergic reaction are obvious, it may be difficult to identify by antibody or skin testing the presence of immune reactivity. Therefore the results of skin testing must be interpreted with caution relative to an individual patient. If the test to penicilloyl–lysine is negative, reactions to other minor antigenic determinants must be tested using benzylpenicillin. In skin test–reactive patients, approximately 70% will demonstrate a wheal and flare reaction, 20% an Arthus reaction, and 10% a delayed reaction. If antibiotic treatment is required, another drug should be given to avoid a possibly serious allergic response to penicillin. However, in some instances, the nature of an infectious disease is such that no drug, other than penicillin, will be effective; yet the patient who requires penicillin treatment is allergic to penicillin.

If penicillin is considered essential, desensitization may be attempted. This is done by injecting small doses of penicillin (10 units) subcutaneously and gradually increasing the dose at 20-minute intervals over a 6-hour period to 400,000 units intramuscularly. Such patients usually tolerate this procedure, but care must be taken to treat anaphylactic shock. After desensitization, penicillin therapy may be continued for at least 6 weeks. The mechanism for desensitization is not clear. Desensitized patients become skin test negative, but demonstrate no change in IgE or IgG antibodies to penicillin.

Allergic Reactions to Cancer Chemotherapeutic Agents

Although clearly less frequent than allergic reactions to antimicrobial agents, the increased use of chemicals to treat cancer has led to an increased recognition of reactions to the drugs used. The reactions to some of the more frequently used chemotherapeutic drugs are given in Table 23-6. In most instances allergic reactions to most of these drugs are infrequent or very rare. The polypeptide L-asparaginase is the drug most likely to produce an allergic reaction, with a 1% mortality rate due to anaphylactic shock. A history of previous use, intravenous administration, and use without other drugs (prednisone, 6-mercaptopurine, and/or vincristine) are factors that increase the risk of allergic reactions to L-asparaginase. The presence of IgG antibodies to L-asparaginase reduces the effective level of the drug, protecting against an anaphylactic reaction, but reducing its effectiveness through a neutralization reaction.

Some drugs produce anaphylactoid reactions due to effects on mast cells not directly mediated through IgE antibody. Anaphylactic reactions due to IgE antibody as well as anaphylactoid reactions due to direct release of vasoactive mediators from mast cells have been found in 1% to 25% of cisplatin recipients, but no deaths from cisplatin allergy have been reported. Cisplatin may also be associated with neutralization and hemolytic reactions. Anthracyclin antibiotics (daunorubicin, doxorubicin, and aclarubicin) may produce severe anaphylactoid reactions on the first exposure, including shock or cardiac arrhythmias, due to direct action on mast cells.

Table 23-6. Allergic Reactions to Cancer Chemotherapeutic Agents

Drug	Type of Reaction	Risk
L-Asparaginase	Anaphylactic, neutralization, immune complex, hemolytic (very rare)	Appreciable
Cisplatin	Anaphylactic, nonspecific release of vasoactive agents, hemolytic	Appreciable
Melphalan	Anaphylactic	Appreciable (IV), infrequent (oral)
Methotrexate	Anaphylactic, immune complex	Infrequent
Bleomycin	Pyrogen release from neutrophils	Infrequent
Cyclophosphamide	Anaphylactic	Infrequent
Cytosine arabinoside	Anaphylactic, immune complex	Very rare
Chlorambucil	Anaphylactic	Very rare
Hydroxyurea	Pyrogen release	Very rare
5-Fluorouracil	Anaphylactic	Very rare
Mitomycin	Anaphylactic	Very rare

Modified from Weiss RB: Hypersensitivity reactions to cancer chemotherapy. In Perry MC, Yarbro JW (eds): Toxicity of Chemotherapy. New York, Grune & Stratton, 1984.

Unsuspected Drug Reactions to Contaminants

Clinically, reactions often are not to a drug itself, but to a contaminating substance in the drug preparation used. Certain vaccines produced in tissue culture may contain trace amounts of penicillin. Many other similar situations have been identified. For instance, in insulin allergy the reaction may be not to insulin but to zinc in the insulin preparation. Some patients develop reactions to insulin, manifested by delayed type hypersensitivity reactions at the injection site. Usually these are self limiting and resolve with continued insulin use. Cases of persistent reactions may be handled by changing to another insulin preparation. However, some patients have persistent reactions to different insulin preparations, due not to insulin but to zinc present in different insulin preparations.

Drug-Induced Lupus Erythematosus

Syndromes resembling systemic lupus erythematosus (SLE) are induced by several drugs including hydralazine, procainamide, isonicotinic acid, and penicillamine (see Chapter 17). The fully developed clinical picture includes arthritis resembling rheumatoid arthritis, fever, skin rashes, hepatomegaly, splenomegaly, and lymphadenopathy. The mechanism of drug-induced SLE is not clear. Antibodies to the drugs have not been shown to cause the syndrome. Antinuclear antibodies are found in many of these patients, suggesting that drug-induced alterations lead to sensitization to nuclear antigens. Since the syndrome goes away when the drug is withdrawn, it appears that drugs may alter nuclear components and that this process is reversible.

Summary

Allergic reactions to drugs include manifestations of each of the six immunopathological mechanisms. Treatment failure may result from rapid clearance of drug–antibody complexes to insulin, clotting factors, antibiotics, or cancer chemotherapeutic agents. Hemolytic anemia, thrombocytopenia, and agranulocytosis are associated with antibodies to many different drugs. Immune complex reactions are responsible for serum sickness–like reactions, inflammatory skin lesions, and glomerulonephritis. Anaphylactic reactions may cause death from shock minutes after drug exposure or produce urticaria and wheezing. Many drugs elicit delayed skin reactions upon injection. Although granulomatous reactions are rare, granulomatous arteritis or hepatitis is associated with exposure to some antibiotics.

Most drugs are small nonimmunogenic haptens that must be covalently bound to carriers to become immunogenic. Immunogenic forms may be present as contaminants in the drug preparation itself or may be found in small amounts in foods or other products (soap, dyes, etc.). Since many drugs also may produce unexpected pharmacological effects, it is often difficult to prove that an allergic mechanism is responsible for a given clinical reaction. Tests for antibodies of different classes and for delayed hypersensitivity (DTH) are often, but not always, associated with drug reactions. The presence of antibody or DTH does not necessarily prove an allergic mechanism for a drug reaction.

The most effective therapy for drug reactions is discontinuation of the drug. Epinephrine or steroids may be required to control severe reactions. Desensitization may be carried out if administration of a specific drug, such as penicillin, is considered essential for treatment of a patient who is allergic to the drug.

References

Drug Allergies

General

Baer RL, Witten VH: Drug eruptions. *In* Year Book of Dermatology. Chicago, Year Book Med, 1961.

Cluff LE, Johnson JE III: Drug fever. Prog Allergy 8:149, 1964.

de Weck AL: Drug reactions. *In* Sampter M (ed): Immunological Diseases, 2nd ed. Boston, Little, Brown, 1971, p415.

Girard JP, Cattin S, Cuevas M: Immunological mechanisms and diagnostic tests in allergic drug reactions. Ann Clin Res 8:74, 1976.

Jick H: Drug surveillance: the Boston Collaborative program. Hosp Pract 9:145, 1974.

Parker CW: Mechanisms of drug allergy. N Engl J Med 292:511, 1975.

Sherman WB: Drug allergy. South Med J 64:22, 1971.

Van Arsdel DP: Drug allergy: an update. Med Clin North Am 65:1089, 1981.

Penicillin

Ahlstedt S: Penicillin allergy — can the incidence be reduced? Allergy 39:151, 1984.

Ahlstedt S, Kristofferson A: Immune mechanisms for induction of penicillin allergy. Prog Allergy 30:67, 1982.

Graybill JR, et al: Controlled penicillin anaphylaxis leading to desensitization. South Med J 67:62, 1974.

Levine BB: Immunochemical mechanisms involved in penicillin hypersensitivity in experimental animals and in human beings. Fed Proc 24:45, 1965.

Levine BB, Zolov DM: Prediction of penicillin allergy by immunological tests. J Allergy 43:231, 1969.

Naclerio RM, Mizrahie A, Adkinson NF: Immunologic observations during desensitization and in evidence of clinical tolerance to penicillin. J Allergy Clin Immunol 7:294, 1983.

Tagami H, et al: Delayed hypersensitivity in ampicillin-reduced toxic epidermal necrolysis. Arch Dermatol 119:910, 1983.

Voss HE, Redmond AP, Levine BB: Clinical detection of the potential allergic reaction to penicillin by immunologic tests. JAMA 196:679, 1966.

Cancer Chemotherapy

Weiss RB: Hypersensitivity reactions to cancer chemotherapeutic agents. Ann Intern Med 94:66, 1981.

Weiss RB: Hypersensitivity reactions to cancer chemotherapy. *In* Pevy MC, Yarbro JW (eds): Toxicity of Chemotherapy. Orlando, Fla., Grune & Stratton, 1984, p101.

Drug-Induced Lupus Erythematosus

Blomgren SE: Drug-induced lupus erythematosus. Semin Hematol 10:345, 1973.

Seigal M, Lee SL, Peress NS: The epidemiology of drug-induced systemic lupus erythematosus. Arthritis Rheum 10:407, 1967.

Weinstein A: Drug-induced systemic lupus erythematosus. Prog Clin Immunol 4:1, 1980.

PART 3

IMMUNITY

Immunity is protection against or exemption from a given deleterious action or effect. The same immune mechanisms that are responsible for the diseases discussed in the preceding section (immunopathology) also mediate specific resistance to infection (acquired immunity) (see table on following page). Thus immune mechanisms are "double-edged swords," protecting against infectious diseases on the one hand, and causing tissue damage and disease on the other hand. These immune mechanisms most likely evolved, and were selected for, as a means of protection from the destructive effects of parasitic organisms and their products or as a means of resisting the growth of neoplastic cells (see Chapter 29).

Immunopathology and Immunity

Immune Effector Mechanism	Destructive Reaction "Allergy"	Protective Function "Immunity"	Protective Immunity Examples
Neutralization	Insulin resistance, pernicious anemia, myasthenia gravis, hyperthyroidism	Toxin neutralization, blockade of virus receptors	Diphtheria, tetanus, cholera, botulism
Cytotoxic	Hemolysis, leukopenia, thrombocytopenia	Bacteriolysis, opsonization	Bacterial infection, staphylococci, streptococci, etc.
Immune complex	Vasculitis, glomerulonephritis, serum sickness, rheumatoid diseases	Acute inflammation, opsonization, polymorphonuclear leukocyte activation	Bacterial infections, staphylococci, streptococci, pneumococci, etc.
Anaphylactic	Asthma, urticaria, anaphylactic shock, hay fever	Focal inflammation, increased vascular permeability, increased gastrointestinal secretion and motility, expulsion of inhaled organisms by sneezing	Intestinal parasites, bacterial infections
Delayed hypersensitivity	Contact dermatitis, autoallergies, viral exanthems, postvaccinial encephalomyelitis	Intracellular parasites, destructon of virus-infected cells, immune surveillance of tumors	Tuberculosis, syphilis, herpes simplex, smallpox
Granulomatous	Berylliosis, sarcoidosis	Isolation of organisms in granulomas	Tuberculosis, filariasis, schistosomiasis, leprosy, helminths, fungi

Modified from Sell S: Introduction to symposium on immunopathology: "Immune Mechanisms in Disease." Hum Pathol 9:24, 1978.

24 | Immune Resistance to Infection

Reactions to Infectious Agents

Innate Immunity

Human survival depends upon an ability to resist a wide variety of infections (viral, bacterial, fungal, others). As presented in Chapter 1, the mechanisms of resistance include nonspecific innate characteristics and specific immune reactions. The skin and mucous membranes represent mechanical barriers to invasion by infectious agents. Each species also has inherent internal resistance to many infectious agents by virtue of such factors as pH, temperature, and metabolic products. These factors are immunologically nonspecific in that they operate against antigenically unrelated agents. Other factors that inhibit growth of infectious agents may be released by certain cells after stimulation. Interferons are examples of soluble substance induced by a variety of stimulatory events that inhibit or interfere with viral infections. In addition to this innate resistance, which does not require previous contact with the specific infectious agent, there is an acquired immunity dependent upon specific immune mechanisms.

Acquired Immunity

A specific immunity usually follows recovery from an infectious disease. The primary infection results in a state of decreased susceptibility to a subsequent attack by the organism that was responsible. This is a naturally developing state of specific active immunity (acquired immunity). Resistance to an antigenically unrelated organism is not affected. Prophylactically specific acquired immunity may be induced intentionally by immunization (see Chapter 25).

Specific active immunity is mediated through immunoglobulin antibody or cellular sensitivity. The importance of these immune mechanisms in maintaining the integrity of the person is best illustrated by those diseases in which immune reactions are depressed or absent (see Chapter 26). Such immune-deficient persons are unable to mount a defense against a variety of infectious agents that usually cause no disease or

565

symptoms in individuals with normal immune capacity. The type of protective mechanism differs with different infectious agents (Table 24-1). In general, the mechanisms mediated by

Table 24-1. Major Immune Defense Mechanisms for Infectious Diseases

Type of Infection	Major Immune Defense Mechanism
Bacterial	Antibody
Viral	Delayed and antibody
Mycobacterial	Granulomatous (delayed)
Protozoal	Delayed and antibody
Worms	Anaphylactic and granulomatous
Fungal	Delayed (granulomatous)

humoral antibody (immunoglobulin) are effective against infectious agents that exist extracellularly, whereas cellular mediated reactions (delayed hypersensitivity and granulomatous reactions) are effective against intracellular parasites.

Natural Immunity

Antibodies to certain infectious agents appear in the sera of "normal" persons who have had no known contact with the antigen. The formation of "natural" antibodies most likely results from contact with cross-reacting antigens in intestinal flora, contact with ingested organisms in food, or subclinical infections. Such natural antibodies are usually of the IgM class of immunoglobulin and are often directed against organisms found in the gastrointestinal tract (enteric bacteria).

Specific Protective Immunity to Infection

The immune mechanisms responsible for protection against infectious agents are the same mechanisms responsible for immune-mediated disease. In this chapter the effect of immune mechanisms in defense against infection is presented in general, and then the contrasting role in protection and pathogenesis of the different immune effector mechanisms in selected specific infections is described. The selected infections—tetanus, malaria, rheumatic fever, allergic bronchopulmonary aspergillosis, smallpox, leprosy, syphilis, filariasis, and strongyloides—are chosen to illustrate how immune mechanisms protect against infection but also cause disease: the "double-edged sword" of immunopathology.

Bacterial Infections

Specific immunity to the destructive effects of bacteria or bacterial products is usually mediated by humoral antibody. The mechanisms of antibody-mediated protection against bacterial infections are illustrated in Figure 24-1. Some bacteria produce disease not by direct effects of the organism but by the release of products called *toxins*, which may have severe destructive effects distant from the site of infection. Destructive bacterial toxins are rendered harmless by reaction with antibody (neu-

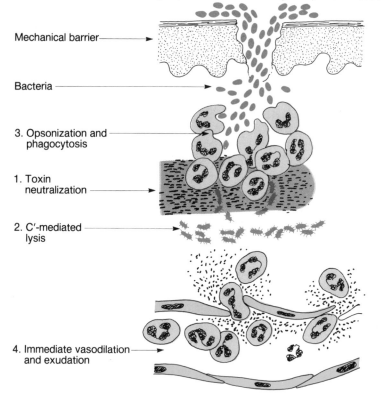

Figure 24-1. Antibody-mediated mechanisms of protection against bacterial infections. Bacterial infections may be resisted by each of the antibody-mediated immune mechanisms, including (1) neutralization of bacterial toxins, (2) cytotoxic lysis by antibody and complement, (3) acute polymorphonuclear infiltration (Arthus reaction) and opsonization of bacteria leading to increased phagocytosis, and (4) acute anaphylactic vascular events permitting immediate exudation of inflammatory cells and fluids.

tralization reaction). Destruction of infecting organisms is accomplished by the activation of complement following the reaction of antibody with the organism. This leads to increased susceptibility of the organism to phagocytosis (toxic complex reaction) or destruction by lysis (cytotoxic reaction). Enhanced states of phagocytosis (see Activated Macrophages, Chapter 12) may increase the effectiveness of antibody-mediated protection. Activation of mast cells by IgE-mediated reactions serves to increase vascular permeability (endothelial cell contraction), permitting egress of bloodborne antibody or inflammatory cells into the site of infection.

Viral Infections

Immune resistance to viral infections is mediated mainly by cellular sensitivity, but humoral antibody also plays a role by preventing virus from attaching to cell receptors (Fig. 24-2). Viruses live within the host's cells, and can spread from cell to cell without contacting extracellular fluid. To be effective in attacking intracellular organisms, an immune mechanism must have the capacity to react with cells in solid tissue. This is a general property of cell-mediated reactions, but not of antibody-mediated reactions. Many cells infected with a virus will, at some stage of the infection, express viral antigens on the cell surface. It is at this stage that specifically sensitized cells can

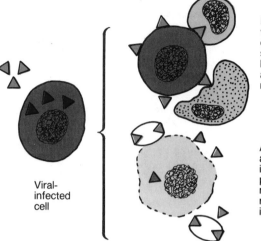

Figure 24-2. Cellular and antibody-mediated mechanisms of protection against viral infections. Sensitized lymphocytes may destroy virus-infected cells that express viral antigens on the surface, whereas antibody can react with released viral particles and prevent their attachment to uninfected cells, thus inhibiting spread of the infection.

Destruction of virus-infected cell by sensitized lymphocyte or activated macrophage

Antibody prevents attachment of infective viral particles to new cells when released from infected cell

Viral-infected cell

recognize and destroy the virus-infected cell either by direct killing or by attraction and activation of macrophages. Adverse effects of this reaction occur if the cell expressing the viral antigens is important functionally, as is the case for certain viral infections of the central nervous system (see Chapter 19). Humoral antibody can prevent the entry of virus particles into cells by interfering with the ability of the virus to attach to a host cell, and secretory IgA immunoglobulin antibody can prevent the establishment of viral infections of mucous membranes. However, once the virus is within cells, it is not susceptible to the effects of antibody. Patients with deficiencies in antibody production alone usually do not have serious viral infections but develop life-threatening bacterial infections. Patients with defects in delayed hypersensitivity develop serious virus infections (see Chapter 26).

Mycobacterial Infections

Mycobacterial infections such as tuberculosis and leprosy are resisted by cellular mechanisms, including granulomatous hypersensitivity. At one time it was thought that the disease of tuberculosis required the effect of delayed hypersensitivity. The term hypersensitivity was coined because animals with cellular immune reactivity to tubercle bacilli developed greater tissue lesions after inoculation than did animals injected for the first time. The granulomatous lesions seen in tuberculosis do depend upon immune mechanisms for their formation. However, these lesions are not really the cause of the disease but an unfortunate effect of the protective mechanisms; the granulomatous inflammatory reaction to the infective mycobacteria results in destruction of normal tissue. In the lung, for instance, extensive damage may be done by the formation of large granulomas in response to a tuberculosis infection, resulting in cavitation or in respiratory failure. The granulomatous immune response produces the lesion, but the mycobacterium causes the disease.

Protozoal Infections

The mechanism of protection against protozoal infections, as with viral infections, depends on the location of the agent in the host. Protozoa are unicellular organisms that may be located intracellularly, extracellularly in the blood, both intracellularly and in the blood, or primarily in the gastrointestinal tract. Intracellular protozoans such as *Leishmania* are eliminated by delayed and granulomatous reactions similar to the response evoked by leprosy. In certain types of leishmaniasis the organism is limited to focal inflamed areas of the skin. This response has histologic characteristics of a delayed hypersensitivity reaction. If this delayed hypersensitivity is lost, dissemination of the organisms may occur. Trypanosomiasis is an example of a bloodborne extracellular parasite that may also be found intracellularly; the major defense appears to be via humoral antibody. Malaria protozoa multiply intracellularly, but disseminate through release into the bloodstream. Malarial immunity is mediated by IgG antibody, which can effectively attack the blood-borne organism but is not effective against the intracellular stage. Therefore, humoral immunity is effective only during a short period of the malarial protozoal life cycle. Even highly immune infected persons may be unable to clear the parasites completely because of the inability of antibody to affect the intracellular stages. The number of organisms present in the body may be controlled by antibody, and the host lives in balance with his/her infection. Preventive immunity to malaria may be mediated by antibodies to the sporozoite form introduced by the mosquito vector or by preventing initial infection of hepatocytes (see below for details). *Entamoeba histolytica* is an intestinal protozoan infection of man. Although antibodies are produced, the protective effect of these antibodies remains to be demonstrated.

Helminth (Worm) Infections

The response to worm infections also depends on the location of the agent. Worms are located in the intestinal tract and/or tissues. Tapeworms, which exist only in the intestinal lumen, promote no protective immunological response. On the other hand, worms with larval forms that invade tissue do stimulate an immune response. The tissue reaction to *Ascaris* and *Trichinella* consists of an intense infiltration of polymorphonuclear leukocytes, with a predominance of eosinophils. Anaphylactic antibodies (IgE) are also frequently associated with helminth infections, and intradermal injection of worm extracts elicits a wheal and flare reaction. Children infested with *Ascaris lumbricoides* have attacks of urticaria, asthma, and other anaphylactic or atopic types of reactions presumably associated with dissemination of *Ascaris* antigens. An eosinophilic pulmonary infiltrate (pneumonia) may be found associated with migration of helminth larvae through the lung. The possible protective role of anaphylactic sensitivity is not clear, but it has been found in experimental models that expulsion of parasitic worms from the gastrointestinal tract occurs following the induction of peristalsis and diarrhea from intestinal anaphylactic reactions to worms.

Fungal Infections

Cellular immunity appears to be the most important immunologic factor in resistance to fungal infections, although humoral antibody certainly may play a role. The importance of cellular reactions is indicated by the intense mononuclear infiltrate and granulomatous reactions that occur in tissues infected with fungi and by the fact that fungal infections are frequently associated with depressed immune reactivity of the delayed type (opportunistic infections). *Chronic mucocutaneous candidiasis* refers to persistent or recurrent infection by *Candida albicans* of mucous membranes, nails, and skin. Patients with this disease generally have a form of immune deviation, that is, a depression of cellular immune reactions with high levels of humoral antibody, similar to lepromatous leprosy.

Insect Stings

Immune reactions to insect stings are generally believed to be responsible for most of the irritating skin reactions that follow. Individuals vary markedly in their immune reactions to insect stings. Clearly, the reaction of a given person to an insect sting depends on the dominant type of immune response. Most people react to insect stings, including mosquito bites, by acute cutaneous anaphylactic reactions, and desensitization or hyposensitization can be achieved. Systemic shock and death from wasp or bee stings, while infrequent, may develop in hyperreactive individuals. Two possible protective functions of anaphylactic reactions to insect stings are possible: (1) immediate avoidance behavior by the recipient serves to reduce antigen contact, and (2) anaphylactic reactions may help prevent toxic complex reactions or delayed hypersensitivity reactions. Since potentially fatal anaphylactic reactions require much less antigen contact than other allergic reactions, the latter mechanism seems unlikely. In fact, hyposensitization via the production of blocking IgG antibodies is attempted clinically to reduce the possibility of anaphylactic reactions to insect bites (see Chapter 18). An anaphylactic reaction to insect stings may be protective in producing avoidance behavior. However, in all likelihood, anaphylactic reactions to insect bites are not protective reactions but examples of potentially protective immune reactions being applied inappropriately.

Summary of Role of Immune Mechanisms in Protection Against Infections

From the preceding discussion, it can be appreciated that each of the six types of allergic reactions responsible for immune disease also has important functions in resistance to infection.

1. Neutralization of inactivation of biologically active toxins by antibodies is highly desirable. This is precisely what is accomplished by immunization with diphtheria toxoid.
2. Cytotoxic or cytolytic reactions are directed against the infecting organisms, leading to their death or lysis.
3. The inflammatory effect of antigen–antibody complexes in the Arthus mechanism results in stickiness of leukocytes, platelets, and endothelium and increases permeability. These effects promote defense by localization and diapedesis of leukocytes. At the dose level of a usual infection, this effect is not harmful to the host. Precipitating antibody and complement, as means of enhancing phagocytosis (opsonization), are responsible for protection against many bacterial infections.
4. The effect of histamine release (the anaphylactic mechanism) at the usual dose level results in slight vasodilation and increased capillary permeability, both effects interpreted in classic pathology as aiding defense. Smooth muscle contraction and diarrhea induced by the anaphylactic mechanism may cause expulsion of intestinal parasites.
5. Delayed hypersensitivity at the dose level occurring in infection results in local mobilization and activation of phagocytes and effective destruction of infecting agents.
6. Granulomatous hypersensitivity may serve to isolate or localize insoluble toxic materials or organisms.

Immune Effector Mechanisms in Specific Infections

Neutralization: Tetanus

Tetanus is caused by a highly fatal endoneurotoxin (tetanospasmin) released by the anerobic gram-negative bacillis *Clostridium tetani*. Tetanus toxin is synthesized as a single polypeptide chain of MW 150,000. Upon secretion, cleavage by a *C. tetani* "nickase" results in a two-chain molecule joined by a single disulfide bond, with a heavy chain of MW approximately 100,000 and a light chain of MW 50,000. The heavy chain is able to bind to cell surface gangliosides and is taken into the cell. In the cell the light chain is cleaved by cellular enzymes to produce a peptide fragment that blocks an elongation factor (EF2) required for protein synthesis. One activated light chain is able to block all EF2 activity in a cell. This effectively destroys, inhibits, or blocks protein synthesis and the function of the cell.

Spore forms of the organism are ubiquitous in soil and can infect a seemingly trivial wound. Natural defenses are essentially limited to local healing processes. The organisms multiply locally and produce endotoxin. The endotoxin is released when organisms are destroyed in the necrotic wound tissue, and travels via the blood or by retrograde axonal transmission to the spinal cord. The toxin increases reflex excitability in motor neurons by blocking the function of inhibitory neurons. This results in rigidity and reflex spasms, with death most often due to respiratory failure. The incubation period is usually less than 14 days. The length of the incubation period is critical in determining the outcome (60% fatality if less than 9 days; 25% if greater than 9 days).

The major immune defense mechanism of the host is neutralization of the toxin by specific antibody that blocks binding of the toxin to neurons (Fig. 24-3). Unfortunately in the natural

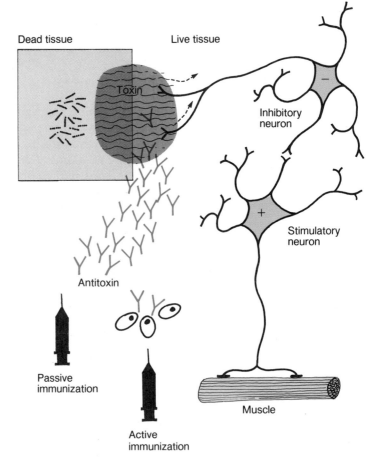

Figure 24-3. Neutralization of tetanus toxin by antitoxin. Antitoxin blocks entry of toxin into neurons. *Clostridium tetani* releases endotoxin when the organisms die in necrotic tissue. The endotoxin is taken up by axons and delivered to nerve cells, where it inactivates protein synthesis. The loss of activity of inhibitory neurons permits hyperactivity of stimulatory neurons and muscle spasm. Antitoxin provided by active or passive immunization prevents toxin from reaching inhibitory neurons.

infection, the potency of the toxin is so great that even fatal doses of tetanospasmin are not usually sufficient to stimulate antibody production. However, in high-incidence countries such as Ethiopia up to 30% of adults have toxin-neutralizing antibody, presumably from natural exposure. Since the organism cannot survive in living tissue because it is anaerobic, *C. tetani* benefits if the infected individual dies, at which point the entire body can be colonized. Primary therapy is directed toward keeping the wound clean and debrided to avoid the anaerobic conditions favoring growth of *C. tetani.* Secondary therapy is to neutralize tetanospasmin by antibody.

In 1890 von Behring and Kitasato demonstrated protective immunization using repeated small doses of tetanus toxin. Their report included the finding that the protection was due to a new factor present in the serum of immunized individuals *(antitoxin).* This classic report laid the foundation for subsequent development of immunoprophylaxis of infectious diseases using bacterial products. Antitoxin produced in horses was prepared and used to treat patients with tetanus or those with wounds that could accommodate *C. tetani.* Unfortunately, treated patients often developed another serious disease, serum sickness, caused by production of antibody to the horse antitoxin (see Chapter 16).

In 1925 Ramon introduced chemically modified toxin *(toxoid)* for active immunization. Active immunization with toxoid has greatly reduced the incidence of tetanus. Humans have taken advantage of the potential provided by nature to activate specific immunoprevention. It should be noted that antibodies directed against the *C. tetani* itself would not be useful, since the organism lives only in dead tissue and antibody cannot reach the site of infection. Although the number of cases in the United States has been drastically reduced because of an active immunization program, there are still about 200 cases per year.

For toxin to be active it must be internalized into the neuron, presumably at the axon level. Antitoxin binding to toxin prevents entry of the toxin into the cell. This may be accomplished by alteration of the tertiary structure of the toxin molecule. Once the toxin is bound to the neuron or internalized, antitoxin is ineffective. Neutralization of tetanus toxin is a powerful, specific, and effective mechanism of protection. Artificial immunization with tetanus toxoid provides prolonged, but not permanent protection. Defenses must be boosted by immunization if exposure to toxin is expected (see Chapter 25).

Cytotoxicity: Malaria

Hippocrates first recognized different types of malaria by different periods of fever. During the middle ages the disease was attributed to bad air, *"malair"* (Torti, 1753). Although the role of immune mechanisms in the pathogenesis of malaria is incompletely understood, IgG antibodies appear to play an important part through the activation of cytotoxicity directed against the infected host cells (Fig. 24-4). In endemic areas, natives develop resistance to malarial strains that is associated with specific humoral antibodies. Neonates in endemic areas are resistant as a result of placentally transferred maternal anti-

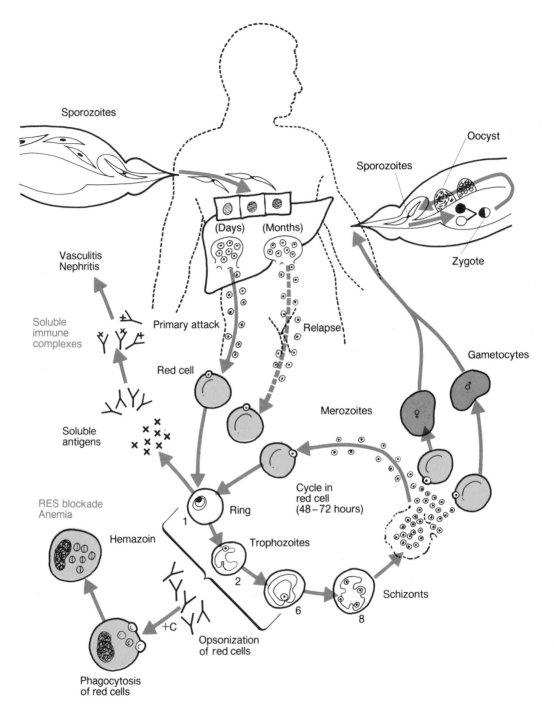

body. A peak of susceptibility occurs at about 1 year of age. However, infection at this age is less severe than in persons who first contract infection as adults. Malaria organisms exist primarily within erythrocytes during an established infection.

◀ **Figure 24-4.** Immune mechanisms in malaria. Malaria is transmitted from the salivary glands of mosquito to the blood by sporozoites that enter host liver cells and develop into intracellular stages. Merozoites are released into the circulation and reinfect other liver cells and red blood cells. Micro- and macrogamites are produced, which are taken up by mosquitos where they develop, after fusion and formation of an oocyst in the stomach, into sporozoites. Malaria antigens are found not only in organisms, but also on the surface of infected cells. Antibodies to these antigens are able to lyse organisms or infected cells, producing anemia or liver cell necrosis. Soluble antibody–antigen complexes formed may produce immune complex lesions (glomerulonephritis). The production of large numbers of opsonized red cells and particulate antigen results in accumulation of phagocytosed material in macrophages (hemazoin pigment), reticuloendothelial blockade, and immune dysfunction. Malarial organisms are able to change antigens expressed on the cell surface, avoid destruction by antibody, and set up another cycle of infection (antigenic variation). Protective immunity may be effected by antibodies to sporozoites, which prevent infection. Protective immunity could be mediated by antibody directed to extracellular stages: (1) sporozoites, (2) merozoites, (3) zygotes. (Modified from Brown HW: Basic Clinical Parasitology, 3rd ed. New York, Appleton–Century–Crofts, 1969; and Miller, *In* Greenwalt and Jamieson (eds): Transmissible Disease and Blood Transfusion. New York, Grune & Stratton, 1975.

Whereas antibody is a protective response in malaria, it is also responsible for many lesions of the disease (Table 24-2). Some

Table 24-2. Protective and Destructive Effects of Antibodies in Malaria

PROTECTIVE

Block infection of cells
Opsonization of organisms
Antibody-mediated lysis of organisms
Lysis of infected cells

DESTRUCTIVE

Autoerythrocyte antibody (anemia)
Immune complexes (nephritis, vasculitis)
Erythrophagocytosis (reticuloendothelial system blockade)
Immunoevasive mechanisms (antigenic variation)

of the major manifestations of malaria (anemia, fever, nephritis, and vasculitis) appear to be associated with an antibody-mediated cytotoxic, or immune complex reaction. The erythrocytes of patients with malaria become coated with IgG or IgM and have an increased susceptibility to phagocytosis and destruction by splenic macrophages. The macrophages in the spleen and liver may be loaded with malaria pigment (hemazoin) from phagocytosed and degraded red blood cells. Although this reaction may help to eliminate infected cells, it also contributes to the anemia. During malarial paroxysms, parasites are released from intracellular (intraerythrocyte) locations, resulting in the formation of immune complexes in antigen excess. Glomerulonephritis, the nephrotic syndrome, and multiple vasculitides are presumed to be consequences.

Finally, the preoccupation of macrophages with erythrophago-cytosis may contribute to the immunosuppression observed in association with malaria.

The ability to produce an effective vaccine against malaria is complicated by species-specific antigens, by the stage-specific antigens that are produced during the malarial life cycle, and by antigenic variation during infection. Different species of malaria have different antigens, so that antibody to one malarial species may not protect against other species. In addition, antibodies blocking one stage of infection are not effective at another. In endemic areas adults resistant to malaria infection have antibodies to blood stages as well as to sporozoite antigens. It has been possible to induce effective preventative immunity using irradiated sporozoites but not with blood stages. However, it is not feasible to produce anywhere near the numbers of sporozoites, which require culture in infected mosquitos, needed to prepare a practical vaccine. Recently it has been shown that different malarial species share a common sporozoite antigen demonstrated by reaction of antibodies to the sporozoite. This antigen consists of 12 tandem repeated subunits of 12 amino acids. As visualized by electron microscopy, antibody not only causes the whole surface of the sporozoite to appear rough, but also induces a tail-like precipitate that extends a considerable distance from the organism. This is termed the *circumsporate* (CSP) reaction. Immunization with this antigen and passive transfer of monoclonal antibodies to this antigen have resulted in effective protective immunity in animals. Using gene cloning techniques the complementary DNA (cDNA) for the 12-amino acid (12-AA) dodecapeptide antigen has been prepared, and trials of vaccination using circumsporate antigen produced by vector-translated cDNA are now underway. Antibodies to the sporozoite antigen act by preventing establishment of malarial infection following inoculation of sporozoites by infected mosquitos. Another possibility is to immunize to micro- and macrogametes. If these antibodies were present in an individual bitten by a mosquito, they could prevent infections of the mosquito by micro- and macrogametes present in the blood of other infected individuals, and thus prevent spread of malaria.

In Summary

1. Cytotoxic mechanisms appear responsible for major immune reaction against malaria-infected erythrocytes, leading to destruction of red blood cells as well as deposition of pigment in the reticuloendothelial system (RES), formation of immune complexes during secondary lesions, and immunosuppression.

2. Antigenic variation of blood stages of malaria and variation in antigens in blood stages of different malarial species pro-

vide barriers in development of an effective vaccine to these stages.

3. Antibodies to sporozoites may provide protection immunity by blocking infection of liver cells, but are not effective naturally (too late). Sporozoite antigen produced by cloned DNA is now being tested in clinical trials.

4. Human antibodies to micro- and macrogametes could provide passive immunity in mosquitos and prevent spread of malaria.

Immune Complex: Rheumatic Fever

Rheumatic fever is an acute systemic sequel to infection caused by Group A β-hemolytic streptococci (see Chapter 17). Although antistreptococcal antibodies neutralize toxins and opsonize organisms, lesions are believed to result from the formation of antibodies produced to streptococcal antigens, which cross-react with antigens present in the tissues of the host (molecular mimicry) (Fig. 24-5). Antibodies to a number of

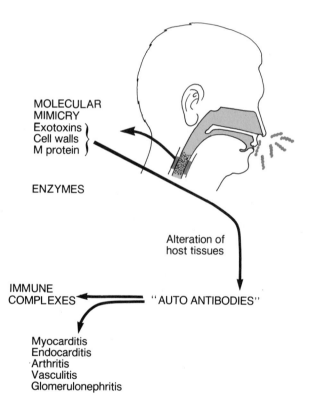

Figure 24-5. The immune response to streptococcal group A antigens and rheumatic fever. Antibodies produced to streptococcal antigens cross-react with host tissue antigens. These "autoantibodies" as well as soluble immune complexes are responsible for the lesions of rheumatic fever (myocarditis, endocarditis, arthritis, vasculitis, and glomerulonephritis).

streptococcal antigens are found in the serum (see Chapter 17). Because antistreptococcal M protein antibodies cross-react with heart muscle, they may be responsible for carditis; T cell cytotoxic activity for myocardial cells may also play a role. Some patients with rheumatic fever develop involuntary and irregular jerking movements (St. Vitus' dance, chorea). The chorea of rheumatic fever has been associated with autoantibodies to basal ganglia, which can be absorbed with streptococcal cell walls. Other lesions of rheumatic fever are most likely the result of immune complex formation, in particular erythema marginatum (vaculitis in the dermis) and glomerulonephritis. Rheumatic nodules are small, rubbery granulomas and most likely the end result of vasculitis caused by the deposition of immune complexes containing antigens resistant to degradation, leading to accumulation of macrophages and the formation of granulomas. The major chronic effect of rheumatic endocarditis is scarring of the heart valves, particularly the mitral and aortic valves (healed rheumatic endocarditis). Healed rheumatic endocarditis is still a major cause of deformation of heart valves requiring surgery. Antibodies to streptococcal products serve to inactivate streptococcal organisms and products as well as to initiate acute protective inflammatory reactions (immune complex mechanism). Cross-reaction of antistreptococcal antibodies with host tissues and formation of soluble complexes of antibodies and streptococcal antigens may cause immune complex–mediated inflammatory reactions distant from the site of infection.

Anaphylaxis: Allergic Bronchopulmonary Aspergillosis

Anaphylactic reactions to fungal or bacterial antigens are not uncommon and may be responsible for some acute asthmatic attacks and dermal reactions. For example, several laundry detergents contain enzymes from *Bacillus subtilis*, which may elicit acute allergic reactions. A more serious problem is allergic reaction to fungi in the tracheobronchial flora (e.g., *Aspergillus fumigatus*).

The syndrome of allergic bronchopulmonary aspergillosis includes wheezing, fever, occasional expectoration of golden-brown plugs that contain mycelia, systemic eosinophilia, elevated serum IgE concentrations, and the presence of antibodies to *Aspergillus* spp. in the serum. The syndrome is caused by prolonged anaphylactic reactions to *Aspergillus* antigens (Fig. 24-6). Allergic aspergillosis most likely begins with the inhalation and trapping of aspergillal conidia in the viscous secretions present in the bronchi of an asthmatic. The spores germinate and form mycelia; antigens released from mycelia react with IgE on mast cells in the bronchial walls, resulting in greatly increased mucus secretion and bronchospasm. Allergic bronchopulmonary aspergillosis differs from most other forms of asthma in that the supply of inciting antigen is continuously replenished by replication within the bronchi and bronchioles. Anaphylactic reaction to *Aspergillus* in bronchi may lead to formation of mucus plugs containing fungi, may produce protracted construction of bronchial smooth muscle, and may cause death by asphyxiation.

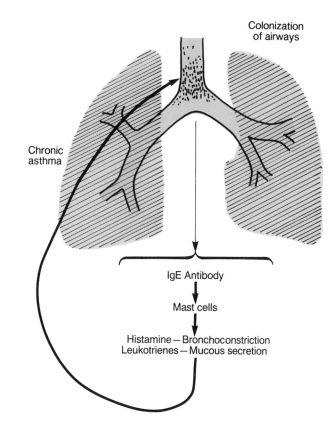

Figure 24-6. Allergic bronchopulmonary aspergillosis. Anaphylactic reaction to aspergillus infection in the bronchi causes secondary pathological effects leading to repeated asthmatic attacks and plugging of airways with thick mucus plugs.

The criteria for diagnosis of allergic bronchopulmonary aspergillosis are listed in Table 24-3. Almost all affected patients will react with a wheal and flare skin response to dermal injection of *Aspergillus* antigens (IgE). Many patients also have precipitating IgG antibodies and may have pulmonary vasculitis presumably due to immune complexes. Nonallergic patients may develop *Aspergillus* infections that usually present as single

Table 24-3. Major and Minor Diagnostic Criteria in 50
Patients with Allergic Bronchopulmonary Aspergilloses

Criteria	Number of patients fulfilling criteria
MAJOR	
Recurrent pulmonary densities	50
Eosinophilia of sputum and blood	50
Asthma	50
Allergy to *Aspergillus fumigatus*	50
MINOR	
Recovery of *A. fumigatus*	34
A. fumigatus antibody in serum	44
History of recurrent pneumonia	43
History of mucous plugs in sputum	33

lesions (fungus ball) in areas of previously damaged lung tissue. Invasive aspergillosis in which mycelia actually extend into tissue is different from allergic bronchopulmonary aspergillosis and is seen in patients with immune deficiency diseases.

Delayed Hypersensitivity

Smallpox

As presented in Chapter 19, the development of delayed hypersensitivy is responsible for protective active immunity against smallpox, as well as to other viral exanthems such as measles and chicken pox. Vaccination against smallpox is accomplished by inoculation into the skin of a related virus (vaccinia) that usually produces only a local lesion. The local lesion, called a *take*, is produced by a delayed hypersensitivity reaction to viral antigens that are shared with the virulent smallpox virus. The take reaction consists of a focal necrotic reaction produced by infiltrating lymphocytes and macrophages killing virus-infected epithelial cells (Fig. 24-7). Please see Chapter 25 for more details on smallpox immunization (vaccination).

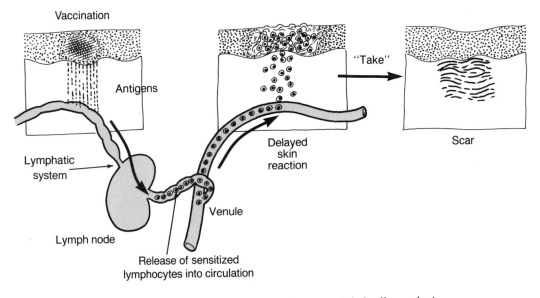

Figure 24-7. Vaccination against smallpox. Introduction of vaccinia virus into the skin results in proliferation of organisms in epithelial cells followed by development of delayed hypersensitivity and destruction of infected cells. Viral antigens are carried by lymphatics to draining lymph nodes where primary T cell response results in production of sensitized cells. The sensitized cells return to attack virus-infected epithelial cells, producing a delayed skin reaction (take). The presence of delayed reactivity signifies a state of protective immunity to reinfection.

Syphilis

The host–parasite relationship in syphilis has been the subject of study for 500 years since syphilis was introduced into Europe by sailors returning with Columbus. By 1498 syphilis was ravaging Europe, killing up to 30% of infected individuals in the acute (primary) stage. The association of syphilis with sexual activity became readily apparent and is believed by some to have been the major factor in the change of sexual mores that occurred in the sixteenth and seventeenth centuries, giving rise to Puritanism. The social effects of syphilis in the fifteenth century resemble the effects of AIDS in the twentieth century.

The natural history of the disease syphilis has changed, presumably as the less resistant population was killed off. Today we recognize primary, secondary, latent, and tertiary disease, each of which is determined largely by the immune response of the host. The evolution of the primary lesion, the chancre, the first clinical manifestation of primary syphilis, follows closely the pattern of a delayed hypersensitivity reaction in the skin. It lasts from 1 to 5 weeks, is initiated by sensitized T cells reacting with antigen, and is resolved by phagocytosis and digestion of organisms by macrophages (Fig. 24-8). Protection against rein-

Figure 24-8. Progression of the primary chancre of syphilis. Infection with *Treponema pallidum* occurs by inoculation through abraded skin. Following inoculation there is systemic dissemination of the organisms as well as local proliferation of the site of infection. Hyperplasia of draining lymph nodes (lymphadenopathy) signifies an active immune response. Both sensitized cells and humoral antibody are produced. The primary lesion, which is a firm, elevated skin lesion with central necrosis, is a manifestation of a delayed hypersensitivity reaction. T cells infiltrate first, followed by macrophages, which phagocytose and destroy the infecting organisms. Viable organisms remain in "protective niches" in the body, giving rise to secondary, latent, and tertiary disease.

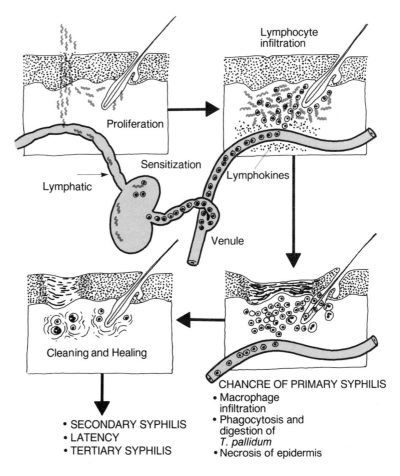

Proliferation

Sensitization

Lymphatic

Lymphocyte infiltration

Lymphokines

Venule

Cleaning and Healing

CHANCRE OF PRIMARY SYPHILIS
• Macrophage infiltration
• Phagocytosis and digestion of *T. pallidum*
• Necrosis of epidermis

• SECONDARY SYPHILIS
• LATENCY
• TERTIARY SYPHILIS

fection may be partially mediated by antibody neutralization of organisms, or by macrophage activated by a delayed hypersensitivity reaction killing the organism. Immunity to infection (*chancre immunity*) is only established by active infection for at least 3 months. The relative contributions of different immune mechanisms to chancre immunity are not clear at this time.

The skin and mucous membrane lesions of secondary syphilis, which appear 2 weeks to 6 months after primary infection, appear to be mixed delayed hypersensitivity and antibody-mediated immune complex reactions at sites of dissemination and replication of *Treponema pallidum*. The cellular reaction is similar to that of primary lesions, although plasma cells and vasculitis may be more prominent. Many systemic effects of secondary syphilis are the result of immune complexes. The lesions heal spontaneously, and the patient enters a period of latency.

In latent syphilis there is no clinical evidence of infection. However, some *T. pallidum* survive the immune attack of the host and remain viable. There does not appear to be any abnormality of the immune system; indeed, persons with latent syphilis are resistant to reinfection; that is, they are immune, yet are infected (concomitant immunity).

The destructive lesions characteristic of tertiary syphilis are granulomatous reactions (gummas), which occur in areas where spirochetes apparently persist during latency, for example, brain, skin, bone, or viscera. As no differences in immune potential distinguish patients who develop tertiary disease from those who do not, it is not known why some patients move from latency to tertiary disease. Development of tertiary lesions could result either from an increased state of hypersensitivity causing more intense inflammation or from a decreased state of reactivity permitting organisms to proliferate and initiate a destructive reaction.

At present no vaccine for syphilis is available. Attempts are being made to construct a "vaccinia" vector that includes cDNA encoding for *T. pallidum* antigens. The major problem is that although there are over 100 antigens in *T. pallidum*, those that might be effective in induction of protective immunity have not been identified.

Granulomatous Hypersensitivity: Leprosy

The clinical manifestations of leprosy are determined by the immune response of the patient. The protective function of granulomatous reactivity is exemplified by the spectrum of leprosy. The high resistance of tuberculoid leprosy is associated with delayed hypersensitivity and the formation of granulomas, whereas the low resistance characteristic of lepromatous leprosy is associated with the presence of high levels of humoral antibodies. The role of immune effector mechanisms in the pathogenesis of leprosy is presented in detail in Chapter 21.

The tendency for some individuals to produce the "wrong" form of immune response, such as occurs in lepromatous leprosy, is a form of *immune deviation*. Thus, cellular hypersensitivity manifested as tuberculoid granulomas is protective; humoral antibody is not. A similar situation exists in other diseases such as chronic mucocutaneous candidiasis, other fungal diseases, and sarcoidosis where antibody titers are associated with progressive disease. It is not clear why certain individuals respond "inappropriately," but it is believed to be related to genetic control of immune responsiveness.

Mixed Mechanisms

Filariasis

Filaria are roundworms with complex life cycles that live in the subcutaneous or lymphoreticular tissues. Filiform larvae are transmitted to man by a biting insect that serves as the intermediate host. The larvae penetrate the skin and may pass into the lymphatic system. All seven filariids known to infect humans may evoke allergic reactions (Table 24-4); however, only three

Table 24-4

Species	Site of Infection	Immune Effector Mechanism	Distribution
Wucheria bancrofti	Lymphatic	Multiple	Tropics
Brugia malayi	Lymphatic	Multiple	Southeast Africa
Onchocerca volvulus	Subcutaneous	Cellular	Africa, South and Central America
Loa loa	Subcutaneous	Anaphylactic	Africa
Dipetalonema perstans	Subcutaneous	Anaphylactic	Africa, South America
Dracunculus medinesis (nonfilarial)	Connective tissue	Anaphylactic	Tropics

cause serious disease: *Wuchereria bancrofti, Brugia malayi,* and *Onchocerca volvulus.*

The manifestations of filariasis clearly reflect the state of immune responsiveness of the host (Table 24-5). Chronic,

Table 24-5

Disease State	Age of Infection	Immune Mechanism
Asymptomatic microfilaremia	Infants	Tolerance
Occult filariasis	Infants	IgG antibody
Tropical eosinophilia	Adult, acute	Anaphylactic
Lymphadenitis	Adult, chronic	Delayed hypersensitivity
Lymphatic obstruction	Adult, chronic	Granulomatous

asymptomatic filaremia is associated with specific hyporesponsiveness to filarial antigens. It is a host–parasite relationship that permits prolonged production of microfilaria, which are cleared from the circulation by the lungs, liver, and spleen without evoking symptoms.

In occult filariasis, there are neither symptoms nor microfilaria in the blood. IgG antibodies may be responsible for the rapid, apparently complete clearance of organisms from the blood, and an asymptomatic latency is established.

However, immune responses that apparently cure the infection may actually lead to disease. Thus, filarial fevers are an indication that an immune response has been activated, most likely involving immune complexes. The manifestations of tropical eosinophilia—attacks of bronchial asthma with interstitial inflammation of the lungs—are consistent with an IgE response and the formation of immune complexes. A cellular (granulomatous) response is implicated in the pathogenesis of lymphadenitis and lymphatic obstruction leading to massive edema (elephantiasis).

The development of the different, more benign host–parasite relationships is related to the age at which exposure to the parasite occurs. When previously unexposed adults are infected, there is a tendency to develop acute inflammation with pain, urticaria, angioedema, and marked lymphangitis, which disappear without sequelae if exposure is terminated. However, if exposure continues, the disease progresses rapidly from temporary to permanent lymphatic obstruction. Thus, continued exposure to the organism in sensitized individuals is required for the development of lymphatic obstruction by granulomas formed around killed microfilaria. In contrast, residents of endemic regions who contract filaria early in life develop less frequent and less severe manifestations of the disease. In some as yet unknown way, the immune response of such persons is either specifically suppressed or restricted to IgG antibody production, resulting in an asymptomatic carrier state or occult filariasis. Adults from outside the endemic area tend to produce IgE antibody or cellular hypersensitivity when infected. This intriguing host–parasite relationship clearly deserves further study.

Strongyloides Hyperinfection

An example of the role of delayed hypersensitivity (granulomatous reactivity) and anaphylactic mechanisms in controlling intestinal nematode infection is the occurrence of "hyperinfection" by *Strongyloides stercoralis* in immunosuppressed individuals. Infestations with *S. stercoralis* were first noted in

Figure 24-9. The life cycle of *Strongyloides stercoralis* provides three routes of human infection: (1) infection by invasive filiform larvae excreted into the soil, (2) maturation of invasive filiform larvae from free-living organisms in the soil, and (3) autoinfection from filiform larvae that mature in the gastrointestinal tract of the host. Filiform larvae invade skin, enter the venous circulation, and pass to the alveolar capillaries. In the lung the adolescent worms mature into adult male and female worms. The adult worms pass to the gastrointestinal tract presumably by being coughed up and swallowed. The females lodge in mucosa of the gastrointestinal tract, set up housekeeping, and lay many eggs; the male is no longer needed and most likely is passed out in the feces. In the gastrointestinal tract eggs may mature to rhabdiform larvae and to filiform larvae. All of these forms may be passed into the soil. In addition, filiform larvae may invade the intestinal mucosa, particularly at the terminal colon, permitting autoinfection. ▶

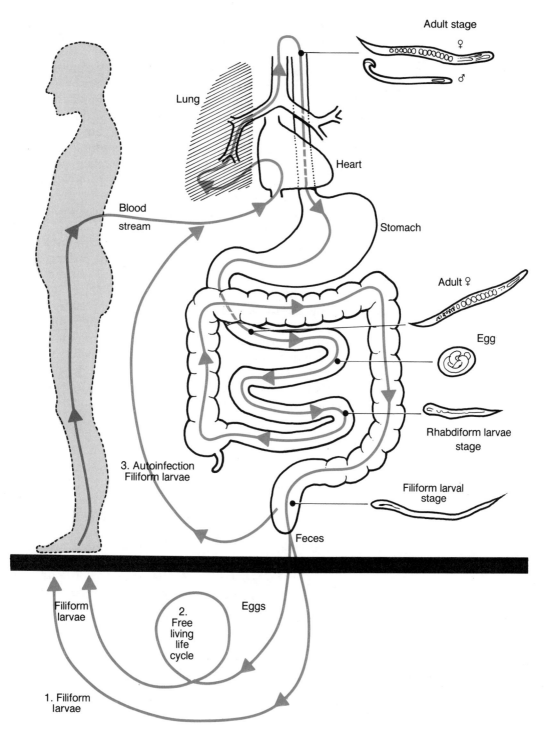

Adult stage

♀

♂

Lung

Heart

Blood
stream

Stomach

Adult ♀

Egg

Rhabdiform larvae
stage

3. Autoinfection
Filiform larvae

Filiform larval
stage

Feces

Filiform
larvae

2.
Free
living
life
cycle

Eggs

1. Filiform
larvae

French soldiers returning from Vietnam in 1876. It is estimated that 100–200 million people in the tropics and subtropics have *S. stercoralis* infections. *S. stercoralis* is also found in the southeastern United States. In one study, stools from 4% of patients in a New Orleans hospital were found to contain eggs or larvae.

Unique among the intestinal nematodes of man is the ability of invasive larvae of *S. stercoralis* to mature within the gastrointestinal tract (Fig. 24-9). This allows autoinfection. However, infected individuals with normal immune function remain essentially asymptomatic; the immune system provides a barrier to autoinfection. In immunosuppressed individuals, however, hyperinfection occurs.

Hyperinfected individuals are most likely asymptomatic bearers of *S. stercoralis* until natural disease (Hodgkin's disease, lymphoma, debilitation, leprosy, etc.) or immunosuppressive therapy (steroids, cytotoxic drugs) results in depressed immunity. It is believed that anaphylactic and delayed hypersensitivity mechanisms are primarily responsible for maintenance of the asymptomatic state. Evidence for this is the association of poor prognosis with absence of eosinophilia, and the finding of hyperinfection in patients with lepromatous leprosy who have a selective deficiency in delayed hypersensitivity. In hyperinfected patients there is a failure to develop granulomas in infected organs; such granulomas are characteristic of lesions in infected individuals with normal immune function.

The apparent pathogenesis of hyperinfection is depicted in Figure 24-9. The major factors are loss of intestinal barriers to invasion of filiform larvae secondary to immune deficiency, and decreased intestinal motility allowing more time for filiform larvae to develop from eggs and rhabdiform larvae. Patients with *Stronglyoides* hyperinfection develop inflammatory changes in the intestine associated with diarrhea and ileus. Massive infiltration leads to severe inflammation in the lung, and larvae may be seen in the liver, lung, brain, and meninges. Also associated is sepsis by enteric organisms leading to fatal meningitis. Invasion of the *Strongyloides* larvae opens the way for organisms in the gut to enter the body of an already immunosuppressed individual.

Evasion of Immune Defenses

Infectious organisms have evolved "ingenious" ways to avoid immune defense mechanisms (Table 24-6). Organisms may locate in niches not accessible to immune effector mechanisms or mask themselves by acquiring host molecules. They may change their surface antigens, hide within cells, produce factors that inhibit the immune response, or fool the immune system into responding with an ineffective effector mechanism.

Coevolution of the human host and its infectious organisms results in an eventual mutual coexistence with most envi-

Table 24-6. Some Mechanisms of Evasion of Immune Defenses by Infectious Agents

Mechanism	Example
Localization in protective niches	Latent syphilis, herpes simplex
Imitation of host antigens	Schistosomiasis
Antigenic modulation, loss of cell surface antigens	Malaria, trypanosomiasis, leishmaniasis
Immunosuppression	Malaria, tuberculosis (anergy), AIDS virus
Intracellular location	Histoplasmosis, viruses
Inappropriate immune response	Lepromatous leprosy, chronic mucocutaneous candidiasis
Extracorporeal location	*Clostridium tetani, Ascaris lumbricoides*

ronmental organisms. The best evidence of this is the loss of this coexistence when the immune mechanisms do not function properly. Then organisms that do not normally cause disease become virulent. The lesson of AIDS demonstrates that new infectious organisms become dominant when introduced into a previously unexposed population. Previous examples of this are the devastating effects of tuberculosis and smallpox introduced to previously unexposed American Indians and of syphilis introduced into Europe in the 1490s. The genetic diversity of immune responsiveness in populations is responsible for both the inability of some individuals to develop an immune response to a new infectious agent and the ability of other individuals to make a protective response and survive. If genetic diversity in immune responsiveness were not present, a new infectious agent could annihilate a genetically unresponsive population. In a fully evolved, mature relationship, host and infectious agent coexist without detrimental effects.

Summary

The "double-edged sword" of immune reactivity is illustrated by the role of immune effector mechanisms in resistance to infectious agents and the contribution of immune mechanisms to tissue lesions and disease. Each immune effector mechanism has a defensive function for the host. Antibody-mediated effector mechanisms generally operate against bacteria or bacterial products; cellular effector mechanisms protect against viral or fungal diseases. Neutralization or inactivation of biologically active bacterial toxins is clearly protective. This is what is accomplished by active immunization with diphtheria or tetanus toxoids. Cytotoxic reactions are effective in killing bacteria or preparing bacteria for phagocytosis by opsonization. The inflammatory effect of immune complexes produces stickiness of leukocytes and platelets to vascular endothelium and increased permeability. These reactions promote defense by localization, diapedesis, and activation of polymorphonuclear leukocytes.

Table 24-7. Postulated Specific Immune Defense Mechanisms in Some Infectious Diseases

Disease	Agent	Site of Infection	Defense Mechanism
VIRUSES (RNA)			
Influenza	Paramyxovirus	Lung	Antibody blocks cell attachment
Mumps	Paramyxovirus	Parotid gland	DTH, kills infected cells
Measles (rubeola)	Paramyxovirus	Skin, systemic	DTH, kills infected cells
Rabies	Rhabdovirus	Brain cells	DTH, kills infected cells
Polio	Picornavirus	Systemic, neurons	Antibody blocks cell attachment
Yellow fever	Flavivirus	Viscera	Antibody blocks cell attachment
VIRUSES (DNA)			
Herpes	Herpesvirus	Skin, mucous membranes	?DTH
Smallpox	Poxvirus	Skin	DTH, kills infected cells
Hepatitis B	Hepatitis B virus	Liver	Antibody block cell attachment
RICKETTSIA			
Rocky Mountain spotted fever	*Rickettsia rickettsii*	Vascular endothelium	DTH, kills infected cells
Typhus	*Rickettsia prowazekii*	Vascular endothelium	DTH, kills infected cells
BACTERIA			
Botulism	*Clostridium botulinum*	Exotoxin	Neutralization by antibody
Tetanus	*Clostridium tetani*	Exotoxin	Neutralization by antibody
Diphtheria	*Corynebacterium diphtheriae*	Exotoxin	Neutralization by antibody
Pertussis	*Bordatella pertussis*	Endo- and exotoxin	Neutralization, opsonization
Cholera	*Vibrio cholerae*	Enterotoxin	IgA neutralization of toxin
Staphylococcus	*Staphylococcus aureus*	Connective tissue, pyogenic abscess	Antibody neutralization of toxin, opsonization
Streptococcus	*Streptococcus β-hemolytic*	Connective tissue, cellulitis	Antibody neutralization of toxin, opsonization
Pneumonia	*Streptococcus pneumoniae,*	Pneumonia	Antibody opsonization, cytotoxicity
Meningitis	*Neisseria meningitidis*	Meninges	Antibody opsonization
Gonorrhea	*Neisseria gonorrhoeae*	Mucous surface	Antibody opsonization, protease neutralization
Influenza	*Hemophilus influenza*	Lung, endotoxin	Antibody opsonization, neutralization
Infantile diarrhea	*Escherichia coli*	GI tract, endotoxin	Antibody blocks cell attachment, neutralization, opsonization

Disease	Organism	Location	Immune mechanism
Typhoid fever	*Salmonella typhosa*	GI tract, systemic endotoxin	Antibody neutralization, DTH macrophage activation
Actinomycosis	*Actinomyces* spp.	Connective tissue, other	Immune complex opsonization, granulomatous
MYCOBACTERIA			
Tuberculosis	*Mycobacterium tuberculosis*	Lung	Granulomatous, DTH
Leprosy	*Mycobacterium leprae*	Dermis	Granulomatous, DTH
SPIROCHETES			
Syphilis	*Treponema pallidum*	Connective tissue	DTH, ?antibody opsonization
FUNGI			
Aspergillosis	*Aspergillus* spp.	Lung	Immune complex, granulomatous
Candidiasis	*Candida albicans*	Skin, mucous membranes	DTH, granulomatous
Coccidioidomycosis	*Coccidioides immitis*	Lung	DTH, granulomatous
Cryptococcus	*Cryptococcus neoformans*	Lung	Granulomatous
Histoplasmosis	*Histoplasma capsulatum*	Inside macrophages	DTH, macrophage activation
PROTOZOA			
Ambeiasis	*Entomoeba histolytica*	GI mucosa	Immune complex, inflammation
Malaria	*Plasmodium* spp.	Inside cells, free in blood	Cytotoxic, immune complex opsonization
Leishmaniasis	*Leishmania* spp.	Inside macrophages	DTH, activated macrophages
Toxoplasmosis	*Toxoplasma gondii*	Intracellular	Immune complex opsonization
Chagas' disease	*Trypanosoma cruzi*	Free in blood, intracellular	Cytotoxic opsonization
Sleeping sickness	*Trypanosoma rhodesiense, Trypanosoma gambiense*	Free in blood	Cytotoxic, immune complex opsonization
Giardiasis	*Giardia lambdia*	GI tract	IgA antibody
HELMINTHS			
Schistosomiasis	*Schistosoma* spp.	Veins	Atopic, granulomatous
Fascioliasis	*Fasciola* spp.	Biliary ducts	Atopic, granulomatous
Trichinosis	*Trichinella spiralis*	In muscle	Atopic, DTH
Strongyloidiasis	*Strongyloides stercoralis*	GI tract	Atopic, DTH
Filariasis	*Wuchereria bancrofti* *Onchocerca volvulus*	Lymphatics Dermis	Atopic, granulomatous Granulomatous, immune complex
Taeniasis	*Taenia*	GI tract	?Atopic

DTH, delayed type hypersensitivity; GI, gastrointestinal.

Anaphylactic mechanisms serve to open up capillaries, permitting extravasation of blood/bone components into tissues and delivery of inflammatory cells or antibodies to sites of infection. Spasmodic and massive diarrhea (gastrointestinal anaphylaxis) may effect expulsion of intestinal parasites. Delayed hypersensitivity reactions result in local mobilization of lymphocytes and attraction and activation of macrophages, effects clearly necessary for defense against viral, fungal, and mycobacterial infections. Granulomatous hypersensitivity functions to isolate insoluble toxic material or microorganisms. A list of postulated specific effector mechanisms for selected infectious diseases is given in Table 24-7. In many infectious diseases more than one mechanism may be active, particularly if the organism exists in different stages.

Examples of the destructive capacity of immune responses to some selected infectious agents have also been presented. Tissue lesions caused by immune reactions to infectious agents usually occur when an inappropriate mechanism is activated. Thus, in leprosy, antibody causes problems due to immune complex formation but has no protective effect against the intracellular bacilli; granulomatous reactivity is protective but may cause tissue damage if activated after large numbers of organisms have already been disseminated. The relative contributions of different immune mechanisms to the pathogenesis of other infectious diseases reflect even more variations in the interplay between immune effector mechanisms in protection and pathogenesis.

References

General

Austen KF, Cohn Z: Contribution of serum and cellular factors in host defense reactions. Engl J Med 268:933, 1963.

Braude AI: Infection and Immunity. *In* Giallium A (ed): Clinical Physiology, New York, McGraw-Hill, 1957, p773.

Capron A, Dessaint JP: Effector and regulatory mechanisms in immunity to schistosomes: A hieratic view. Annu Rev Immunol 3:455, 1985.

Chaparas SD: Immunity in tuberculosis. Bull WHO 60:447, 1982.

Ellner JJ, Mahmoud AAF: Phagocytes and worms: David and Goliath Revisited. Rev Infect Dis 4:698, 1982.

Gillis HM: Selective primary health care: strategies for control of disease in the developing world. XVII. Hookworm infection and anemia. Rev Infect Dis 7:111, 1985.

Hirsch JG: Host resistance to infectious disease: A centennial. Adv Host Defense Mechanisms 1:1, 1982.

Keusch GT: Immune Responses in parasitic diseases. Rev Infect Dis 4:751, 1982.

Mendes, E: *Immunopathology of Tropical Diseases.* São Paulo, Brazil, Sawyer, 1982.

Mitchell GF, Anders RF: Parasite antigens and their immunogenicity in infected hosts. *In* Sela M (ed), The Antigens, Vol 4. New York, Academic Press, 1982, p69.

Moller G (ed): The Immune Response to Infectious Diseases. Transplant Rev 19, 1974.

Moller G (ed): Immunoparasitology. Immunol Rev 61, 1982.

Nahamias AJ, O'Reilly RF (eds): Immunology of Human Infection. New York, Plenum, 1981.

Sell S: Immunopathology of infectious diseases. *In* Hoeprich, PD (ed): Infectious Diseases, 3rd ed. Hagerstown, Md., Harper & Row, 1983, p57.

Sissons JGP, Oldstone MBA: Killing of virus-infected cells by cytotoxic lymphocytes. J Infect Dis 142:114, 1980.

Tetanus

Blake PA, Feldman RA, Buchanan TM, Brooks GF, Bennett JV: Serologic therapy of tetanus in the United States, 1965, 1971. JAMA 235:42, 1976.

Brooks VB, Curtis DR, Eccles JC: Mode of action of tetanus toxin. Nature 175:120, 1955.

Fraser DW: Preventing tetanus in patients with wounds. Ann Intern Med 84:95, 1976.

LaForce FM, Young LS, Bennett JV: Tetanus in the United States: Epidemiologic and clinical features. N Engl J Med 280:569, 1969.

Nielsen PA, Ablondi FB, Querry MV, et al: Antigenic and immunogenic studies on purified tetanus toxoid. J Immunol 98:1248, 1967.

Proceedings of the IV International Conference on Tetanus, Dakar, Senegal, April 6–12, 1975. Lyon, France, Foundation Merieux, 1975.

Rubbo SD: A re-evaluation of tetanus prophylaxis in civilian practice. Med J Aust 2:105, 1965.

Malaria

Allison AC, Eugui EM: The role of cell mediated immune responses in resistance to malaria with special reference to oxidant stress. Annu Rev Immunol 1:361, 1983.

Boyd MF (ed): Malariology. Philadelphia, Saunders, 1949.

Clyde DF, McCarthy VC, Miller RM, Woodward WE: Immunization of man against falciparum and vivax malaria by use of attenuated sporozoites. Am J Trop Med Hyg 24:397, 1975.

Deans JA, Cotton S: Immunology of malaria. Annu Rev Microbiol 34:25, 1983.

Freeman RR, Trejdosiewicz AJ, Cross G: Protective monoclonal antibodies recognizing stage-specific merozoite antigens of a rodent malaria parasite. Nature 284:366, 1980.

Howard RJ: Antigenic variation of bloodstage malaria parasites. Philos Trans R Soc Lond Ser B 307:141, 1984.

Neva FA: Malaria: Recent progress and problems. N Engl J Med 277:1241, 1967.

Nussenzweig R, Nussenzweig V: Development of sporozoite vaccines. Philos Trans R Soc Lond Ser B 307:117, 1984.

Rener J, Carter R, Rosenberg Y, Miller LH: Anti-gamete hybridoma antibodies synergistically block transmission of malaria. Proc Nat Acad Sci USA 77:6797, 1980.

Spitz S: The pathology of acute falciparum malaria. Milit Surg 99:555, 1946.

Young JF, Hockmeyer WT, Gross M, et al: Expression of plasmodium falciparum circumsporate proteins in E. coli for potential use in the human malaria vaccine. Science 228:958, 1985.

Rheumatic Fever

Breese BB, Hall C (eds): Beta Hemolytic Streptococcal Diseases. New York, Wiley, 1978.

Ginsburg I: Mechanisms of cell and tissue injury induced by group A streptococci: relation in post-streptococcal sequelae. J Infect Dis 126:294–340,419–456, 1972.

Haverkorn MJ (ed): Streptococcal Disease and Immunity. New York, American Elsevier, 1974.

Markowitz M, Gordis L: Rheumatic Fever, 2nd ed. Philadelphia, Saunders, 1972.

Kaplan MH, Suchy ML: Immunologic relation of streptococcal and tissue antigens. II. Class reaction of antisera to mammalian heart tissue with a cell wall constituent of certain strains of group A streptococci. J Exp Med 119:643, 1964.

Rammelkamp CH Jr: Epidemiology of streptococcal infections. Harvey Lect 51:113–142, 1955.

Stollerman GH: Rheumatic Fever and Streptococcal Infections. New York, Grune & Stratton, 1975.

Stollerman GH: The relative rheumatogenicity of strains of group A streptococci. Mod Concepts Cardiovasc Dis 44:35, 1975.

Stollerman GH: Streptococcal vaccines and global strategies for prevention of rheumatic fever. Am J Med 68:636, 1980.

Zabriski JB: Mimetic relationships between group A streptococci and mammalian tissues. Adv Immunol 7:147, 1967.

Aspergillus

Aisner J, Schimpff SC, Wiernick PH: Treatment of invasive aspergillosis: relation of early diagnosis and treatment to response. Ann Intern Med 86:539–543, 1977.

Carbone PP, Seymour MS, Sidransky H, Frei E: Secondary aspergillosis. Ann Intern Med 60:556–567, 1964.

English MP, Henderson AH: Significance and interpretation of laboratory tests in pulmonary aspergillosis. J Clin Pathol 20:832–834, 1967.

Harvey C, Blacket RB, Read J: Mucoid impaction of the bronchi. Aust Ann Med 6:16, 1957.

Henderson AH, English MP, Vecht RJ: Pulmonary aspergillosis. Thorax 23:513, 1968.

Hinson KFW, Moon AJ, Plummer NS: Bronchopulmonary aspergillosis. Thorax 7:317, 1952.

Imbeau SA, Nichols D, Flaherty D, et al: Allergic bronchopulmonary aspergillosis. J Allergy Clin Immunol 62:243, 1978.

Patterson R, Greenberger PA, Radin RC, Roberts M: Allergic broncho-pulmonary aspergillosis: staging as an aid to management. Ann Intern Med 96:286, 1982.

Pepys J: Hypersensitivity diseases of the lungs due to fungi and organic dusts. *In* Kallos P, Hasek M, Interbitzen TM, Miescher P, Waksman BH (eds): Monographs in Allergy, Vol 4. New York, Karger, 1969.

Young RC, Bennett JE, Vogel CL, Carbone PP, DeVita VT: Aspergillosis: the spectrum of disease in 98 patients. Medicine 49:147, 1970.

Smallpox

Behbehani AM: The small pox story: life and death of an old disease. Microbiol Rev 47:455, 1983.

Breman JG, Arita I: The confirmation and maintenance of smallpox eradication. N Engl J Med 303:1263, 1980.

Dixon CW: Smallpox. London, Churchill, 1962.

Esposito JJ, Obijeskie JF, Nakano JH: The virion and soluble antigen proteins of variola, monkeypox and vaccinia viruses. J Med Virol 1:95, 1977.

Foege WH: Editorial: should the smallpox virus be allowed to survive? N Engl J Med 300:670, 1979.

Jenner E: An inquiry into the causes and effects of the variolae vaccine. London, Low, 1798.

Plotkin SA, Plotkin SL: Vaccination: one hundred years later. *In* Koprowski H, Plotkin SA (eds), World's Debt to Pasteur. New York, Liss, 1985, p83.

Ricketts TF, Byles JB: The Diagnosis of Smallpox, Vol I. London, Cassell, 1908.

World Health Organization. The Global Eradication of Smallpox: Final Report of the Global Commission for the Certification of Smallpox Eradication. Geneva, 1980.

Syphilis

Chesney AM: Immunity in syphilis. Medicine 5:463, 1926.

Dennie CC: A History of Syphilis. Springfield, Ill., Thomas, 1962.

Jones JA: Bad Blood. New York, Free Press/Macmillan, 1981.

Lederer SE: The right and wrong of making experiments on human beings: Udo J. Wile and syphilis. Bull Hist Med 58:380, 1984.

Schell RF, Muscher DM (eds): Pathogenesis and Immunology of Treponemal Infection. New York, Dekker, 1983.

Sell S, Norris SJ: The biology, pathology, and immunology of syphilis. Int Rev Exp Pathol 24:203–276, 1983.

Turner TB, Hollander DH: Biology of the treponematoses. Geneva, WHO, 1957.

Leprosy

Bjune G, Closs O, Barnetson RS: Early events in the host–parasite relationship and immune response in clinical leprosy—its possible importance for leprosy control. Clin Exp Immunol 54:289–297, 1983.

Bullock WE: Studies on immune mechanisms in leprosy. I. Depression of delayed allergic response to skin test antigens. N Engl J Med 278:298, 1968.

Cochrane RG, Davey TF (eds): Leprosy in Theory and Practice, 2nd ed. Baltimore, Williams & Wilkins, 1964.

Drutz DJ, Chen TS, Lu WH: The continuous bacteremia of lepromatous leprosy. N Engl J Med 287:159, 1972.

Godal T: Immunological aspects of leprosy—present status. Prog Allergy 25:211, 1978.

Rees RJW: The significance of the lepromin reaction in man. Prog Allergy 8:224, 1964.

Rees RJW: Enhanced susceptibility of thymectomized and irradiated mice to infection with Mycobacterium leprae. Nature 211:657, 1966.

Ridley DS: Histologic classification and the immunological spectrum of leprosy. Bull WHO 51:451, 1974.

Skinsness OK: Notes on the history of leprosy. Int J Leprosy 41:220, 1973.

Skinsness OK: Immunopathology of leprosy: The century in review. Pathology, pathogenesis and development of classification. Int J Leprosy 41:329, 1973.

Turk JL, Bryceson ADM: Immunological phenomena in leprosy and related diseases. Adv Immunol 13:209, 1971.

Wagner O: Immunological aspects of leprosy with special reference to autoimmune diseases. Bull WHO 41:793, 1969.

Filariasis

Conner DH, Palmieri JR, Gibson DW: Pathogenesis of lymphatic filariasis in man. Parasitenkunde 72:13, 1986.

Galindo L, Von Lichtenberg F, Baldison C: Bancroftian filariasis in Puerto Rico: infection pattern and tissue lesions. Am J Trop Med 11:739, 1962.

Lie KJ: Occult filariasis and its relationship to pulmonary tropical eosinophilia. Am J Trop Med 11:646, 1962.

Nelson GS: The pathology of filarial infections. Helminth 35:355, 1966.

Ottesen EA: Immunopathology of lymphatic filariasis in man. Immunopathology 2:373, 1980.

Turner JH: Studies in filariasis in Malaya: the clinical features of filariasis due to Wuchereria malayi. Trans Roy Soc Trop Med Hyg 55:107, 1961.

Strongyloides

Cruz T, Rebokas C, Rochas H: Fatal strongyloidiasis in patients receiving corticosteroids. N Engl J Med 27:1093, 1966.

Gill CV, Bell DR: Strongyloides stercoralis infection in former Far East prisoners of war. Br Med J 2:572, 1979.

Poltera AA: Fatal strongyloidiasis in Uganda. Ann Trop Med Parasitol 68:81, 1974.

Purtillo DT, Meyers WM, Conner DH: Fatal strongyloidiasis in immunosuppressed patients. Am J Med 56:488, 1974.

Rivera E, Maldonado N, Velez-Garcia E, Grillo AJ, Malaret G: Hyperinfection syndrome with strongyloides stercoralis. Ann Intern Med 72:199, 1970.

Evasion of Immune Defenses

Bernards A: Antigenic variation of trypanosomes. Biochim Biophys Acta 824:1, 1984.

Bloom BR: Games parasites play: how parasites evade immune surveillance. Nature 279:21, 1979.

Davidson RA: Immunology of parasitic infections. Med Clin North Am 69:751, 1985.

Donelson JE, Turner MJ: How the trypanosome changes its coat. Sci Am 252:44, 1985.

Halsted SB: Immune enhancement of viral infection. Prog Allergy 31:301, 1982.

Medici MA: The immunoprotective niche — a new pathogenic mechanism for syphilis, the systemic mycoses and other infectious diseases. J Theor Biol 36:617, 1972.

Navel J, Behin R: Immunology of leishmaniasis. *In* Levandowski M, Hutner SH (eds), Biochemistry and Physiology of Protozoa, Vol 4. New York, Academic Press, 1981, p385.

Warren KS: The present impossibility of eradicating the omnipresent worm. Rev Infect Dis 4:955, 1982.

25 | Immunization

Since prehistoric times primitive physicians noted that a previous natural exposure to an infectious agent or product thereof would produce a state of specific resistance to reinfection (immunity). Many satisfactory procedures for intentionally inducing immunity have been developed and are used prophylactically, while others are in the process of being made available for general or specific use. Because of active immunization, many infections that were considered part of growing up in the Western world 10 or 20 years ago have become so infrequent that physicians trained in the last few years have had no experience with these natural infections personally or professionally. In addition, passive immunity also has been applied successfully in more limited situations.

Passive Immunity

The transfer of immune products (humoral or cellular) from a sensitized person to a nonimmunized person produces a temporary passive state of specific immunity in the recipient.

Humoral Antibody

For humoral antibody, this may be accomplished by injection of a serum-containing antibody from immunized animals or by injection of pooled human immunoglobulin in which specific antibody is present (Table 25-1). Horse antiserum has been used following exposure to toxins of botulism, diphtheria, gas gangrene, and tetanus. Although the horse antitoxin neutralizes the toxins or the infectious agent, the administration of horse serum frequently leads to serum sickness, because the host responds to the horse serum proteins by forming precipitating antibody (see Chapter 16). Therefore, horse serum should be used only in life-threatening circumstances and only after careful testing fails to detect a preexisting allergy to horse serum. Pooled human immunoglobulin is effective after exposure to hepatitis, measles, or rubella (German measles) during the first trimester of pregnancy. Although cellular immunity may be

Table 25-1. Immune Globulin Preparations Available for Passive Immunization and Indications for Use[a]

Pooled Human Immune Globulin	Specific Human Immune Globulin	Specific Equine Immune Globulin
Humoral immune deficiency	Hepatitis B	Black widow spider venom
Hepatitis A	Pertussis	Botulism toxin
Measles	Rabies	Diphtheria toxin
	Rh isoimmunization	Snake venoms
	Tetanus	
	Vaccinia	
	Varicella zoster	

[a] For emergencies call Centers for Disease Control, 404-329-3311 (day) or 404-329-3644 (night).

required to eliminate virus-infected cells, passively transferred antibody is effective if administered shortly after exposure to hepatitis virus, and for measles, polio, rabies, smallpox, and varicella. Passive immunity occurs naturally in fetal life. Maternal antibodies cross the placenta and provide specific immunity for the newborn until about 3 to 4 months of age, when the infant begins to produce its own antibody (see Chapter 26).

Cellular Immunity

The passive transfer of cellular immune reactions using living cells is generally not satisfactory in humans because of immune rejection of the transferred cells. Passive transfer of cellular sensitivity may be accomplished if the recipient is unable to reject transferred living lymphoid cells or through use of a product of sensitized cells known as *transfer factor*. The former is possible with transfers between identical twins. Cellular reactivity may also be transferred if lymphoid cells are given to a recipient who is incapable of reacting because of an immunological deficiency. However, the transferred cells may react to the recipient's tissues (see Graft versus Host Reactions, Chapter 19). Successful cell transfer depends on histocompatibility matching of donor and recipient. Transfer factor has been used with limited success in a number of human immune deficiency diseases such as chronic mucocutaneous candidiasis. (For a further discussion of the use of lymphoid cells or cell products as therapy for immune deficiencies, see Chapter 26.)

Active Immunity

Active immunity occurs upon recovery from a naturally acquired infection. Active immunity may be induced intentionally by inoculation, ingestion, or inhalation of a modified form of an infectious organism or a product of an organism so that the immunizing material retains the antigenicity of the intact organism but does not have the capacity to cause disease. The types of artificial immunogens that have been used include low doses of a product of the organism, altered products such as chemically modified toxins (toxoid), antibody-neutralized toxin, killed organisms, low doses of virulent organisms given by nonpathogenic or relatively innocuous routes, living attenuated (avirulent) strains, and organisms altered in such a way that they can infect but cannot complete a complex life cycle (e.g., immunization of cattle against lungworm). Attenuated strains are produced by culturing virulent organisms in vitro or in unnatural hosts so that the organisms are no longer pathogenic for the natural host but retain the antigenic specificity of the virulent strains. The use of adjuvants to enhance specific active immunization is discussed in Chapter 27.

Prophylactic Immunization

Some diseases for which active prophylactic immunization is available are listed in Table 25-2. Diseases for which immunization is widely employed include diphtheria, whooping cough (pertussis), tetanus, measles (rubeola), poliomyelitis, rubella, and mumps. Immunizations in clinical practice are scheduled as a compromise between immunization efficiency and convenience of administration, that is, to obtain safe, adequate protection with a minimum number of visits to the doctor. Most immunizations usually require two to three applications and occasional booster injections. Children are usually immunized with diphtheria toxoid, killed pertussis organisms, and tetanus toxoid by three injections of the combined antigens (DPT) between 2 and 6 months of age, with another booster at 18 to 24 months. Infants younger than 2 months of age develop poor immune responses. One inoculation with attenuated measles and mumps virus and two or three oral doses of attenuated poliovirus are given between 7 and 11 months of age or along with DPT immunization. Pertussis vaccination has been associated with a substantial decline in the prevalence of whooping cough. A clear decline in the prevalence of whooping cough had occurred prior to the introduction of pertussis vaccination in the 1940s. There is brain damage associated with approximately 1 in 300,000 injections. However, the continued use of pertussis vaccination is recommended as it is projected that far more children would suffer serious complications from pertussis infection if vaccination were not done. For more detailed immunization recommendations, see Tables 25-3 and 25-4.

Smallpox Variolation and Vaccination

Vaccination against smallpox (variola) represents one of the most spectacular successes in control of an infectious disease. Smallpox was once one of the greatest lethal and disfiguring diseases of man. In ancient China smallpox killed so many children that names were not given to infants until they had survived smallpox. So many children died that families would run out of favorite names. The Chinese noted that milder forms of smallpox could be induced using infected tissue from people with a relatively benign course of

Table 25-2. Prophylactic Immunization for Human Infectious Diseases

Disease	Antigen Preparation	Indication	Immunization Route	Results
TOXOIDS				
Diphtheria	Formaldehyde-treated toxin	All children	Intramuscular	Satisfactory
Botulism	Formaldehyde-treated toxin	On exposure	Intramuscular	Needs improvement
Tetanus	Formaldehyde-treated toxin	All children	Intramuscular	Satisfactory
KILLED ORGANISMS				
Pertussis	Thiomersalate-treated	All children	Intramuscular	Needs improvement
Typhoid	Acetone-treated or heat-killed	Travelers[a]	Subcutaneous, intramuscular	Needs improvement
Cholera	Phenol-treated	Travelers[a]	Subcutaneous	Needs improvement
Plague	Formalin-killed	On exposure	Subcutaneous	Needs improvement
Hepatitis B	Purified HBsAg from plasma/formaldehyde-treated	Exposed individuals	Intramuscular	Needs improvement
POLYSACCHARIDES				
Meningococcus	Polysaccharide (A and C)	Endemic areas (Africa)	Subcutaneous	Needs improvement/short duration of protection in infants
Pneumococcus	Polysaccharide (14 types)	Susceptible individuals	Intramuscular	Needs improvement/antigenicity variable
Hemophilus influenzae	Capsular polysaccharide, A or B (polyribosomal phosphate) type B (approved by FDA April 1985)	Infants and children	Intramuscular	Needs improvement
Smallpox	Vaccinia (cowpox) virus	Military	Intradermal or subcutaneous	Needs improvement/...

ATTENUATED ORGANISMS

Poliomyelitis	Monkey tissue culture (live)	All children	Oral	Satisfactory
Measles (rubeola)	Chicken tissue culture (live)	All children	Subcutaneous	Satisfactory
Mumps	Chicken tissue culture (live)	All children	Subcutaneous	Satisfactory
Rubella	Human tissue culture (live)	All children	Subcutaneous	Satisfactory
Yellow fever	Egg tissue culture	Travelers[a]	Subcutaneous	Needs improvement
Influenza	Egg tissue culture (4 strains) purified antigens	High-risk group	Subcutaneous	Needs improvement
Varicella	Tissue culture/attenuated strain	Children with leukemia	Subcutaneous	Needs improvement
Adenovirus	Live virus/enteric capsules	Military	Oral	Needs improvement
Tuberculosis	Bacillus Calmette–Guérin	High-risk group	Intradermal	Needs improvement

KILLED PARTIALLY ATTENUATED ORGANISMS

Typhus	Chick embryo culture	Travelers[a]	Subcutaneous	Satisfactory
Rabies	Human tissue culture/inactivated with β-propriolactone	On exposure	Intramuscular	Satisfactory
Cutaneous leishmaniasis	Controlled route and dose	Virulent organisms, exposed children	Intradermal	Needs improvement

[a] Travelers to areas where disease is endemic.

Table 25-3. Recommended Immunization Schedules for Infants

Age	Immunization
2 months	DTP, OPV
4 months	DTP, OPV
6 months	DTP, OPV
12 months	TB test
15 months	Measles, rubella, mumps
1½ years	DTP, OPV
4–6 years	DTP, OPV
14–16 years	TD, repeated every 10 years

[a] DTP, diphtheria and tetanus toxoid combined with pertussis vaccine; OPV, trivalent oral polio vaccine; TD, combined tetanus and diphtheria toxoids (adult type).
Modified from Krugman S, Katz SL: Childhood immunization procedures. JAMA 237:2228, 1977.

Table 25-4. Recommended Immunization Schedules for Older Children Not Previously Immunized

When Seen	15 months–5 years	6 years or older
First visit	DTP, OPV, TB test	OPV, TB test
1 month later	Measles, rubella, mumps	Measles, rubella, mumps[b]
2 months later	DTP, OPV	TD, OPV
4 months later	DTP, OPV	—
10–16 months later	DTP, OPV	
Preschool	DTP, OPV	
Age 16 years	TD, repeat every 10 years	TD, repeat every 10 years

[a] DTP, diphtheria and tetanus toxoid combined with pertussis vaccine; OPV, trivalent oral polio vaccine; TD, combined tetanus and diphtheria toxoids (adult type).
[b] Rubella immunization should not be given during pregnancy.
Modified from Krugman S, Katz SL: Childhood immunization procedures. JAMA 237:2228, 1977.

the disease. The Chinese developed the first method of artificial active immunization. A powder made from smallpox crusts was made into a snuff that was inhaled into the nose. Although this produced fatal smallpox in up to 1 in 50 exposed individuals, the course of the disease induced in most individuals was generally much milder than that in the naturally acquired disease. The introduction of *variolation* against smallpox in the Western world is largely attributed to the efforts of Lady Mary Wortley Montagu, who was the wife of the British Ambassador to Turkey. She learned of the practice of variolation in Constantinople. Infected tissue from individuals with mild forms of smallpox was injected into young uninfected people. The inoculated individuals developed mild disease, and recovered. She returned to England and persuaded King George I to conduct "clinical trials" on prisoners at Newgate Prison. The trials were successful and variolation become a regular practice in England until later replaced by vaccination. In the United States variolation was introduced by Zabdiel Boylston in Boston in 1721 through the urging of Cotton Mather. During the Revolutionary War smallpox broke out among the American army late in 1775, and disaster threatened. However, the disease was controlled by variolation and by September 1776, the army was again prepared to take the field free of smallpox.

In 1770 Edward Jenner noted that milkmaids, who contracted cowpox, had a mild smallpox-like disease, but never developed the much more prevalent disease of smallpox. In 1796 he inoculated a healthy young boy with cowpox (vaccinia) from the sore of a dairy maid. The boy developed cowpox, which healed, and was subsequently found to be resistant to challenge with smallpox. In 1807 a National Vaccine Establishment was set up in London and by 1840 compulsory vaccination was established by law and variolation was made illegal.

The vaccinia virus has low pathogenicity for man and contains antigens that cross-react with smallpox virus. Dermal inoculation induces delayed type hypersensitivity that results in a typical delayed skin reaction at the site of inoculation approximately 8 days after application. This long-lasting cellular sensitivity protects the vaccinated person against smallpox. The term *vaccination*, now used to cover all kinds of protective immunization, is derived from the vaccinia virus. Through the application of worldwide vaccination programs, the once great killer disease of smallpox has been eliminated. A few cases of smallpox were reported in Somalia in 1976 and the last known case was diagnosed in October 1977. Extensive investigations are now underway to determine if any human infections still occur. Inoculation with vaccinia virus leads to complications such as postvaccinial encephalitis or disseminated vaccinia in a small but significant number of vaccinated individuals. Because the untoward consequences of vaccination are now more significant than the naturally occurring disease, vaccination against smallpox has been discontinued in many parts of the world. In December 1979 an independent scientific commission certified global eradication of smallpox. The causative virus is now maintained in six known laboratories for scientific study. However, the possibility that smallpox could be used for biological warfare has led to recommendations that military personnel continue to be vaccinated.

Immunization for Other Infectious Diseases

Immunization for diseases such as cholera, typhoid, typhus, and yellow fever is not done routinely, but is indicated for a person traveling to areas where the disease is endemic. For example, use of acetone-treated or heat-killed organisms for typhoid vaccination has resulted in great reduction of cases in the military but induces marked local inflammation and febrile reactions. Attempts are being made to improve this vaccine through the use of attenuated organisms. Work is now underway to produce and evaluate immunogens for gonorrhea, syphilis, hepatitis A, mycoplasma, rotaviruses, streptococci, respiratory syncytial virus, and cytomegalovirus. Attempts have been made to immunize patients with treated organisms grown from cultures of the patient's own tissues (autogenous vaccines), but such procedures have not been clinically rewarding. The sine qua non for production of a vaccine is the availability of an experimental animal host or in vitro culture to produce an attenuated strain or enough of the agent for chemical modification. The breakthrough in the production of both attenuated and killed poliomyelitis vaccines was the development of in vitro conditions for culture of the virus. Regardless of the care taken to produce specific antigens for immunizations, it is virtually impossible to rule out dangerous contaminating materials. Although it was impossible to know at the time, the original Salk polio vaccine was contaminated with simian virus 40, which may be responsible for the production of slow virus infections.

Respiratory Disease Viruses

Immunization to acute virus-induced respiratory diseases, including the common cold, remains an as yet unattained goal. The status of vaccines for respiratory disease viruses of man is given in Table 25-5. The difficulties in developing such vaccines are exemplified by influenza, for which the most data are available. Immunization against influenza viruses is complicated because different strains show antigenic variations. When the influenza vaccine used contains the prevalent strain of virus the incidence of influenza in immunized individuals is reduced 75% to 90%. Influenza vaccine immunity is short-lived and yearly boosters must be given to maintain protection. Yearly immunization for elderly and other high-risk groups is recommended. Complications of immunization to influenza virus are exemplified by the epidemics of "swine flu" and "Russian flu" in the 1970s. A crash program was set up to produce a vaccine that would be effective against the new antigenic variation occurring in the swine flu virus. This required the cultivation of a large number of virus particles. A recombinant virus (X-53) was made up of the swine flu, a low-yield virus, and a high-yield laboratory virus (PR8G) by coculturing the two viruses in chick embryos. Isolates of viral particles containing most of the core RNA of the high-yield laboratory virus and the surface antigens (and the RNA coding for the surface antigens) of the swine flu virus were made. This permitted rapid production of the large number of viruses needed for the immunization program.

Although the necessary number of doses of the vaccine were prepared in time, two factors led to discontinuation of its use. First, the expected pandemic of swine flu never really materialized, and, second, the number of complications at least partially attributed to the vaccine was not acceptable. These included unexplained sudden death in the elderly (perhaps not statistically significant from the expected death rate) and development of the Guillain–Barré

Table 25-5. Status of Vaccines for Respiratory Tract Viruses of Man

Family	Genes	Clinical Effects	Vaccine	Status	Problem
Orthomyoviridae	Influenza virus (A, B, and C)	Acute respiratory diseases (adults and children)	Formalin-killed virus	Needs improvement	Antigenic drift, expensive
Paramyxoviridae	Paramyxovirus (types 1–4)	Croup, URI,[a] pneumonia (infants and children)	Formalin-killed virus	Unsatisfactory	No protective effect
	Pneumovirus (respiratory syncytial virus)	Pneumonia (infants)	Attenuated	Unsatisfactory	Lacks protective effect, intensifies infection
Picornaviridae	Rhinovirus (111 serotypes)	Common cold	Monovalent killed virus	Unsatisfactory	Many serotypes
	Enterovirus (70 serotypes)	Common cold, pneumonia, others	None available		Heterogeneity of genus
Coronaviridae	Coronavirus (3 types)	Coldlike illness	None available		Very great technical difficulties
Adenoviridae	Mastadenovirus (36 serotypes)	Pneumonia, URI,[a] acute respiratory disease, cystitis, keratoconjunctivitis	Formalin-killed	Needs improvement effective for types 4 and 7	Multiple serotypes

[a] Upper respiratory infection.

syndrome (see Chapter 20) in a small number of recipients (approximately ten cases per million doses). Although this was not a satisfactory experience, it is possible that future influenza epidemics could be controlled by careful administration of appropriate flu vaccines. The use of newly formulated swine flu vaccines between 1978 and 1981 has not been associated with an increased incidence of Guillain–Barré syndrome above that seen in an unimmunized population.

The concept of artificially providing partial protection against an infection, which will limit its extent but not prevent it, is illustrated by influenza vaccines. Influenza NA glycoprotein (NA) and hemagglutination (HA) antigens have been compared for protective effects. Both induce neutralizing antibody. Anti-HA prevents infection by blocking the ability of virus to bind to cells. Anti-NA is neutralizing only in high doses and does not prevent disease but limits cyclic infection in vivo. Thus, influenza vaccination that produces anti-HA may prevent infection temporarily when active, whereas anti-NA will not prevent infection, but will limit infection, prevent serious illness, and allow longer-lasting active immunity of infection to be established. In the long run it is possible that the partial protection provided by anti-NA may be more effective than the temporary "full protection" provided by anti-HA, since the full immunity provided by immunization to HA will decrease more rapidly than the full immunity established with immunity of infection.

Hepatitis

Other viral vaccines with promise are those for hepatitis and rabies. Attempts to culture hepatitis virus in vitro have not yet been successful. Several vaccines have been prepared by isolating hepatitis B viral particles from the blood of carriers and preparing surface antigens by biochemical procedures. These vaccines have been successfully tested in chimpanzees and are now being used in humans. There is no vaccine for hepatitis A or non-A, non-B forms of hepatitis virus. Hepatitis antigens produced by recombinant DNA technology may provide a solution to this problem.

Rabies

Since the development of the first rabies vaccine by Louis Pasteur in 1885 there have been serious problems in effectiveness and dangerous complications. Rabies virus vaccines had been prepared from viruses cultured on chick embryo cultures that were then inactivated. Although the neurological complications (autoallergic encephalomyelitis) are rare compared with those arising from the use of viruses obtained from the nervous system of infected animals, the potency of the chick embryo vaccine is not satisfactory.

In 1980 a new rabies vaccine produced in human diploid cultured cells became available. This vaccine produces antibody titers 10–20 times higher than those of the chick embryo vaccine. Only 5 injections of the cultured vaccine, in contrast to 14–21 injections of the duck vaccine, are required and the frequency of allergic reactions is far lower. Use of the duck vaccine has been discontinued. Exposed individuals are given passive immunization with human rabies immune globulin on Day 0 followed by the new vaccine on Days 0, 3, 7, 14, and 28.

Polio

Formalin-killed (Salk) and attenuated (Sabin) vaccines are available for immunization against polio. In evaluation of immunization to polio, factors in addition to protection of the immunized individual must be considered. Oral immunization by ingestion of attenuated virus induces local immunity within the gastrointestinal tract and may prevent passage of the virus through fecal contamination, while injection of killed virus is relatively ineffective in this regard. Polio infections are contracted naturally by swallowing of virus-contaminated materials. In an unprotected person, the virus passes into the bloodstream, leading to a systemic infection. Disease occurs when the virus attacks the anterior horn cells of the medulla and spinal cord. Antibody induced by injection prevents the systemic spread of the virus, but the gastrointestinal phase may still occur. On the other hand, oral immunization leads to local immunity in the gastrointestinal tract, presumably due to production of secretory antibody. This prevents the gastrointestinal phase of infection and limits spread of the virus. Persons inoculated with the killed virus may be protected from disease but can still serve as carriers to disseminate the virus during an epidemic. If a substantial portion of a population has received the oral vaccine, even the unimmunized portion of the population is protected from epidemic disease. The incidence of paralytic poliomyelitis in the United States from 1951 to 1978 is given in Table 25-6. Although some controversy exists in regard to the efficiency of intramuscular injections of killed polio vaccine and of oral administration of attenuated poliovirus, oral vaccine is recommended by most authorities at this time, administered for the first time between 2 months of age and the preschool period.

Table 25-6. Correlation of Paralytic Poliomyelitis and Vaccine Use in the United States, 1951–1978

Period	Vaccine	Total Number	Average Number/Year	Average Number/ Million/Year
1951–1955	None	111,040	22,208	135
1956–1960	IPV only	22,970	4,594	26
1961–1965	IPV and OPV	2,341	468	2.4
1973–1978	OPV only	55	9	0.004

IPV, formalin-inactivated polio vaccine; OPV, oral (attenuated) line polio vaccine.
Modified from Sabin AE: Paralytic poliomyelitis: old do nas and new perspectives. Rev Infect Dis 3:543–564, 1981.

Measles

Measles and other diseases such as rubella and mumps could theoretically be eliminated by effective global vaccination programs. Not only have attenuated measles vaccines been effective in reducing active measles infections, but the incidence of late occurring disease manifestation believed to be related to measles, such as subacute sclerosing panencephalitis (see Chapter 20), has also dropped dramatically after institution of measles vaccination.

Helminths

Helminths (worms) are the most prevalent infectious agents of humans, yet no vaccine is available for any of these agents. For example, programs aimed at eliminating schistosomiasis have been unsuccessful. The problem may be addressed at three points in the life cycle of the organisms: (1) prevention of parasite contact between the intermediate host (snail) and the definitive host (human) in the water, by sanitation and protected water supplies; (2) destruction of the intermediate host (snail); and (3) prevention of infection in the human by vaccination or chemotherapy. To eradicate this disease, attack at all three levels is required. Control of the intermediate host (snail) has not proven feasible by itself and treatment of water supplies remains costly and not possible at this time in all infected areas. Chemotherapy, particularly of infected children, who may pass thousands of schistosome eggs in their stools per day, could drastically reduce transmission of the disease since the drugs hycanthone or metriforiate provide more than 90% reduction in worm burdens, thus greatly reducing the chances of spreading infections. Unfortunately a vaccine for schistosomiasis does not yet exist.

Oral Vaccines

Oral or inhalation administration of vaccines has been proposed to deliver antigens in order to induce effective local immunity. Over 100 years ago, on the basis of immunization against chicken cholera, Louis Pasteur suggested that vaccination by the oral route might be more effective against enteropathogenic bacteria than vaccination by intramuscular or subcutaneous inoculation. Such an approach has been attempted using *Vibrio cholera*, typhoid, and dysentery. Local protection may be due to production of mucosal IgA antibody or sensitized cells, and may not be reflected in titers of serum antibodies. As discussed in Chapter 3, there is an extensive gastrointestinal and bronchoalveolar associated lymphoid system in all mammalian species, which responds vigorously to antigens and produces effective antibody- and cell-mediated immunity. The results of limited trials of oral vaccination against adenovirus type 4, cholera, dysentery, and herpes simplex have suggested that mucosal immunity may be enhanced by oral challenge. Inhalation of influenza vaccine has been associated with production of IgA mucosal antibody, but a definite increased protective effect using this route has not been demonstrated.

Complications of Virus Vaccines

Vaccines prepared from live attenuated viruses, such as measles, mumps, rubella, and trivalent oral poliomyelitis vaccines, may cause symptomatic infection in the nervous system in 1 of 10,000 to 1,300,000 vaccine recipients. Vaccines prepared from killed whole organisms may cause demyelinating disease in approximately 1 in 100,000 recipients. An additional complication of vaccination is an allergic reaction to a component of the vaccine. For instance, yellow fever vaccine is prepared in embryonated chicken eggs. Because of the possibility of anaphylactic shock, yellow fever vaccine must be carefully administered to patients who are allergic to eggs or chicken feathers. Influenza vaccine is also produced in eggs, but is highly purified prior to use. Rarely anaphylactic reactions have been attributed to trace amounts of calf serum proteins in measles vaccines.

New Approaches to Vaccine Production

The development of new techniques in molecular biology and immunology offers breakthroughs for the production of immunogens for infectious diseases. The approaches now being used are (1) in vitro synthesis of immunogenic peptides, (2) cloning of DNA for immunogens, and (3) use of anti-idiotypes as immunogens.

Synthetic Vaccines

To synthesize antigenic peptides the amino acid sequences of the epitope recognized by the immune system must be identified, and the peptide must be synthesized and administered to the responding animal in an immunogenic form. The identification of epitope peptides can be accomplished by direct analysis of the amino acid sequence of the protein or deduced from the cDNA sequence for the protein. For instance, the 220-amino-acid primary structure of hepatitis B surface antigen (HBsAg) was determined from the sequence of bases in the cDNA for HBsAg. The tertiary structure was deduced and candidate peptides for epitopes for immunization selected. The selection process includes (1) presence of charged amino acids that permit solubility, (2) predicted presence of sequences on the surface of the antigenic molecule, (3) peptides longer than 10 amino acid residues (small peptides tend to be poorly immunogenic), (4) presence of a proline residue (usually present at bends in the mature polypeptide chain and important for the tertiary conformation), and (5) presence of an amino acid residue that will allow coupling to a carrier, such as cysteine residue. The selected peptides are synthesized by the automated method of Maryfield. The peptides are then tested for immunogenicity by immunization of rabbits or other experimental animals with or without coupling to carriers. In this manner immunogenic peptides of HBsAg, foot and mouth disease virus, and the hemagglutinin antigen of influenza A virus have been identified and tested in animals. So far the results are encouraging, but application to man requires considerably more development. In the case of influenza A hemagglutinin, antibodies to common peptides not in the four dominant strain-specific antigenic domains have been produced. This observation suggests that immunization to a common sequence conserved among different virus strains might be impossible. A major theoretical problem is the ability of these engineered antigens to mimic the conformation of the naturally produced antigenic proteins.

Recombinant Vaccines

Expression of cloned DNA for immunogenic molecules in bacterial and viral vectors offers another method for vaccine production. The hemagglutinin of influenza virus, HBsAg, and antigens of *T. pallidum*, malaria, and other organisms have been produced in plasmids introduced into *E. coli*, yeast, or mammalian tissue culture cells and by insertion into vaccinia virus. Vaccinia and other viruses offer genomes that can be easily manipulated through the use of restriction enzymes to construct recombinants that will synthesize the desired polypeptide product and at the same time provide a highly immunogenic nonpathological carrier.

Idiotype Vaccines

Anti-idiotypic antibodies that react with the paratope of an antibody to an infectious organism may be used to immunize animals to produce an anti-anti-idiotype that reproduces the paratope of the original antibody (see Chapter 7). By such immunization the anti-anti-idiotype will have paratope specificity for the epitope on the original infectious agent. In experimental systems anti-idiotypic antibodies have been used to induce protective antibodies to *Trypanosoma rhodesiense*, and anti-idiotypic antibodies against antiphosphorylcholine known to protect against lethal streptoccal pneumonia infection have been successful in immunizing mice to resist infection. Delayed hypersensitivity to herpes simplex has been induced in mice using rabbit anti-mouse idiotype sera. Finally, monoclonal antibodies to specific epitopes of infectious agents have been shown to be effective in producing temporary protection by passive transfer. Each of these approaches offers great expectations for future development of artificial immunization against infectious diseases.

Antifertility Vaccines

Control of population growth is the major problem in large areas of the world, particularly India and China. Conventional birth control methods are difficult to apply to many of the people who need them the most. Conceptually it is possible to immunize against an antigen that is unique to a reproductive organ and has a fertility-related function that could be blocked by antibody. Potential antigens include reproductive hormones, sperm, embryonic tissue, and/or egg antigens.

Chorionic Gonadotropin. Successful trials in baboons and women have demonstrated that immunization to human chorionic gonadotropin (hCG) can effectively decrease fertility without producing side effects, either in the women immunized or in infants that are born to hCG immunized mothers. However, the immunogenicity is not uniform; many women do not develop effective antibody titers.

Sperm Antigen. A more consistent immunizing protocol or antigenic preparation is lactate dehydrogenase-C4 (LDH-C4), an isozyme of lactate dehydrogenase (LDH) found only in male germinal cells. This enzyme may be purified to crystalline homogeneity, and female rabbits and mice immunized with LDH-C4 have significantly reduced pregnancies. This effect is reversible when serum antibody levels fall after immunization. Other potential sperm antigens are being studied at this time.

Egg Antigens. Although little is known about egg antigens, at least three unique glycoproteins are found in the noncellular gelatinous layer surrounding the mature oocyte, the zona pellucida. Antibodies to these glycoproteins are able to block fertilization in vitro and passive immunization has been effective in decreasing pregnancies in experimental animals.

Embryonic Antigen. Antibodies to embryonic antigens such as the F9 antigen found on the blastocyst of mouse embryos may also reduce fertility, but little is known of human embryonic antigens that could provide effective antifertility immunogens. The use of antifertility vaccines is clearly at an early developmental stage and not yet practical as an effective means of birth control.

Evaluation of Immunization

Evaluation of the effectiveness of a vaccine poses considerable problems. If an experimental animal is available, the vaccine can be tested for its ability to protect the infected animal. In many cases, either an animal model is not available or the experimental disease does not resemble the human disease. The ability of the vaccine to induce antibody formation or delayed hypersensitivity in humans can be tested, but the presence of antibody or cellular sensitivity may not necessarily be correlated with resistance to disease. The only valid method is to test the ability of the vaccine to reduce the incidence or severity of disease in human clinical trials. This requires painstaking planning and evaluation. Protection of the immunized individual may not be the sole criterion of effectiveness; the effect of immunization on populations, "herd immunity," must also be considered.

Liability for Vaccine Manufacture

Vaccine production has become complicated by financial liability of manufacturers for untoward effects of vaccine administration. Large financial payments have been awarded to claimants under the tort legal system. Thus, many manufacturers have decided not to continue producing proven vaccines. The American Academy of Pediatrics has recommended that a manufacturer not be held liable if its product is listed in the Vaccine Compensation Table and if the vaccine has been tested, manufactured, distributed, and labeled in accordance with the requirements of the Food and Drug Administration, and that all claimants file for compensation via a proposed federal no-fault system.

Immunity as a Relative Condition

Specific or nonspecific resistance to infection is a relative state. The effect of different doses of infectious agents or their products on experimental animals clearly demonstrates that administration of sufficiently large numbers of organisms can overcome the resistance of a highly immune animal. In addition, doses of toxins can be given that kill animals with high titers of neutralizing antibody. Thus, immunity to infection is not an absolute condition, but depends on a large number of complex variables, including not only the resistance of the host but also the dose, route of contact, and virulence of the infecting agent. In leprosy, chemotherapy may reduce the organism load in a given person, permitting immune defense mechanisms to achieve the upper hand. In an extensive chemotherapeutic eradication program in Malta, there has been a marked reduction in the incidence of the disease.

Summary

Specific immunity may be conferred passively by transfer of immune serum or cells to a naive recipient, or by active immunization. Passive immunity by transfer of antibody is effective if immediate neutralization of toxin or other agents is needed. Passive transfer of cellular immunity has been generally unsuccessful in man except in specific cases where transfer factor has been beneficial in selected diseases such as chronic mucocutaneous candidiasis.

Active immunization has changed the history of mankind in that a number of previously uncontrolled infectious diseases are now rarely seen or even eliminated. Vaccination against smallpox has eliminated one of history's greatest scourges. Some other diseases now essentially under control by active immunization include tetanus, diphtheria, polio, measles, and mumps.

New approaches to production of vaccines using synthetic antigens, antigens produced by gene cloning, and anti-idiotypic immunogens give promise that improved vaccination methods will lead to control of additional infectious diseases in the future.

References

Passive Immunity

Centers for Disease Control: Immune globulin for protection against viral hepatitis. Recommendations of the immunization practices advisory committee. Ann Intern Med 96:193, 1982.

Dix RD, Pereira L, Baringer JF: Use of monoclonal antibodies directed against herpes simplex virus glycoprotein to protect mice against acute virus-induced neurological disease. Infect Immun 34:192, 1981.

Merler E (ed): Immunoglobulins: Biological Aspects and Clinical Uses. Washington, D.C., National Academy of Sciences, 1971.

Steim ER: Standard and special human immune globulins as therapeutic agents. Pediatrics 63:301, 1979.

Active Immunization

Smallpox

Behbehani AM: The smallpox story: life and death of an old disease. Microbiol Rev 47:455, 1983.

Henderson DA: Smallpox eradication. Proc Soc Lond [Biol] 199:83, 1977.

Jenner E: Inquiry into the Cause and Effects of the Variolae Vacciniae. London, Low, 1798; republished in 1896 by Cassell.

Sabin AB: Eradication of smallpox and elimination of poliomyelitis: contrast in strategy. Jap J Med Sci Biol 34:109, 1981.

von Pirquet CF: Klinische Studien über Vakzination und vakzinale Allergie. Leipzig, Deuticke, 1907.

Others

Baguley DM, Glasgow GL: Subacute sclerosing panencephalitis and Salk Vaccine. Lancet 2:763, 1973.

Baker CJ, Kasper DL: Group B streptococcal vaccines. Rev Infect Dis 7:458, 1985.

Beneson AS: Immunization and military medicine. Rev Infect Dis 6:1, 1984.

Brown IN: Immunologic aspects of malaria infection. Adv Immunol 11:268, 1969.

Cannon DA (ed): Symposium on Immunization in Childhood. Edinburgh, Livingstone, 1960.

Cvjetanovic B: Immunization programmes. WHO Chron 27:66, 1973.

Dudgeon JA: Immunization in times ancient and modern. J Roy Sci Med 73:581, 1980.

Eickhoff TC: Immunization. The adult thing to do. J Infect Dis 152:1, 1985.

Enders JF, Weller TH, Robbins FC: Cultivation of the Lansing strain of poliomyelitis virus in cultures of various human embryonic tissue. Science 109:85, 1949.

Fazekas de St Groth S: Evolution and hierarchy of influenza viruses. Arch Environ Health 21:293, 1970.

Freerksen E, Rosenfeld M: Leprosy eradication project of Malta. First published report after 5 years running. Chemotherapy 23:356, 1977.

Germanier R (ed): Bacterial Vaccines. Orlando, Fla., Academic Press, 1984.

Glenny AT, Hopkins BE: Diphtheria toxoid as an immunizing agent. Br J Exp Pathol 4:823, 1923.

Heggie AD: Immunization against infectious disease. Med Clin North Am 67:17, 1983.

Hennessen W, Regamey RH (eds): Joint WHO/IABS Symposium on the standardization of rabies vaccines for human use produced in tissue culture (Rabies III). Basel, Karger, 1978.

Holt LB: Developments in Diphtheria Prophylaxis. London, Heinemann, 1950.

Katzenellenbogen I: Vaccination against oriental sore: reports of 555 inoculations. Arch Dermatol 50:239, 1944.

Killbourne ED: Influenza as a problem in immunology. J Immunol 120:1447, 1978.

Krugman S, Katz SL: Childhood immunization procedures. JAMA 237:2228, 1977.

Krugman S, Perkins FT: Vaccination against communicable diseases. Am J Dis Child 126:406, 1973.

Lennette EH: Viral respiratory diseases and antivirals. Bull WHO 59:305, 1981.

Melnick JL: Viral vaccines: new problems and prospects. Hosp Pract 13:104, 1978.

Oxman M: Hepatitis B vaccination of high-risk hospital personnel. Anesthesiology 60:1, 1984.

Sabin AB: Paralytic poliomyelitis: old dogmas and new perspectives. Rev Infect Dis 3:543, 1981.

Salk J, Salk D: Control of influenza and poliomyelitis with killed virus vaccines. Science 195:834, 1977.

Schiff P: Modern trends in immunization. Med J Aust 1:551, 1973.

Sever JL: Infectious disease and immunization. Rev Infect Dis 4:136, 1982.

Smith DT: Autogenous vaccines in theory and practice. Arch Intern Med 125:344, 1970.

Stokes J Jr: Recent advances in immunization against viral diseases. Ann Intern Med 73:829, 1970.

Wiktor TJ: Historical aspects of rabies treatment. *In* Koprowski H, Plotkin SA (eds), World's Debt to Pasteur. New York, Liss, 1985.

Evaluation

Anderson LJ, et al: Post exposure trial of a human diploid strain. Rabies vaccine. J Infect Dis 142:133, 1982.

Artenstein MS: The current status of bacterial vaccines. Hosp Pract 8:49, 1973.

Bres P: Immunization in developing countries. Ann Inst Pasteur 136D:293, 1985.

Celers J: Measles immunization: a ten year report. Bull Inst Pasteur 75:327, 1977.

Cochi SL, Biloome CV, Hightower MS: Immunization of U.S. children with hemophilus influenza type B polysaccharide vaccine. JAMA 253:521, 1985.

Creese AL, Henderson RH: Cost benefit analysis and immunization program in developing countries. Bull WHO 58:491, 1980.

Creese AL, et al: Cost-effectiveness appraisal of immunization programmes. Bull WHO 60:621, 1982.

D'Arcy Hart P: Efficacy and applicability of mass BCG vaccination in tuberculosis control. Br Med J 1:587, 1967.

Frenkel JK: Models for infectious disease. Fed Proc 28:179, 1969.

Fulginiti VA: Immunizations. Current controversies. J Pediatr 101:487, 1982.

Gershon AA, et al: Live alternated varicella vaccine efficacy for children with leukemia in remission. JAMA 252:355, 1984.

Perkins FT (ed): Symposium Series in Immunobiological Standardization. 22: International Symposium on Vaccination against Communicable Diseases. Basel, Karger, 1973.

Sabin AB: Present position of immunization against poliomyelitis virus with live virus vaccines. Br Med J 1:663, 1959.

Sisk JE, Riegelman RK: Cost effectiveness of vaccination against pneumococcal pneumonia: An update. Ann Intern Med 104:79, 1986.

Taylor AER (ed): Immunity to Parasites. Oxford, Blackwell, 1968.

New Approaches to Vaccine Development

General

Dorner F, McDonel JL: Bacterial toxin vaccines. Vaccine 3:94, 1985.

Lerner RA, Chanock RM: Modern Approaches to Vaccines: Molecular and Chemical Basis of Virus Virulence and Immunogenicity. Cold Spring Harbor, N.Y., Cold Spring Harbor Laboratory, 1984.

Liew FY: New aspects of vaccine development. Clin Exp Immunol 62:225, 1985.

Mizrahi A, Hertman I, Klingberg MA, Kohn A: New Developments with Human and Veterinary Vaccines. New York, Liss, 1980.

Morin B, Simons K: Subunit vaccines against developed viruses: virosomes, micelles and other protein complexes. Vaccine 3:83, 1985.

Synthetic Vaccines

Brown F: Synthetic viral vaccines. Annu Rev Microbiol 3:221, 1984.

Lerner RA, et al: The development of synthetic vaccines. Hosp Pract 16:55, 1981.

Shinnick TM, et al: Synthetic peptide immunogens as vaccines. Annu Rev Microbiol 37:425, 1983.

Idiotype Vaccines

Bona C, Moran T: Idiotype vaccines. Ann Inst Pasteur 136:21, 1985.

McNamara MK, Ward RE, Kohler H: Monoclonal idiotope vaccine against streptococcus pneumonia infection. Science 226:1325, 1984.

Sacks DL, Kelsoe GH, Sacks DH: Induction of immune responses with anti-idiotypic antibodies: implications for the induction of protective immunity. Springer Semin Immunopathol 6:79, 1983.

Recombinant Vaccines

Arnot DE, et al: Circumsporozoite protein of plasmodium vivax: gene cloning and characterization of the immunodominant epitope. Science 230:815, 1985.

Brown F, Schild GC, Ada GL: Recombinant vaccinia viruses as vaccines. Nature 319:549, 1986.

Burnette WN, et al: Production of hepatitis-B recombinant vaccines. *In* Lerner RA, Chanock RM (eds): Modern Approaches to Vaccines: Molecular and Chemical Basis of Virus Virulence and Immunogenicity. Cold Spring Harbor, N.Y., Cold Spring Harbor Laboratory, 1984.

Godson N: Molecular approaches to malaria vaccines. Sci Am 252:52, 1985.

Macrina FL: Molecular cloning of bacterial antigens and virulence determinants. Annu Rev Microbiol 38:193, 1984.

Antifertility Vaccines

Anderson DJ, Alexander NJ: A new look at antifertility vaccines. Fert Steril 40:557, 1983.

Liability

Aukrust L, Almeland TL, Refsum D, Aas K: Severe hypersensitivity or intolerance reactions to measles vaccine in six children. Allergy 35:581, 1980.

Fenichel GM: Neurological complications of immunization. Ann Neurol 12:119, 1982.

Leinikki PO: Vaccination policies for the 80's. Am Clin Res 14:195, 1982.

Peter G: Vaccine crisis: an emerging social problem. J Infect Dis 151:981, 1985.

Immunity as a Relative Condition

Austin KF, Cohn ZA: Contribution of serum and cellular factors in host defense reactions. N Engl J Med 268:933,934,1056, 1963.

Bienenstock J, Befus AD: Mucosal immunity. Immunology 41:249, 1980.

Braude AI: Resistance to infection. *In* Grollman A (ed): Clinical Physiology. New York, McGraw–Hill, 1957, p773.

Capron A, Dessaint JP, Capron M: Immunoregulation of parasites. J Allergy Clin Immunol 66:91, 1980.

Gladstone GP: Pathogenicity and virulence of micro-organisms. *In* Florey HW (ed): General Pathology, 4th ed. Philadelphia, Saunders, 1970.

Rich AR: The Pathogenesis of Tuberculosis, 2nd ed. Springfield, Ill., Thomas, 1951.

Shulman S: Allergic responses to insects. Annu Rev Entomol 12:323, 1967.

Soulsby EJL: The mechanism of immunity to gastro-intestinal nematodes. *In* Biology of Parasites. New York, Academic Press, 1966.

Stebbings JH: Immediate hypersensitivity: a defense against arthropods. Perspect Biol Med 17:233, 1974.

Turk JL, Bryceson ADM: Immunological phenomena in leprosy and related diseases. Adv Immunol 13:209, 1971.

Wakelin D: Immunity to intestinal parasites. Nature 273:617, 1978.

Wheelock EF, Toy ST: Participation of lymphocytes in viral infections. Adv Immunol 16:123, 1973.

26 | Immune Deficiency Diseases

The occurrence of repeated infections in an individual may reflect a deficiency in defense mechanisms against infection. Such deficiencies must be especially considered if the infecting organism is one that is not usually responsible for human diseases. The type of infection observed is determined by the kind of immune abnormality present. Immune deficiency diseases may be classified as primary or secondary. Primary immune deficiencies result from genetic or developmental abnormalities in the acquisition of immune maturity. Secondary deficiencies result from diseases that interfere with the expression of a mature immune system.

Multiple levels of defensive reactions must be considered in evaluating resistance to infection. Infections may occur with increased frequency in elderly individuals, in debilitated patients, or when natural nonimmune barriers are affected. The depression of pulmonary clearing mechanisms due to the loss of the ciliary activity of bronchial lining cells found associated with exposure to cigarette smoke is an example. In addition there is a genetic disorder resulting in a microtubule defect that affects the mobility of cilia, the immotile cilia syndrome. Affected patients also have immobile sperm and chronic respiratory infections, frequent *Hemophilus influenzae* infection, and abundant mucus secretions. Because of the complexity of immune deficiencies and the diverse clinical presentation of deficiency states, a careful systematic diagnostic workup must be carried out in order to select appropriate therapy.

Development of Immune Maturity

A common ancestral cell for all white cells, including immunologically competent cells, arises from a bone marrow precursor. For potentially immunologically competent cells to mature and obtain the capacity to recognize antigen they must come into contact with, or be affected by, products of endodermal tissue. The embryonal gut-associated (endodermal) lymph-

617

oid tissue, termed the *central* lymphoid tissue, consists of the thymus, tonsils, appendix, Peyer's patches, liver, and in fowl, the bursa of Fabricius. The peripheral lymphoid tissue is the remaining lymphoid tissue, including lymph nodes and spleen. If needed, the reader should refer to Chapter 4 for a detailed exposition of this subject.

Response of Immature Animals

Fetal and neonatal animals may be induced to form antibody or develop high levels of immunoglobulins if given strong antigenic stimuli, but often have a delayed or blunted response to T-dependent antigens. Neonatal animals normally are protected by maternal antibody received by placental transfer or by absorption of colostral antibodies shortly after birth (Fig. 26-1). The newborn animal begins to produce its own antibodies due to natural stimulation. The development of "normal"

Figure 26-1. Serum immunoglobulin levels during normal life. The newborn human has high levels of serum IgG because of maternal transfer of IgG across the placenta. Colostrum provides additional immunoglobulins, particularly gastrointestinal IgA. During infancy, serum IgM becomes elevated within 1 month and serum IgG between 4 and 8 months; serum IgA rises gradually over the first 10 years of life. Neonates also have decreased cellular immune responses most likely due to smaller numbers of T cells in the immature state.

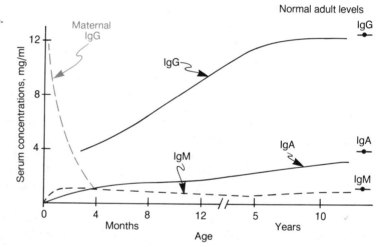

lymphoid tissue and "normal" immunoglobulin levels depends on contact with antigen; germ-free animals that have a markedly reduced antigenic load maintain only very low levels of serum immunoglobulins and have undeveloped, immature lymphoid tissue. However, germ-free animals can respond to appropriate antigenic stimuli.

Hypogammaglobulinemia of Infancy

A temporary functional delay in the production of immunoglobulins by a newborn may cause a transient hypogammaglobulinemia of infancy. Hypogammaglobulinemia occurs when the normal catabolism of placentally transferred maternal IgG commencing after birth is associated with an abnormal delay in the onset of the immunoglobulin synthetic capacity. This temporary immunoglobulin deficiency usually terminates between 9 and 18 months of age. Since it is only temporary, this hypogammaglobulinemia is not considered a primary immune deficiency disease. If it continues, a true permanent immune deficiency disease must be considered.

Neonatal Wasting Syndrome: TORCH

"Wasting" of newborn infants is seen following infection in utero with a number of organisms that are able to cross the placenta from the mother to the fetus (e.g., rubella), or with infection at birth because of organisms in the birth canal (herpes). A newborn infant with low birth weight, microencephaly, eye abnormalities, and liver and other visceral abnormalities may reflect the effects of congenital infection with a number of otherwise unrelated agents given the acronym *TORCH*. TORCH refers to *to*xoplasmosis, *r*ubella, *c*ytomegalovirus, and *h*erpes simplex, in recognition of the infectious organisms most frequently recognized as the causative agents. Other infectious agents, such as *Treponema pallidum* (congenital syphilis) and *Listeria*, may produce similar findings, so that the *O* in *TORCH* may be considered to stand for "other" infectious agents. The chronic infectious state appears to be related to immaturity of the infant's immune system at the time of infection. Such infections are not able to be controlled, resulting in chronic wasting disease. In addition to immune deficiencies, congenitally infected infants frequently also have other developmental abnormalities, that is, blindness, mental retardation, and heart defects.

Primary Immune Deficiencies

Developmental abnormalities result in a permanent loss of immune cells at specific anatomic sites. Such abnormalities may occur at one of the major sites of immune development mentioned above: the ancestral anlage, the thymus-dependent system, or the immunoglobulin-producing system. The levels of development where immune deficiencies may occur are illustrated in Figure 26-2. Essentially, three major primary immune deficits occur: combined antibody and cellular, antibody alone, and cellular alone.

Combined Immune Deficiencies

Anlage Defects

The failure of development of all blood cell lines, presumably because no hematopoietic stem cells are present, is known as reticular dysgenesis. Affected fetuses lack all types of white blood cells and at autopsy have no lymphoid tissue. All have been stillbirths. The genetic defect is unknown.

Severe Combined Immune Deficiencies

Severe combined immune deficiencies (SCID) may have several etiologies, including a failure in development of stem cells and inborn errors of metabolism in which purine synthesizing enzymes are inactive or defective. Severe combined immune deficiencies include Swiss type agammaglobulinemia, thymic alymphoplasia, Wiskott-Aldrich syndrome, and ataxia–telangiectasia. Infants with SCID fail to grow normally and have severe infections. Symptoms may appear within the first few days of life, but in most cases infectious complications do not appear until 4–6 months of age. Maternal transfer of some cellular immune function, as well as immunoglobulin, occurs. Children with severe combined immune deficiencies fre-

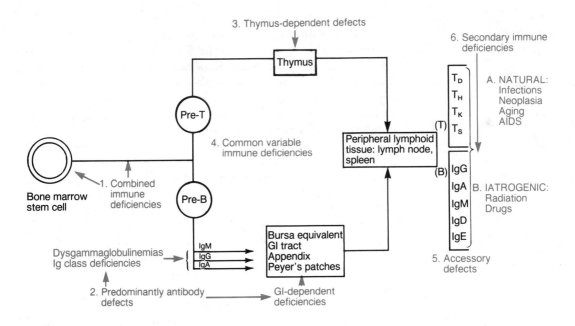

Figure 26-2. Postulated sites of defects in immune diseases. The type and severity of infections seen are related to the deficiency type and the level of development affected. Blocks 1–6 indicate the possible sites of development defects in primary immune deficiencies: (1) combined immune deficiencies, (2) predominantly antibody defects (dysgammaglobulinemias), (3) thymus-dependent defects, (4) common variable deficiencies, (5) defects in accessory systems such as complement or phagocytic capacity, and (6) secondary immune deficiencies that affect an already developed immune system and are due to other disease states or treatment for other diseases (see also Fig. 4-1).

quently develop a skin rash, consistent with a graft versus host reaction, believed to be caused by maternal lymphoid cells. Maternal lymphocytes may cross the placenta during gestation. Normally such placentally transferred cells are rejected by the immune system of the fetus. However, if the fetus is unable to react to them, the foreign cells may proliferate in the immune deficient child and produce a graft versus host reaction. Such cells may also provide some cellular immunity and protect the child from fulminant viral infections during the first 4 to 6 months of life.

Swiss Type Agammaglobulinemia and Thymic Alymphoplasia. All major immunoglobulin groups (IgG, IgA, and IgM) are severely depressed (total <0.25 mg/ml) and there is a striking deficiency of lymphocytes in the blood (<1000/ml). At autopsy only a few plasma cells and lymphocytes are found, and the thymus is atrophic and lacks Hassall's corpuscles. A deficiency in the reactivity of lymphocytes from patients with this disease can be demonstrated by the lack of in vitro stimulation by phytohemagglutinin. SCID occur as an autosomal recessive (Swiss

Table 26-1. Combined Immune Deficiency Diseases

Designation	Usual Phenotypic Expression					Presumed Nature of Basic Defect	Inheritance
	Serum Ig	Serum Antibodies	Circulating B Cells	Circulating T Cells	CMI		
1. Reticular dysgenesis	None	None	None	None	None	No anlage	?
2. Swiss type agamma-globulinemia	Decreased or absent	Absent	Decreased or absent	Decreased or absent	Absent	No lymphoid stem cell	AR
3. Thymic alymphoplasia	Decreased or absent	Absent	Decreased or absent	Decreased or absent	Absent	No lymphoid stem cell	X-linked
4. Wiskott–Aldrich syndrome[a]	Increased IgA, IgE; decreased IgM	Decreased	Normal	Progressive decrease	Progressive decrease	Cell membrane defect affecting all hematopoietic stem cell derivatives	X-linked
5. Ataxia–telangiectasia[a]	Often decreased IgA, IgE, and IgG; increased IgM (monomers)	Variably decreased	Normal	Decreased	Decreased	Unknown: defective T cell maturation	AR

[a] Characteristic associated features: Wiskott–Aldrich syndrome—thrombocytopenia, eczema; ataxia–telangiectasia—cerebellar ataxia, telangiectasia, ovarian dysgenesis, chromosomal instability, decreased α-fetoprotein.

type agammaglobulinemia) or sex-linked (thymic alymphoplasia) defect. The presence of epithelial remnants in the thymus associated with an absence of lymphocytes suggests a defect in the production of prothymocytes as well as of B stem cells, that is, a defect at the level of the lymphoid stem cell that gives rise to both T and B cell lineages.

The features of other severe combined immune deficiencies, including Wiskott–Aldrich syndrome and ataxia–telangiectasia, are listed in Table 26-1.

Wiskott–Aldrich Syndrome. This syndrome is an X-linked recessive, combined immune deficiency with a marked deficiency in IgM and usually depressed cellular immunity resulting in death in early infancy from infections. Serum IgA and IgG levels are usually normal. There is also eczema and thrombocytopenia (low blood platelets), and bleeding may be the first manifestation of the disease.

Ataxia–Telangiectasia. Ataxia–telangiectasia is an autosomal recessive combined immune deficiency disease. The serum IgA is very low, the IgG low or normal, and the IgM usually normal. The lymphoid organs are atrophic or absent. There is also oculocutaneous telangiectasia (dilated and redundant vessels), progressive cerebellar ataxia, and increased lymphoreticular malignancies.

Purine Metabolism and Primary Immune Deficiencies

A small number of children with SCID have enzymatic defects in the purine biosynthesis pathways. Purine interconversions are required for normal maturation of the rapidly dividing cells of the lymphoid system. Blocks in purine biosynthesis may lead to accumulation of deoxynucleosides which are toxic to lymphocytes (Fig. 26-3). These include a T cell deficiency, a B cell deficiency, and a combined deficiency (Table 26-2).

Figure 26-3. Purine metabolism and immune deficiencies (see Table 26-6).

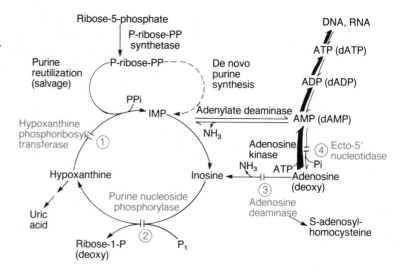

Table 26-2. Clinical Symptoms and Expression of Diseases Associated with Defects in Purine Metabolism

1. HYPOXANTHINE–GUANINE PHOSPHORIBOSYLTRANSFERASE DEFICIENCY (LESCH–NYHAN SYNDROME)

Possible B cell immunodeficiency. There is a marked overproduction of purines and overexcretion of uric acid. These children have severe neurological impairment and self-destructive behavior. Their lymphocytes respond poorly to stimulation with pokeweed mitogen.

2. PURINE NUCLEOTIDE PHOSPHORYLASE (PNP) DEFICIENCY (T CELL IMMUNODEFICIENCY)

Features large quantities of ribonucleosides (inosine and guanosine) as well as 2′-deoxyribonucleosides (2′-deoxyinosine and 2′-deoxyguanosine) in urine, in red cells, and in lymphocytes; a loss of purines that are necessary for lymphocyte proliferation; and severe impairment of DNA synthesis. There is recurrent infection and anemia, severe lymphopenia, pronounced depression of lymphocyte responses to mitogenic and allogeneic cell stimuli, and decreased T cell rosette formation.

3. ADENOSINE DEAMINASE (ADA) DEFICIENCY (T AND B CELL IMMUNODEFICIENCY)

Children have high concentrations of AMP and deoxy-AMP in erythrocytes and lymphocytes (2–10 times normal), and large amounts of 2′-deoxyadenosine are excreted in urine. They have respiratory infections, lymphopenia, and no delayed hypersensitivity response to candida, mumps, and streptokinase–streptodornase. Their lymphocytes respond poorly to phytohemagglutinin, pokeweed mitogen, and allogeneic cells, and they fail to develop isohemagglutinins.

4. ECTO-5′-NUCLEOTIDASE DEFICIENCY (B CELL IMMUNODEFICIENCY)

Children have increased concentrations of toxic deoxyribonucleotides in lymphocyte subpopulations and agammaglobulinemia.

Bare Lymphocyte Syndrome

Rarely, patients with combined immune deficiencies have decreased expression of class I and, less frequently, class II major histocompatibility complex (MHC) determinants on blood mononuclear cells. This defect in MHC expression on lymphocytes apparently interferes with the self recognition mechanisms required for induction of effective immune responses.

Predominantly Antibody Defects (Dysgammaglobulinemias)

A listing of immune deficiencies with diminished production of humoral antibody is given in Table 26-3. The dysgammaglobulinemias include six possible combinations of depressed levels of a major immunoglobulin group or groups associated with normal or elevated levels of the other immunoglobulins: selective IgA or IgG deficiency; selective IgM deficiency; deficiencies of IgG and IgA with normal IgM (type I dysgammaglobulinemia, usually associated with cellular immune deficiency); deficiencies of IgM and IgA with normal IgG (type II dysgammaglobulinemia); and deficiency of IgG and IgM associated with normal or elevated levels of IgA. Some of these are considered to be late-appearing, genetically controlled defects whereas others may be acquired abnormalities of control of the immune response. The classic example, the first recognized immune deficiency, is Bruton's disease.

Bruton's Congenital Sex-Linked Agammaglobulinemia

This disease is also called *infantile sex-linked agammaglobulinemia*. Symptoms appear when transplacentally acquired maternal antibodies disappear from the circulation at 5

Table 26-3. Predominantly Antibody Defects

Designation	Usual Phenotypic Expression					Presumed Pathogenesis/ Differentiation Defect	Inheritance
	Serum Ig	Serum Antibodies	Circulating B Cells	Circulating T Cells	CMI		
1. Bruton's X-linked agammaglobulinemia	All isotypes decreased	Decreased	Usually absent	Normal	Normal	Intrinsic defect in pre-B to B cell differentiation	X-linked
2. Autosomal recessive agammaglobulinemia	All isotypes decreased	Decreased	Decreased	Normal	Normal	Intrinsic defect in pre-B to B cell differentiation	AR
3. Ig deficiency with increased IgM (and IgD)	IgM and IgD increased, IgG and IgA decreased	IgM increased, IgG + IgA decreased	Normal IgM- and IgD-bearing cells, no IgG- or IgA-bearing cells	Normal	Normal	Intrinsic isotype switch defect: failure of IgM$^+$, IgD$^+$ B cell maturation to IgG$^+$, IgA$^+$, IgE$^+$ B cells	X-linked or AR or unknown
4. IgA deficiency	IgA decreased	IgA decreased	Immature serum IgA B cells	Usually normal	Usually normal	Defective IgA ($\pm$ IgG subclass) B cell maturation	Unknown: some AR
5. Selective deficiency of other Ig isotypes	Decrease in IgM, IgE, or IgD	Decrease of the deficient isotype	Normal	Normal	Normal	Differentiation defect of IgM B cell to isotype-specific plasma cell	Unknown

6. κ chain deficiency	Ig(κ) decrease	Decreased	Normal or decreased κ+ B cells	Normal	Normal	Unknown	Unknown
7. Antibody deficiency with normal or hypergammaglobulinemia	Normal	Decreased	Near normal	Normal	Variable	B cell differentiation defect: defective T cell help	Unknown
8. Immune deficiency with thymoma	All isotypes decreased	Decreased	Absent or very low	Variable	Variably decreased	Unknown defect in pre-B cell maturation	None
9. Transcobalamin 2 deficiency	All isotypes decreased	Decreased	Normal	Normal	Normal	Defect in B-12 transport resulting in defective cell proliferation; B cell to plasma cell differentiation	AR
10. Transient hypogammaglobulinemia of infancy	IgG and IgA decreased	Decreased	Normal	Decreased T cell help	Variable	IgG/IgA B cell to IgG/IgA plasma cell differentiation defect: delayed maturation of T cell help, ? other	Unknown (frequent in heterozygous individuals in families with SCID)

CMI, cell-mediated immunity; AR, autosomal recessive; AD, autosomal dominant; SCID, severe combined immune deficiencies.
Modified from WHO Meeting Report: Clin Immunol Immunopathol 28:450–475, 1983.

to 6 months. Affected infants lack all three types of the major immunoglobulins but can develop reactions of the delayed type. The structure of the thymus is normal. There is a striking lack of tonsillar, appendiceal, and Peyer's patch lymphoid tissue, and plasma cells are absent. This disease may be treated with antibiotics or gammaglobulins, but early death is usual. A similar finding associated with autosomal recessive inheritance is known as *autosomal recessive agammaglobulinemia*.

Findings in other dysgammaglobulinemias are listed in Table 26-3.

Dysgammaglobulinemias

Single deficiencies of an immunoglobulin class are often associated with no clinical problems. Selective IgM deficiencies are rare, and are associated with autoimmune disease and increased incidence of pneumococcal pneumonias. IgA deficiencies (<5 μg/dl) are associated with autoantibodies to IgA, allergies, recurrent sinopulmonary infections, and autoimmune diseases. It is the most common immune deficiency (1/800), but most IgA deficient individuals usually are asymptomatic. Symptomatic IgA deficiencies may be those with associated IgG subclass deficiencies. Selective deficiencies of IgG are usually asymptomatic, but may be associated with increased infection with pneumococci, *Hemophilus influenzae*, and *Staphylococcus aureus*.

The hyper-IgM syndrome—increased levels of IgM, but depressed IgA and IgG—is due to a defect in isotype switching from IgM to other classes. This is associated with recurrent pyogenic infections, but fortunately is very rare. Somatic hybridization of cells from patients with failure of IgA and IgG production to cells from mouse lymphocyte lines results in some hybrids that produce human IgA and IgG, demonstrating that the genes for IgA and IgG are present in the cells of patients with these deficiencies. This suggests a defect in a regulatory rather than a structural gene that is required for expression of the IgA and IgG genes.

Thymus-Dependent Defects (T Cell)

Thymic Aplasia

In this syndrome (also known as DeGeorge syndrome) there is absence of the thymus, deficiency of cellular reactions, and a normal immunoglobulin-producing system. The third and fourth pharyngeal pouches fail to develop, resulting in an absent or rudimentary thymus, absent parathyroids, and aortic arch defects. Neonatal tetany occurs due to a lack of parathyroid hormone. Peripheral blood lymphocyte counts and serum immunoglobulin levels are normal. These patients are susceptible to viral and fungal infections.

Thymic Dysplasia

Thymic dysplasia (Nezelof's syndrome) is an autosomal recessive lymphopenia with normal or abnormal immunoglobulins. These patients have a vestigial embryonic thymus associated with diminished cellular immunity, and normal immunoglobulins. No lymphocytes are evident in the lymphoid tissues, although plasma cells are normal. Parathyroid tissue is normal. Wasting disease similar to that observed in neonatally thymectomized mice may be the terminal event. It is possible that a prethymic lymphocyte defect (prothymocyte) is responsible for the deficiency.

Common Variable Immune Deficiencies

Common variable immunodeficiencies (CVI) are listed in Table 26-4. They are late-onset (after 4–5 years) immune deficiencies with different immune defects not associated with an identifiable cause (i.e., not related to drugs, etc.). Clinically the immune defects may be predominantly in antibody, due to (1) abnormalities in B cell numbers or maturation or (2) to defects in T helper cells or increased activity of T suppressor cells or (3) to autoantibodies to T or B cells. In all cases there is a decrease in one or more immunoglobulin classes associated with variable defects in cellular immunity. These defects appear to be abnormalities in control of the immune response.

Defects in Inflammatory Mechanisms

Immunologically mediated defense against bacterial infections involves (1) the reactions of specific antibody with the bacteria, (2) the activation of complement components resulting in chemotaxis and immune phagocytosis, (3) the ingestion of the bacteria by phagocytic cells (polymorphonuclear leukocytes or macrophages), and (4) destruction of the ingested bacteria by products of the phagocytic cells. Therefore, increased susceptibility to bacterial infections may be due to a deficiency in certain complement components or an abnormality in phagocytic cells (phagocytic dysfunction), as well as to a lack of immunoglobulin antibody.

Complement Deficiencies

A listing of complement deficiencies is given in Table 26-5. Activation of complement occurs upon reaction of antibody with antigen. If the antigen is an infectious agent, the complement system may activate phagocytosis (opsonization) or cause lysis of the offending agent. Thus, a deficiency in complement might be expected to be associated with an immune deficient state. Deficiencies in a complement component are extremely rare. Most occur as autosomal recessive inherited abnormalities. Complement deficiencies are also associated with rheumatoid diseases, primarily systemic lupus erythematosus (SLE). Chronic complement consumption may also be associated with glomerulonephritis (hypocomplementemic glomerulonephritis). A deficiency in C1 inhibitor is associated with hereditary angioedema in which massive swelling lesions of the body surface or gastrointestinal tract are believed to be caused by loss of control of early complement components C1, C4, and C2 and increased formation of anaphylatoxin, resulting

Table 26-4. Common Variable Immunodeficiency

Designation	Usual Phenotypic Expression					Presumed Nature of Basic Defect	Inheritance
	Serum Ig	Serum Antibodies	Circulating B Cells	Circulating T Cells	CMI		
1. Common variable immunodeficiency with predominant B cell defect	Decreased	Decreased	Near-normal numbers but abnormal proportions of subtypes	Variable	Variable	Intrinsic defect in cell differentiation of immature to mature B cells	Unknown AR, AD
2. Common variable immunodeficiency with predominant immunoregulatory T cell disorder							
(A) Deficiency of T helper cells	Decreased	Decreased	Normal	Variable	Variable	Immunoregulatory T cell disorder: defect in thymocyte to T helper cell differentiation	Unknown
(B) Presence of activated T suppressor cells	Decreased	Decreased	Normal	Variable	Variable	Immunoregulatory T cell disorder—cause unknown	Unknown
3. Common variable immunodeficiency with autoantibodies to B or T cells	Decreased	Decreased	Decreased	Decreased	Variable	Variable; no differentiation defect known	Unknown

CMI, cell-mediated immunity; AR, autosomal recessive; AD, autosomal dominant.

Table 26-5. Complement Deficiencies

Component	Increased Susceptibility to Infection	Associated with SLE	Comments
C1 esterase inhibitor	No	No	Hereditary angioedema
C1q	Yes	No	Associated with hypogammaglobulinemia
C1r	Yes	Yes	AR
C1s	No	Yes	
C2	Yes/no	Yes	Usually normal, AR antibody infections
C3	Yes	Yes	Very rare, AR infections
C3b inhibitor	Yes	No	Depletion of C3 and C5–9
C4	Yes	Yes	Infections
C5	Yes	Yes	Phagocytic dysfunction, infections
C6	Yes	No	AR infections ⎫
C7	Yes	Yes	AR infections ⎬ especially *Neisseria*
C8	Yes	Yes	AR infections ⎭

SLE, systemic lupus erythematosus; AR, autosomal recessive.

in increased vascular permeability and edema. The increased availability of reliable assays for complement components (C50 hemolysis is used as a screen for complement deficiencies; see below) has made recognition of deficiencies in complement more frequent.

Phagocytic Dysfunction

Phagocytic dysfunction occurs when phagocytic cells cannot ingest bacteria normally or can ingest but cannot kill. Such a dysfunction may be due to an abnormality in the digestive vacuole (lysosome) or to a lack of digestive enzymes in the vacuole (Table 26-6). A summary of the steps in phagocytosis and the postulated levels of phagocytic defects is illustrated in Figure 26-4. These disorders are characterized by increased susceptibility to bacterial infections associated with the accumulation of lipochrome-laden macrophages and granulomas in the affected tissues. The granulomas are caused by a reaction to bacterial products and the debris of the dead and dying phagocytic cells. Macrophages stuffed with material that they are unable to digest accumulate in tissues. Such macrophages are able to phagocytose normally, but process ingested materials less rapidly or efficiently. Job's syndrome was recognized as "cold" abscesses in skin and lymph nodes of fair-skinned red-haired girls of Italian descent. The patience of the biblical character Job was tested in part by afflictions of his daughters.

Table 26-6. Phagocytic Deficiency Syndromes

CHEDIAK–HIGASHI SYNDROME

Features a microtubular defect, with a deficit in phagosome–lysosome fusion.

Large abnormal lysosomes are seen in all white cells. The defect is inherited as an autosomal recessive, and there is a partial defect in heterozygotes. Affected individuals may also have albinism and lymphoproliferative diseases.

CHRONIC GRANULOMATOUS DISEASE OF CHILDREN (CGD)

There is a deficiency in nicotinamide–adenine dinucleotide phosphate oxidase activation, with a failure to develop superoxide free radicals.

It is sex-linked, affecting male children.

Mothers of affected children have a partial defect.

The problem in CGD is that the first line of bacterial killing, oxidative-dependent killing, fails. The neutrophil dies during the battle with the invading microorganism, leaving macrophages to deal with dead cells and the invading organisms. Macrophages (which also lack respiratory burst activity) ingest the debris and kill the microorganisms using nonoxidative defenses (e.g., lysozyme, neutral proteases). This killing is usually successful, but prolonged, leading to the formation of granulomas after each infectious episode.

JOB'S SYNDROME (HYPER IGE SYNDROME)

These patients have a deficiency in glutathione reductase and glucose-6-phosphatase, a deficiency in lysosome function similar to CGD. It is inherited as an autosomal recessive, and parents have normal function. These patients also have high serum IgE levels.

LAF-1, MAC-1 DEFICIENCY

Some individuals lack surface adherence glycoprotein on their phagocytic cells. Such cells have a decreased capacity for phagocytosis and chemotaxis. This is inherited as an autosomal recessive.

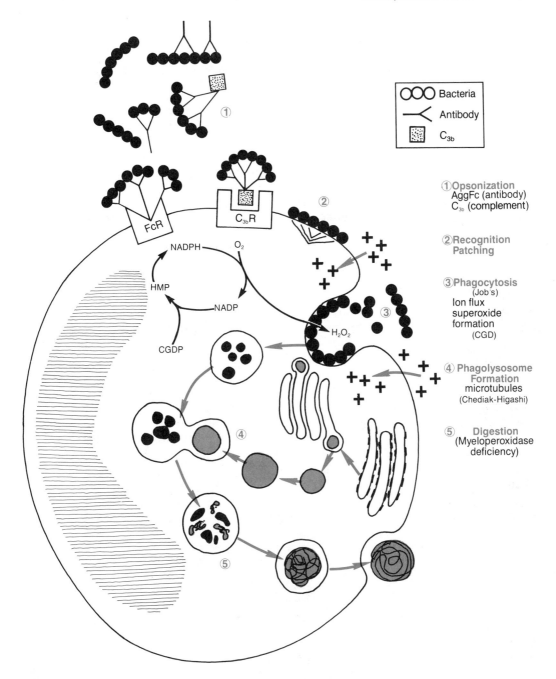

Bacteria

Antibody

C₃b

①Opsonization
AggFc (antibody)
C₃b (complement)

②Recognition
Patching

③Phagocytosis
(Job's)
Ion flux
superoxide
formation
(CGD)

④ Phagolysosome
Formation
microtubules
(Chediak-Higashi)

⑤ Digestion
(Myeloperoxidase
deficiency)

Figure 26-4. Schematic drawings of steps in phagocytosis and postulated levels of defects in phagocytic disorders: (1) Opsonization: aggregated Fc, C3b (defects in antibody or complement). (2) Recognition through receptors (adhesion) and patching. (3) Ingestion (defect in Job's syndrome): Cation influx stimulates transduction of hexose monophosphate shunt and conversion of O_2 to H_2O_2 (defect in chronic granulomatous disease). (4) Fusion of lysosome and phagosome to form phagolysosome (defect in Chediak–Higashi disease): microtubule defect. (5) Digestion of bacteria in phagolysosome (myeloperoxidase deficiency).

It has been suggested that Chediak–Higashi disease (CGD) might be called Jonah's syndrome. The Biblical character Jonah was phagocytosed by a large multicellular organism that was unable to digest him, and he was eventually released. The enzymatic defect in CGD and Job's syndrome can be tested by the inability of isolated polymorphonuclear cells from affected individuals to kill bacteria in vitro or to reduce the dye nitroblue tetrazolium.

Interleukin Deficiencies

Deficiencies in interleukin 1 (IL1) or interleukin (IL2) production may occur secondary to loss of function of macrophage (IL1) or lymphocyte (IL2) populations. However, the clinical significance of interleukin deficiencies has not been extensively documented. IL2 production by blood lymphocytes appears to be depressed in burn patients and may be responsible for depressed cellular immunity in some burn patients.

Secondary Immune Deficiencies

Secondary immune deficiencies may result from naturally occurring disease processes or subsequent to the administration of suppressive agents. In either case the process operates upon an already developed immune system and, therefore, either destroys or interferes with the expression of established defense mechanisms. "Opportunistic" infection with organisms not usually pathogenic for normal individuals is a common terminal event in these patients.

Diseases affecting cellular immune reactions include Boeck's sarcoidosis, leprosy, tuberculosis, measles and other virus infections, diabetes, and cancer. All these processes may affect lymphoid tissue directly or may secondarily alter nonspecific innate defense systems. In diabetes, for instance, vascular changes lead to decreased tissue perfusion, resulting in an increased susceptibility to tissue damage as well as an impaired ability to mount an inflammatory response. In addition, abnormalities in glycogen metabolism depress the phagocytic and digestive capacity of neutrophils and macrophages. Burn patients not only have destroyed epithelial barriers, but also have a decreased ability to produce IL2. Uremic patients have depressed cell-mediated immunity.

Iatrogenic Deficiencies

The mechanisms of action of the so-called immunosuppressive agents are extremely varied (Table 26-7). These agents may affect (1) the specific induction of the immune response (primary response), (2) the expression of humoral antibody formation only, (3) the expression of cellular immunity only, or (4) the expression of both humoral and cellular immunity.

All these agents have systemic effects on cells other than those of the lymphoid system. The damage caused by these agents in vivo is quite variable. In high doses, most cause derangements of any tissue that is metabolically active, for exam-

Table 26-7. Mechanism of Action of Immunosuppressive Agents

Agents	Mechanisms of Action	Examples
Irradiation	Direct destruction of lymphoid cells, toxic for proliferating cells	Whole body, localized, extracorporeal
Steroids	Multiple, direct destruction of lymphoid cells, alterations in protein synthesis and lymphocyte circulation; anti-inflammatory	Hydrocortisone, prednisone
Alkylating agents	React chemically with nucleophilic centers of molecules, in particular DNA, RNA, and proteins; B cells > T cells	Nitrogen mustard, cyclophosphamide, chlorambucil, busulfan
Purine analogs	Incorporated into DNA and RNA and interfere with nucleic acid synthesis; T cells > B cells	Azathioprine, 6-mercaptopurine, thioguanine
Pyrimidine analogs	Inhibition of enzyme activity; active in RNA and DNA synthesis; B cells > T cells	5-Fluorouracil, azaribine, 5-fluoro-2-deoxyuridine, cytosine arabinoside
Folic acid antagonists	Bind to dihydrofolate reductase, thereby interfering with purine, protein, and DNA synthesis	Methotrexate, amethopterin, aminopterin
Methylhydrazines	Formation of hydroxyl radicals causes changes in DNA similar to ionizing radiation	Procarbazine
Hydroxyureas	Kills DNA synthesizing cells, blocks entry of cell into S	Hydroxyurea
Alkaloids	Blocks assembly of the mitotic spindle leading to metaphase arrest; also inhibits RNA and protein synthesis	Vinblastine, vincristine
Enzymes	Hydrolysis of L-asparagine to L-aspartate and ammonia	L-Asparaginase
Antibiotics	Multiple actions: (1) inhibits DNA-dependent RNA polymerase, (2) alkylating agent, (3) DNA binding	Mithramycin, mitomycin, actinomycin C
Antilymphocyte globulin	Alters lymphocyte circulation; lymphocytotoxic, opsonization of lymphocytes, receptor blockage	Horse, goat, rabbit, anti-human lymphocyte globulin
Cyclosporine A	Blocks T cell helper effect, other effects ?	New wonder drug for organ transplantation

Modified from Gerber NL, Steinberg AD: Drugs 11:14–35, 1976.

ple, depression of the bone marrow with subsequent loss of peripheral blood cell elements, or denudation of the lining epithelium of the gastrointestinal tract.

The effect of various drugs on the immune response is best considered in relation to the site of action during an immune response. Immunosuppressive therapy has become of paramount importance in preventing homograft rejection, especially in regard to organ transplantation, and experimental results indicate that such agents may be effective in suppressing various autoallergic reactions. These benefits are counterbalanced by the increased incidence and severity of opportunistic infections. For a more detailed and systematic discussion of the immunosuppressive agents, see Chapter 27.

Infectious Diseases

Infectious diseases produce a generalized debilitation or may be associated with a selective *anergy* to the infectious agent. *Anergy* specifically refers to a loss of skin test delayed type hypersensitivity (DTH) reaction to antigens of infectious organisms. This may represent lymphocyte sequestration or a disproportionate response of a nonprotective immune mechanism. For instance, in leprosy (see Chapter 21), high antibody production (lepromatous leprosy) is associated with progressive disease whereas high DTH and granulomatous reactivity (tuberculoid leprosy) is associated with arrested disease. The "wrong" type of immune response appears to have occurred; that is, protection against leprosy requires cellular immunity; antibody alone is not effective. If the individual infected with leprosy produces antibody but not DTH, protection is not effective. Selected immune responses to infectious agents are discussed futher in Chapter 24.

Chronic Mucocutaneous Candidiasis

Chronic mucocutaneous candidiasis (CMC) patients have histories of candida infections associated with high antibody responses to candida and absent delayed skin test responses to candida antigens. These patients frequently have polyendocrinopathy, suggesting autoimmune destruction of endocrine organs. As in lepromatous leprosy, these patients respond poorly to therapy unless delayed hypersensitivity can be demonstrated. CMC is another example of the type of immune response determining the nature of the disease manifested: that is, antibody is not effective; cellular immunity is.

X-Linked Lymphoproliferative Syndrome (Duncan's Syndrome)

Abnormalities of B cell differentiation and proliferation are found in patients with Epstein–Barr virus (EBV) infections (infectious mononucleosis, Burkitt's lymphoma). EBV infects B cells, leading to polyclonal B cell proliferation on the one hand and lack of differentiation and agammaglobulinemia on the other hand. These patients have variable immune deficiencies. They generally make a poor anti-EBV response. It is thought that there is lack of appropriate T suppressor control of B cells or abnormal T helper function. The syndrome usually affects males between ages 3 and 23.

The finding of a number of X-linked immune deficiencies (Table 26-8) implies a gene complex controlling immune development or expression on the X chromosome. This could be relevant to the high incidence of AIDS in males, although other

Table 26-8 X-Linked Immune Deficiencies

Bruton's agammaglobulinemia
Severe combined immune deficiencies, Swiss type
Wiskott–Aldrich syndrome
Hyper IgM syndrome
X-linked lymphoproliferative syndrome
Chronic granulomatous disease of children
Acquired immune deficiency syndrome

factors, such as use of drugs or sexual practices, may be more important.

Acquired Immune
Deficiency Syndrome

The disease *acquired immune deficiency syndrome (AIDS)* was first recognized in the United States in 1978 when 4 cases were diagnosed in New York City. Since that time the number of cases per year has increased almost exponentially so that over 20,000 cases will be identified in 1986 in the United States. As with many infectious diseases that are introduced into a previously unexposed population, AIDS is characterized by an extremely high death rate.

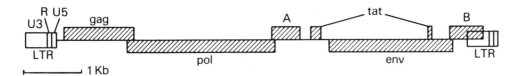

Figure 26-5. Organization of the AIDS retrovirus. The hatched boxes represent the various open reading frames that make up the core proteins (gag), the reverse transcriptase (pol), the envelope glycoproteins (env), and various regulatory genes (tat, A, and B) of the AIDS virus. The regions indicated by the open boxes represent the long terminal repeats (LTR). This region contains additional regulatory sequences for transcription of viral RNA, including the promotor region. (Modified from Rabson A, Martin MA: Molecular organization of the AIDS virus. Cell 40:477–480, 1985.)

The full-blown disease features essentially a wasting syndrome as a result of a variety of opportunistic infections with or without Kaposi's sarcoma (see below). The evolution of AIDS-related lymphadenopathy is discussed in Chapter 28. Acquired immune deficiency syndrome occurs in a high incidence in young homosexual males and intravenous drug abusers. The classic, but not invariable, presentation is of oral candida infection or of enlarging perianal ulcers containing herpes simplex (genital herpes). This is often followed by a prolonged course characterized by weight loss, fever, lymphadenopathy, multiple cutaneous nodules, and evidence of other opportunistic infections including cytomegalovirus, *Pneumocystis carinii, Mycobacterium avium,* and *Candida albicans* as well as syphilis and gonorrhea. Preceding AIDS is AIDS-related complex (ARC), which consists of fever, weight loss, and enlarged lymph nodes (lymphadenopathy) in homosexual men. The diagnosis of ARC also includes the presence of serum antibody to AIDS-related virus antigens. There is a marked depression in cellular immunity and peripheral blood lymphocytes show a reversal of T helper/T suppressor ratios (CD4/CD8), due to low numbers of CD4-positive cells, not only in AIDS patients but also in ARC and in apparently well homosexually active men. Male homosexuals are at a high risk for AIDS and may also have antibody to AIDS virus. However, neither lower numbers of CD4 cells nor antibody to AIDS virus is an accurate prognostic indicator. Recently autoantibody to CD4-positive cells has been found in some homosexual men, but much more frequently in ARC and AIDS, and may be a more accurate prognostic indicator.

The causative agent of AIDS has been shown to be a retrovirus that infects CD4 cells and may also be neurotropic, causing central nervous system abnormalities in some patients. The etiologic virus was called *lymphadenopathy virus (LAV)* by the French who first described the association, and *HTLV-III* by Americans who have shown that antibodies to the virus cross-react with HTLV-I. Another virus, *AIDS-associated retrovirus (ARV)*, has been described in San Francisco. The term *human immunodeficiency virus (HIV)* has replaced the three names previously used.

History and physical

	Inflammation	Phagocytosis	Humoral antibody	Cellular sensitivity
Screening tests	White blood cell count and differential C50 hemolytic complement	White blood cell count and morphology	Immunoelectrophoresis Serum Ig levels	Skin tests T_4/R_8 ratios
Diagnostic tests	Complement levels Inhibitor levels	Phagocytic index Bactericidal tests NBT test Cell surface glycoproteins Lymph node biopsy	Serum IgE Secretory IgA B cell levels Isohemagglutinins Purine metabolizing Enzymes	SRBC rosettes Mitogen responses X ray for thymus Lymph node biopsy
Experimental tests	Complement fragment assays	Chemotactic assays C reactive protein Specific phagocytic enzymes	Skin tests Responses to immunization Ig synthesizing capacity	Interleukin levels Serum inhibitors Sensitization to DNCB Skin graft rejection

Figure 26-6. Evaluation of immune deficiency.

The DNA sequences of the HIV family show general agreement in size and arrangement (Fig. 26-6). The DNA provirus contains a pair of long terminal repeats: a *gag, pol,* and *env* sequence similar to animal retroviruses, coding for group-specific antigen *(gag)*, reverse transcriptase *(pol)*, and virus envelope glycoproteins *(env)*. In addition, HIV contains two unique sequences—A, between *pol* and *env,* and B, between *env* and the long terminal repeat—which may determine the biological properties of the virus. HIV, on the basis of its dramatic cytopathic effect in tissue culture (induction of syncytia and formation of giant cells in infected CD4 cells followed by death of cultured cells in 3–4 weeks) and its ability to produce a slowly progressive disease and to infect brain cells, has many features in common with lente viruses (visna of sheep and equine infectious anemia virus). By DNA hybridization studies HIV is clearly different from HTLV-I and HTLV-II, and more related to lente viruses. There are substantial differences in the restriction endonuclease fragments of different HIV, suggesting considerable heterogeneity in this family of viruses. ARV is different from LAV and HTLV-III, which are very similar if not the same. Most differences lie in the *env* coding sequences.

HIV infects CD4-positive cells in vitro and in vivo. Although the pathogenesis of AIDS is not fully understood, the most likely hypothesis is that the causative virus directly inhibits functions of T helper cells. There is some evidence that the loss of T helper cell functions may be related to the production of an autoantibody that reacts with T helper cells, whether or not they are infected with virus. The loss of T helper cells results in an immune deficiency. There may also be an increase in T suppressor activity. Abnormalities in maturation of other cells in the hematopoietic system (myelodysplasia) are also seen in AIDS.

AIDS is associated with an unusual form of cancer called Kaposi's sarcoma. Previously, Kaposi's sarcoma was more typical of elderly men, in whom it appears as multicentric vascular skin nodules on the lower extremities and pursues a benign course. In young homosexuals, Kaposi's sarcoma takes a much more aggressive form with involvement of lymph nodes and internal organs, with death occurring in a short period of time (approximately 1 year) after diagnosis. Kaposi's sarcoma is composed of atypical spindle cells, with prominent capillary-like spaces containing erythrocytes, suggesting a vascular origin. In some sections large giant cells with cytoplasmic and/or nuclear inclusions may be seen. The association of unusual infections, abnormal routes of entry, and a change in the behavior of an unusual tumor provides exciting possibilities for analysis of the possible relationships among infection, immune deficiency, and cancer.

Transmission of the disease appears to depend upon the transfer of virus-infected cells, perhaps CD4 lymphocytes. The populations at risk are those subject to such transfer. This includes recipients of blood or blood product transfusions; intravenous drug abusers using contaminated needles or syringes; fetuses in utero of infected mothers, who are usually asymptomatic; and homosexuals with exchange of infected body fluids, including seminal fluid. Males are much more susceptible to symptomatic infection than females. The reasons for this are not clear, but the importance of asymptomatic female carriers in spread of the disease is becoming obvious, particularly in congenital AIDS.

Therapy of AIDS is directed toward treatment of the opportunistic infections with antiviral, antifungal, or antibacterial agents and treatment of neoplastic complications by conventional methods. Effective treatment of the underlying defect has been unsuccessful. Immune modulating agents such as interferon, interleukin 2, bone marrow transfer (in identical twins), and cyclosporine have been claimed to have some effect, but such claims either have not been confirmed or the effect is temporary and clinically disappointing. Recently, azidothymidine (AZT), an inhibitor of reverse transcriptase that blocks retrovirus replication, has been recommended for AIDS therapy. AZT appears to alleviate some symptoms of AIDS but is clearly not a cure.

Cancer

Cancer causes depressed immunity in many ways. Perhaps the most significant is the general debilitation seen in terminal cancer patients. In addition, cancer patients are often treated with drastic chemotherapy or irradiation, further compromising immunity and setting the stage for opportunistic infections. Although "immunosuppressive" factors isolated from cancer tissue have been shown to suppress immune reactivity in vitro, the role of such factors in clinical immunosuppression remains poorly defined.

Leukemias and Lymphomas

Selected immune effects may be seen with tumors of the white blood cells and lymphoid organs. In leukemia, the normal inflammatory function of the white blood cells is depressed because the neoplastic cells force out the normal population by occupying "living space." Neoplastic leukemia cells are unable to provide the same function as normal cells. Thus the lymphocytes of chronic lymphocytic leukemia (CLL) do not function properly. However, some acute lymphocytic leukemia (ALL) cells may function as suppressor T cells. The addition of small numbers of some ALL cells to normal peripheral blood lymphocytes inhibits lipopolysaccharide (LPS)-induced Ig synthesis. In addition, autoantibodies to lymphocytes, particularly T cells, may be associated with lymphoproliferative disease and cause abnormalities in T cell function. (See Chapter 28.)

Other lymphoproliferative neoplasias may affect both cellular and humoral immunity, either by occupying the bone marrow and forcing out normal products (living space) or by producing abnormalities in immune control systems. In Sezary's syndrome there is a malignant proliferation of T helper cells. When graded numbers of Sezary cells are added to B cells the amount of immunoglobulin synthesized as a result of LPS stimulation increases. However, at high T/B ratios, normal T cells suppress B cell Ig synthesis and this may occur in later stages of the disease. In addition, Sezary cells cannot provide the T cell help that is required for a specific immune response.

Multiple Myeloma

Suppression of normal antibody levels is seen particularly with plasma cell tumors, *multiple myelomas*. These tumors produce large amounts of nonantibody monoclonal immunoglobulin. The high levels of circulating myeloma immunoglobulin increase the catabolic rate of normal immunoglobulin so that there is less functional antibody.

Malcirculation of Lymphocytes

Lymphocytopenia (low numbers of blood lymphocytes), particularly of T cells, is frequently found in diseases such as Hodgkin's disease, Crohn's disease, hepatitis, rheumatoid arthritis, multiple sclerosis, and tuberculosis. The lymphopenia in these diseases may be due to sequestration of lymphocytes in tissues so that the number of lymphocytes in the blood is lower. In Hodgkin's disease large numbers of T cells are present in the spleen; the blood lymphocytes respond poorly to T cell mitogens, whereas the spleen lymphocytes respond normally. There also appears to be a selective sequestration of T helper cells in the spleen. Splenectomy of patients with Hodgkin's disease may be associated with correction of the lymphopenic condition. T cells may be sequestered in the lesions of Crohn's disease, chronic hepatitis, rheumatoid arthritis, and tuberculosis. Such maldistribution of lymphocytes may lead to depressed immune responsiveness in other organ systems, such as anergy in tuberculosis and Hodgkin's disease.

Opportunistic Infections

The clinical manifestations of immune deficiency diseases are due to infections, often with organisms that are not usually pathogenic in a normal individual. Because many patients have immune deficiency secondary to another disease, they are exposed to organisms in the hospital and acquire the infection in the hospital. Such infections are termed nosocomial. A partial listing of pathogens in the immune-compromised host and the sources of infection is given in Table 26-9. Most infections are acquired from the patient's own flora, but *Aspergillus and Zygomyces* infections are nosocomial. Some infections may be traced to application of devices, such as urinary catheters or endotracheal tubes, in particular *Staphylococcus epidermidis* and *Corynebacterium*. Such hospital manipulations may help establish infections with host organisms by breaching mechanical barriers.

Evaluation of Immune Deficiency

The primary clue to the diagnosis of an immune deficiency disease is obtained by history and physical examination; clinical tests serve for confirmation, definition of the type and severity of the defect and as a guide for therapy. The clues to immune deficiency are the type, severity, cause, and frequency of infections in a patient. Also important is the presence of other factors such as drug therapy and cancer. The laboratory evaluation of immune deficiency disease is summarized in Figure 26-6.

A patient with a history of recurrent infections must be critically examined for a potential defect in defense against infectious agents. The age, condition, and clinical and family history of the patient are vital in establishing the necessity for

Table 26-9. Some Nosocomial Pathogens in the
Immunocompromised Host

| | Source of Infection | |
	Endogenous	Exogenous
BACTERIA		
Staphylococcus aureus	++	+
Staphylococcus epidermidis	++	0
Corynebacterium	++	0
Gram-negative rods *(E. coli, Pseu-domonas, Klebsiella)*	++	+
FUNGI		
Candida, yeasts	++	0
Aspergillus	0	++
Zygomyces	0	++
VIRUSES		
Herpes simplex	++	0
Varicella zoster	+	+
Cytomegalovirus	+	+
PARASITES		
Pneumocystis carinii	++	±
Toxoplasma	++	±
Cryptosporidia		

Modified from Young LS: Infection in the compromised host. Hosp Pract 16:73–84, 1981.

further laboratory workup. Because of the complexity of find-ings in primary or secondary immune deficiencies a systematic series of tests should be performed to permit adequate evalua-tion. Some of the tests indicated are presented below. From the type of recurrent infection one can obtain a clue to the type of deficiency. If mainly viral or fungal, a defect in delayed hyper-sensitivity (T cell function) must be suspected. Recurrent bacterial infections indicate a defect in humoral antibody, in production of polymorphonuclear neutrophils, or in comple-ment. Various nonimmunological factors can be tested by measuring general inflammatory indices, such as white blood count, or serum factors, such as complement or various inhibi-tors. Phagocytic capacity should be determined to rule out a phagocytic defect. Humoral antibody capacity can be mea-sured by determining serum immunoglobulin concentrations, by the presence of preformed antibody or the number of B lymphocytes (EAC rosettes), by the response to antigens that elicit antibody, such as immunization to diphtheria, pertussis, and tetanus (DPT), or by the response to specifically selected antigens such as keyhole-limpet hemocyanin (KLH). Skin tests may also demonstrate anaphylactic or Arthus reactivity. De-layed reactivity can be determined by the transformation response of blood lymphocytes to mitogens such as phytohemagglutinin or concanavalin A, as well as to selected specific antigens. The production of lymphocytic mediators, such as macrophage inhibitory factor or interleukin 2, as well as the presence of serum inhibitors of transformation, can be measured. In addition, the number of blood lymphocytes that form rosettes with unsensitized sheep red blood cells indicates the percentage of T cells and reactivity of monoclonal antibodies to T cell surface markers used to phenotype T cell subpopulations. In vivo tests for delayed hypersensitivity include skin tests to antigens such as the purified protein derivatives of tubercle bacilli, coccidioidin, and others; the ability to induce contact reactivity to dinitrochlorobenzene (DNCB) or other haptens; skin graft rejection; X-ray examination for the thymic shadow; and, when necessary, lymph node biopsy. From the results of a selection of these tests one can define the nature of the defect leading to recurrent or unusual infections and institute appropriate therapy.

The effect of B cell polyclonal activators upon immunoglobulin synthesis by blood lymphocytes has permitted a systematic analysis of patients with common variable immune deficiency (CVI) (Fig. 26-7). Peripheral blood lymphocytes

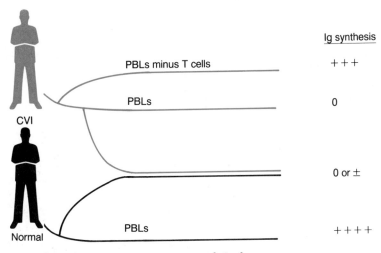

Figure 26-7. Induction of Ig synthesis by mitogens in lymphocyte cultures of some patients with common variable immunodeficiency. Peripheral blood lymphocytes (PBL) of an immune-deficient patient will not synthesize Ig if exposed to mitogen (polyvalent stimulants). Removal of T cells from PBL allows a patient's blood B cells to respond. If a patient's PBL are added to cultures of PBL from a normal person, the Ig synthesis normally found is suppressed. Such an observation is consistent with T suppressor cells in the blood of an immune-deficient patient causing suppression of the B cell system.

(PBL) from normal adults usually respond to stimulation with pokeweed mitogen or LPS (bacterial lipopolysaccharide) in vitro with substantial Ig synthesis. On the other hand, the PBL from patients with CVI produce little or no Ig after stimulation, suggesting that B cells either are not present or do not respond normally to LPS stimulation. There may be a number of reasons for this lack of response. For instance, in some CVI patients suppressor T cells may be inhibiting Ig synthesis. Peripheral blood lymphocytes of some patients with common variable immune deficiency suppress the in vitro production of immunoglobulins of lymphocytes from normal individuals, but mixtures of lymphocytes from two normal individuals produce normal amounts of immunoglobulins in vitro. The immunoglobulin synthesis by normal lymphocytes is also suppressed when they are cocultured with purified T cells from a hypogammaglobulinemic patient but not when cocultured with T cells from a normal individual. Thus, an abnormality in number or activity of suppressor cells may prevent the normal synthesis and release of immunoglobulins in these patients.

Other immune abnormalities have been uncovered in patients with CVI using this approach, as well as in patients with immune deficiencies secondary to leukemia or multiple myeloma. The results of the analysis of a number of patients with late-appearing immune deficiencies are summarized in Figure 26-8.

Figure 26-8. Immune abnormalities in some late-appearing common variable immune deficiencies. Sites of abnormality include (1) lack of pre-B cell, (2) a B cell differentiation arrest, (3) a block in secretion of immunoglobulin, (4) a decrease in T cell help, (5) an increase in T cell suppression, and (6) suppressive effects of macrophages (see Table 26-4).

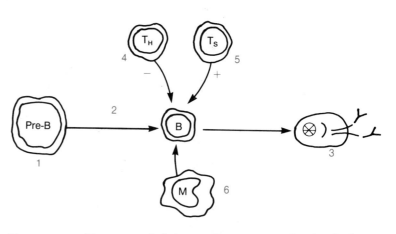

Therapy

Treatment of immune deficiency diseases may be divided into three approaches:

1. Treatment of the infectious agent by antibodies.
2. Treatment of the underlying disease, if present.
3. Specific replacement of the immune defect.

In this chapter only replacement therapy is presented in more detail.

Passive Antibody

Since immunoglobulin deficiencies are caused by a lack of antibody, a lack of immunologically competent cells, or both, attempts have been made to correct these deficiencies by replacing the missing defense system (Table 26-10). For many years, the antibody deficiency syndromes have been treated

Table 26-10. Replacement Therapy for Immune Defects

1. Immunoglobulin deficiencies—passive immune globulin
2. Thymus deficiencies—thymus transplants
3. Combined variable
   Transfer factor: Wiskott–Aldrich; mucocutaneous candidiasis
   Thymic factors: thymosin; thymopoietin; factor thymic serique; restores E rosettes and some in vitro results but convincing clinical trials not accomplished
   Bone marrow: stem cells, problem—graft versus host reaction; HLA matching; other procedures to prevent graft versus host reaction
   Fetal thymus and liver: anecdotal reports of success difficult to evaluate

with partial success by injections of pooled normal immunoglobulins. Whereas such injections give some protection, they do not provide the high levels of specific antibody that are produced in response to an infectious organism by a normal person and do not provide any cellularly mediated immunity.

Passive Cells

Attempts have been made to treat immunological deficiencies of the cellular and combined cellular and immunoglobulin types by bone marrow or thymus transplantation or transfer of cell products. Such transplants must be selected carefully to correct the specific immune deficiency with a minimum potential of unwanted effects, in particular graft versus host reactions. Patients with only cellular deficiencies, such as DeGeorge's syndrome, have been successfully treated with thymus transplants. Patients with combined immune deficiencies may be reconstituted by transfer of bone marrow cells that contain stem cells. Reconstitution of immune reactivity is due to proliferation of donor cells that repopulate the host tissue. Bone marrow transplantation may also provide a longer-lasting replacement for patients with only immunoglobulin deficiencies.

Thymus Transplants

Fetal thymus transplants have been reported to restore cellular immunity in a few patients with combined immune deficiencies; these people have then been maintained with passive gamma globulin to cover humoral antibody deficiency. The responding cells in patients treated with transplantation of the thymus are of donor origin, indicating the presence of T cell precursors in the transplanted thymus. But B cell precursors are not present, and humoral antibody production is not restored. The thymus must be selected from fetuses before the fourteenth week of gestation. Under these circumstances, only minimal graft versus host reactivity has been observed. Therefore fetal thymus grafts may be attempted for severe combined immune deficiency when bone marrow grafting is impossible.

Thymic Factors

The thymus produces soluble factors that induce T cell maturation. In 1963 it was noted by two different groups that thymic tissue implanted in diffusion chambers into thymectomized mice could restore T cell function. However, in vivo effects of injections of extracts of thymic tissue were generally ineffective in inducing T cell function in thymectomized mice. Thymic extracts added to undifferentiated stem cells (T cell precursors), such as lymphocytes from nude mice, which congenitally lack a thymus but produce presumptive T cell precursors in bone marrow, induce expression of the cell surface markers of mature T cells and T cell helper function in vitro. The thymus factor is produced by thymic epithelial cells, as demonstrated by reconstitution of thymectomized mice by implants of epithelial cells in millipore chambers. (For more details on thymic factors see Chapter 4.)

Clinical trials are now being carried out to determine if thymic factors have a therapeutic effect in humans. In vivo and in vitro treatment with thymosin will increase the percentage of E rosettes (presumptive T cells) in immune-deficient patients, and cases claiming clinical improvement as a result of thymosin injection have been reported. However, a convincing systematic clinical trial has not yet been completed, so that it is not yet possible to decide if thymic factors will be therapeutically helpful. In most patients who received thymosin, thymosin treatment was only part of a rigorous therapy regimen employing other agents, so it is impossible to judge the effect of thymosin alone. It must be stressed that thymic factors cannot be expected to have an effect on patients with severe combined immunodeficiency who lack stem cells upon which a humoral thymus factor can act, but may be able to induce maturity in patients who lack thymus epithelial cell function. In fact, thymic humoral factors do not increase rosettes in patients with severe combined immunodeficiency; however, after bone marrow transplantation, induction of T cell rosettes may be possible.

Transfer Factor

Transfer factor, a dialysate of an extract from peripheral blood lymphocytes, has been used to treat certain immune deficient patients. This factor has been used in diseases such as Wiskott–Aldrich syndrome and mucocutaneous candidiasis, which have a variable course with temporary spontaneous improvement. Therefore, the clinical improvement noted in many cases cannot be unequivocally attributed to the effect of transfer factor. However, the number of cases in which a definite clinical response has been seen has now increased to a point where an effect of transfer factor on some cell-mediated reactions must be considered valid. Transfer factor therapy appears to be most applicable for patients with a specific infection, such as candidiasis, coccidiomycosis, or histoplasmosis, but consistent beneficial results have not been obtained. In these cases, the administration of transfer factor obtained from the blood lymphocytes of individuals with a positive skin reaction to antigens of the infectious agent may induce a prompt reaction in infected individuals. Transfer factor is only useful in patients with a limited deficiency and not a stem cell deficiency; transfer factor may push arrested cells to limited differentiation, but cannot replace an absent cell type.

Bone Marrow Transplantation

Stem cell function may be replaced by transfer of bone marrow cells (see Chapter 4). The transplantation of living immunocompetent cells to an immune-deficient recipient is possible because the recipient is unable to reject the transplanted cells. However, the transplanted immunocompetent cells may react to the recipient tissues and death may result from a graft versus host reaction (see Chapter 19). Therefore, attempts must be made to circumvent this reaction in order to treat immune-deficient patients with living immunocompetent cells. A variety of methods have proved to be at least partially feasible.

1. The use of donor cells from an identical twin will not produce a graft versus host reaction, but this source is not usually available and is not useful in hereditary immune deficiencies.
2. The use of donor cells from an HLA-identical sibling will be identical for both serologic and lymphocytic defined histocompatibility antigens; such transplants should not produce a graft versus host reaction.
3. Cells from an HLA- and mixed lymphocyte reaction (MLR)–identical unrelated donor may also be used. In these situations, a temporary graft versus host reaction may occur that passes and results in the establishment of survival of the donor cells in the host environment (chimera). The immune competence is due mainly to donor cells with a variable contribution by recipient cells. In severe combined immune deficiency, bone marrow transplants from HLA-identical siblings result in 60% long-term survival, whereas HLA-identical unrelated donor marrow results in only 30% long-term survival.
4. The use of very low doses of mismatched donor cells may produce a similar effect (akin to the "sneaking through" phenomenon described for tumor cells in Chapter 29). That is, a very low dose of allogeneic bone marrow cells may produce a mild graft versus host reaction that resolves and results in the establishment of a chimeric state. The practical application of this procedure remains untested.
5. Treatment of the recipient with immunosuppressants (see Chapter 27) such as cyclophosphamide or antilymphocyte serum may reduce the graft versus host reaction and permit

survival of the recipient and the donor cells.

6. Treatment of donor cells with antilymphocyte serum specific for T cells may also reduce graft versus host reactions but permit survival of stem cells that can repopulate the host.

7. Blocking factors (see Immune Enhancement, Chapter 29), including humoral antibody from the donor that reacts with antigens of the recipient, may interfere with the graft versus host reaction. Blocking factors have been described in patients who have survived graft versus host reactions, but immune manipulation of the recipient to induce blocking antibody is not yet feasible.

8. Bone marrow cells may be fractionated in an attempt to remove the cells responsible for the graft versus host reaction while retaining the stem cells required for reconstitution of the recipient. Such fractionation by density gradient centrifugation has proved feasible in experimental animals but has been disappointing in human trials.

9. Specific killing of donor cells that recognize recipient cells and treatment of the cultures with doses of radiolabeled thymidine that will kill cells that are stimulated to synthesize DNA (mixed lymphocyte culture). After the reactive cells have been destroyed, the remaining cells that can react to antigens other than those of the recipient can be transferred, thus eliminating the graft versus host reaction. Preliminary trials using this technique are not conclusive.

10. Monoclonal antibodies or lectins specifically directed to T cell populations responsible for graft versus host reactions are now being tested for their ability to remove graft versus host activity from bone marrow cells. A recent development is the use of monoclonal antibodies conjugated to toxic drugs to deliver a fatal dose of the drug to selected cells in the mixture.

Using a variety of the above techniques, a number of successful transplants of bone marrow cells have been made to immune-deficient individuals with not only some spectacular successes but also some disappointing failures. The fact that there are so many methods to reduce or prevent graft versus host reactions indicates that the status of bone marrow transplantation is still less than satisfactory.

An additional factor in determining the effectiveness of stem cell transfers is the necessity of self recognition of T and B cells in order for cooperation to occur. Unless donor and recipient are adequately HLA matched, it is possible that the T and B cells that develop from the engrafted donor stem cells may not be able to cooperate. At first glance it would seem that after transfer, a given population of stem cells from both the developing T and B cells would be of donor origin. However, in experimental systems the ability of T cells to recognize self depends not on the origin of the pre-T (stem) cell but on the thymic environment in which T cell maturation takes place (adaptive differentiation). Thus, if type X stem cells, containing both T and B precursor potential, are engrafted into a type Y recipient, the type X pre-T cells will mature in the environment of the type Y thymus and acquire the capacity to recognize Y and not X as self. On the other hand, the type X pre-B cells will mature as type X cells. The person so reconstituted will have X type T cells that recognize Y and cannot cooperate with X type B cells.

Liver Transplants

In one case, an allograft of fetal liver to a 3-month-old boy with severe combined immune deficiency and adenosine deaminase (ADA) deficiency restored both T and B cell functions as well as ADA activity and clinical improvement. One year later, the child died with a fatal immune complex glomerulonephritis, which could have resulted from reaction to exogenous antigen or from a graft versus host reaction.

Summary

Primary immune deficiency diseases are genetically controlled or developmental abnormalities in the maturation of the immune system. The type of deficiency manifested depends upon the level of maturational arrest that the abnormality affects. Secondary immune deficiencies are the result of naturally occurring diseases or administration of immunosuppressive agents that operate upon a mature immune system. The type of deficiency observed depends upon the location of the defect for the given disease or the mechanism of action of the immunosuppressive agent. Defects may occur in antibody formation, cellular immunity, and accessory systems (complement, phagocytosis) and in mechanical barriers or other nonspecific innate immune mechanisms. Patients with immune defects acquire pathogenic infections with organisms that are not usually pathogens in normal individuals (opportunistic infections). Replacement of the specific defect or therapy of the infection or an underlying disease causing the immune defects may be effective.

References

Development and Maturation of the Immune System

See also Chapter 4.

Abney ER, Cooper MD, Kearney JF, Lawton AR, Parkehouse RME: Sequential expression of immunoglobulin on developing mouse B lymphocytes: a systematic survery that suggests a model for the generation of immunoglobulin diversity. J Immunol 120:2041, 1978.

Cooper MD, Lawton AR III: The development of the immune system. Sci Am 231:58, 1974.

Cooper MD, Lawton AR III, Kincaide PW: A two stage model for development of antibody-producing cells. Clin Exp Immunol 11:143, 1972.

Cooper MD, Peterson RDA, South MA, Good RA: The functions of the thymus system and the bursa system in the chicken. J Exp Med 123:75, 1966.

Goldstein AL, Thurman GB, Cohen GH, Rossio JL: The endocrine thymus: potential role for thymosin in the treatment of autoimmune disease. Ann NY Acad Sci 274:390, 1976.

Good RA, Gabrielsen AE (eds): The thymus. *In* Immunobiology. New York, Harper & Row, 1964.

Jankovic BD: The development and function of immunologically reactive tissue in the chicken. Wiss Z Friedrich-Schiller Univ 17:137, 1968.

Kumuro K, Boyse EA: Induction of T lymphocytes from precursor cells in vitro by a product of the thymus. J Exp Med 138:479, 1973.

Law LW: Studies of thymus function with emphasis on the role of the thymus in oncogenesis. Cancer Res 26:551, 1966.

Levey RH, Tranin N, Law LW: Evidence for function of thymic tissue in diffusion chambers implanted in neonatally thymectomized mice. Preliminary report. J Nat Cancer Inst 31:199, 1963.

McIntire KR, Sell S, Miller JFAP: Pathogenesis of the postneonatal thymectomy wasting syndrome. Nature 204:151, 1964.

Miller JFAP, Marshall AHE, White RG: The immunological significance of the thymus. Adv Immunol 2:111, 1965.

Miller JFAP, Osoba D: Current concepts of the immunological function of the thymus. Physiol Rev 47:437, 1967.

Moller G (ed): B Cell Growth and Differentiation Factors. Immunol Rev 78, 1984.

Osoba D, Miller JFAP: Evidence for a humoral thymus factor responsible for the maturation of immunological faculty. Science 199:653, 1963.

Osoba D, Miller JFAP: The lymphoid tissue and immune response of neonatally thymectomized mice bearing thymic tissue in millipore diffusion chambers. J Exp Med 119:177, 1964.

Parrott DM, DeSousa MAB, East J: Thymus-dependent areas in lymphoid organs of neonatally thymectomized mice. J Exp Med 123:191, 1966.

Raff MC: Two distinct populations of peripheral lymphocytes in mice distinguishable by immunofluorescence. Immunology 19:637, 1970.

Schlesinger DH, Goldstein G, Scheid MP, Boyse EA: Chemical synthesis of a peptide fragment of thymopoietin II that induces selective T cell differentiation. Cell 5:367, 1975.

Smith RT, Meischer P, Good RA: The Phylogeny of Immunity. Gainesville, Fla., University of Florida Press, 1966.

Waksman BH, Arnason BG, Jankovic BD: Role of the thymus in immune reactions in rats. III. Changes in the lymphoid organs of thymectomized rats. J Exp Med 116:187, 1962.

Warner NL, Szenberg A: The immunological function of the bursa of Fabricius in the chicken. Annu Rev Microbiol 18:253, 1964.

Primary Immune Deficiencies

Afzelius BA: The immobile-cilia syndrome: a microtubule associated defect. CRC Crit Rev Biochem 19:63, 1985.

Ammann AJ: Selective IgA deficiency: presentation of 30 cases and a review of the literature. Medicine (Baltimore) 50:223, 1971.

Barton RW, Goldschneider I: Nucleotide-metabolizing enzymes and lymphocyte differentiation. Mol Cell Biochem 28:135, 1979.

Bortin MM, Rimm AA: Severe combined immunodeficiency disease. Characterization of the disease and results of transplantation. JAMA 237:591–600, 1977.

Cohen A, Hirschhorn R, Horowitz SD, Rubinstein A, Polmer SH, Hong R, Martin DW Jr: Deoxyadenosine triphosphate as a potentially toxic metabolite in adenosine deaminase deficiency. Proc Nat Acad Sci USA 75:472, 1978.

Davignon D, Martz E, Reynolds T, Kürzinger K, Springer TA: Monoclonal antibody to a novel lymphocyte function–associated antigen (LFA-1): mechanism of blockade of T lymphocyte–mediated killing and effects on other T and B lymphocyte functions. J Immunol 127:590, 1981.

DeGraff PA, et al: The primary response in patients with selective IgA deficiency. Clin Exp Immunol 54:778, 1983.

Dickler HB, Adkinson NF Jr, Fisher RI, Terry WD: Lymphocytes in patients with variable immunodeficiency and panhypogammaglobulinemia. J Clin Invest 53:834, 1974.

Eibl MN, Mannhalter JW, Zielinski C, Ahmad R: Defective macrophage–T-cell interaction in common variable immunodeficiency. Clin Immunol Immunopathol 22:316, 1982.

Fudenberg HH, Good KA, Goodman HC, Hitzig W, Kinkel HG, Roitt IM, Rosen FS, Rowe DS, Seligmann M, Soothill JR: Primary immunodeficiencies. Report of a World Health Organization committee. Pediatrics 47:927, 1971.

Good RA, Bergsma D (eds): Immunologic Deficiency Diseases in Man, Vol 4, No 1. New York, Nat Foundation Press, 1968.

Good RA, Kelly WD, Rotstein J, Varco RL: Immunological deficiency diseases. Prog Allergy 6:187, 1962.

Kellems RE, Yeung CY, Ingolia DE: Adenosine deaminase deficiency and severe combined immune deficiencies. Trends Genet 1:278, 1985.

Knudsen BB, Dissing J: Adenosine deaminase deficiency in a child with severe combined immunodeficiency. Clin Genet 4:344, 1973.

Kohl S, Springer TA, Schmalstieg FC, Loo LS, Anderson DC: Defective natural killer cytotoxicity and polymorphonuclear leukocyte antibody-dependent cellular cytotoxicity in patients with LFA-1/OKM-1 deficiency. J Immunol 133:2972, 1984.

Lederman HM, Winkelstein JA: X-linked agammaglobulinemia: An analysis of 96 patients. Medicine 64:145, 1985.

Levitt D, Haber P, Richl K, Cooper MD: Hyper IgM immunodeficiency: a primary dysfunction of B lymphocyte isotype switching. J Clin Invest 72:1650, 1983.

Luckasen JR, Sabad A, Gajl-Peczalska KJ, Kersey JH: Lymphocyte bearing complement receptors, surface immunoglobulins and sheep erythocyte receptors in primary immunodeficiency diseases. Clin Exp Immunol 16:535, 1974.

Lurie HI, Duma RS: Opportunistic infections of the lungs. Hum Pathol 1:233, 1970.

Mayer L, et al: Evidence for a defect in "switch" T cells in patients with immunodeficiency and hyperimmunoglobulin M. N Engl J Med 314:409, 1986.

Nahmias AJ, et al: The TORCH complex: prenatal infections associated with toxoplasma, rubella, cytomegalo- and herpes simplex viruses. Pediatr Rec 5:405, 1971.

Peterson RDA, Cooper MD, Good RA: The pathogenesis of immunological deficiency diseases. Am J Med 38:579, 1965.

Rosen FS, Janeway CA: The gamma globulins. II. The antibody deficiency syndrome. N Engl J Med 275:709, 1966.

Rosen FS, et al: Primary immunodeficiency diseases: WHO meeting report. Clin Immunol Immunopathol 28:450, 1983.

Schur PH, Borel H, Gelfand EW, Alper CA, Rosen FS: Selective gamma G globulin deficiencies in patients with recurrent pyogenic infections. N Engl J Med 283:631, 1970.

Seligman M, Fudenberg HH, Good RA: Editorial: a proposed classification of primary immunologic deficiencies. Am J Med 45:817, 1968.

Sell S: Immunological deficiency diseases. Arch Pathol 86:95, 1968.

Teplitz RL: Ataxia telangiectasia. Arch Neurol 35:553, 1978.

Touraine JL, Betuel H, Souillet G, Jenne M: Combined immunodeficiency disease associated with absence of cell surface HLA-A and B antigens. J Pediatr 93:47, 1978.

Touraine JL, Incefy CS, Touraine F, L'Esperance P, Siegal FP, Good RA: T lymphocyte differentiation in vitro in primary immunodeficiency diseases. Clin Immunol Immunopathol 3:228, 1974.

Waldman TA, Broder S: Suppressor cells in the regulation of the immune response. Prog Clin Immunol 3:155, 1977.

Waldman TA, et al: Disorders of B cells and helper T cells in pathogenesis of the immunoglobulin deficiency of patients with ataxia telangectasia. J Clin Invest 71:282, 1983.

Wara DW, Goldstein AL, Doyle NE, Ammann AJ: Thymosin activity in patients with cellular immunodeficiency. N Engl J Med 292:70, 1975.

Wong B: Parasitic diseases in immunocompromised hosts. Am J Med 76:479, 1984.

Windhorst DB, Page AR, Holmes B, Quie RG, Good RA: Pattern of genetic transmission of leukocyte defect in fatal granulomatous disease of childhood. J Clin Invest 47:1026, 1968.

Complement

See also Chapter 12.

Adinolfi M: Human complement: onset and site of synthesis during fetal life. Am J Dis Child 131:1015, 1977.

McClean RH, Winkelstein JA: Genetically determined variation in the complement system. J Pediatr 105:179, 1984.

Ross SC, Densen P: Complement deficiency states and infections: epidemiology, pathogenesis and consequences of neisserial and other infections in an immune deficiency. Medicine 63:243, 1984.

Phagocytic Defects

Bennett JM, Blume JM, Wolff SM: Characterization and significance of abnormal leukocyte granules in the beige mouse: a possible homologue for Chediak–Higashi Aleutian trait. J Lab Clin Med 72:235, 1969.

Davis SD, Schallar S, Wedgewood RJ: Job's syndrome: recurrent "cold" staphylococcal abscesses. Lancet 1:10134, 1966.

Douglas SD, Fudenberg HH: Host defense failure: the role of phagocytic dysfunction. Hosp Pract 4:29, 1969.

Gabig TG, Babior BM: The killing of pathogens by phagocytes. Annu Rev Med 32:313, 1981.

Good RA, Quie PG, Windhorst DB, Page AR, Rodey GE, White J, Wolfson JJ, Holmes BH: Fatal (chronic) granulomatous disease of children: a hereditary defect of leukocyte function. Semin Hematol 5:215, 1968.

Landing BH, Shirkey HS: A syndrome of recurrent infection and infiltration of viscera by pigmented lipid histiocytes. Pediatrics 20:431, 1957.

Padgett GA: The Chediak–Higashi syndrome: a review. Adv Vet Sci Comp Med 12:240, 1968.

Page AR, Berendes H, Warner J, Good RA: The Chediak–Higashi syndrome. Blood 20:339, 1962.

Roberts R, Gallin JI: The phagocyte cell and its disorders. Ann Allergy 50:330, 1983.

Interleukins, Lymphokines, and Monokines

Friedman RM, Vogel SN: Interferons with special emphasis on the immune system. Adv Immunol 34:97, 1983.

Lopez-Botet M, et al: Relationship between IL2 synthesis and the proliferative response to PHA in different primary immunodeficiencies. J Immunol 128:679, 1982.

Secondary Immunodeficiencies

See also Chapters 27–29.

Alper CA, Rosen FS, Janeway CA: The gamma globulins. II. Hypergammaglobulinemia. N Engl J Med 275:652, 1966.

de Sousa M: Lymphocyte maldistribution and immunodeficiency. Hosp Pract 15:71, 1980.

Fisher RJ, et al: Persistent immunologic abnormalities in long term survivors of advanced Hodgkins disease. Am Intern Med 92:595, 1980.

Jeannet M, Rubinstein A, Pelet B: Studies on non HL-A cytotoxic and blocking factor in a patient with immunological deficiency successfully reconstituted by bone marrow transplantation. Tissue Antigens 3:411, 1973.

Moller G (ed): Immunologic Unresponsiveness in Adults. Immunol Rev 80, 1984.

Scharff MD, Uhr JW: Immunological deficiency disorders associated with lymphoproliferative diseases. Semin Hematol 2:47, 1965.

Ward PA, Berenberg JL: Defective regulation of inflammatory mediators in Hodgkins disease. Supernormal levels of a chemotactic inhibitory factor. N Engl J Med 290:76, 1974.

Young LS: Infections in the compromised host. Hosp Pract 16:73, 1981.

AIDS

Corran JW, et al: The epidemiology of AIDS: current status and future prospects. Science 229:1352, 1985.

Devita VT, Hellman S, Rosenberg SA: AIDS, etiology, diagnosis, treatment and prevention. Philadelphia, Lippincott, 1985.

Gluckman JS, Klatzman D, Montagner L: Lymphadenopathy-associated-virus and acquired immunodeficiency syndrome. Annu Rev Immunol 4:97, 1986.

Jaffe HW, et al: The acquired immunodeficiency syndrome in a cohort of homosexual men. Ann Intern Med 103:210, 1985.

Lane HC, Fauci AS: Immunologic reconstitution in the acquired immunodeficiency syndrome. Ann Intern Med 103:714, 1985.

Lane HC, Fauci AS: Immunologic abnormalities in the acquired immunodeficiency syndrome. Annu Rev Immunol 3:477, 1985.

Lane HC, et al: Quantitative analysis of immune function in patients with the acquired immunodeficiency syndrome. N Engl J Med 313:79, 1985.

Rabson AB and Martin MA: Molecular organization of the AIDS retrovirus. Cell 40:477, 1985.

Richert CM, et al: Autopsy pathology in the acquired immune deficiency syndrome. Am J Pathol 112:357, 1983.

Wong-Staal F, Gallo RC: Human T-lymphotopic retroviruses. Nature 317:395, 1985.

Diagnosis of Immunodeficiencies

Asherson GL, Webster ADB: Diagnosis and Treatment of Immunodeficiency Disease. St. Louis, Mosby, 1980.

Bellanti JA, Schlegel RJ: The diagnosis of immune deficiency diseases. Pediatr Clin North Am 18:49, 1971.

Miller ME: Clinical aids in diagnosis of immunologic disease. Clin Pediatr 8:189, 1969.

Moore EC, Meuwissen HJ: Immunologic deficiency disease. Approach to diagnosis. NY State J Med 73:2437, 1973.

Waldman TA, Broder S: Polyclonal B-cell activities in the study of the regulation of immunoglobulin synthesis in the human system. Adv Immunol 32:1, 1982.

Therapy

Ammann AJ, Wara DW, Salmon S, Perkins H: Thymus transplantation: permanent reconstitution of cellular immunity in a patient with sex-linked combined immunodeficiency. N Engl J Med 289:5, 1973.

Asanuma YA, Goldstein AL, White A, et al: Reduction in the incidence of wasting diseases in neonatally thymectomized mice by injection of thymosin. Endocrinology 86:600, 1970.

Ascher MS, Gottlieb AA, Kirkpatrick CH: Transfer Factor. Basic Properties and Clinical Application. New York, Academic Press, 1976.

Beatty PG, et al: Marrow transplantation from related donors other than HLA-identical siblings. N Engl J Med 313:765, 1985.

Buckley RH: Reconstitution: grafting of bone marrow and thymus. *In* Amos B (ed): Progress in Immunology. New York, Academic Press, 1971, p1061.

Buckley RH, Amos B, Kremer WB, Stickel DL: Incompatible bone-marrow transplantation in lymphopenic immunologic deficiency. Circumvention of fatal graft-vs-host disease by immunologic enhancement. N Engl J Med 285:1035, 1971.

Cleveland WW, Fogel BJ, Brown WT, Kay HE: Foetal thymic transplant in a case of DeGeorge syndrome. Lancet 2:1211, 1968.

Good RA: Progress toward a cellular engineering. JAMA 214:1289, 1970.

Dekoning J, Van Bekkum DW, Dicke KA, Dooren LJ, Van Rood JJ, Radl J: Transplantation of bone marrow cells and fetal thymus in an infant with lymphopenic immunologic deficiency. Lancet 1:1223, 1969.

Incefy GS, Boumsell L, Touraine JL, L'Esperance P, Smithwick E, O'Reilly R, Good RA: Enhancement of T lymphocyte differentiation in vitro by thymic extracts after bone marrow transplantation in severe combined immunodeficiencies. Clin Immunol Immunopathol 4:258, 1975.

Lawrence HS: Transfer factor. Adv Immunol 11:195, 1969.

Lawrence HS: Selective immunotherapy with transfer factor. *In* Bach FH, Good RA (eds), Clinical Immunobiology, Vol 2. New York, Academic Press, 1974, p116.

Salmon SE, Mogerman SN, Perkins H, Smith BA, Lehrer RI, Shinefield HR: Transplantation of treated lymphocytes in lymphopenic immunologic deficiency. Am J Dis Child 123:111, 1972.

Santos GW: Application of marrow grafts in human disease. Am J Pathol 65:653, 1971.

Spitler LE, Levin AS, Fudenberg HH: Transfer factor. *In* Bach FH, Good RA (eds): Clinical Immunobiology Vol 2. New York, Academic Press, 1974, p154.

Thierfelder S, et al: Antilymphocyte antibodies and marrow transplantation. IV. Two of nine anti-thy-1 antibodies used for pretreatment of donor marrow suppressed graft versus host reactions without added complement. Exp Neonatal 13:948, 1985.

Thomas ED: Bone Marrow Transplantation. *In* Bach FH, Good RA (eds): Clinical Immunobiology, Vol 2. New York, Academic Press, 1974, p2.

Thomas Ed: Marrow transplantation for malignant diseases. J Clin Oncol 1:517, 1983.

Van Bekkum DW: Use the abuse of hemopoietic cell grafts in immune deficiency diseases. Transplant Rev 9:3, 1972.

27 | Immune Modulation

The immune response may be affected at various levels by many different agents, either specifically or nonspecifically. Modulation of the immune response may involve induction, expression, amplification, or inhibition of the afferent, central, efferent, or accessory phase of the immune response (Fig. 27-1). In preceding chapters, modification of induction of immunity by specific antigen (Tolerance, Chapter 11), alteration of immune response by specific immunization (Desensitization and Hyposensitization, Chapter 18), prevention of Rh sensitization (Chapter 15), and pharmacological intervention in accessory mechanisms (Chapter 12) have been presented in some detail. In this chapter, modulation of the immune response will focus on specific and nonspecific effects on induction and expression of the immune system in general, rather than on accessory mechanisms such as mast cell degranulation or complement activation.

Immunomodulation may be specific, limited to a given antigen, or nonspecific, with a general effect on immune responses (Table 27-1). Major attempts have been made to enhance or inhibit immune responses in humans and experimental animals. Therapeutic stimulation of the immune response is desirable for some persons, such as patients with immune deficiencies, whereas suppression of the immune response is sought for others, such as transplant recipients or patients with autoallergic diseases. Specific immunomodulation may be actively achieved by administration of antigen in a form or by a route that induces a certain type of immune response, suppresses activity (tolerance), or changes activity from one form to another (immune deviation). Immunization vehicles may be used to increase or modify response to a given antigen (adjuvants). In addition, specific immunomodulation may be produced passively by transfer of immune products (cells or antibody) or by factors that affect specific responsive-

655

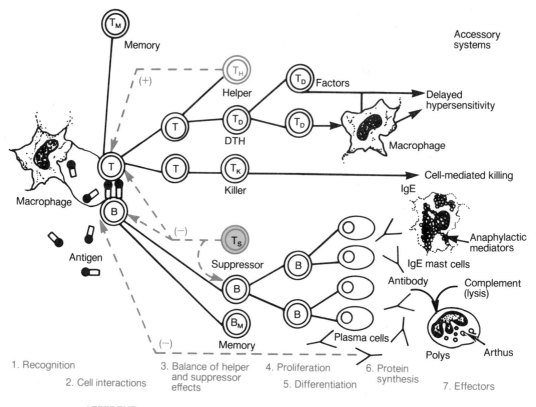

1. Recognition
2. Cell interactions
3. Balance of helper and suppressor effects
4. Proliferation
5. Differentiation
6. Protein synthesis
7. Effectors

AFFERENT   CENTRAL   EFFERENT

Figure 27-1. Immune modulation. Levels of activity that may be affected by specific or nonspecific agents: afferent — (1) antigen recognition, (2) lymphoid cell interactions; central — (3) helper and suppressor cell functions, (4) proliferation of responding cell populations, (5) differentiation of effector cells, (6) synthesis of immune products such as lymphokines or specific antibody; and efferent — (7) T cell-mediated reactions and accessory effector systems (macrophage, mast cell, and complement activity). Administration of specific antigen in different forms may result in a productive immune response on one hand and specific tolerance on the other hand. In some instances a response may be changed from one form (primarily cellular) to another (primarily antibody). Adjuvants may enhance the immune response and antimetabolic drugs may effectively inhibit it. Naturally occurring factors may also increase or decrease certain components of the response. There are several inherent mechanisms for limiting the extent of an immune response, such as suppressor T cells, feedback inhibition by specific antibody, exhaustion of mast cells (desensitization), consumption of complement, catabolism of immunoglobulin, and others. Attempts to control immune responses therapeutically are complicated by effects that are difficult to control. For instance, immunosuppression of graft recipients frequently leads to increased susceptibility to infection. However, effective means of controlling some immune responses are available (e.g., prevention of sensitization of Rh⁻ mothers to Rh⁺ antigens), and with better understanding of the immune response, greater application of immune intervention for a number of diseases is expected.

ness (i.e., transfer factor). Nonspecific immunostimulation may be achieved by administration of agents such as interferon or interleukins that increase some component of the immune

Table 27-1. Classification of Immunomodulation

STIMULATION
  Specific
    1. Active immunization (antigen plus adjuvant)
    2. Passive transfer (cells, antiserum, transfer factor)
  Nonspecific (bacillus Calmette–Guérin, levamisole, polynucleotides, endotoxin, interleukins, interferon)

SUPPRESSION
  Specific
    1. Tolerance (suppressor cells, clonal elimination, desensitization, anti-idiotype)
    2. Hyposensitization
  Nonspecific
    1. Radiation, drugs, antilymphocyte serum
    2. Suppressive factors (immunoregulatory globulin)

response not involving specific antigen recognition. Such agents generally act on some accessory cell type, such as the macrophage or natural killer cells. Nonspecific suppression of the immune response may be achieved by agents that interfere with the induction or expression of an immune response. Such agents include radiation, drugs (steroids, antimetabolites), and immune reagents such as antilymphocyte or antimacrophage serum. The effect of immune modulating agents is dependent on dose and, in particular, on the relationship of antigen stimulation to the time of administration of the agent. For instance, radiation given before antigen may increase the magnitude of the immune response, whereas radiation given after antigen, during the proliferation of antigen activated cells, will greatly inhibit the response. Cyclophosphamide at moderate daily doses leads to suppression of immune functions, including T and B cell depletion, impairment of NK activity, and blocking of T and B cell differentiation. However, at low doses, cyclophosphamide has a selective effect on suppressor cells, resulting in enhancement of antibody and effector T cell production. Immune modulation has achieved its greatest therapeutic effectiveness in immunization procedures for preventing infectious disease (see Chapter 25), in prolonging allografts (particularly renal grafts; see Chapter 19), in preventing immunization, as in prophylaxis for erythroblastosis fetalis (Chapter 15), and in desensitization for allergic reactions (Chapter 18). Immunotherapy of cancer, which has been less successful but is under active study, is discussed in Chapter 29.

Stimulation of Immune Responses

Specific Active Immunization

The most effective way to increase the specific immune response to a given antigen is to administer the antigen (immuno-

Adjuvants

gen) along with an agent that will enhance the reactivity of the lymphoid system. Such agents are termed *adjuvants*. The mechanism of action of adjuvants is not well understood, but they are believed to attract macrophages and reactive lymphocytes to the site of antigen deposition, to localize antigens in an inflammatory site (depot effect), to delay antigen catabolism, to activate the metabolism of antigen processing cells, and to stimulate lymphoid cell interactions. Adjuvants also produce a nonspecific increase in immune reactivity; much of the immunoglobulin produced by adjuvant–antigen stimulation is not a specific antibody. Injection of adjuvant with or without antigen can produce a sustained hyperglobulinemia. Effective adjuvants include oils, mineral salts, double-stranded nucleic acids, products of microorganisms, and a variety of other agents.

Water–Oil Emulsions

The most widely used adjuvant for experimental immunization is Freund's adjuvant. This adjuvant consists of a water or saline in oil emulsion. Typically, soluble antigen is dissolved in saline and emulsified in equal parts of an oil, such as Bayol F (42.5% paraffin, 31.4% monocyclic naphthalene, and 26.1% polycyclic naphthalene) or Arlacel A (mannite monolate). The addition of killed mycobacteria greatly increases the adjuvant activity. Emulsions without mycobacteria are called incomplete (incomplete Freund's adjuvant) and emulsions containing mycobacteria are termed complete (complete Freund's adjuvant). The glycolipid and peptidoglycolipid portions (wax D) of the mycobacteria are responsible for the increased effect of complete Freund's adjuvant. In producing antisera in animals, it is common to use complete Freund's adjuvant for the initial immunization and incomplete Freund's adjuvant for booster immunizations. Repeated immunization with complete Freund's adjuvant can lead to severe necrotic reactions at the site of the injection because of extreme hypersensitivity to the mycobacterial component. To be fully effective, adjuvants must be injected intradermally or subcutaneously. Adjuvant immunizations are particularly effective in producing antibody responses to small doses of immunogen and in inducing primed T cells. In some instances, complete Freund's adjuvant induces extremely active delayed hypersensitivity responses. Freund's adjuvant is noted for its ability to induce cellular autoallergic reactions (see Chapter 20) and to stimulate antibody responses in low responder animals, probably through activation of T helper cells.

Mineral Salts (Alum)

Solutions of antigens precipitated with mineral salts such as calcium phosphate, silica, or alum (aluminum potassium sulfate, $AlK(SO_4)_2 \cdot 12H_2O$, or aluminum phosphate, $AlPO_4$) produce granulomas at the site of injection and in draining lymph nodes. The alum-induced immune granuloma functions similarly to those produced by Freund's adjuvant. Alum-precipitated immunogens have been used in man to increase the extent of an immune response for prophylactic immunization to antigens such as diphtheria toxoid.

Microbial Extracts

Endotoxins. Microbial endotoxins or cell walls may produce a marked increase in immune responses. The endotoxins most active are intracellular lipopolysaccharides produced by gram-negative bacteria. They can function as adjuvants when administered systemically, but are more effective if injected locally along with antigens. Many of these endotoxins are capable of stimulating immunoglobulin synthesis and proliferation by B cells in vitro and of attracting and enhancing phagocytosis by macrophages. Endotoxins increase antibody production when given in vivo and have little, if any, effect on delayed hypersensitivity. Endotoxins seem to activate B cells nonspecifically (polyclonal activation), but will enhance a specific antibody response if a given antigen is present. The mechanism of action of endotoxin is not clear. Endotoxin may increase some responses and decrease others. In different systems, endotoxin may act on B cells directly, activating B cells and blocking T cell help; may substitute for T cell help in the absence of T cells, or may activate T cell help in the presence of T cells.

Cell Wall Extracts. The cell walls of certain bacteria (mycobacteria) and fungi also serve to enhance immune reactivity. In general, the effect is less than, but similar to, that of complete Freund's adjuvant. These agents also produce a marked nonspecific activation of the effector arm of immune responses that involve macrophages. They attract and activate macrophages, thus increasing phagocytosis at the site of antigen-induced inflammation.

Synthetic immunostimulants derived from bacterial cell walls are exemplified by peptidoglycan derivatives such as muramyl dipeptide (MDP). MDP is a simple dipeptide deriva-

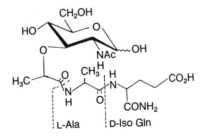

tive of muraminic acid and is the minimal molecule capable of replacing myocobacterial cell walls in complete Freund's adjuvant in increasing antibody production and for inducing delayed hypersensitivity. However, this compound is toxic and produces fever, leukopenia, and platelet lysis in animals. Synthetic disaccharide peptides, such as disaccharides from lactobacilli coupled to the dipeptide L-alanyl-D-isoglutamine, may be even more active than MDP and less toxic. Other artificial saccharides, lipids, and peptidolipids structurally related to MDP are also being tested for possible clinical use. The primary action of adjuvants is on macrophage activation, resulting in increased T and B cell proliferation, presumably through IL1 production.

Mycobacteria and other organisms also produce 6,6'-diesters of trehalose called *mycolic acids* (or *cord factors*), which have various α-branched β-hydroxy acids. These and related

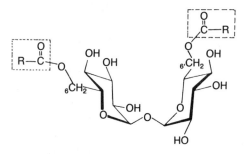

glycolipids contain a balance of lipophilic and hydrophilic groups and interact with cell membranes. They are chemotactic for macrophages and function as adjuvants in attracting and activating macrophages.

Attempts are now underway to produce derivatives of adjuvant molecules and test combinations of molecules to achieve maximum immunostimulation with minimum toxicity for use in vaccines.

Polynucleotides

Double-stranded polynucleotides, such as polyinosine–polycytidylic acid [poly(IC)] or polyadenylic–polyuridylic acid [poly(AU)], are also potent adjuvants and immunostimulants. They appear to act through activation of antigen-reactive T cells. Polynucleotides are not effective in T cell–depleted animals. The mechanism of action is believed to be through elevation of cyclic AMP in antigen-reactive T cells. Polynucleotides may also serve to activate macrophages nonspecifically, perhaps through stimulation of T cell factors.

Nonspecific Immunostimulation

Many of the agents mentioned above, such as oils, salts, endotoxins, mycobacterial cell walls, and polynucleotides, produce a generalized increase in immune responsiveness by nonspecifically activating the effector arm of immune responses (nonspecific immunostimulation) as well as by functioning as adjuvants in the induction of antigen-specific immune responses in the presence of specific antigen. These agents may also act nonspecifically to activate T cells, B cells, macrophages, or complement. Such stimulation has been widely used in attempts to potentiate or stimulate immune responses to tumors (see Chapter 29). Agents that are most effective in this regard are bacillus Calmette–Guérin (BCG), *Corynebacterium parvum*, *Listeria monocytogenes*, and *Bordatella pertussis*, as well as polynucleotides and levamisole. Other agents include products of activated cells such as interleukins and interferon. These are classified as biological response modifiers, a general term used for biological products that alter the defensive responses of an individual.

Macrophage Activators

BCG, *C. parvum*, and *L. monocytogenes* act primarily on macrophages. Following injection of these organisms, macrophage activity is increased in the following ways: content of lysosomal enzymes, adherence to glass, rate of phagocytosis, and bactericidal activity. Such macrophages are called *activated* or *armed*. In general, nonspecific stimulators act by enhancing the activities of the macrophage in the effector arms of the immune response, thus primarily increasing the magnitude of expression of delayed hypersensitivity reactions and resistance to intracellular bacterial infections. This action may be mediated through activation of T cells to release macrophage activating factors, but there is evidence that macrophage activation need not always require T cells. Animals treated with BCG, *C. parvum*, and *L. monocytogenes* demonstrate an increased resistance to antigenically unrelated organisms and an enhanced ability to reject some transplanted syngeneic tumors (see Chapter 29). Levamisole is able to restore the phagocytic and T cell responses of compromised animals, but has little stimulatory effect on normal animals. Given just before tumor transplantation, levamisole decreases growth of transplantable tumors in animals, but timing of the administration is critical. Increased tumor growth may occur if levamisole is given 5 days before the tumor begins to grow. Clinically, levamisole has been reputed to have a beneficial effect in immune deficiency diseases, cancer, and other diseases, but the results of systematic clinical trials are not yet available. Injections of *B. pertussis* result in a marked lymphocytosis because of increased recirculating and decreased homing of small lymphocytes; pertussis-treated animals also tend to produce IgE type antibody and demonstrate an increased sensitivity to anaphylactic mediators.

Lymphokines and Monokines

Products of lymphocytes or macrophages may act on other cells as effector molecules (lymphokines or monokines) or may act on other white cells to increase or decrease immune reactivity (interleukins; see Chapter 11). Some lymphokines or interleukins that have potential for use as modulators of immunity are listed in Table 24-2. Thymic humoral factors and transfer factor are discussed under immune deficiency diseases (Chapter 26). Thymic humoral factors are able to induce T cell differentiation in vitro, and some anecdotal reports suggest a beneficial effect in treatment of patients with T cell deficiencies. Transfer factor, a lysate of lymphocytes from patients who are highly sensitive to a given antigen, have been used to control or modify selected diseases such as chronic mucocutaneous candidiasis. In this disease there is preferential production of humoral antibody over development of delayed hypersensitivity. Transfer factor appears to be able to restore delayed hypersensitivity to candida in some patients and results in clinical improvement. Both of these factors give inconsistent results. Of the factors listed in Table 27-2 only interferons and

Table 27-2. Lymphokines and Interleukins: Action and Therapeutic Use

Lymphokine	Function	Possible Therapeutic Use	Clinical Status
Thymic hormones	Stimulate T cell differentiation	Thymic deficiencies	Anecdotal, inconsistent
Transfer factor	Transfers specific T cell sensitivity	Specific T cell deficiencies	Anecdotal, inconsistent
Macrophage maturing factors	Activate macrophages	Nonspecific tumor immunity	Not used
Interferons[a]	Inhibit proliferation, activate NK cells, increase immune response	Nonspecific tumor immunity, virus infections	Clinical trials underway
Lymphotoxin	Kills target cells	Tumor therapy	Not used
Suppressor factors	Inhibit T or B cell functions	Transplantation, autoimmunity	Not used
Interleukin 1	Activates T cells	Cancer, virus infections	Not used
Interleukin 2[a]	Activates LAK cells	Cancer	Clinical trials underway
Eosinophil-chemotactic factor	Attracts eosinophils	Parasitic infection	Not used
Vascular permeability factors	Contract endothelial cells	Cancer	Not used
Tumor migration inhibitory factor	Inhibits migration of cancer cells in vitro	Cancer	Not used
Tumor necrosis factor	Toxic or static for cancer cells in vitro	Cancer	Experimental

[a] For more detailed information see Chapter 27.

interleukin 2 are now being actively studied in clinical trials (see Chapter 29).

Interferons. Interferons are a family of glycoproteins produced by lymphocytes and other cells (see Chapter 12). Interferons available for clinical use include both natural products from cultured cells and interferons produced by recombinant

DNA techniques. Most clinical studies have been done using interferon α, but now highly purified interferons α, β, and γ are each being tested in clinical trials (Table 27-3). Interferon α is

Table 27-3. Interferons Used for Clinical Trials

Source		Purity
Alpha		
Natural	Virus-activated lymphocyte	Variable
Lymphoblastoid	cultures	Variable
Recombinant α_2, A, or D	Cultured lymphoma cells	Pure
	E. coli, plasmid cyclic DNA	
Beta		
Natural	Cultured fibroblasts or	Variable
Recombinant β_1 or B	SV40 transformed cells	Pure
	E. coli, plasmid cDNA	
Gamma		
Natural	Activated lymphocytes,	Variable
Recombinant 1	lymphocyte lines	Pure
	E. coli, plasmid cDNA	

produced by virus-infected lymphocytes within 6 hr of infection, β by fibroblasts, and γ by mitogen or antigen activated lymphocytes. α exists in up to 25 different forms; β and γ also exist in different forms, but how many is not yet known. Recombinant and natural α interferons appear to be very similar. In clinical trials interferon α has had little or no effect on epithelial tumors, but has been associated with remissions in about 10% of patients with lymphoma, myeloma, and melanoma. Preliminary work with interferons β and γ has given similar results. Untoward side effects at high doses include fever, intolerable fatigue, weight loss, and malaise. The mechanism of action of interferons remains unclear. Interferons may have a direct cytostatic effect on some tumors and may act by this mechanism rather than by specific effects on the immune system. More promising preliminary results have been obtained in viral infections. Inhalation of interferon may prevent upper respiratory viral infections or modulate symptoms of colds and flu-like virus infections.

Interleukin 2. Interleukin 2 (IL2) is produced by activated T lymphocytes and stimulates a number of activities in other lymphocytes including activation of helper and cytotoxic T cells, B cells, and natural killer (NK) cells (see Chapter 10). IL2 administered to animals has a very short half-life in serum (approximately 2 min) and little or no effect on tumors. In addition, IL2 has not been effective in treatment of immune deficiency diseases. However, clinical trials in which the blood lymphocytes from cancer patients are treated with IL2 in vitro and then injected back into the same patient are now underway.

Suppression of Immune Responses

Specific Immunosuppression

Tolerance

The subject of specific tolerance is presented in detail in Chapter 11 and is only briefly repeated here. Specific tolerance, the lack of ability to mount an immune response to a given antigen while maintaining the ability to respond to other antigens, is particularly desirable in treatment of specific allergies or in preparation for organ transplantation. In these situations, it is the goal of therapy to eliminate or suppress the undesirable immune response to the allergen or transplantation alloantigen but not induce a general immunosuppression. Although tolerance has been demonstrated repeatedly in experimental animals, the application to humans has proved difficult, if not impossible. Hypothetically, tolerance could be induced in two ways: by blocking or eliminating the specifically reacting cells (clonal elimination), or by suppressing the reactive cells by specific immune controlling products. This latter effect may be produced by specific suppressor cells, by products (suppressor factors) of cells, or by specific immunoglobulin antibody that provides a feedback mechanism to limit further production of antibody. Tolerance may be induced in experimental animals either by antigen exposure or by passive transfer. In some cases, specific tolerance may be induced in atopic individuals by administration of atopic antigens (see Chapter 18). In addition, tolerance may also be produced in some transplant recipients who survive for a long time. In such cases, it may be possible to withdraw nonspecific immunosuppressive therapy without serious rejection occurring. The mechanism for this phenomenon is not clear, however, and other mechanisms, such as masking of graft antigens, may be operating.

Hyposensitization

Hyposensitization (see Chapter 18) is replacement of expression of one effector mechanism by another. This is achieved by injection immunotherapy of atopic persons. Expression of anaphylactic or atopic reactions requires reaction of antigen with IgE antibody on effector (mast) cells. If IgG antibody is also present, competition of the IgG with mast cell–bound IgE antibody may eliminate the anaphylactic symptoms. This process of changing the expression of immune reactivity by changing the specific immune product is termed *immune deviation*.

Desensitization

Desensitization is accomplished by "using up" antibody by increasing doses of antigen given under controlled conditions (also see Chapter 18). If antigen administration is discontinued, the immune state will be reestablished. Desensitization may be effective in decreasing anaphylactic and delayed hypersensitivity reactions.

Nonspecific Immunosuppression

A variety of procedures, physical agents, and drugs have been used to suppress immune reactivity. The objective is to interfere with either the induction or the expression of an immune response. The mechanisms include physical removal of serum or certain cell populations, killing of cells, interference with metabolism of reactive cells, blocking of cell surface receptors, or alteration of the tissue distribution of reactive cells. In addition, depending on the immune mechanism involved, blocking of effector mechanisms may be achieved by drugs that lower complement, interfere with mediators, depress mast cell sensitivity, block end organ responses to anaphylactic mediators (atopic reactions), or interfere with accessory cell (polymorphonuclear, macrophage) activity (Fig. 27-1).

Plasmapheresis

Therapeutic plasmapheresis is the process whereby plasma containing antibodies, immune complexes, hormones, drugs, or other substances soluble in plasma is removed from the circulation and replaced by a harmless substance. In immune-mediated diseases this process can be used to remove circulating antibodies or antibody–antigen complexes. Plasmapheresis has been used to supplement treatment of antibody- or immune complex–mediated diseases such as systemic lupus erythematosus, anti-glomerular basement membrane (anti-GBM) glomerulonephritis, factor VIII deficiency, myasthenia gravis, and pemphigus. In general, plasmapheresis is successful if the process of autoantibody or immune complex formation is self limited, as is the case in anti-GBM glomerulonephritis. In the other diseases removal of antibody usually produces an immediate beneficial effect. However, the short-term effects of plasmapheresis may be followed by a rebound of increased antibody formation and more severe disease manifestations. Thus plasmapheresis may be used to control acute life-threatening situations, such as respirator-dependent myasthenia gravis, but to be effective in the long term, it must be followed by the use of immunosuppressive drugs to establish a sustained remission of disease.

Mechanical Removal of Cells

Extirpation of specific lymphoid organs may lead to loss of immune responsiveness. Neonatal thymectomy of most mammals produces a loss of responsiveness of the T cell system, whereas bursectomy of chickens produces a loss of B cell function. Removal of circulating lymphocytes by chronic thoracic duct drainage has also resulted in depression of T cell functions, mainly by removal of long-lived T cells. In animals, this technique has been used to prolong allograft survival. These procedures are not readily applicable to modulation of immune responses in humans.

*Immunosuppressive
Agents*

The mechanism of action of immunosuppressive agents is extremely varied (Table 27-4). These agents may affect the specific induction of both humoral and cellular immune responses (primary response), humoral antibody formation only, cellular immunity only, or expression of a given effector mechanism, or may produce nonspecific depression of accessory cells involved in inflammation. They may cause the establishment of specific tolerance, or the failure of expression of a primary response to a given antigen, even though memory is induced so that a secondary response occurs upon reexposure to the same antigen. The enhancement of an immune response following the administration of an "immunosuppressive" drug is believed to be caused by a decrease in the number of suppressor cells so that when antigen is given, a greater-than-normal immune response may be observed. All these agents have systemic effects on cells other than those of the lymphoid system that seriously limit their usefulness. In high doses, most cause derangements of any tissue that is metabolically active (e.g., depression of the bone marrow with subsequent loss of peripheral blood cell elements or denudation of the lining epithelium of the gastrointestinal tract).

The effect of various drugs on the immune response is best considered in relation to the stage of interference in the response (Fig. 27-1). Immunosuppressive therapy has become of paramount importance in preventing homograft rejection, especially in regard to organ transplantation, and experimental results indicate that such agents may be effective in prevention of suppression of various autoallergic reactions, but the incidence and severity of opportunistic infections and neoplasms are substantially increased.

Clinically, various combinations of irradiation, steroids (prednisone), antimetabolites (azathioprine), alkylating agents (cyclophosphamide), cyclosporine, and antilymphocyte serum have been used effectively to prevent graft rejection, modify graft versus host disease and control autoimmune diseases. The most widely used immunosuppressive regimen for graft recipients, prednisone and azathioprine, is now being replaced with a relatively new drug, cyclosporine. In selected instances total lymphoid irradiation and antilymphocyte globulin are also used. The effect of cyclophosphamide is difficult to control and it must be used carefully and selectively. Antilymphocyte globulin (ALG) may allow reduction in dose or use of other drugs, but the clinical effectiveness of ALG has been disappointing.

Prolonged immunosuppression has two major complications: increased susceptibility to infections and increased risk of cancer. Infection with a variety of opportunistic organisms is seen in graft recipients, particularly bacterial and candida infections immediately after suppression because of a loss of granulocytes; viral infections, especially cytomegalovirus, after 1 to 3 months of treatment; and *Pneumocystis carinii* and herpes zoster after 3 months. Increased risk of cancer may be caused by loss of immune surveillance or loss of control of the immune system due to alterations in suppressor and inducer activity. Increases in B cell malignancies in immunosuppressed patients may result from a loss of suppressor activity combined with increased antigenic stimulation provided by an organ graft or opportunistic infection leading to polyclonal B cell activation.

Irradiation. The effects of irradiation have been studied extensively in animals. Large doses of radiation (900–1200 rads) destroy the host's capacity to muster an immune response by destroying both unstimulated immunologically competent cells and memory cells, so that both the primary and the secondary responses may be lost. Smaller doses (300–500 rads) affect primary immune responses more than secondary responses. If induction of the antibody response is carried out at a suitable time prior to sublethal irradiation, primary antibody production may actually be greatly enhanced, presumably because of the disproportionate proliferation of antigen-induced proliferating cells; depletion of other nonsensitized cells permits more living space into which sensitized cells could expand. On the other hand, low to moderate doses of irradiation affect helper activity much more than suppressor activity, so that increased T suppressor function may result in a tolerance-like state.

In general, the proliferative phase of the immune response is most sensitive to radiation, so that suppression by radiation will be most effective if given when antigen-induced proliferation is occurring. Both T cells and B cells are susceptible to irradiation, but phagocytic capacity is relatively radioresistant. The precursors of the effector population, such as unstimulated T or B cells, are radiosensitive, whereas effector cells are resistant. For instance, T cell help for a primary response is extremely radiosensitive, but T cell help of primed animals (secondary T cell help) is radioresistant. Thus, primary responding immune-competent cells are radiosensitive but memory cells are relatively resistant.

Although whole body irradiation has been used in the past on human transplant recipients to suppress rejection reactions, whole body irradiation is no longer given because of the many harmful effects on other cell systems. Therapy involving extracorporeal irradiation of the blood is difficult to manage; the procedure is expensive and only circulating lymphocytes are exposed. Whole body irradiation has been modified to *total*

Table 27-4. Stages of Immune Response and Effect of Immune Modulating Agents

Agent	Example	Mechanism of Action	Stage of Immune Response (see Figure 25-1)						
			(1) Antigen Processing	(2) Cell Interaction	(3) Suppressor/ Helper Function	(4) Proliferation	(5) Differentiation	(6) Protein Synthesis	(7) Accessory or Effector System
Irradiation	Whole body, total lymphoid, extracorporeal	Blocks proliferation, lymphocytolytic	Decreases number of macrophages	Loss of cells	Helper > suppressor	+++ T > B	May block B cell isotype switch	Indirect	Decreases T cytotoxic cells, macrophages
Steroids	Hydrocortisone, prednisone, etc.	Alter mRNA and protein synthesis	Decrease antigen processing and binding by macrophages	Sequestration of lymphocytes	Suppressor > helper	++ T > B	May block B cell isotype switch	Decrease IL2 and lymphokine production	Vasoconstriction, inhibits inflammatory response and PMN margination
Alkylating agents	Cyclophosphamide, nitrogen mustard, busulfan, cis-platin	React chemically with nucleophilic portions of DNA, RNA and proteins	Decrease phagocytosis, number of macrophages	Loss of cells in tissue	Suppressor ≫ helper (especially for DTH)	B > T	Block T_H and B cell differentiation	Decrease lymphokine production	Decrease NK activity, phagocytosis
ANTIMETABOLITES									
Purine analogues	Azathioprine, 6-mercaptopurine	Incorporated into DNA and RNA							
Pyrimidine analogues	5-Fluorouracil, cytosine arabinoside	Inhibit DNA and RNA synthesizing enzymes							
Folic acid antagonists	Methotrexate, aminopterin	Bind to dihydrofolate reductase, inhibit DNA synthesis	Decrease number of macrophages	Loss of cells secondary to inhibition of proliferation	Suppressor ≫ helper	++++ T > B	Block B cell differentiation, helper cells may be resistant	Indirect	Decrease numbers of inflammatory cells
Methylhydrazines	Procarbazine	Formation of hydroxyl radicals, radiomimetic							

Hydroxyureas	Hydroxyurea	Kills DNA synthesizing cells	Decrease binding by macrophages	Decrease lymphocyte–macrophage interaction	Suppressor > helper	+++ T > B	Synchronize cells, can make tolerant	Inhibit protein synthesis	Block lysis of target cells by T cytotoxic cells
Alkaloids	Vinblastine, vincristine	Block mitotic spindle	Decrease phagocytosis and processing by macrophages		Helper > suppressor	++ B > T	Block B cell differentiation		Decrease complement synthesis, decrease phagocytosis
Inhibitors of protein synthesis	Antibiotics, actinomycin D, puromycin	Inhibit DNA-dependent RNA polymerase, DNA binding etc.						Block antibody and lymphokine production	?
Cyclosporine	Cyclosporine	Blocks cell activation, IL2 receptors	?	Lymphocyte depletion in tissues	Helper ≫ suppressor	+++ T ≫ B	Blocks T cell effector	Decreases IL production	
Nonsteroidal anti-inflammatory agents	Indomethacin, aspirin	Inhibit prostaglandin synthesis	0	0	Block prostaglandin E inhibition of suppressor cells	Block prostaglandin inhibition of proliferation	0	Decrease IL production	Decrease DTH, NK, decrease inflammation, decrease collagenase release from macrophages
Interferon	α, β, γ	Acts on cell surface, stimulates proliferation and differentiation	Increases phagocytosis, increases binding to macrophages	Increases interactions	Increases helper activity	Increases at low doses, decreases at high doses	Increases differentiation of B cells, T effector cells	Increases antibody and lymphokine production	Synergizes with lymphokines, increases NK activity
Antilymphocyte serum	Heterologous ALG, monoclonal antibodies	Lymphocytotoxicity	"Blindfolding" of receptors	Lymphocyte depletion	May be made specific	Indirect	Decreases production of factors	0	Blocks effector cell recognition of target
Adjuvants	Mycobacterial cell walls, muramyl dipeptides, BCG	Increase numbers and metabolic activity of macrophages at site of infection	Increase antigen processing	Increase lymphocyte–macrophage interactions	Increase helper cells	Increase polyclonal B cells	Increase production of factors, IL1	Stimulates macrophage protein synthesis	Macrophage activation

IL, interleukin; NK, natural killer; DTH, delayed type hypersensitivity; PMN, polymorphonuclear leukocytes; BCG, bacillus Calmette–Guérin; ALG, antilymphocyte globulin.

lymphoid irradiation (TLI) with application to prolonging allograft survival by induction of specific tolerance. In addition, clinical trials of TLI for control of autoimmune diseases are now underway. TLI delivers high doses of radiation to lymphoid tissues while protecting radiosensitive nonlymphoid tissues. Lead shielding sharply limits the radiation to lymph nodes, thymus, and spleen, while protecting kidneys, lungs, brain, bone marrow, gastrointestinal tract, etc. This procedure was developed in the 1960s by Henry Kaplan of Stanford for the treatment of Hodgkin's disease and other lymphomas. Patients who are treated with TLI have immune suppression as effective as do those treated by steroids, cytotoxic drugs, and antilymphocyte serum, with a much lower incidence of bacterial or viral infections. This is most likely due to the protection of the stem cell population in the bone marrow. In addition, there appears to be selective generation of suppressor cells following TLI so that exposure to antigen following TLI can result in specific tolerance-like conditions, particularly in generation of cytotoxic T cells. Thus TLI theoretically has great potential, perhaps in combination with other forms of therapy, to control graft rejection or autoimmune disease, by favoring specific control of immune reactions by T suppressor cells.

Ultraviolet light irradiation, in experimental systems, produces depressed delayed hypersensitivity responses by two mechanisms: loss of antigen presenting cells (Ia^+ macrophages) and induction of specific T suppressor cells. Clinical applications of this phenomenon have not yet been identified.

Steroids. Corticosteroids produce multiple effects in animals, and it is difficult to determine which effect may be most important for a given therapeutic result. Corticosteroids act through cytoplasmic receptors that are present in essentially all nucleated mammalian cells. Steroids are derivatives of cholesterol, are fat soluble, pass freely through the cell membrane, combine with cytosol receptors, are transported to the nucleus, bind to segments of DNA, cause derepression of certain genes, and result in synthesis of new mRNA species and thus new proteins. The major action of steroids is as an anti-inflammatory agent. It is not clear how the biochemical steps described above cause this effect. Steroids may act by stimulating lipocortin (lipomodulin, macrocortin) release from various cell populations. Lipocortin has the ability to modulate phospholipase A_2 in inflammatory cells and decrease activation of arachidonic acid metabolites. Lipocortin is a polypeptide stored in white blood cells and is rapidly released following exposure to steroids. Lipocortin in vitro inhibits the release of radiolabeled fatty acids from phosphatidylcholine, the substrate for phospholipase. Careful studies indicate that steroids have little effect on the specific induction of immune responses at the central level except at very high doses. Three major effects of steroids may be considered: leukocyte circulation, leukocyte function, and vasoconstriction. Steroids may affect the effector stage of the immune response by affecting the tissue distribution of lymphocytes and macrophages or decreasing the phagocytic capacity of macrophages. Steroids also appear to inhibit production of interleukins (IL1 and IL2) and block chemotaxis of inflammatory cells. Steroids are potent vasoconstrictors and limit access of inflammatory cells to sites of inflammation in tissues. Steroids may also decrease receptors on phagocytic cells. In asthma, steroids may also act as a β-agonist potentiator, contributing to bronchodilation and inhibiting the migration of eosinophils. Steroids also inhibit synthesis of prostaglandins to reduce late stages of chronic inflammation. Steroids appear to inhibit phospholipid lipase, resulting in decreased formation of arachidonic acid. Thus, the beneficial effect of steroids in many immune diseases appears to be as a modulator of inflammation rather than an effect on specific immunity. Humans are more resistant than some experimental animals (mice, rats, and rabbits) to the effects of steroids so that close extrapolation of experimental results in these species is not possible. Although much needs to be clarified regarding the mechanism of action of steroids, they are widely used to control severe immunopathological processes, particularly autoallergic diseases, graft rejection, and asthma, but considerable caution is needed because of the dangerous side effects.

Alkylating Agents   These drugs are called radiomimetic because the effect of their administration resembles the effect of irradiation. They are generally chemically active agents that combine with DNA and interfere with cell proliferation. Included are nitrogen mustard, cyclophosphamide, tetramine, busulfan, cisplatin, and mustard gas. The action of these drugs is only temporary, and immune reactions return when therapy is discontinued. The effects on DNA may be the most important. Alkylation of the DNA of resting lymphocytes may have little or no effect until the cells are stimulated to proliferate. Lymphoid cells have the capacity to repair the lesions produced so that if the drug is given long before antigen exposure, cellular proliferation following antigen exposure will proceed normally. However, if given at the time of antigen-induced proliferation, alkylating agents can greatly reduce, and may even eliminate, the responding cells, leading to tolerance by clonal elimination. High doses of alkylating agents generally suppress secondary B cell responses more than secondary T cell responses because of the higher metabolic activity of antibody-producing cells. Cyclophosphamide is a potent inhibitor of antibody formation at doses that have little effect on skin graft rejection, although other T cell functions may be suppressed.

Cyclophosphamide is the alkylating agent most widely used. In addition to affecting DNA synthesis, cyclophosphamide and other alkylating agents can inhibit glycolysis, respiration, RNA synthesis, protein synthesis and a variety of enzyme functions. Cyclophosphamide appears to act principally on B cells directly and on precursors of suppressor T cells that are more sensitive than B cells. The effect on a primary antibody response is much greater than on a secondary response. At moderate doses cyclosphosphamide may inhibit antibody responses by action on B cells. At low doses enhancement of antibody production by action on suppressor T cells or on suppressor macrophages is observed. Augmentation of delayed hypersensitivity reactions may also be obtained.

The effect of cyclophosphamide in humans is obviously dose dependent and has been difficult to evaluate. High doses result in lymphopenia and inhibition of B cell responses that is greater than inhibition of T cell responses. In general, established delayed hypersensitivity is resistant. Suppressor cells for delayed hypersensitivity appear to be sensitive at lower doses of cyclophosphamide than are T helper cells for antibody production by B cells. This may explain the finding that cyclophosphamide given before antigen enhances delayed hypersensitivity, but suppresses antibody production if higher doses are given.

Antimetabolic Drugs

Antimetabolites interfere with the synthesis of RNA, DNA, or protein and prevent cell division and proliferation.

Purine Analogs. The mechanism of action of these drugs is multiple. Azathioprine inhibits RNA and DNA synthesis, but also interferes with enzyme and coenzyme activity, purine conversions, and incorporation of purine into amino acids. Very large doses may severely depress not only bone marrow function, but also antibody production, cellular immunity, and even secondary responses. At lower doses, the secondary response is not affected. The effects of 6-mercaptopurine and azathioprine, which is metabolized to 6-mercaptopurine, on antibody formation are determined by the timing of the drug administration with respect to antigenic stimulus, the dose of the drug, the dose of the antigen, and the nature of the antigenic challenge. By varying these parameters in experimental animals, one may obtain suppression of all classes of antibody, selective suppression of IgG antibody, enhancement of IgM synthesis, or enhancement of both IgM and IgG antibody.

The suppressive effects of azathioprine are most impressive if given 24 hours after antigen injection, because of its antiproliferative effect or action on early events in the immune response. T cells appear to be the principal cells affected, because alkylating agents are particularly effective in inhibition of T rosette formation, mixed lymphocyte reactions, graft rejections, and delayed hypersensitivity reactions, including experimental autoallergic diseases, whereas specific antibody responses are relatively spared.

Pyrimidine Analogs. These agents interfere with RNA and DNA synthesis, and experimentally, doses can be given that suppress humoral immunity while sparing T cell reactions, such as skin graft rejection or contact sensitivity. Pyrimidine analogs are used extensively in cancer chemotherapy and may contribute significantly to the decreased resistance to bacterial infections observed in such patients.

Folic Acid Antagonists. Folic acid antagonists prevent the conversion of dihydrofolic acid to tetrahydrofolic acid by binding to the enzyme dihydrofolate reductase. This, in turn, blocks methylation of deoxyribonucleic acid and thymidylic acid (required for DNA synthesis) and interferes with transport of carbon fragments for purine and protein synthesis. In appropriate doses, these agents can partially suppress immune reactions without causing bone marrow suppression, but this side effect has limited the clinical usefulness of folic acid antagonists in controlling immune responses. In addition, methotrexate is excreted by the kidney so that toxic levels may be achieved at low doses if given to patients with impairment of renal function, such as renal transplant recipients.

Other Antimetabolites. Other antimetabolites may affect immune responses in a variety of ways (see Table 27-4). Actinomycins inhibit RNA synthesis by combining specifically with the guanine base of the DNA molecule without markedly inhibiting DNA synthesis. This results in a reduction in RNA synthesis at the time of the primary injection of antigen. Agents that inhibit protein synthesis without preventing RNA synthesis (puromycin, streptomycin, erythromycin, chloramphenicol) have very little inhibitory effect on primary immunization unless large doses are given. With doses of chloramphenicol large enough to block protein synthesis and depress antibody formation during the primary response, the development of an anamnestic response on reexposure is not affected, indicating interference not in induction but at a later stage in antibody production. Aminoacridines intercalate between both RNA and DNA. Administration of acriflavine greatly suppresses primary immune responses. No apparent interference with cell replication is observed. Dimeric alkaloids (vinblastine, vincristine) completely inhibit antibody formation and cellular reactivity when given at the same time as antigen. They also appear to inhibit proliferation of lymphoid cells. In addition, vincristine has a nonspecific anti-inflammatory effect. The mechanism of action of these drugs is not well understood, although interference with gene expression is most likely.

Antibiotics may cause an increase in incidence and severity of clinical infections with unusual organisms (*Candida albicans, Aspergillus*). The mechanisms by which antibiotics operate to decrease resistance to these organisms include overgrowth of organisms not susceptible to the given antibiotic because of a decrease or absence of competing susceptible organisms, inhibition of immune responses, and inhibition of phagocytosis. In large doses, the tetracyclines may have a marked effect on all types of immune reactivity.

Cyclosporine

The immunosuppressive effects of cyclosporine, a metabolite of a soil fungus, *Trichoderma polysporum* Rifai, now called *Tolycopaladium inflatum*, were first noted in 1972 as inhibition of antibody (hemagglutinin) formation following treatment of mice in vivo during immunization with sheep erythrocytes. The active compound is a cyclic polypeptide containing 11 amino acids, one of which is a unique amino acid. This amino acid contains nine carbon atoms and the C9 is *N*-methylated. In experimental models cyclosporine exerts its effect early during activation of lymphocytes, primarily T cells, without significant toxicity, and the effect is reversible. These findings suggested to investigators that cyclosporine might be a useful clinical immunosuppressive drug. The success of cyclosporine in experimental organ transplantation showed that it is effective in prolonging allograft survival with a minimal number of side effects or infectious complications.

Clinical trials using cyclosporine have been highly successful. In 1981 the preliminary results of two groups suggested a marked improvement in 1-year survival rate of cadaveric donor kidneys. Subsequently a number of studies have supported these preliminary conclusions. Cyclosporine has also been effective in reducing graft versus host disease, increasing takes, and reducing infections in human bone marrow transplant recipients. In addition, cyclosporine has made orthotopic liver allografting a feasible procedure in humans and it is also being used for pancreas and heart transplantation. The exact reason for the better clinical effect is not exactly clear, since the mechanism of action has not been clearly defined. Cyclosporine appears to interfere less with nonlymphoid cell function, in particular other hematopoietic bone marrow cells, and permits reduction in dose of other agents (such as steroids). This results in more specific immune control with fewer infections. Since most grafted patients actually die from infection rather than graft rejection, the ability to produce more limited immune suppression, allowing fewer infections, appears to be critical.

In human transplant recipients receiving cyclosporine the major problem is nephrotoxicity. In renal transplant patients the differentiation between an allograft rejection reaction and cyclosporine toxicity has been difficult and is controversial. Both are associated with glomerulitis and a diffuse cellular infiltrate. The fact that nephrotoxicity occurs in patients receiving cyclosporine for bone marrow or liver transplantation strongly supports the conclusion that toxicity does exist separately from renal graft rejection.

The mechanism of action of cyclosporine has been studied extensively in vitro. Cyclosporine blocks T cell activation by mitogens and by antigens. Cyclosporine may block IL1 and IL2 production, or the ability to respond to IL2. Cyclosporine also inhibits mixed lymphocyte reactions (proliferation) and generation of cytotoxic cells, but not the effector function of primed killer cells. Natural killer activity, antibody-dependent cell-mediated cytotoxicity, nonspecific accessory cell function, neutrophil function, and wound healing are not affected, so that the immunosuppressive effect is primarily directed to T cell activation, and the effect is reversible in most, but not all, systems. Cyclosporine is also able to block B cell activation, but T cells are more sensitive. T suppressor cells for MLR responses and T helper cells for T suppressor cell induction appear to be relatively resistant, but T helper cells for B cell responses are sensitive.

Nonsteroidal Anti-inflammatory Drugs

Nonsteroidal anti-inflammatory drugs act to suppress inflammation mediated by prostaglandins and leukotrienes (eicosanoids; see Chapter 12). The effect of nonsteroidal anti-inflammatory drugs on immune responses is mainly through inhibition of cyclooxygenase and decreased prostaglandin E production from arachidonic acid. Prostaglandin E acts as an inhibitor of cellular immune responses, so that depressed delayed hypersensitivity reactions can be restored by administration of cyclooxygenase inhibitors. Indomethacin increases cell-mediated immune responses in patients with decreased activity, sometimes restoring delayed hypersensitivity in anergic patients. Suppressor T cells have a high density of prostaglandin E receptors. Cyclooxygenase inhibitors depress immunoglobulin synthesis, presumably by reversal of prostaglandin E inhibition of suppressor cells.

Endogenous prostaglandin E_2 can induce or increase autoantibody production through inhibition of suppressor cell activity. Cyclooxygenase inhibitors may act to decrease autoantibody production in patients with diseases such as rheumatoid arthritis by releasing prostaglandin E–induced inhibition of suppressor cells, thus damping antibody-producing B cells.

Antilymphocyte Serum

Antilymphocyte serum is an antiserum that contains antibody activity directed against lymphocytes. Antilymphocyte globulin is a purified fraction of antilymphocyte serum containing the antibody-active immunoglobulin portion of antilymphocyte serum. Xenogeneic (heterologous) antilymphocyte serum is produced by immunizing an animal of one species (rabbit) with lymphoid cells obtained from another species (thymus or spleen of mouse). With proper selection of the lymphocyte source and care in preparation, an antiserum can be obtained that reacts specifically with lymphocytes from the donor animal. The reactivity of this antiserum may be demonstrated in vitro by its ability to agglutinate lymphocytes and to lyse lymphocytes in the presence of complement (lymphocytotoxicity).

In Vivo Effects. The effect of antilymphocyte serum (ALS) upon in vivo immune reactions is best understood by consideration of the role of the lymphocyte in different stages of the immune response. Antilymphocyte serum blocks cellular reactions, presumably by cytotoxic destruction of the lymphocytes (sensitized cells). This effect appears to be specific, as other tissues are not affected. Antilymphocyte serum may also prevent a primary response to antigen, presumably by an effect on precursor cells, and if administered in large enough doses, may even suppress or eliminate a second-set graft rejection or secondary antibody responses (loss of immune memory). The serum does not reduce reactions mediated by humoral antibody in animals that are already immunized (Arthus reaction) or nonimmune inflammatory reactions that are induced by cotton wool or turpentine. Antilymphocyte sera specific for different functional lymphocyte populations have been developed. Antisera to T cells generally kill T cells and inhibit T cell functions in vitro and in vivo, whereas antisera to B cells may prevent maturation of antibody-forming cell precursors and thus inhibit antibody formation. Such antisera have been used to define further the role of different lymphoid cell populations in immune reactions.

Mechanism of Action. The mechanism of action of antilymphocyte serum is not completely understood. There is difficulty in comparing the results of one investigator with those of another, because of differences in source, preparation, and injection of antigen (lymphocytes) used for antiserum production; in fractionation of antiserum; in dosage, route, or duration of treatment; and in differences in the immune responses tested. The possible mechanisms of immunosuppression by antilymphocyte serum include direct destruction of lymphocytes (lymphocytotoxicity), resulting in lymphopenia; opsonization of lymphocytes with clearance of affected cells by the reticuloendothelial system; coating of lymphocytes with antibody so that the lymphocytes can no longer react with antigen (blindfolding); stimulation of proliferation of lymphocytes that do not have the ability to react with antigen (sterile activation); specific cytotoxic effect upon one class of lymphocytes (long-lived) with the ability to recognize antigen, with little or no effect on

nonspecific short-lived lymphocytes (selective lymphocytotoxicity); inactivation of a thymic factor responsible for development of immunologically competent cells (thymus effect);
direction of immunologically reactive cells toward producing
an immune response to the injected serum and away from a
response to other antigens (antigenic competition); or coating
of the target organ (skin graft) with antibodies so that the antigens of the target organ are not recognized by the recipient
(target organ coating). None of the above satisfactorily explains
all the immunosuppressive effects of antilymphocyte serum. In
spite of the voluminous experimental data indicating that this
material may profoundly affect the immune responses of experimental animals, a statistically significant effect of antisera to
human lymphocytes on allograft survival in human recipients
has been difficult to demonstrate. However, recent results indicate a prolongation of skin and kidney graft survival in some
recipients treated with antilymphocyte globulin, and a higher
success rate of bone marrow grafts in patients treated prior to
transplantation. In these patients, antilymphocyte globulin
eliminates immunocompetent cells and reduces graft versus
host reactions.

Antipolymorphonuclear
Leukocyte Serum

Antipolymorphonuclear leukocyte serum has also been applied
to experimental situations. Antineutrophil serum reduces nonimmune neutrophil-mediated inflammation induced by urate
crystals, as well as antibody-induced skin reactions and
glomerulonephritis. Antineutrophil serum produces a rapid
neutropenia through reticuloendothelial clearance, with subsequent reduction of cells available for inflammatory reactions. Antieosinophil serum has been used to inhibit passive
cutaneous anaphylactic reactions in guinea pigs, suggesting
that eosinophils may play a role in some anaphylactic reactions.

Antimacrophage Serum

Experimentally, xenogeneic antiserum to macrophages has
also been used to inhibit antibody formation, presumably by
interfering with antigen processing or phagocytosis. In addition, antimacrophage serum may interfere with the effector
arm of delayed hypersensitivity, as exemplified by prolongation
of skin allograft survival, passive transfer of delayed hypersensitivity, and a small decrease in adjuvant-induced arthritis. Antimacrophage serum may eliminate macrophages directly by
killing or through clearing by the reticulendothelial system,
resulting in a lowering of peripheral mononuclear cells. Application of antimacrophage or antipolymorphonuclear serum to
human diseases has not yet been proven feasible.

Monoclonal Antibodies

The problems relating to variability in different preparations of
xenogeneic ALG in immune modulation may be circumvented
by monoclonal antibodies. Monoclonal antibodies to helper/

inducer T cells have been shown to reduce circulating lymphocytes in clinical trials and to prolong graft survival in monkey. However, a clear-cut clinical effect has not yet been demonstrated.

Monoclonal antibodies to T cells have been used more successfully in vitro to remove functioning T cells from bone marrow cell populations. Three methods have been employed to remove cells mediating graft versus host reactions: T lymphocyte depletion by lectin agglutination using soybean agglutinin, by antibody and complement cytotoxicity, and by antibody–toxin (ricin) conjugates. Such treatment can prevent serious graft versus host reactions in bone marrow recipients receiving allogeneic transplants from HLA-mismatched donors.

The major limitation to the use of monoclonal antibodies at the present time is the production of antibody by the patient to the monoclonal antibodies, which are mouse immunoglobulins. This results in clearance of the monoclonal antibody and obliteration of the beneficial effect. Efforts are now underway to identify human cell lines that could be used to generate human- anti-human monoclonal antibodies that would circumvent this problem (for further discussion of the application of monoclonal antibodies to cancer therapy, see Chapter 29).

Clinical Application of Immunosuppressive Agents

In practical terms, six major immunosuppressive agents are now used clinically: steroids, alkylating agents, purine analogs, folic acid antagonists, cyclosporine, and antilymphocyte globulin. The effectiveness of these agents in immune-mediated diseases other than transplantation and immune deficiencies is shown in Table 27-5. The effectiveness of cyclosporine in the treatment of autoimmune diseases is not yet known. Immunosuppression is well-established therapy for graft recipients and certain autoallergic or immune complex–mediated diseases. In many other diseases, immunosuppressive therapy is of questionable merit. Although individual reports may claim a beneficial effect of immunosuppressive drugs, in many situations the efficacy of such treatment has not been critically evaluated. Antimetabolites may be used to decrease the dose of steroids required for maintenance. The "steroid saving" effect may be of great benefit in some patients. Careful monitoring of the immune reactivity of immunosuppressed patients must be performed to ensure that immune reactivity is not reduced to the point where opportunistic infections will become manifest. Such infections were common during the first few years of renal transplantations; most transplant recipients did not die from rejection crises but from infections. With careful monitoring of recipients and titration of immunosuppressive drugs, a substantial improvement in survival of renal allograft recipients has taken place.

Table 27-5. Clinical Use of Immunosuppressive Drugs

Disease Treated	Steroids	Alkylating Agent (Cyclophosphamide)	Purine Analog (Azathioprine)	Folic Acid Antagonist (Methotrexate)	ALG[a]
Neutralization					
Hemophilia (anticoagulants)	+[b]	+	−	−	−
Myasthenia gravis	+	−	−	−	−
Cytotoxic					
Autoallergic hemolytic anemia	++	+	−	−	−
Idiopathic thrombocytopenic purpura	++	+	−	−	−
Toxic complex					
Nephrotic syndrome (minimal)	++	+	−	−	−
Chronic glomerulonephritis	+	++	−	−	−
Systemic lupus erythematosus	++	++	+	−	−
Rheumatoid arthritis	++	++	++	++	−
Progressive systemic sclerosis	+	−	−	++	−
Psoriasis	++	−	+	++	−
Pemphigus	++	++	+	+	−
Dermato(poly)myositis	++	+	+	−	−
Anaphylactic					
Asthma, chronic	+	−	−	−	−
Delayed hypersensitivity					
Organ transplantation	++	+	++	+	+
Bone marrow transplantation	−	−	−	−	−
Multiple sclerosis	+	−	−	−	−
Ulcerative colitis	++	++	++	+	−
Regional enteritis	++	+	+	−	−
Sjögren's syndrome	+	−	−	−	−
Thyroiditis	−	−	−	−	−
Chronic active hepatitis	+	−	−	−	−
Granulomatous					
Wegener's granulomatosis	+	++	+	−	−

[a] ALG, antilymphocyte globulin.
[b] ++, effective; +, questionably effective; −, not effective.

Modified from Gerber NL, Steinberg DO: Drugs 11:14–112, 1976.

Immunosuppressive Factors

A number of serum proteins and cellular extracts may nonspecifically suppress immune induction or expression. Although many reports have convincingly demonstrated effects in vitro, the significance of the effects of these proteins in vivo is not clear. It is theoretically possible that some of these factors could be used passively to suppress immune reactivity. As a group, these proteins have been termed immunoregulatory globulins. Included are α_2-globulin (immunoregulatory α-globulin), α_2-macroglobulin, pregnancy-associated α-macroglobulin, α-fetoprotein, very low density lipoprotein, and C reactive protein. Immunoregulatory α-globulin has been studied extensively. Among the reactions inhibited are mitogen and antigen proliferation responses, plaque-forming cell responses, delayed hypersensitivity skin reactions, allograft rejections, and immunity to syngeneic tumors. The effect of α_2-macroglobulin (α_2M) on immune reactivity is probably because of the ability of α_2M to inhibit the activity of proteases and inactivate inflammatory mediators, such as kallikrein and plasminogen activator. Pregnancy-associated α-macroglobulin is a serum protein that increases dramatically during pregnancy and decreases just as dramatically after birth. The addition of this protein to lymphocyte cultures in vitro markedly suppresses mitogen-induced T cell responses. This protein appears to be different from α_2-macroglobulin, but the precise relationship is not clear, because sensitive assays indicate its presence in many normal sera. Another pregnancy-associated protein, α-fetoprotein, has also been reported to have immunosuppressive properties in vitro although conflicting reports have appeared. The possible role of pregnancy-associated α-macroglobulin and α-fetoprotein in protecting the fetus from maternal immune rejection has attracted considerable attention, but has not yet been demonstrated convincingly. A species of low density lipoprotein found in human sera suppresses lymphocyte stimulation in vitro and inhibits antibody formation in mice. C reactive protein is an α_2-glycoprotein in serum, which increases in concentration in humans with various acute febrile illnesses. It is called C reactive protein because of its ability to precipitate the C polysaccharide of pneumococcal cell walls and polycations. Following this reaction, C reactive protein is able to fix complement via the classical pathway. C reactive protein selectively binds to the T lymphocytes of humans, inhibits E rosette formation, and suppresses the proliferation response to allogeneic cells (mixed lymphocyte reaction).

In summary, several non-antigen-specific immunosuppressive serum factors have been identified and partially characterized. Immunoregulatory α-globulin, α_2-macroglobulin, low density lipoprotein inhibitor, and C reactive protein may help control the extent of an inflammatory process or immune reaction. Pregnancy-associated α-globulin and α-fetoprotein could help block allorejection of the fetus. However, convincing evidence for a significant therapeutic role of these proteins has yet to be reported.

Summary

Modulation of the immune response may be antigen specific or nonspecific. The immune response may be affected at different stages of the immune response: afferent, central, efferent, or accessory mechanisms. Stimulation of an active specific immune response may be enhanced by a variety of adjuvants. Specific passive immunization may be accomplished by transfer of humoral antibody or specifically sensitized lymphocytes. Macrophage activation, lymphokines, and interleukins can nonspecifically increase the immune response at the level of either induction or expression.

Suppression of immune responses may also be specific or nonspecific. Specific mechanisms involve tolerance, hyposensitization, or desensitization using specific antigen. Nonspecific suppression may be accomplished with a number of agents including irradiation, steroids, alkylating agents, antimetabolic drugs, cyclosporine, antilymphocyte globulin, or monoclonal antibodies.

Immune suppression is necessary for success of allografts and may be useful in control of certain autoimmune diseases. Clinically, immune stimulation of reponses is desired in patients with immune deficiency diseases or cancer. Specific active immunization has been most effective in protection of normal individuals against infectious diseases (Chapter 25). When a specific defect can be replaced, such as immunoglobulin antibody in patients with humoral immune deficiencies or thymic grafts in patients with thymus deficiencies, specific passive immunity is effective (Chapter 26). Clinical trials for immune modifiers in cancer have been less rewarding (Chapter 29).

Specific immune suppression involving antibody feedback has been spectacularly successful in preventing erythroblastosis fetalis (Chapter 15), and antigen injection therapy is often helpful in decreasing allergic symptoms in hay fever (Chapter 18). Combinations of irradiation, steroids, antimetabolic agents, cyclosporine, and antilymphocyte globulin are used to control graft rejections, but frequently result in complicating opportunistic infections. Monoclonal antibodies may provide more precise and effective modulation of immune responses. Although many beneficial effects have resulted from clinical application of immune modification, many other approaches to immunotherapy, particularly in cancer treatment, have been disappointing.

References

See Chapter 25

Specific Active Immunization

Braun W, Rega MJ: Adenyl cyclase–stimulating catecholamines as modifiers of antibody formation. Immunol Commun 1:523, 1972.

Chase MW: Immunization of mammals other than man. *In* Williams CA, Chase MW (eds): Methods in Immunology and Immunochemistry. New York, Academic Press, 1967, p197.

Freund J: The mode of action of immunological adjuvants. Adv Tuberc Res 7:130, 1956.

Hamaoka T, Katz D: Mechanism of adjuvant activity of poly A:U on antibody responses to hapten–carrier conjugates. Cell Immunol 7:246, 1973.

Holt LB: Developments in Diphtheria Prophylaxis. London, Heinman, 1950.

Ishizuka M, Braun W, Matsumoto T: Cyclic AMP and immune responses. I. Influence of poly AU and cAMP on antibody formation in vitro. J Immunol 107:1027, 1971.

Lederek E: Synthetic immunostimulants derived from the bacteria cell wall. J Med Chem 23:819, 1980.

Munoz J: Effect of bacteria and bacterial products on antibody responses. Adv Immunol 4:397, 1964.

Persson U, Moller E: The effect of lipopolysaccharide on the primary immune response to the hapten NHP. Scand J Immunol 4:571, 1975.

Reed CE, Benner M, Lockey SD, Enta T, Makino S, Carr RH: On the mechanism of the adjuvant effect of Bordatella pertussis vaccine. J Allergy Clin Immunol 49:1741, 1972.

Skidmore BJ, Chiller JM, Morrison DC, Weigle WO: Immunologic properties of bacterial lipopolysaccharide (LPS): correlation between the mitogenic, adjuvant, and immunologic activities. J Immunol 114:770, 1975.

Warren HS, Vogel FR, Chedid LA: Current states of immunological adjuvants. Annu Rev Immunol 4:369, 1986.

White RG: The adjuvant effect of microbial products on the immune response. Annu Rev Microbiol 30:579, 1976.

Nonspecific Immune Stimulation

See also Chapter 29.

Andersson J, Sjoberg O, Moller G: Induction of immunoglobulin and antibody synthesis in vitro by lipopolysaccharides. Eur J Immunol 2:349, 1972.

Bast RC Jr, Zbar B, Borsos T, Rap HJ: Medical progress: BCG and cancer. N Engl J Med 29:1413, 1458, 1974.

Chirigos MA: Immunotherapeutic agents: their role in cellular immunity and their therapeutic potential. Springer Semin Immunopathol 8:327, 1985.

Christie GH, Bomford B: Mechanisms of macrophage activation by Corynebacterium parvum. I. In vitro experiments. II. In vivo experiments. Cell Immunol 17:141, 1975.

Claman HN: Anti-inflammatory effects of corticosteroids. Clin Allergy Immunol 4:317, 1984.

Cone RE, Johnson AG: Regulation of the immune system by polynucleotides. IV. Amplification of proliferation of thymus-influenced lymphocytes. Cell Immunol 3:283, 1972.

Douglas RM, Moore BW, Miles HB, et al: Prophylactic efficiency of intranasal alpha2 interferon against rhinovirus infections in the family setting. N Engl J Med 314:65, 1986.

Durum SK, Schmidt JA, Oppenheim JJ: Interleukin 1: an immunological perspective. Annu Rev Immunol 3:363, 1985.

Hoffman MK, Weiss O, Koenig S, Hirst JA, Oettgen HF: Suppression and enhancement of the T cell–dependent production of antibody to SRBC in vitro by bacterial lipopolysaccharide. J Immunol 114:738, 1975.

Johnson HG, Johnson AG: Regulation of the immune system by synthetic polynucleotides. II. Action on peritoneal exudate cells. J Exp Med 133:649, 1971.

Keller R: Mechanisms by which activated normal macrophages destroy rat tumor cells in vitro. Cytokinetics, non-involvement of T lymphocytes and effect of metabolic inhibitors. Immunology 27:285, 1974.

Kirchner H: Interferons, a group of multiple lymphokines. Springer Semin Immunopathol 7:347, 1984.

Lane FC, Unanue ER: Immunologic events during Listeria monocytogenes infection in mice: adjuvanticity and immunogenicity of macrophage bound antigens. J Immunol 110:105, 1964.

Mackaness GB: The immunological basis of acquired cellular resistance. J Exp Med 120:105, 1964.

Murahata RI, Mitchell MS: Modulation of immune response by BCG: a review. Yale J Biol Med 49:283, 1976.

Nelson DS: Immunobiology of the Macrophage. New York, Academic Press, 1976.

Oldham RK: Biologicals for cancer treatment: interferons. Hosp Pract 20:71, 1985.

Rabinovitch M, Majias RE, Russo M, Abbey EE: Increased spreading of macrophages from mice treated with interferon inducers. Cell Immunol 29:86, 1977.

Rosenberg S: Lymphokine activated killer cells: a new approach to immunotherapy of cancer. J Nat Cancer Inst 75:595, 1985.

Smith KA: Interleukin 2. Annu Rev Immunol 2:319, 1984.

Talmadge JE, Chirigos MA: Comparison of immunomodulary and immunotherapeutic properties of biologic response modifiers. Springer Semin Immunopathol 8:1, 1985.

Specific Immunosuppression

Tolerance

See Chapter 11.
Nossal GJV: Cellular mechanism of immunologic tolerance. Annu Rev Immunol 1:33, 1983.

Desensitization

See Chapter 18.
Ishizaka K: Regulation of IgE synthesis. Annu Rev Immunol 2:159, 1984.

Nonspecific
Immonosuppression

Aisenberg AC, Murray C: Transfer studies in cyclophosphamide-induced tolerance. Cell Immunol 7:143, 1973.

Anderson RE, Warner NL: Ionizing radiation and the immune response. Adv Immunol 24:215, 1976.

Bach SF: The pharmacological and immunological basis for the use of immunosuppressive drugs. Drugs 11:1, 1976.

Benjamin E, Sulka E: Antikörperbildung nach experimenteller Schädigung des Hämatopoetischen durch Röntgenstrahlen. Wien Klin Wochenschr 21:10, 1908.

Bertino JR: The mechanism of action of the folate antagonists in man. Cancer Res 23:1286, 1963.

Braun DP, Harris JE: Modulation of the immune response by chemotherapy. Pharmacol Ther 4:89, 1981.

Chalmers AH, Burgoyne LA, Murray AW: Antineoplastic and immunosuppressive drugs. I. Biochemical and clinical pharmacological considerations. Drugs 3:227, 1972.

Claman HN: Anti-inflammatory effects of corticosteroids. Clin Allergy Immunol 4:317, 1984.

Claman HN: Corticosteroids and lymphoid cells. N Engl J Med 287:388, 1972.

Dyminski JW, Argyris BF: Prolongation of allograft survival with antimacrophage serum. Transplantation 8:595, 1969.

Elion GB: Significance of azathioprine metabolites. Proc R Soc Med (Lond) 65:257, 1967.

Fauci AS: Mechanism of corticosteroid action on lymphocyte subpopulations. I. Redistribution of circulating T and B lymphocytes to the bone marrow. Immunology 28:669, 1975.

Feldman JD, Unanue ER: Role of macrophages in delayed hypersensitivity. II. Effects of antimacrophage antibody. Cell Immunol 2:275, 1971.

Fox IJ, Perry LL, Sy MS, et al: The influence of ultraviolet light irradiation on the immune system. Clin Immunol Immunopathol 17:141, 1980.

Gabrielsen AE, Good RA: Chemical suppression of adaptive immunity. Adv Immunol 6:92, 1967.

Goodwin JS: Immunologic effects of nonstandard anti-inflammatory drugs. Am J Med 77:7, 1985.

Hadden JW, Merriam LK: Immunopharmacologic basis of immunotherapy. Clin Physiol Biochem 3:111, 1985.

Hengst JCD, Cempe RA: Immunomodulation by cyclophosphamide. Clin Immunol Allergy 4:199, 1984.

Heppner GH, Griswold DE, Di Lorenzo J, Poplin EA, Calabresi P: Selective immunosuppression by drugs in balanced immune responses. Fed Proc 33:1882, 1974.

James K: The preparation and properties of antilymphocyte sera. Prog Surg 7:140, 1969.

Jasin HE, Lennard D, Ziff M: Studies on antimacrophage globulin. Clin Exp Immunol 8:801, 1971.

Jones JF: Plasmapheresis in the treatment of immunological diseases. Clin Immunol Allergy 5:13, 1985.

Kripke ML: Immunologic mechanism in UV radiation carcinogenesis. Adv Cancer Res 34:69, 1981.

Lands WEM: Mechanisms of action of anti-inflammatory drugs. Adv Drug Res 14:147, 1985.

Lee K, Langman RE, Paekau VH, Diener E: The cellular basis of cortisone-induced immunosuppression of the antibody response. Studies of its reversal in vitro. Cell Immunol 17:405, 1975.

Lurie HI, Duma RS: Opportunistic infections of the lungs. Hum Pathol 1:233, 1970.

Mevleman J, Katz P: The immunologic effects and use of glucocorticoids. Med Clin North Am 69:805, 1985.

Miller JJ, Cole LS: Resistance of long-lived lymphocytes and plasma cells in rat lymph nodes to treatment with prednisone, cyclophosphamide, 6-mercaptopurine and actinomycin D. J Exp Med 126:109, 1967.

Moeller G (ed): Immunosuppressive Agents. Immunol Rev 65, 1982.

Norbury KC: Immunotoxicologic evaluation: an overview. J Am Coll Toxicol 4:279, 1985.

Panijel J, Cayeux P: Immunosuppressive effects of macrophage antiserum. Immunology 14:769, 1968.

Rinehart JJ, Sagoue AL, Balcerzak SP, Ackerman GA, LoBuglio AF: Effects of corticosteroid therapy on human monocyte function. N Engl J Med 292:236, 1975.

Schleimer RP: The mechanism of anti-inflammatory steroid action in allergic diseases. Am Rev Pharmacol Toxicol 25:381, 1985.

Schwartz RS: Therapeutic area of immune suppression and enhancement. Hosp Pract 16:93, 1981.

Shevach EM: The effect of cyclosporin A on the immune system. Annu Rev Immunol 3:397, 1985.

Simpson DM, Ross R: Effects of heterologous anti-neutrophil serum in guinea pigs: hematologic and ultrastructural observations. Am J Pathol 65:79, 1971.

Strober S: "Managing" the immune system with total lymphoid irradiation. Hosp Pract 16:77, 1981.

Strober S: Natural suppressor cells. Neonatal tolerance and total lymphoid irradiation: exploring obscure relationships. Annu Rev Immunol 2:219, 1984.

Taliaferro WH: Modification of the immune response by radiation and cortisone. Ann NY Acad Sci 69:745, 1957.

Turk JL, Parker D, Poulter LW: Functional aspects of the selective depletion of lymphoid tissue by cyclophosphamide. Immunology 23:493, 1972.

White DJG (ed): Proceedings of a Conference on Cyclosporin A. New York, Elsevier, 1982.

Clinical Applications

See also Nonspecific Immunosuppression above.

Gerber NL, Steinberg AD: Clinical use of immunosuppressive drugs, Parts I, II. Drugs 11:14(I),90(II), 1976.

Monaco AP, Campion J-P, Kapnick SJ: Clinical use of antilymphocyte globulin. Transplant Proc 9:1007, 1977.

Salvatierra O, Potter D, Cochrum KC, Amend WJC, Duca R, Sachs BL, Johnson RWJ, Belzer FO: Improved patient survival in renal transplantation. Surgery 79:166, 1976.

Schwartz RS: Immunosuppressive drugs. Prog Allergy 9:246, 1965.

Schwartz RS: Specificity of immunosuppression by antimetabolities. Fed Proc 25:165, 1966.

Sell S: Antilymphocytic antibody: effects in experimental animals and problems in human use. Ann Intern Med 71:177, 1969.

Starzl TE, Porter KA, Andres G, Halgrimson CG, Hurwitz R, Giles G, Terasaki PI, Penn I, Schroter GT, Lilly J, Starkie SJ, Putnam CW: Long term survival after renal transplantation in humans. Ann Surg 172:437, 1970.

Stenzl KH, Whitsell JC, Stubenbord WT, Fotino M, Riggio RP, Sullivan JF, Lewy JE, Cheigh JS, Rubin AL: Kidney transplantation: improvement in patient and graft survival. Ann Surg 180:29, 1974.

Symoens J, Rosenthal M: Levamisole in the modulation of the immune response: The current experimental and clinical state. J Reticuloendothel Soc 21:175, 1977.

Weiner M, Piliero SJ: Nonsteroid antiinflammatory agents. Annu Rev Pharmacol 10:171, 1970.

Wolstenholme GEW (ed): Antilymphocytic Serum. Boston, Little, Brown, 1967.

Immunosuppressive Factors

Abernethy TS, Avery OT: The occurrence during acute infections of a protein not normally present in the blood. I. Distribution of the reactive protein in patients' sera and the effect of calcium on the flocculation reaction with the C-polysaccharide of pneumococcus. J Exp Med 73:173, 1941.

Chase P: The effects of human serum proteins on phytohemagglutinin and concanavalin A–stimulated human lymphocyte cultures. Cell Immunol 5:544, 1972.

Curtiss LK, DeHeer DH, Edgington TS: In vivo suppression of the primary immune response by a species of low density serum lipoprotein. J Immunol 118:648, 1977.

Gallin JT, Kaplan AP: Mononuclear cell chemotactic activity of kallikrein and plasminogen activator and its inhibition by C1 inhibitor and α_2 macroglobulin. J Immunol 113:1928, 1974.

Mortensen RF, Osmand AP, Gewurz H: Effects of C-reactive protein on the lymphoid system. I. Binding to thymus dependent lymphocytes and alteration of their functions. J Exp Med 141:821, 1975.

Mowbray JF: Effect of large doses of an α_2-glycoprotein fraction on the survival of rat skin homografts. Transplantation 1:15, 1963.

Ptak W, Guminska M, Stachurska B, Czarnik Z: Inhibitory effect of α-globulins of different origin on the cell mediated immune response in mice. Int Arch Allergy 53:145, 1977.

Stimson WH: Studies on the immunosuppressive properties of a pregnancy associated α-macroglobulin. Clin Exp Immunol 25:199, 1976.

28 | Lymphoproliferative Diseases

Immunoproliferative (lymphoproliferative) diseases include both benign (self-limited, reversible) and malignant (progressively growing) increases in numbers of cells belonging to lymphoid cell populations (lymphocytes and macrophages). The term malignant lymphoma was first proposed by Billroth in 1871 to differentiate malignant tumors from inflammatory reactions or benign hyperplasias. The suffix *oma* means "mass (or lump)"; thus *lymphoma* means "an increase in mass of a lymphoid organ." *Leukemia* means "white blood," describing the effect of large numbers of leukemic white blood cells on the color of the blood. Thus *lymphoma* is used for malignant proliferation of white cells in lymphoid organs, *leukemia* for malignant increases in white cells in the blood. Lymphomas and leukemias are progressively growing tumors that mimic in appearance normal lymphoid cells. Until recently, classification and understanding of these diseases were based mainly on morphological observations and clinical correlations. The identification of cell surface markers for different lymphocyte populations has led to a much better understanding of lymphocyte differentiation and to reclassification of immunoproliferative diseases on the basis of T cell, B cell, or macrophage (histiocyte) lineage. This reclassification, in conjunction with investigations with animal models of immunoproliferation, is being applied to give a better appreciation of these diseases in humans. Older classifications are confusing because the terminology incorrectly presumed a cell type of origin on the basis of morphology. For instance, the terms *reticulum cell sarcoma* and *histiocytic lymphoma*, implying a macrophage origin, have been used in the past for some tumors that are now known to express B cell markers. These are now classified as large-cell forms of diffuse B cell lymphoma.

687

Lymphoid Tissue Structure and Lymphoproliferative Disease

Maturation of Blood-Forming Cells

To understand the morphology, growth patterns, manifestations, and tissue distribution of the human lymphoproliferative diseases, the localization of normal lymphoid cells in lymphoid organs and phenotypic markers reflecting differentiation of lymphocytes must be considered (see Chapters 2–4). The precursors of lymphoid cells arise mainly in the bone marrow. Before maturation, these cells do not express T and B cell markers. A diagram of the normal maturation of blood cells, including lymphocytes as well as other blood cell lineages, and the putative site of the block in differentiation in lymphomas is illustrated in Figure 28-1. A block in the differentiation of malig-

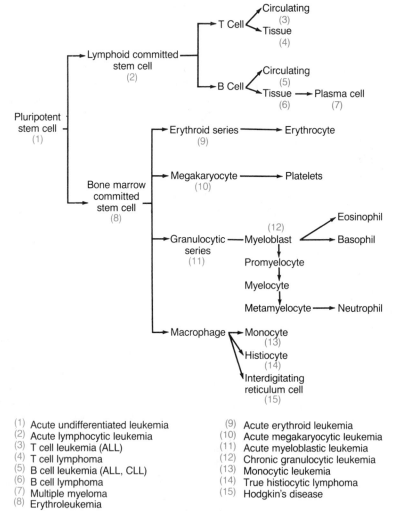

Figure 28-1. Maturation of blood-forming cells and postulated site of maturation arrest in lymphomas and leukemias. Pluripotent stem cells are present in the bone marrow and give rise to other cell types by differentiation to "end" cells. Mature cells in each series normally die at the same rate as new cell types in each series are produced, resulting in a relatively constant number of each cell type. In lymphomas and leukemias differentiation of a given cell lineage is arrested so that increasing numbers of a given cell type appear. This process is not normally reversible by physiological mechanisms, although it may be controlled by chemotherapy. ALL, acute lymphocytic leukemia; CLL, chronic lymphocytic leukemia. (See Chapter 4 for a detailed description of the development of the immune system.)

(1) Acute undifferentiated leukemia
(2) Acute lymphocytic leukemia
(3) T cell leukemia (ALL)
(4) T cell lymphoma
(5) B cell leukemia (ALL, CLL)
(6) B cell lymphoma
(7) Multiple myeloma
(8) Erythroleukemia
(9) Acute erythroid leukemia
(10) Acute megakaryocytic leukemia
(11) Acute myeloblastic leukemia
(12) Chronic granulocytic leukemia
(13) Monocytic leukemia
(14) True histiocytic lymphoma
(15) Hodgkin's disease

nant lymphocytes results in the accumulation of large numbers of relatively homogeneous, less mature cells as compared with normal. As a result of the differentiation block, cells in a given lineage that normally would differentiate into cells that would die and be turned over to make way for newly formed cells (terminally differentiate) do not die and continue to accumulate in tissues. This results in the "forcing out" of normal cells, leading to loss of function of blood cells and resulting disease manifestations such as bleeding (loss of platelets), susceptibility to infection (loss of lymphocytes and granulocytes), and wasting.

Tissue Localization of Lymphoid Cells

In this chapter the emphasis is on tumors of the lymphoid cells, that is, lymphocytes and monocytes (macrophages). Most lymphocytic tumors (lymphomas) are of B cell lineage; tumors of T cells and macrophages occur less frequently. Tumors of lymphoid cells usually are located in lymphoid organs in areas where cells of the same lineage are normally found (Fig. 28-2). T cell precursors circulate to the thymus, develop into mature T

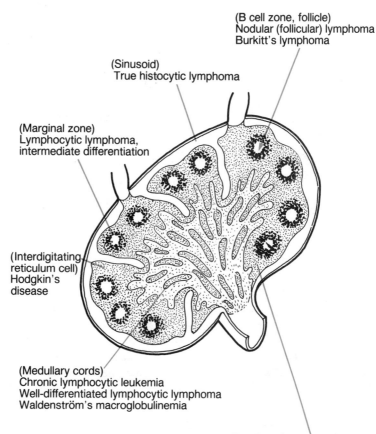

Figure 28-2. Structure of lymph node and origin of lymphomas: drawing of lymph node illustrating anatomic localization of B cells (follicles), T cells (diffuse, paracortex, and deep cortex), and macrophages (medullary cords). B cell tumors arise in the cortex and are often follicular in structure, but sometimes diffuse. T cell lymphomas arise in the paracortex and deep cortex and are always diffuse. Tumors of macrophages arise in the medulla and are diffuse. In general, the structure of the tumor reflects the normal morphology of the cell type from which it arises. (Modified from Mann RS, Jaffe ES, Berard CW: Malignant lymphomas—a conceptual understanding of morphologic diversity. Am J Pathol 94:105–192, 1979.)

(B cell zone, follicle)
Nodular (follicular) lymphoma
Burkitt's lymphoma

(Sinusoid)
True histocytic lymphoma

(Marginal zone)
Lymphocytic lymphoma,
intermediate differentiation

(Interdigitating reticulum cell)
Hodgkin's disease

(Medullary cords)
Chronic lymphocytic leukemia
Well-differentiated lymphocytic lymphoma
Waldenström's macroglobulinemia

(T cell zone, paracortex)
Sézary's syndrome
Mycosis fungoides
Lymphoblastic lymphoma
Acute lymphoblastic leukemia

cells, and then migrate from the thymus to localize in T-dependent zones (lymph node paracortex, spleen periarteriolar sheath, etc.) in peripheral organs. B cells arise in bone marrow or fetal liver and localize in B cell zones (lymph node follicles, spleen follicles), with mature immunoglobulin-producing plasma cells found in medullary zones (lymph node medulla or splenic red pulp cords). Macrophages are found in follicular zones and are prominent in medullary zones. In addition to these, a substantial proportion of cells without markers (null cells) are found at different tissue sites. Of particular importance is the fact that these cells normally circulate and are found in peripheral blood. Thus, it is to be expected that neoplastic cells derived from these cells will often be found in blood and lymph. The tissue localization of lymphoproliferative diseases usually reflects the normal tissue distribution of the respective cell type and the nature of the cell types involved.

Nonmalignant Lymphoproliferation

Physiological stress may result in reversible increased production of a given cell type (hyperplasia). At high altitudes the production of erythrocytes increases, resulting in higher numbers of erythrocytes; during a chronic infection, production of granulocytes increases. With removal of the stimulus for hyperplasia, production returns to normal and the number of cells dying exceeds production until normal cell numbers are reached.

Benign (nonmalignant) hyperplasia of lymphoid tissue usually occurs in response to inflammatory stimuli or infections. Clinically, self-limited hyperplasias must be distinguished from malignant tumors. Both benign and malignant lymphoproliferative diseases may present with enlarged lymph nodes or spleen associated with fever, so that it is not always simple to differentiate benign from malignant lymphadenopathy or splenomegaly (enlarged lymph nodes or spleen). If an obvious source of infection is present, such as inflamed tonsils associated with cervical lymphadenopathy or enlarged inguinal nodes with genital syphilis, and if this responds to appropriate therapy by antibiotics, malignancy may be considered unlikely. However, in many instances, it is necessary to obtain a lymph node biopsy to rule out malignancy. If an invasive procedure is to be performed, every effort should be made to obtain a satisfactory diagnostic tissue specimen. It is important to obtain the largest nodes accessible to the surgeon, not just some nodal tissues, because frequently not all nodes in a group are involved. Histologically, inflammatory hyperplasias are not monoclonal or limited to one cell type, as are most lymphomas. The cells involved are a mixture of T, polyclonal B, null, and polymorphonuclear cells and macrophages. Malignant tumors demonstrate a relative uniformity of cell type and replacement of normal structures, whereas hyperplasias contain a mixture of cell types and an exaggeration of normal structure.

Suppurative Lymphadenitis

Suppurative lymphadenitis is an inflammatory reaction in the lymph node draining a zone of acute infection. Usually polymorphonuclear leukocytes are found early after onset; macrophages appear later. The basic structure of the lymph node is not altered. Tonsillitis is a form of suppurative lymphadenitis.

Postvaccinial and Viral Lymphadenitis

The lymph nodes draining the site of vaccination (tetanus, diphtheria, others) or viral infection show a mixed cellular response, particularly an increased paracortical component with a large number of blast cells and, in some instances, even giant cells. In some cases, it may be very difficult to distinguish this response from malignant lymphomas by histologic examination. These responses are also seen in immunized animals and represent the response of lymphoid tissue to antigenic stimulation or viral infection.

AIDS-Related Lymphadenopathy

Generalized enlargement of lymph nodes has been noted to precede the appearance of opportunistic infections characteristic of the AIDS syndrome. (See Chapter 26 for a more detailed description of AIDS.) AIDS is caused by the human immunodeficiency virus (HIV) family. These retroviruses infect helper T cells, as well as other cell types, particularly in the brain (neurotrophic). Antibody to virus antigen is found in over 90% of affected individuals. The presence of antibody is an important adjunct to the diagnosis of pre-AIDS. These patients also have a decrease in the number of cells expressing the CD4 phenotype in peripheral blood cells. Histologically the nodes in pre-AIDS show polyclonal follicular (B cell) and diffuse (T cell) hyperplasia. As the disease progresses there is a mixture of hyperplasia and hypoplasia in the same node. Finally, marked lymphocyte depletion is seen in lymph nodes in fatal AIDS and is believed to represent the end stage lesion. The findings are qualitatively similar to those seen in other viral infections, such as infectious mononucleosis, but are often more extensive. In some patients the polyclonal B cell proliferation resembles B cell lymphoma histologically.

Drug-Induced Lymphadenopathy

Ingestion of anticonvulsant drugs (diphenylhydantoin, mephenytoin) may lead to a lymphoid cell reaction that mimics lymphoma, including skin rash, fever, and lymphadenopathy. There may be loss of normal architecture with a pleomorphic cell infiltrate, including blasts, eosinophils, neutrophils, and plasma cells. Without the clinical history of drug exposure, differentiation from lymphoma may be difficult, and the term *pseudolymphomatous lymphadenitis* has been used to emphasize the resemblance of these lesions to lymphoma.

Sinus Histiocytosis With Massive Lymphadenopathy (Rosai–Dorfman Disease)

Massive cervical lymphadenopathy, fever, and leukocytosis may be associated with dilation of lymph node subcapsular and medullary sinusoids that become filled with proliferating histiocytes, which phagocytose normal lymphocytes. This may persist for some years, but is entirely self limited. The etiology is unknown, but most likely represents a response to a chronic inflammatory or antigenic stimulus.

Lymphodermatitis (Dermatopathic Lymphadenitis)

Lymphadenopathy may occur with a variety of infectious diseases, such as tuberculosis, sarcoidosis, cat scratch disease, or various dermatologic conditions, and following injection of radiographic contrast media (lymphangiography). Usually the enlarged lymph nodes show some form of inflammation, including granulomas, histiocytosis, follicular hyperplasia, and polymorphonuclear exudation.

Giant Lymph Node Hyperplasia

Giant lymph node hyperplasia (Castleman's disease) is a benign, usually localized lesion of unknown etiology. There are two varieties: hyaline vascular and plasma cell. The hyaline vascular type consists of small follicles containing hyalinized blood vessels in the center. Between the follicles is a mixture of capillaries and lymphoid cells. The plasma cell variety has sheets of plasma cells in the interfollicular tissue. The lesions are usually mediastinal, but may occur in other locations such as mesentery or axillary. Most of the proliferating cells are polyclonal B cells.

Infectious Mononucleosis

Infectious mononucleosis (IM) is a benign lymphoproliferative disease related to the malignant B cell tumor, Burkitt's lymphoma. It is common in young adults, sometimes reaching epidemic proportions when young adults from different backgrounds and, for the most part, different sexes, are placed together, as in college ("kissing disease"). It is associated with, and most likely caused by, infection with Epstein–Barr virus (EBV), the virus that is also found with Burkitt's lymphoma and nasopharyngeal carcinoma. These diseases may represent different racially or environmentally determined responses to the same infectious agent, but such a relationship has not been critically established. The symptoms of infectious mononucleosis follow an incubation period of about 20 to 30 days and consist of fatigue, general malaise, and loss of appetite. Occasionally, high fever, lymphadenopathy, pharyngitis, and hepatosplenomegaly are found, all of which usually last for a few weeks. Antibodies to EBV antigens appear in the serum of patients during the course of the disease.

The peripheral blood of patients with infectious mononucleosis contains a peculiar cell known as an *atypical lympho-cyte*. These are large lymphocytes with enlarged nuclei and abundant cytoplasm. Sometimes autologous rosettes with the patient's red blood cells (RBC) are formed. Most of the atypical cells have properties of T cells (they form rosettes with sheep RBC, react with anti-T cell sera), whereas others have B or no cell markers. Atypical lymphocytes of infectious mononucleosis may be immunocompetent cells reacting immunologically to EBV infection. These atypical lymphocytes have been shown to be actively synthesizing DNA and it is postulated that they represent heterogeneous T and B blast cells responding to antigens and are not infected proliferating cells. In contrast, the proliferating (EBV-infected) cells of Burkitt's lymphoma are homogeneous (monoclonal) B cell populations. Heterogeneous atypical lymphocytes are also found in the blood after organ transplantation or immunization, in patients with rheumatoid or autoallergic disease, in association with malignant tumors, during drug reactions, and in the presence of other bacterial or viral infections. Although it is tempting to speculate that infectious mononucleosis is a benign form and that Burkitt's lymphoma is a malignant form of EBV infection, absolute proof of this relationship has not been obtained.

Permanent cell lines are relatively easy to obtain using the blood lymphocytes of patients with infectious mononucleosis. These cell lines are invariably infected with EBV and often have chromosome 8 → 14 translocations. The cells are usually diploid and display monoclonal surface and cytoplasmic immunoglobulin (B cells). Therefore the cells that grow out are infected B cells and not the atypical lymphocytes seen in peripheral blood. EBV infects only B cells, apparently because a receptor for the virus is related to the C3 receptor found on B cells and not on T cells. T cells from patients with IM are often able to kill B cell lines expressing EBV antigens. Therefore, atypical T lymphocytes may actually be cytotoxic reactive cells to infected B cells. Very rarely is infectious mononucleosis a fulminant fatal disease similar to acute lymphoblastic leukemia, and IM features a polyclonal instead of monoclonal increase in "transformed" B cells. It may be that in this acute form of the disease, multiple cells are undergoing transformation at about the same time, resulting in more than one type of B cell in the tumor. In the absence of the immune mechanisms of T cell cytotoxicity, these cells might proliferate rapidly and produce an overwhelming diffuse lymphoproliferative disease.

Human Lymphomas

Human lymphoproliferative diseases consist of T cell, B cell, macrophage, and null (cells without markers) malignant lymphomas, as well as benign "inflammatory" hyperplasias of different cell types. It is of practical clinical importance to separate non-Hodgkin's from Hodgkin's lymphoma, because the response to therapy and clinical course of Hodgkin's disease and other lymphomas is critically different. The cellular origin of Hodgkin's disease has been the subject of controversy, but recent evidence suggests that these tumors arise from a particular macrophage subpopulation, the interdigitating reticulum cells (see below), whereas non-Hodgkin's lymphomas usually are derived from lymphocytes. Also of critical importance is the characterization of the growth potential and clinical course as acute or chronic.

Non-Hodgkin's Lymphomas

Three major findings determine the ability to predict the growth behavior of a malignant lymphoma: the pattern of tissue replacement, the morphology of the cells, and the extent of organ involvement. A general principle of neoplastic disease is that cancer tissue is a caricature of the normal tissue from which it arises. Lymphomas are tumors of lymphoid organs, and the morphological structure reflects the cellular organ. The most useful working morphological classification of non-Hodgkin's lymphomas reflects this relationship (Table 28-1). Non-Hodgkin's lymphomas may assume a nodular (follicular) or a diffuse form. Nodular lymphomas reflect the morphology of lymphoid follicles and are composed of B cells. Diffuse lymphomas appear as sheets of cells without follicular structure and may be of B cell, T cell, null, or true histiocytic (macrophage) origin. Nodular tumors have a much better prognosis than diffuse tumors.

The second major morphological feature is the size of the cells that make up the tumor. Tumors made up of small lymphocytes have a better prognosis than tumors made up of large lymphocytes. Tumors made up of mixture of large, intermediate, and small cells have an intermediate prognosis.

The third major prognostic factor is the extent of organ involvement by the tumor. This is known as clinical staging and is described in more detail below.

The morphological features are incorporated into the classic classification of non-Hodgkin's lymphomas proposed by Henry Rappaport in 1956 (Table 28-1). In this classification

Table 28-1.
Morphological Classification of Non-Hodgkin's Lymphomas

Topography	Nodular or diffuse
Cell type	Lymphocyte, well differentiated
	Lymphocytic, poorly differentiated
	Histiocytic[a] (reticulum cell sarcoma)
	Mixed histiocytic and lymphocytic
	Undifferentiated (blast)

[a] *Histiocytic* refers to large cells and does not necessarily imply macrophage origin.
Modified from Rappaport H, et al: Cancer 9:792, 1956.

histiocytic refers to a large lymphocytic type of tumor, now known usually to be composed of lymphocytes and not histiocytes. Rappaport used the term *histiocytic lymphoma* because the large cells looked like tissue histiocytes. Over the last 30 years this classification has provided a valuable method of evaluating non-Hodgkin's lymphomas.

B Cell Tumors

These include chronic lymphocytic leukemia (90% of cases), several kinds of nodular or diffuse lymphoma, and tumors of plasma cells (e.g., multiple myeloma). The cells of these tumors reflect their B cell origin by expressing either cell surface immunoglobulin, cytoplasmic monoclonal immunoblobulin, or rearranged Ig genes. These may all be considered to be tumors arising from cells at different stages of B cell development and thus reflect the tissue distribution and surface characteristics of normal B cells at similar stages. The incidence of B cell tumors is much higher in elderly individuals (50–70 years of age) than in people younger than 50 years of age. It has been postulated that B cell tumors may arise because of a lack of control by the appropriate suppressor cells. Thus, a loss of T cell control of B cell proliferation with aging may result in uncontrolled B cell proliferation. Monoclonal immunoglobulins are sometimes found in other diseases, such as with nonlymphoid tumors, and in elderly persons. The significance of these elevations remains uncertain. The presence of a monoclonal immunoglobulin (gammopathy) in an otherwise normal person suggests that covert lymphoma is present and will become manifest if the person lives long enough.

Follicular Center Cells. In 1971 Robert Lukes and Robert Collins attempted to refine the cellular classification of non-Hodgkin's lymphomas. They recognized that the cells of most non-Hodgkin's lymphomas resembled cells seen in germinal centers, and postulated that these cells represented different stages of the cell cycle of B cells, whether lymphoma was nodular or diffuse. This concept is presented in Figure 28-3. Most non-Hodgkin's lymphomas are B cell type and the idea that the morphology of these tumors reflects the cell cycle position of the majority of the cells in the tumor is probably correct. Lukes and Collins also postulated that the shape of the nuclei of the cells of a lymphoma reflected the stage of maturation of the cells in the tumor and that there is evolution of B cell lymphomas from small noncleaved → small cleaved → large cleaved → large noncleaved associated with progression to more aggressive behavior. Unfortunately, the fine morphological characteristics used in this classification are subject to subtle changes in tissue fixation and processing and are not easily defined, even by experienced pathologists. Thus the reproducibility of this classification at different centers has not been uniform. In the 1970s a number of classification systems of non-Hodgkin's lymphomas were proposed, generating consid-

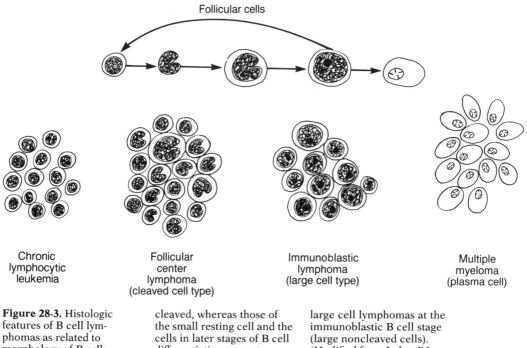

Follicular cells

| Chronic lymphocytic leukemia | Follicular center lymphoma (cleaved cell type) | Immunoblastic lymphoma (large cell type) | Multiple myeloma (plasma cell) |

Figure 28-3. Histologic features of B cell lymphomas as related to morphology of B cells. During the cell cycle B cells change from small round cells to large "blast cells" and divide to form small cells. Differentiation results in production of plasma cells. The nucleus of the early activated B cell is cleaved, whereas those of the small resting cell and the cells in later stages of B cell differentiation are not cleaved. Chronic lymphocytic leukemia represents a maturation arrest at the small noncleaved stage, multiple myeloma at the plasma cell stages, follicular lymphomas at the activated B cell stage (cleaved), and large cell lymphomas at the immunoblastic B cell stage (large noncleaved cells). (Modified from Lukes RJ, Collins RD: Lukes–Collins classification and its significance. Cancer Treat Rep 61:971–979, 1977; Taylor CR: Classification of lymphomas. Arch Pathol Lab Med 102:549–554, 1978.)

erable interest and confusion. These classifications, while still useful, have largely been superseded by the use of other cellular markers, but morphological classification of small, large, intermediate, and mixed cell types is still critical in determining the prognosis of lymphoma. Small cell types usually progress very slowly, but do not respond to chemotherapy. Large cell types progress more rapidly, but about 50% are curable by chemotherapy.

Phenotypic Markers. The stage of maturation arrest in the B cell linage may be deduced from the phenotypic expression of immunoglobulins produced by B cell tumors (Fig. 28-4). The major distinguishing feature of B cell tumors is monoclonality, that is, the presence or production of only one class of immunoglobulin and/or one light chain type by all the cells of the tumor. In contrast, the B cells or plasma cells that make up normal or benign lymphoproliferation are mixtures of cells with different Ig classes and light chains. A simple test for monoclonality is immune labeling of tissue for κ and λ light chains of immunoglobulin. If all of the cells contain one light

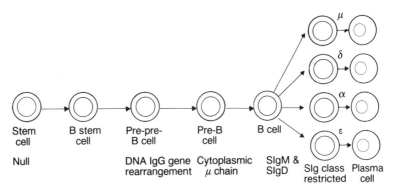

Stem cell | B stem cell | Pre-pre-B cell | Pre-B cell | B cell

Null | | DNA IgG gene rearrangement | Cytoplasmic μ chain | SIgM & SIgD | SIg class restricted | Plasma cell

Figure 28-4. Stages of maturation arrest in B cell lymphomas. The designation of B cell lineage in leukemia or lymphoma may be deduced from the presence of rearranged IgG genes (pre-pre-B cell), the presence of cytoplasmic μ-chain in the absence of surface Ig (pre-B cell), the presence of surface immunoglobulin restricted to one class (monoclonal), or the presence of plasma cells restricted to one class and one light chain.

chain type, then the criterion for monoclonality is met. If some cells express κ-chain and others λ-chain (usually 60:40 ratio) then polyclonality is established. However, rarely some polyclonal B cell proliferations behave like malignant lymphomas.

As described in Chapter 6, the first step in B cell differentiation that can be detected is rearrangement of the immunoglobulin genes. First, genes encoding the heavy chain rearrange, beginning with the diversity region (D), then the joining region (J), and the variable region (V). The DNA between these segments is deleted. The second event is rearrangement between the V and J regions of the κ light chain and then after both κ genes are rearranged, the λ light chain genes rearrange. B cell lymphoma rearrangements can be differentiated from normal polyclonal rearrangements by the presence of a single band on polyacrylamide gel fractionation of DNA digested with appropriate restriction enzymes. Selected enzymes cut the DNA at specific points in the sequence of bases. Polyclonal DNA contains multiple gene arrangements that produce a diffuse, nondistinct pattern when labeled with a specific cDNA probe for the Ig genes (Fig. 28-5). In contrast, the DNA

Figure 28-5. Autoradiography of polyacrylamide gel electrophoresis of *Bam*HI restriction endonuclease fragments of DNA from fibroblasts (germ line), normal B cells (polyclonal), and B cell lymphoma tissue (monoclonal). The presence of κ region sequences is detected using a radiolabeled cDNA for κ light chain. Monoclonal rearranged κ genes appear as a single tight band compared with the rearranged germ line genes. *Bam*HI will produce many different-sized fragments because of digestion occurring at different positions in the Ig gene polyclonal fragments, and these fragments yield a diffuse pattern.

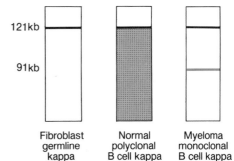

121kb

91kb

Fibroblast germline kappa | Normal polyclonal B cell kappa | Myeloma monoclonal B cell kappa

from a clonal proliferation will be cleaved at the same site, giving rise to discrete bands. In this manner, clonal B cells that make up only 2–5% of a heterogeneous tissue sample may be detected, and diagnosis of lymphoma within a mixture of polyclonal cells can be made accurately. In addition, undifferentiated carcinomas or atypical hyperplasias of lymphocytes can be differentiated from B cell lymphomas. Correlation of Ig gene rearrangements with cell surface markers has shown that B cell lymphomas with μ but not κ gene rearrangement express HLA-DR antigens (detected by monoclonal antibody) but not the common leukemia antigen (CALLA), whereas cells with both μ and κ gene rearrangements are HLA-DR positive and CALLA positive. Thus these phenotypic markers may also be used to deduce the stage of B cell maturation. Similarly, rearrangement of T cell receptor β-chain may be used to detect T cell lymphomas.

Multiple Myeloma. The final step in differentiation of B cells is the plasma cell that synthesizes and secretes immunoglobulin. Tumors of plasma cells almost always arise in the bone marrow and are termed *multiple myelomas* because of many sites (multiple) of masses (*-oma*) of the tumor cells found in the bone marrow (*myel-*). The cells of multiple myeloma are plasma cells that usually contain or secrete a single type of immunoglobulin molecule (monoclonal). These may belong to any of the major immunoglobulin classes and may demonstrate antigen-binding capacity. A variant form of myeloma that produces IgM and that has slightly different morphological and clinical features is termed *Waldenström's macroglobulinemia.*

Monoclonal immunoglobulin refers to a uniform, homogeneous, molecular species of immunoglobulin, in contrast to the heterogeneous array of immunoglobulins present in normal persons. Homogeneous immunoglobulin present in patients with multiple myeloma is often referred to as myeloma paraprotein. Electrophoretic or immunoelectrophoretic analysis of sera from myeloma patients reveals a characteristic peak of protein in about 80% of cases (myeloma spike). The myeloma proteins are usually complete immunoglobulin molecules. In some cases, one part of the molecule (e.g., light chain or heavy chain) may be produced in excess or may be the only myeloma paraprotein found. The light chain paraprotein is usually rapidly cleared from the circulation by filtration through the kidney and appears in the urine as Bence Jones protein. Bence Jones protein (light chains) classically precipitates in acidified urine when heated to 50–60°C, and redissolves at 100°C (see also Chapter 27). Free, excess heavy chains may also be the only secreted myeloma paraprotein identified in the serum of affected patients (H-chain disease). In about 1% of cases, no myeloma paraprotein can be detected, even though myeloma plasma cells are present in the bone marrow and contain monoclonal immunoblobulin. κ light chains are present in myeloma proteins at a slightly higher frequency than the λ type (55% versus 45%), and patients with κ type myeloma proteins tend to have longer survival. The degree of elevation of a paraprotein in a given patient may be used to monitor therapeutic effects (e.g., chemotherapy). Symptoms related to the excess immunoglobulin may appear: hyperviscosity of the blood because of the high intrinsic viscosity of the myeloma protein, insolubility in the cold (cryoglobulinemia), or formation of immunoglobulin complexes by paraprotein interactions. These lead to circulatory disturbances and microvascular occlusions. IgM production is associated with a cell type that is generally less differentiated than the plasma cell. This disease is called *Waldenström's macroglobulinemia*. The cell type is more like that seen in chronic lymphocytic leukemia.

In summary, the B cell tumors may also be considered as occurring at various stages of B cell development, from small lymphocytes to large "blast" cells to well-differentiated plasma cells, with multiple myeloma representing the most differentiated stage. Although the most impressive cellular component of multiple myeloma is the differentiated plasma cell, clearly tumor cells in different stages of the cell cycle and at different levels of differentiation may be present in the malignant population, including dividing, less differentiated plasma cells. The cells in myelomas, like B cell tumors, have surface immunoglobulin. Since the immunoglobulin produced by these cells is monoclonal, each surface Ig-bearing cell will contain immunoglobulin with antigens specific for that molecule (idiotype).

The myeloma idiotype not only serves as a marker for all cells in the myeloma, but also may be used as a target for specific immunotherapy. In experimental models, immunization of mice with a myeloma idiotype can produce resistance to transplanted myeloma cells bearing the idiotype. There appears to be more than one mechanism for control of myeloma cell growth. The resistance may be mediated by antibodies to the idiotype (antibody-directed complement-dependent killing, opsonization, or antibody-dependent cell-mediated immunity) or by T cells (specific T suppressor cells for the idiotype or T killer cells directed to the idiotype). In human clinical trials mouse monoclonal antiidiotypic infusion has had limited success. Most recipients demonstrate no effect, whereas approximately 2 of 10 appear to have a definite antibody-related remission. Clinical trials using drug-conjugated anti-idiotypic antibodies are now underway. Biological problems in anti-idiotypic therapy include the ability of some tumors to switch idiotype expression and escape idiotype-directed control mechanisms, the ability of tumor cells to modulate cell surface expression of antigenic molecules, and, if mouse monoclonal anti-human idiotypic antibodies are used, a host response, resulting in neutralization of human anti-mouse immunoglobulin.

Chronic Lymphocytic Leukemia. Chronic lymphocytic leukemia is a protracted disease consisting of a marked increase in small lymphocytes in the bone marrow and blood. Lymph node and spleen involvement may occur late in the disease, with diffuse infiltration of small lymphocytes. The tumor cells express monoclonal surface immunoglobulin or rearranged Ig gene's in 90% of cases. The disease most likely starts in the bone marrow. Later in the course of disease, large numbers of mature lymphocytes extend from the bone marrow to the blood and visceral organs to give the appearance of diffuse lymphocytic lymphoma. The course of the disease is relatively long and patients with this disease often die of infection or from some unrelated disease.

B Cell Lymphomas. Two major patterns of B cell lymphoma are recognized morphologically: follicular and diffuse. The cells of these lymphomas bear monoclonal surface immunoglobulin (sIg$^+$) or rearranged Ig genes. Follicular lymphomas may contain both small and large lymphocytes in different proportions and are usually found in lymph nodes and spleen. The growth pattern mimics the nodular arrangement of cells in lymphoid follicles, thus the designation as follicular or nodular (see Fig. 28-3). In contrast to normal lymph follicles, which are found in the cortex of a lymph node, neoplastic follicles are found throughout the node with obliteration of the normal

Normal follicle

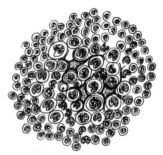

Follicular lymphoma

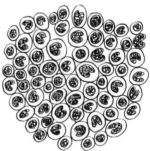

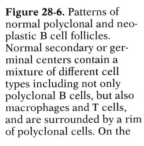

Figure 28-6. Patterns of normal polyclonal and neoplastic B cell follicles. Normal secondary or germinal centers contain a mixture of different cell types including not only polyclonal B cells, but also macrophages and T cells, and are surrounded by a rim of polyclonal cells. On the other hand, malignant B cell tumors may form follicles or replace the node structure diffusely with a homogenous cell type. Malignant follicles are made up of cells of a single clonal line, do not contain T cells or macrophages, and are not surrounded by a rim of polyclonal cells. Malignant follicles efface the other components of the lymph node (paracortex, medulla) and extend diffusely into adjacent tissue with loss of the structure of capsule and subcapsular sinus, whereas these areas, although relatively less conspicuous, are preserved in nonmalignant hyperplasia.

node architecture (Fig. 28-6). Diffuse B cell lymphocytic lymphoma consists of small- to medium-sized lymphocytes, which diffusely infiltrate and replace lymph node and spleen structures. The variations in follicular and diffuse patterns of B cell lymphomas and the progression from follicular to diffuse are illustrated in Fig. 28-7. Diffuse large cell lymphoma consists of

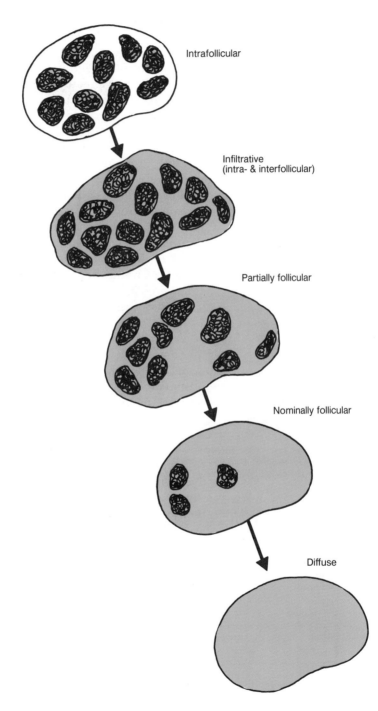

Figure 28-7. B cell lymphoma exists in variations from follicular to diffuse patterns. Increased malignancy or the progression toward more aggressive tumor is associated with a change from more follicular to more diffuse as well as with cell size and morphology. Small, cleaved, follicular tumors have the best prognosis. Large, noncleaved, diffuse tumors have the worst prognosis. Approximately 30% of patients observed carefully demonstrate progression from less to more malignant forms.

large cells, sometimes resembling reticulum cells or macrophages, which replace lymphoid organs as sheets of malignant cells. This tumor has a much worse prognosis than the diffuse lymphocytic (small cell) tumor.

Burkitt's Lymphoma. Burkitt's lymphoma features the presence of cytoplasmic and surface Ig, receptors for C3, and, in many but not all cases, surface viral antigens of the EBV. Burkitt's lymphoma was first identified in African children residing in high-rainfall areas of Africa, where mosquitos are abundant. Cases of Burkitt's lymphoma have now been identified throughout the world, and the relationship to the self-limiting disease infectious mononucleosis, which is common in Western nations, has attracted considerable attention. In African patients, the jaw is involved with a diffuse rapidly growing lymphoid tumor composed of blast cells. In Americans, abdominal, pelvic, and bone marrow involvement is more common. Chemotherapy with cyclophosphamide can produce sustained remissions in 80% of patients with African Burkitt's lymphoma. These tumors are also very responsive to radiotherapy and may undergo spontaneous remission. This supports the concept of a viral etiology, because virally induced tumors of animals are often self limiting or responsive to therapy in adults, but grow progressively in newborns.

The presence of EBV antigens on the cell surface provides a relatively strong potential tumor antigen to which the human host may respond. Both cell-mediated and humoral antibody responses may occur to EBV antigens in patients with Burkitt's lymphoma. Some antigens are found on Burkitt's lymphoma cells that are not viral antigens but are new antigenic specificities unique to early EBV transformed cells. Since antibodies to these antigens are found before antibodies to viral antigens, they have been termed *early EBV antigens*. Antibody responses are complicated in that high antibody titers to "early antigen" expressed on Burkitt's lymphoma cells are associated with relapses, whereas responses to viral capsid antigens may be protective. Antibodies to capsid antigens are found in tumor-free relatives of patients with Burkitt's lymphoma. A reduction of antibody to early antigens is associated with the development of delayed hypersensitivity to early antigens. The relationship of antibody against capsid antigens or appearance of delayed hypersensitivity in the course of the disease remains uncertain, but is believed to be protective (see Infectious Mononucleosis, above).

Hairy Cell Leukemia (Leukemic Reticuloendotheliosis). This disease is characterized by the appearance of an unusual mononuclear cell in the peripheral blood, associated with splenomegaly and a decrease in other cellular elements of the blood.

The disease progresses slowly and severe infections appear to be related to the decreased number of normally functioning monocytes in the blood. The hairy cell is of the size of normal, nonlymphocytic mononuclear cells, has hairy-looking convoluted cytoplasm, has monoclonal cytoplasmic and surface Ig, and is capable of phagocytosis. Thus, it is a B cell with some features of macrophages and most likely represents an immature B cell type. T cell variants of hairy cell leukemia have also been reported, but rearrangements of Ig genes have been found in all cases of hairy cell leukemia so far studied in this manner.

T Cell Tumors

These include thymoma, lymphoblastic lymphoma, acute lymphoblastic leukemia (20–30%), mycosis fungoides (Sezary's syndrome), and ~30% of diffuse non-Hodgkin's lymphomas.

T Cell Markers. Monoclonal antibodies to T cell populations are now being applied to define T cell tumors. These monoclonal antibodies identify T cell differentiation markers as defined in Chapter 4 (see Table 4-2). Previously, phenotypic markers, such as E rosette formation, lack of surface Ig, presence of terminal deoxytransferase (TdT), lack of surface HLA-D antigens, and reactivity with heteroantisera to T cells were used. Of these, E rosettes and TdT remain the most useful markers. In addition, T cell malignancies may be phenotyped by monoclonal antibodies (Table 28-2). Many of these, such as CD1, CD5, transferrin receptor, T_{10}, HLA-A, -B, and -C, HLA-DR, and CALLA, are not particularly useful for delineation of T cell lineage since they also appear on non-T cell tissue. Others, such as E rosette receptor and antigens defined by CD3, CD4, CD6, CD8, and CD9, are essentially T cell specific. These markers define T cell lineage and stage of maturation arrest areas (see Fig. 4-4). However, as yet, the clinical relevance of the phenotypic identification of T cell tumors is not clear. The phenotypic characterization of some clinical types of T cell malignancies is summarized in Table 28-3. Again the major feature of malignancies is the monoclonal nature of the malignant cells (all have the same markers) as compared with normal nonmalignant polyclonal T cell populations. Phenotypic characterization may be carried out on cell suspensions, for example from leukemic blood or effusions, as well as on frozen tissue sections. The future application of such analysis depends upon clinical correlations yet to be made.

In studies of cells of chronic lymphocytic leukemia (CLL), it was found that most CLL cells express not only a monoclonal immunoglobulin, but also a T cell marker (CD5). The significance of this observation is not clear. Either CLL represents a stage of development of lymphoid neoplasms with shared T and B cell phenotype or CD5 is not specific for T cells (see Table 28-3).

Table 28-2. Lymphoid or T Cell Antigens Defined by Monoclonal Antibodies Used in the Study of T Cell Malignancies

Antigen (Monoclonal Antibodies)	Antigen size (MW)	Reactivity
CD1 (NA1/34, OKT$_6$, Leu6)	48,000–42,000	Cortical thymocytes, epidermal Langerhans cells
CD5, T$_1$ (Leu 1, 10.2, L17F12, T101, 16B2, DUSKW3-1 A-50)	65,000	Thymocytes, mature cells, subset of malignant B cells
CD2, E rosette receptor (9.6, OKT$_{11}$, Leu5, 35.1)	50,000	Thymocytes, mature T cells
CD3 (OKT$_3$, UCHT-1, Leu4)	19,000	Subset of thymocytes, all mature T cells
CD4 (OKT$_4$, Leu3a)	62,000	Cortical thymocytes, inducer/helper T cells
CD8 (OKT$_8$, Leu2a)	33,000	Cortical thymocytes, suppressor/cytotoxic mature T cells
9.3 (9.3)	44,000	Subset of thymocytes, inducer T cells
CD9 (3A1, 4A, Leu9, 4G6, 5A12, WT-1)	40,000	Thymocytes, 85% of mature T cells
CD6 (T$_{12}$, 12.1), T411	100,000	Mature T cells
Transferrin receptor (5E9, OKT$_9$, B3/25)	90,000	Antigen of cell activation
p80 (A1G3)	80,000	Mature T cells
T$_{28}$ (T$_{28}$)	28,000	Mature T cells
T$_{10}$	44,000	Antigen of cell activation
CD10, CALLA (J-5), BA-3	95,000	Subset of normal B cells, mature granulocytes, kidney tubular epithelium
HLA-DR (Ia-like)	33,000	Monocytes, macrophages, T cells, B cells, activated T cells
HLA-A, -B, -C (3F10, W6/32)	44,000 12,000	Thymocytes and mature T cells, many normal tissue types
3-40	35,000–40,000	T ALL cells, some non-B, non-T ALL cells, some AML cells, thymic epithelium, many normal tissues
3-3	35,000–40,000	T ALL cells, normal connective tissue

ALL, acute lymphoblastic leukemia; AML, acute myelogenous leukemia.
Modified from Harden EA, Polker TJ, Haynes BF: Monoclonal antibodies: probes for the study of malignant T cells. In Sell S, Reisfeld R (eds): Monoclonal Antibodies in Cancer. Crescent Manor, N.J., Humana Press, 1985.

Thymoma. Tumors of the thymus are extremely rare and may be classified into three major types: lymphoid, epithelial, and mixed. Most tumors are mixed and it is believed that the lymphocyte component is not malignant. The lymphoid cell component is generally considered to be a nonmalignant proliferation of lymphocytes accompanying the malignant epithelial cells. Tumors of the epithelial cells of the thymus are usually composed of spindle or cuboidal epithelial cells, and mixed tumors contain elements of both. Thymic tumors

Table 28-3. Phenotypic Characterization of Some Clinical Types of T Cell Malignancies[a]

Clinical or Histologic Diagnosis	Phenotypic Characterization
T acute lymphoblastic leukemia	Heterogeneous antigen profile; most express immature T cell phenotype
T chronic lymphocytic leukemia	Mature T cell phenotype (CD4$^+$ or CD8$^+$), CD5$^+$, sIg$^+$
T lymphoblastic lymphoma	Heterogeneous antigen profile; most express immature T cell phenotypes
IgG Fc receptor positive (T$_G$) lymphoproliferative disease	Mature T cell phenotype CD9$^-$, CD4$^-$, CD1$^-$
Cutaneous T cell lymphoma	PBL[b]: mature helper phenotype (CD9$^-$, CD4$^+$, CD8$^-$, CD1$^-$)
Mycosis fungoides/Sezary's syndrome	Skin: mature helper phenotype type (CD9$^+$, CD4$^+$, CD8$^-$, CD1$^-$)
T cell type of hairy cell leukemia	CD4$^+$, CD8$^-$, mature T cell phenotype
HTLV-associated Japanese, Caribbean and American adult T cell leukemia/lymphoma	Skin and PBL: mature helper phenotype (CD9$^-$, CD4$^+$, CD8$^-$, CD1$^-$)
T cell non-Hodgkin's lymphoma	Mature T cell phenotype

[a] Phenotypes in this table, when given, are the usual phenotypes for the clinical/histologic syndrome. In most cases, minor variations or alternative phenotypes have been reported.
[b] PBL, peripheral blood lymphocytes.
Modified from Harden EA, Polker TJ, Haynes BF: Monoclonal antibodies: probes for the study of malignant T cells. In Sell S, Reisfeld R (eds): Monoclonal Antibodies in Cancer. Creascent Manor, N.J., Humana Press, 1985.

present as masses in the anterior mediastinum and may be associated with a number of systemic autoallergic diseases, including myasthenia gravis, pancytopenia, multiple myeloma, thyroiditis, and dermatomyositis. In most cases, with or without systemic manifestations, the tumor is limited to the thymus; metastatic extension of thymomas (malignant thymoma) is extremely rare. Most T cells in thymomas have the phenotype of cortical (immature) thymocytes (CD1$^+$). The term *lymphocytic lymphoma of the thymus* may be used in the rare instances when invasion of the capsule or widespread disease consisting of mainly small lymphocytes indicates malignancy. This may be a true thymic T cell tumor.

Acute Lymphoblastic Leukemia. T cell acute lymphoblastic leukemia begins in the bone marrow, has a rapid course, and involves the peripheral blood and lymphatics extensively. Approximately 15% to 25% of the tumors bear T cell markers; others bear B cell markers or no markers. Those patients with T cell acute leukemia have a much worse prognosis and respond poorly to chemotherapy, compared with patients with non-T cell acute leukemia. T cell leukemias are usually TdT positive and acid phosphatase positive. T cell differentiation markers are heterogeneous, but are generally of immature T cells and thymocytes.

Lymphoblastic Lymphoma. A rare T cell tumor, usually occurring in adolescents, this lymphoma mimics the virus-induced T cell tumors of mice. It usually begins in the thymus and rapidly extends and infiltrates diffusely (T zones) into lymph node, spleen, bone marrow, skin, and other organs and may have a terminal leukemic phase. In humans, this tumor may resemble diffuse cleaved B cell lymphoma morphologically, but can be identified by the presence of T cell markers. This tumor has also been termed *lymphoblastic sarcoma* when extensive involvement with immature lymphocytes occurs. T cell lymphoblastic lymphomas are E rosette positive and sIg and Ia negative. T cell differentiation markers are usually of thymocyte type, but some tumors express a more differentiated phenotype.

Mycosis Fungoides and Sezary's Syndrome. Both are tumors of T cells. Mycosis fungoides begins in the skin and the disease may be grouped into three stages: skin involvement as an inflammatory-like condition that presents as dermatitis, parapsoriasis, or erythroderma; infiltrated dermal plaques; and gross tumors. The length of survival depends upon the stage of the disease: 8–12 years for stage 1, 3–5 years for stage 2, and 1–3 years for stage 3. Tumors in the skin appear as solid masses with terminal extensions into visceral organs. Sezary's syndrome is a leukemic variant. The same cutaneous features as seen in mycosis fungoides are present, but tumor cells are also present in blood (leukemia). Most often these cells have T cell properties and may be able to function as helper cells and stimulate immunoglobulin production by B cells. The cells also bear the helper phenotype: $CD4^+$, $CD8^-$. Although the thymus is not usually involved, it is probable that mycosis fungoides and Sezary's cells are T cell tumors arising from T cells present in the skin. It has been proposed that antigen persistence on intraepithelial macrophage-like cells, the Langerhans cells, may result in chronic exposure to contact antigens, leading to excess intraepithelial stimulation as well as involvement of the dermis and draining lymph nodes.

Chronic Lymphocytic Leukemia. CLL cells express B cell phenotypes, but as mentioned above, may also react with a monoclonal antibody for T cells and for E rosettes. Approximately 2% of CLL are restricted to T cells as defined by E rosette formation, lack of sIg, and mature T cell phenotype as defined by monoclonal antibodies (TdT^-, $CD1^-$, $CD3^+$).

HTLV-Associated Adult T Cell Leukemia/Lymphoma. In 1980 the association of a human retrovirus with human T cell tumors was described: human T cell leukemia/lymphoma virus (HTLV$_1$). This tumor appears in high frequency in Japan, the Caribbean basin, and the southern United States. The virus infects CD4$^+$ cells and produces a highly malignant tumor that is CD4$^+$ CD8$^-$. Although these cells bear the helper (CD4) phenotype, they function as suppressor cells for B cell function in vitro. These tumors also bear HLA-B5 antigens simultaneously, presumably due to shared antigens between HLA-B5 and HTLV$_1$.

Diffuse Lymphomas. Most diffuse lymphomas are of B cell type, but approximately 30%, usually of a large cell type, are sIg negative and may express CD4 or CD8 phenotype.

Macrophage Tumors

Histiocytosis X is used for tumors of macrophages. Histiocytosis X is a family of diseases including Letterer–Siewe disease, Hand–Schuller–Christian disease, and eosinophilic granuloma of bone. These tumors consist of space-occupying lesions filled by mature histiocytes with abundant cytoplasm. Hand–Schuller–Christian disease and eosinophilic granuloma occur in bone, with the former also occurring predominantly in spleen and lymph node. Letterer–Siewe disease involves the skin, lymph nodes, pituitary, and spleen. The cells in these diseases contain a distinctive rod-shaped inclusion also found in intraepithelial monocytes (Langerhans' cells). Note that in the Rappaport classification the term *histiocytic lymphoma* has been used for a B cell tumor, not a true histiocytic (macrophage) tumor. True histiocytic lymphomas are believed to arise from fixed histiocytes; Letterer–Siewe disease cells may arise from Langerhans' cells.

Hodgkin's Disease

Hodgkin's disease is a malignant tumor of lymphoid organs composed of mixed cell types. Hodgkin's disease has been known in one form or another for over 150 years; however, the original description by Hodgkin in 1872 of seven patients with "tumors of the absorbant glands" included lesions now known to be tuberculosis. Whereas significant advances have been made in the diagnosis and treatment of Hodgkin's disease, the etiology remains unknown. Major theories of the nature of Hodgkin's disease include that it is a form of lymphoma, an inflammatory response, or a viral infection. Until more is known about its etiology, it is best to consider Hodgkin's disease a lymphoma. As stated above, two general classifications of lymphomas are Hodgkin's and non-Hodgkin's lymphomas.

Histopathological Classification

The major feature of Hodgkin's disease is the pleomorphism (different cell types) of the tumor lesions, in contrast to the more homogeneous cell types of the non-Hodgkin's lymphomas. Tentative agreement of the classification of Hodgkin's disease was reached at a conference in Rye, New York, in 1966. This classification scheme is important because the histologic forms of each type correlate with the clinical course (Table 28-4). Because of the different cell types seen in Hodgkin's

Table 28-4. Histopathological Classification of Hodgkin's Disease

Type	Feature	Relative Prognosis
Lymphocyte predominance	Mainly small lymphocytes, Few R–S[a] cells	Most favorable
Nodular sclerosis	Lymphoid nodules separated by fibrous bands	Favorable
Mixed cellularity	Numerous R–S cells in pleomorphic stroma	Guarded
Lymphocyte depletion	Diffuse irregular fibrosis, anaplastic R–S cells	Least favorable

[a] R–S, Reed–Sternberg cells.
From Lukes RJ, et al: Cancer Res 26:1311, 1966.

lymphomas there has been controversy as to which is the cell line responsible for the tumors and which are nonneoplastic reactive cells. Monoclonal antibodies to markers of different cellular lineage have been applied to this problem. Marker studies indicate that the other cell types in Hodgkin's disease lesions are polyclonal whereas the Reed–Sternberg cells are monoclonal. The characteristic large binuclear cell of Hodgkin's disease was described independently in the United States by Dorothy Reed, a pathology resident at Johns Hopkins University, and by the famous German pathologist Professor C. Sternberg. In the United States these cells were referred to as Reed–Sternberg cells; in Europe, Sternberg–Reed cells (Fig. 28-8). The present evidence strongly indicates the cell of origin

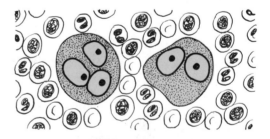

Figure 28-8. Reed–Sternberg cells are large multinucleated "giant" cells considered essential for the diagnosis of Hodgkin's disease.

of Hodgkin's disease to be a particular subset of macrophages known as *interdigitating reticulum cells* (Table 28-5). Cells in the monocyte–macrophage lineage exist in the body in different tissue locations and most likely have different, but related functions: Reed–Sternberg cells and interdigitating cells have morphological similarities; express similar levels of HLA-DR

Table 28-5. Classification of Macrophage–Histiocyte–Derived Tumors

Histiocyte Type	Normal Tissue Distribution	Putative Tumor or Tumor-like Lesion
Free histiocytes	Circulating monocytes	Monocytic leukemia
Fixed histiocytes	Reticuloendothelial cells	True histiocytic lymphoma
Dendritic histiocytes	Follicular zones, lymph node cortex	?Hand–Schuller–Christian disease
Interdigitating reticulum cells	T cell zone, lymph node paracortex	Hodgkin's disease
Langerhans' cells	Intraepithelial	Letterer–Siewe
Macrophage stem cell	Bone marrow	?Eosinophilic granuloma

antigen, esterase, and acid phosphatase; do not react with monoclonal antibodies shared by other cells in the monocyte series, but (both) do react with monoclonal antibody LeuM1, which identifies an epitope on interdigitating reticulum cells.

The histopathological classification is based on the relative proportion of lymphocytes, fibrosis, and Reed–Sternberg cells in relation to other cells (neutrophils, eosinophils, plasma cells) in the pleomorphic tumor. Reed–Sternberg cells are of particular diagnostic significance for Hodgkin's disease (Fig. 28-9).

Lymphocyte predominant	Nodular sclerosis	Mixed type	Lymphocyte depleted

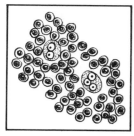 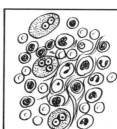 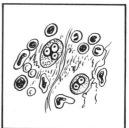

Figure 28-9. Histologic classification of Hodgkin's disease. Lymphocyte predominant: many small lymphocytes with occasional Reed–Sternberg cells. Nodular sclerosis: bands of connective tissue separating cells; Reed–Sternberg cells located in halo-like spaces (lacunar cells). Mixed type: different cell types including lymphocyte, eosinophils, plasma cells, monocytes, and Reed–Sternberg cells. Lymphocyte depleted: few lymphocytes, some fibrosis and acellular areas (hyaline), atypical histiocytes and Reed–Sternberg cells.

Staging

The clinical course of Hodgkin's disease is also dependent on the extent of the disease when first diagnosed. Prognosis generally becomes worse as the extent of the disease increases (Fig. 28-10).

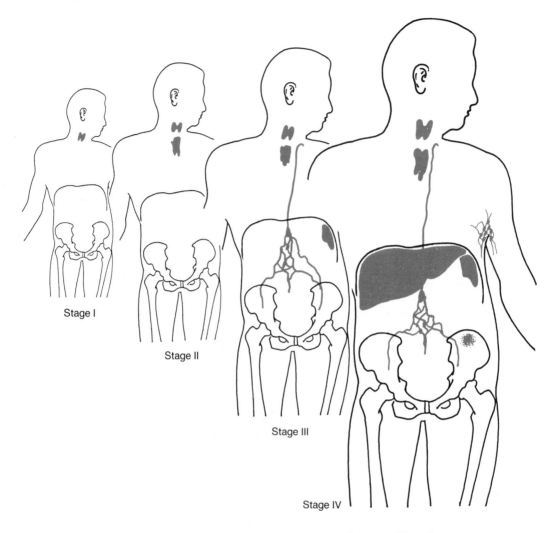

Stage I

Stage II

Stage III

Stage IV

Figure 28-10. Clinical staging of Hodgkin's disease. Staging correlates well with prognosis and helps in deciding the selection of therapy. The same clinical staging is also applicable to non-Hodgkin's lymphomas. Stage I: involvement of a single lymph node region; Stage II: involvement of two or more lymph node regions on the same side of the diaphragm; Stage III: involvement of lymphatic structures on both sides of the diaphragm; Stage IV: diffuse or disseminated involvement.

Treatment

The treatment of Hodgkin's disease with high-dose irradiation to the total lymphoid tissue has led to substantial increases in survival times and essential cure of some patients. In addition, combined drug chemotherapy has yielded up to 80% complete remission, even in patients with far advanced disease, and has induced remission in patients who relapse after radiotherapy. Hodgkin's disease patients frequently demonstrate immunodeficiencies, particularly of the cellular immune system, and may develop infectious complications.

Angioimmunoblastic Lymphoadenopathy

This particular lesion is associated with clinical findings similar to those seen in Hodgkin's disease (fever, sweats, weight loss, skin rash, etc.). There may also be gammaglobulinemia (polyclonal). Histologically, there is a marked increase in small blood vessels (particularly endothelial hyperplasia) in the involved nodes, with numerous blasts and plasma cells, epithelial cells, and large numbers of dying and degenerating cells. The lesion resembles a florid proliferation of the B cell system, although T cells may also be involved. Most patients demonstrate a rapid downhill course, with death occurring after 1 to 2 years. It is not yet clear if this condition is truly a malignant tumor. Some investigators consider this to be a nonneoplastic progressive immune reaction, but the progressive clinical course is consistent with malignancy. A variant is angioimmunoblastic lymphodenopathy with dysproteinemia. These patients usually have partial or complete displacement of lymph nodes, with diffuse lymphoplasmacytic proliferation, and evidence of autoimmune or immune complex disease.

Transplantation-Associated Lymphoproliferation

Patients who are heavily immunosuppressed — in particular, recipients of cardiac or hepatic grafts — are at risk for developing an unusual lymphoproliferation lesion. The cells resemble those of large cell lymphoma, often occur outside of lymphoid organs (muscle and fat), and may progress rapidly. Although the disease progresses with the features of a true malignancy, marker studies demonstrate a polyclonal B cell proliferation that frequently contains EBV. However, studies on the immunoglobulin gene arrangements in these lesions indicates one major cell population (monoclonal), and thus these could be true malignancies.

Treatment of Leukemia and Lymphomas

Treatment of leukemia and lymphomas is accomplished by administration of selected antimetabolic or cytotoxic drugs. In many instances complete cures can be affected by the proper choice of drug, dosage, and timing. Other modes of therapy include irradiation, irradiation with bone marrow transfer, or monoclonal antibodies (see Chapter 27). It is not in the scope of this text to present this subject in more detail.

Animal Models of Lymphoid Tumors

Animal models of lymphoma and leukemia support the concept of tissue localization of different tumor cell types. Most of the animal tumors are caused by tumor viruses. However, the tumor cells may express properties of different lymphocyte lineage and demonstrate related growth patterns in vivo. Lymphoid tumors in mice, chickens, cats, and guinea pigs are considered (Table 28-6).

Mice

Malignant tumors of both T and B cells occur in mice. A large

Table 28-6. Animal Models of Lymphoid Tumors

Animal	Type	Organ of Origin	Site of Proliferation	Etiology
Mouse	T cell	Thymus	Paracortex of lymph nodes	MuLV
	Null	Spleen/lymph node	Diffuse	MuLV
	B cell	Spleen/lymph node	Cortex of lymph nodes	MuLV
	Myelomas	Intraperitoneal	Intraperitoneal	Inflammatory stimulus (mineral oil)
Chicken	T cell	Thymus	Paracortex	DNA virus
	B cell	Bursa of Fabricius	Cortex	RNA virus
Cat	T cell	Thymus	Blood	FeLV
	B cell	Gastrointestinal tract	Gastrointestinal tract	FeLV
Guinea pig	B cell	Transplantable leukemia	Blood, cortex	

MuLV, murine leukemia virus; FeLV, feline leukemia virus.

number of T cell tumors occur spontaneously in some strains of mice (AKR) or may be induced in mice by radiation and contain murine leukemia virus (MuLV). These tumors almost always start in the thymus, bear T cell surface markers, migrate to proliferate in T cell zones of lymphoid organs upon transplantation, and are similar to diffuse lymphoblastic T cell lymphoma of humans. A small number of MuLV-induced tumors do not express T cell markers (null cell tumors). These tumors proliferate diffusely, show no preference for T cell zones in the lymph node, and selectively invade the red pulp of the spleen.

Malignant tumors of differentiated B cells (immunoglobulin-secreting plasma cells) occur spontaneously in C_3H mice and may be induced by injection (particularly intraperitoneally) of inflammatory agents (such as mineral oil) into BALB/c mice. In this manner, a large number of transplantable plasma cell tumors have been produced. These tumors and their products have been used extensively to study plasma cell tumor growth characteristics, effects of therapy, and mechanisms of immunoglobulin synthesis and assembly, and have been a major source of homogeneous immunoglobulin use for determining the structure of immunoglobulin.

The observation that plasma cell tumors may be induced in mice by inflammation suggests that such stimuli may play an etiologic role in human plasma cell tumors (multiple myeloma). Plasma cell tumors may be caused by chronic stimulation of the B cell system associated with decreased T cell control. The finding that most immunoglobulin-producing tumors produce only one class and type of immunoglobulin has been used as an argument that these tumors are in fact derived from a single clone (monoclonal). However, a number of instances of single myeloma cells of both mice and humans producing more than one class of Ig have been reported.

Chickens	Lymphoid tumors of chickens include a DNA virus–induced tumor with T cell markers (Marek's disease) and an RNA virus–induced lymphoma, which is most likely a B cell tumor (lymphoid leukosis). Both of these diseases combine features of a virus infection and a lymphoid neoplasm. In Marek's disease, tumor incidence is decreased by thymectomy and increased by bursectomy. The former result is believed to be caused by a loss of T cells that can be infected by virus, and the latter effect by a decrease in the humoral immune response to the virus infection. The tumor cells are mainly T cells. There is a multifocal diffuse lymphoid proliferation in the gonads, liver, and lymphoid organs, consisting of small and medium lymphocytes, blast cells, and other mononuclear cells. The disease may be prevented by immunization with a related nonpathogenic turkey virus. T cells may play a dual role in this disease as cells that are infected by the virus—the predominant tumor cell—and as immunologically reactive cells that mount a cellular immune response to viral antigens. Both thymus and bursa become infected with virus, suggesting that the original target tissue is not T or B cell dependent, but clearly 70% or more of the tumor cells that develop later are T cells.

In contrast, the RNA virus–induced tumor (lymphoid leukosis) appears to require B cells. Bursectomy results in a decrease in tumor incidence, presumably by removing B cells that become infected. This tumor usually begins in the bursa of Fabricius as a polyclonal proliferation of B cells. Eventually one clone outgrows the rest so that at a later stage of the disease, a monoclonal B cell tumor with surface Ig is produced. The tumor than spreads to lymph nodes, spleen, and liver, but not to the thymus. Histologically, the tumor has the appearance of a "nodular" lymphoma (B cell zones), and upon transplantation the cells preferentially home to B cell zones (bursa of Fabricius) of the recipient animal.

Cats	A lymphoproliferative disease of the cat is caused by feline leukemia virus (FeLV), which shows some similarities to murine leukemia virus. The lymphoid tumors produced fall into two distinct patterns: thymic and alimentary. The thymic form is similar to the T cell murine leukemia, with major involvement of the thymus and peripheral blood, as in acute leukemia, whereas the alimentary form occurs primarily in the gastrointestinal tract. The thymic form is of T cell origin, and the alimentary form of B cell origin.

Guinea Pigs	The L_2C leukemia is an acute B cell tumor of guinea pigs. The cells of L_2C leukemia have receptors for C_3 and express surface IgM, with a characteristic idiotype. This tumor is transplantable in strain 2 guinea pigs, in which it produces an acute leukemia

with extension into spleen, lymph nodes, liver, and Peyer's patches. The thymus and bone marrow are not usually involved, but the brain frequently is, and central nervous system complications are frequent. This tumor is unlike most human B cell leukemias, but resembles some rare human leukemias.

These animal models help us to understand human lymphomas, but in fact many more different kinds of lymphoid tumors have been studied in man as the result of extensive diagnostic studies on individual tumors. Because of the nature of human immunoproliferative diseases and the necessity to classify and follow each patient individually, most of the information on the human deals with morphological appearance, growth patterns, clinical course, response to therapy, and, more recently, immunological and gluetic markers.

Etiology of Lymphoproliferative Diseases

The etiology of cancer remains one of the major questions in medical science. A number of theories, including malignant mutations, abnormal development, and embryonic reversion, have been proposed. Two major mechanisms seem likely for lymphoid tumors: inadequately controlled responses of the immune system and viral infection.

Loss of Immune Regulation

Loss of normal immunoregulatory mechanisms has been postulated as a possible cause of lymphoid tumors. Patients who are administered drugs that depress immune responses, such as recipients of allografted organs, display an extremely high incidence of lymphoid malignancies but a normal incidence of other nonlymphoid tumors. Thus, patients receiving immunosuppressive therapy may reflect loss of the ability to regulate proliferation of clones of cells that would normally be suppressed by immune regulatory (T suppressor) cells. Further support for this concept is the observation that the incidence of many of the lymphoid tumors increases with aging. Aging is also associated with involution of the thymus, autoantibody production, and other evidence of loss of immunoregulation. In addition, the incidence of lymphoid tumors, particularly those of B cell origin, is increased in patients with naturally occurring immune deficiency diseases such as ataxia–telangiectasia. It is postulated that immune deficiencies are associated not only with losses of responding cells (T helper and B cells), but also with losses of controlling cell populations (suppressor or regulatory cells). This imbalance permits inadequately controlled proliferation of the remaining lymphoid cells.

Viral Infection

Although many tumors of animals are known to be caused by viral infection, a viral etiology for most human cancers has been difficult to demonstrate. Many of the virus-induced tumors of animals are lymphoid (see above). These are usually fast-growing tumors that are more frequent in young than old animals. Virus-induced tumors of animals are similar to the acute lymphoid tumors of children. Burkitt's lymphoma is the most likely example of an acute virus-induced neoplasm of young humans. Thus, two major etiologies of leukemia and lymphoma appear likely: virus infection for the acute, rapidly growing malignancies of children, and loss of immune regulation for the chronic, more slowly growing tumors of the elderly.

Chromosomal Translocations

Cells from lymphomas and leukemias demonstrate a variety of nonrandom chromosome translocations that may bring "promotor" areas of one gene into juxtaposition with "protooncogene" DNA sequences. The activation of these protooncogenes may play a key role in producing neoplastic activation of the cells. For example, in Burkitt's lymphoma, the *myc* oncogene in chromosome 8 is transposed to the Ig heavy chain locus on chromosome 14, resulting in activation of the oncogene. This and other such translocations are illustrated in Figure 28-11.

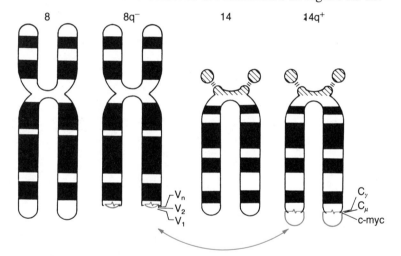

Figure 28-11. Diagram of the t(8:14) translocation in Burkitt's lymphoma cells. The *c-myc* gene on chromosome 8 translocates next to the Cμ and Cγ genes on chromosome 14. (From Erikson J, et al: Transcriptional activation of the translocated *c-myc* oncogene in Burkitt lymphoma. Proc Soc Exp Med Biol 80:820, 1983.)

Infection and Lymphoproliferative Diseases

Patients with lymphoproliferative disease are subject to an increased incidence of clinically significant infections. This may be caused by the nature of the disease or, secondarily, by the type of treatment usually employed, chemotherapy or irradiation. Abnormalities of immune function are fequently found in patients with lymphoproliferative diseases. These include increased production of abnormal immunoglobulins, found with immunoglobulin-secreting tumors, and a variety of autoantibodies as well as depressed immune reactivity. Some reasons for increased susceptibility to infections in these diseases are (1) replacement of normally functioning immune cells with tumor cells that function poorly, (2) production of secreted products that inhibit inflammatory or immune reactions, (3) appearance of cells (suppressor cells) that suppress normal immune function, and (4) loss of normal homeostatic mechanisms (loss of suppressor cells), permitting overproduction of some immune products and underproduction of others. See Chapter 24 for further information.

Summary

Both benign and malignant proliferation of lymphoid cells may lead to enlargement of lymph nodes and spleen, increases in lymphoid cells in the peripheral blood, and systemic symptoms (fever, sweats, and weight loss). Benign lymphoproliferative lesions are usually made up of a heterogeneous population of lymphoid cells that may cause enlargement of lymphoid organs, but the basic structures of the organs (cortex, follicles, medulla) are usually, but not always, maintained. Malignant lymphoid tumors result from an arrest in maturation of a single cell lineage and usually consist of a homogeneous cell type that replaces or destroys the normal architecture of the organ. Strict morphological criteria are not adequate for acceptable diagnosis of lymphoproliferative disease; immune characteristics and phenotypic markers of the cell type provide additional information in regard to diagnosis and prognosis. In many instances, the growth pattern of the tumor reflects the cell type of origin (B cells produce follicular tumors, T cells produce diffuse tumors), but considerable deviation from predicted growth patterns occurs in individual patients.

References

Lymphoid Tissue Structure and Lymphomas

Baird S, Raschke W: The pattern of involvement of murine lymphoid tissues by primary lymphomas of different cell lineage. Hum Pathol 9:47, 1978.

Lukes RJ, Collins RD: New observations in follicular lymphoma. Gann Monogr Cancer Res 15:209, 1973.

Mann RB, Jaffe ES, Berad CW: Maligniant lymphomas — a conceptual understanding of morphologic diversity. Am J Pathol 94:105, 1979.

Warnke R, Levy R: Immunopathology of follicular lymphomas: a model of B-lymphocyte homing. N Engl J Med 298:481, 1978.

Weissman IL, Warnke R, Butcher EC, Rouse R, Levy R: The lymphoid system. Its normal architecture and the potential for its understanding by the study of lymphoproliferative diseases. Hum Pathol 9:25, 1978.

Classification of Lymphomas

Bennett MH, Farrer-Brown J, Henry K, Jeliffe AM: Classification of non-Hodgkin's lymphomas. Lancet 2:405–406, 1974.

Bloomfield CD, Peczalska G: The clinical relevance of lymphocyte surface markers in leukemia and lymphoma. Curr Top Hematol 3:175, 1980.

Dorfman RF: Classification of non-Hodgkin's lymphomas. Lancet 2:961, 1974.

Gajl-Peczalska JK, Bloomfield CD, Coccia DF, Sosin H, Brunning RD, Kersey JH: B and T cell lymphomas, analysis of blood and lymph nodes of 87 patients. Am J Med 59:674, 1975.

Jones SE, et al: Non-Hodgkin's lymphomas. IV. Clinicopathologic correlation in 405 cases. Cancer 31:806, 1973.

Lennert K, Mohri N, Stein H, Kaiserling E: The histopathology of malignant lymphomas. Brit J Haematol (Suppl) 31:199, 1975.

Lukes RJ, Botler JJ: The pathology and nomenclature of Hodgkin's disease. Cancer Res 26:1311, 1966.

Lukes RJ, Collins RD: Immunologic characterization of human malignant lymphoma. Cancer 34:1488, 1974.

Lukes RS, Craver LF, Hall TC, Rappaport H, Rubin P: Report of the nomenclature committee. Cancer Res 26:1311, 1966.

Nathwahi BN: A critical analysis of the classification of non-Hodgkin's lymphomas. Cancer 44:347, 1979.

O'Connor GT, Sobin LH: EORTC-CNS: international colloquium on lymphoid neoplasms. Biomedicine 26:385, 1977.

Parker JW: Immunologic basis for the identification of malignant lymphomas. Am J Clin Pathol 76:270, 1979.

Rappaport H: Tumors of the hematopoietic system. *In* Atlas of Tumor Pathology, Sect 3, Fasc 8. Washington, D.C., Armed Forces Institute of Pathology, 1966.

Taylor CR: Classification of lymphomas: new thinking on old thoughts. Arch Pathol Lab Med 102:549, 1978.

Tsukimoto I, Wong KY, Lampkin BC: Surface markers and prognostic factors in acute lymphoblastic leukemia. N Engl J Med 294:245, 1976.

Whiteside TL, Rowlands DT Jr: T-cell and B-cell identification in the diagnosis of lymphoproliferative disease: a review. Am J Pathol 88:754, 1977.

Nonmalignant Lymphoproliferation

Castleman B, Iverson L, Menrenden P: Localized mediastinal lymph node hyperplasia resembling cancer. Cancer 9:8221, 1956.

Frizzera G, Moran EM, Rappaport H: Angio-immunoblastic lymphadenopathy: diagnosis and clinical course. Am J Med 59:803, 1975.

Keller Ar, Hochholzer L, Castleman B: Hyaline-vascular and plasma-cell types of giant lymph node hyperplasia of the mediastinum and other locations. Cancer 29:670, 1972.

Koo CH, et al: A typical lymphoplasmacytic and immunoblastic proliferation in lymph nodes of patients with autoimmune disease (autoimmune-disease – associated lymphadenopathy). Medicine 63:274, 1984.

Kyle RA, Bayzd ED: Benign monoclonal gammopathy: a potentially malignant condition. Am J Med 40:426, 1965.

Lukes RS, Tindle BH: Immunoblastic lymphadenopathy. N Engl J Med 292:1, 1975.

Neiman RS, Dervan P, Haudenschild C, Jaffe R: Angioimmunoblastic lymphadenopathy. Cancer 41:507, 1978.

Rosai J, Dorfman PF: Sinus histiocytosis with massive lymphadenopathy: a newly recognized benign clinicopathologic entity. Arch Pathol 87:63, 1969.

Saltzstein SL, Ackerman LV: Lymphadenopathy induced by anticonvulsant drugs mimicking clinically and pathologically malignant lymphomas. Cancer 12:164, 1959.

AIDS-Related Lymphadenopathy

Devita VT, Hellman S, Rosenberg SA: AIDS: Etiology, Diagnosis, Treatment and Prevention. Philadelphia, Lippincott, 1985.

Ewing EP, Chandler FW, Spira TJ, Brynes RK, Chan WC: Primary lymph node pathology in AIDS and AIDS related lymphadenopathy. Arch Pathol Lab Med 109:977, 1985.

Hoxie JA, et al: Persistent noncytopathic infection of normal human lymphocytes with AIDS-associated retrovirus. Science 229:1400, 1985.

Ioachim HL, Lerner CW, Tapper ML: The lymphoid lesions associated with the acquired immune deficiency syndrome. Am J Surg Pathol 7:543, 1983.

Krueger GRF, et al: Immunopathology of AIDS: observations in 75 patients with pre-AIDS and AIDS. Pathol Rec Pract 180:463, 1985.

Niedt GW, Schinella RA: Acquired immunodeficiency syndrome: clinicopathologic study of 56 autopies. Arch Pathol Lab Med 109:727, 1985.

Reichert CM, O'Leary TJ, Levens DL, et al: Autopsy pathology in the acquired immune deficiency syndrome. Am J Pathol 112:357, 1983.

Infectious Mononucleosis

Henle G, Henle W, Diehl V: Relation of Burkitt's tumor–associated herpes-type virus to infectious mononucleosis. Proc Nat Acad Sci USA 59:94, 1968.

Pattengale PK, Smith RW, Perlin E: Atypical lymphocytes in acute infectious mononucleosis: identification by multiple T and B lymphocyte markers. N Engl J Med 291:1145, 1974.

Royston I, Sullivan JL, Periman PO, Perlin E: Cell-mediated immunity to Epstein–Barr virus transformed lymphoblastoid cells in acute infectious mononucleosis. N Engl J Med 293:1159, 1975.

Sheldon PJ, Papamichail M, Hemsted EH, Hoborow EJ: Thymic origin of atypical lymphoid cells in infectious mononucleosis. Lancet 1:1153, 1973.

Shiftan TA, Mendelsohn J: The circulating "atypical" lymphocyte. Hum Pathol 9:51, 1978.

B Cell Tumors

Aisenberg AC, Bloch KJ: Immunoglobulins on the surface of neoplastic lymphocytes. N Engl J Med 187:272, 1975.

Bollum FJ: Terminal deoxynucleotidyl transferase as a hematopoietic cell marker. Blood 54:1203, 1979.

Burke JS, Byrne GE, Rappaport H: Hairy cell leukemia (leukemic reticuloendotheliosis): a clinical pathologic study of 21 patients. Cancer 33:1399, 1974.

Dameshek W: Chronic lymphocytic leukemia—an accumulative disease of immunologically incompetent lymphocytes. Blood 29:566, 1967.

Fu SM, Winchester RJ, Rai KR, Kunkel HG: Hairy cell leukemia: proliferation of a cell with phagocytic and B-lymphocyte properties. Scand J Immunol 3:847, 1974.

Hubbard SM, Chabner BA, DeVita VT, et al: Histologic progression in non-Hodgkin's lymphopenia. Blood 59:258, 1982.

Korsmeyer SJ, Greene WC, Cossman J, et al: Rearrangements and expression of immunoglobulin genes and expression of Tac antigen in hairy cell leukemia. Proc Nat Acad Sci USA 80:4522, 1983.

Korsmeyer SJ, Hieter PA, Sharrow SO, et al: Normal human B cells display ordered light chain gene rearrangements and deletions. J Exp Med 156:975, 1983.

Levy R, Warnke R, Dorfman R, Haimovich J: The monoclonality of human B-cell lymphomas. J Exp Med 145:1014, 1977.

Rappaport H, Winter WS, Hicks EB: Follicular lymphoma: a re-evaluation of its position in the scheme of malignant lymphoma. Based on a survey of 253 cases. Cancer 9:792, 1956.

Salsano F, Fraland SS, Natvig JB, Michaelsen TE: Some idiotypes of B-lymphocyte IgD and IgM: formal evidence for monoclonality of chronic lymphocytic leukemia cells. Scand J Immunol 3:841, 1974.

Seshadri RS, Brown EJ, Zipursky A: Leukemic reticuloendotheliosis: a failure of monocyte production. N Engl J Med 295:181, 1976.

Waldmann TA, Korsmeyer S: Hierarchy of immunoglobulin gene rearrangements and deletions in human lymphoid leukemias. *In* Murphy SB, Gilbert JR (eds): Leukemia Research: Advances in Cell Biology and Treatment. New York, Elsevier, 1983.

Multiple Myeloma

Broder S, Humphrey R, Durm M, et al: Impaired synthesis of polyclonal (non-paraprotein) immunoglobulins by circulating lymphocytes from patients with multiple myeloma: role of supressor cells. N Engl J Med 293:887, 1975.

Durie BGM, Salmon SE: Cellular kinetics, staging and immunoglobulin synthesis in multiple myeloma. Annu Rev Med 26:283, 1975.

Fudenberg HH, Wang AC, Pink JRL, Levin AS: Studies of an unusual biclonal gammopathy: implications with regard to genetic control of normal immunoglobulin synthesis. Ann NY Acad Sci 190:501, 1971.

Grey HM, Kohler PF: Cryoimmunoglobulins. Semin Hematol 10:87, 1973.

Kopp WL, Beirne GS, Borus RO: Hyperviscosity symptoms in multiple myeloma. Am J Med 43:141, 1967.

Kyle RA, Elveback LR: Management of prognosis of multiple myeloma. Mayo Clin Proc 51:751, 1976.

Lindstrom FD, Williams RC Jr: Serum anti-immunoglobulins in multiple myeloma and benign monoclonal gammopathy. Clin Immunol Immunopathol 3:503, 1975.

Morse HC, Neiders ME, Lieberman R, Lawton AR, Asofsky R: Murine plasma cells secreting more than one class of immunoglobulin heavy chain. II. SAMM368-A plasmacytoma secreting IgG$_2$b-K and IgA-K immunoglobulins which do not share idiotypic determinants. J Immunol 118:1682, 1977.

Salmon SE: Immunoglobulin synthesis and tumor kinetics of multiple myeloma. Semin Hematol 10:135, 1973.

Seligmann M, Brouet JC: Antibody activity of human myeloma globulins. Semin Hematol 10:163, 1973.

Shustic C, Bergsagel DE, Pruzanski W: K and λ light chain disease: survival rates and clinical manifestations. Blood 48:41, 1976.

Soloman A: Homogeneous (monoclonal) immunoglobulins in cancer. Am J Med 63:169, 1977.

Waldenstrom J: The occurrence of benign, essential monoclonal (M type), nonmacromolecular hyperglobulinemia and its differential diagnosis. Acta Med Scand 176:345, 1964.

Van Camp BGK, Shuit HRE, Hijmans W, Radl S: The cellular basis of double paraproteinemia in man. Clin Immunol Immunopathol 9:111, 1978.

Burkitt's Lymphoma

Burkitt DP, Wright DH: Burkitt's lymphoma. Edinburgh/London, Livingston, 1970.

Epstein MA, Achong BG, Barr YM: Virus particles in cultured lymphoblasts from Burkitt's lymphoma. Lancet 1:702, 1964.

Klein G: The biology and serology of Epstein–Barr virus (EBV) infections. Bull Cancer (Paris) 63:399, 1976.

Mann RB, Jaffe ES, Braylan RC, Manba K, Frank MM, Zieglar JL, Berard CW: Nonendemic Burkitt's lymphoma: a B cell tumor related to germinal centers. N Engl J Med 295:685, 1976.

Nkrumah F, Henle W, Henle G, Herberman R, Perkins V, Depue R: Burkitt's lymphoma: its clinical course in relation to immunologic reactivities to Epstein–Barr virus and tumor related antigens. J Nat Cancer Inst 57:1051, 1976.

T Cell Tumors

Broder S, Edelson RL, Lutzner MA, Nelson DL, MacDermott RR, Durm M, Goldman CK, Meade BD, Waldman TA: The Sezary syndrome: a malignant proliferation of helper T cells. J Clin Invest 58:1297, 1976.

Castleman B: Tumors of the thymus gland. In Atlas of Tumor Pathology, Sect V, Fasc 19. Washington, D.C., Armed Forces Institute of Pathology, 1955.

Clendenning WE: Mycosis fungoides: history, clinical features and controversies. Bull Cancer (Paris) 64:167, 1977.

Goding JW, Burns GF: Monoclonal antibody OKT-9 recognizes the receptor for transferrin on human acute lymphocytic leukemia cells. J Immunol 127:1256, 1981.

Gramatzki M, et al: Immunologic characterization of a helper T cell lymphoma. Blood 59:702, 1982.

Guillan RA, Zelman S, Smalley RL, Iglesias PA: Malignant thymoma associated with myasthenia gravis, and evidence of extrathoracic metastases. Cancer 27:823, 1971.

Kaplan J, Mastrangelo R, Peterson WD Jr: Childhood lymphoblastic lymphoma. A cancer of thymus derived lymphocytes. Cancer Res 34:521, 1974.

Korsmeyer SJ, et al: Immunoglobulin gene rearrangement and cell surface antigen expression in acute lymphocytic leukemias of T cell and B cell precursor origins. J Clin Invest 71:301, 1983.

Mann RB, Jaff ES, Braylan RC, Eggleston JC, Ransom L, Kaizer H, Berand CW: Immunologic and morphologic studies of T cell lymphoma. Am J Med 58:307, 1975.

Miller RA, et al: Sezary syndrome: a model for migration of T lymphocytes to skin. N Engl J Med 303:89, 1980.

Rowden G, Lewis MG: Langerhans' cells: involvement in the pathogenesis of mycosis fungoides. Br J Dermatol 95:665, 1976.

Seligmann M, Preud'homme JL, Brouet JC: B and T cell markers in human proliferative blood diseases and primary immunodeficiencies with special reference to membrane bound immunoglobulins. Transplant Rev 16:85, 1973.

Sen L, Borella L: Clinical importance of lymphoblasts with T cell markers in childhood acute leukemia. N Engl J Med 292:828, 1975.

Waldmann TA: Advances in diagnosis of hemotologic malignancies. Hosp Pract 21:69, 1986.

Waldmann TA, David MM, Bonglovann KF, Korsmeyer SJ: Rearrangements of genes for the antigen receptor on T cells as markers of lineage and clonality in human lymphoid neoplasms. N Engl J Med 313:776, 1985.

Winkelmann K (ed): Symposium on the Sezary cell. Mayo Clin 49:513, 1974.

Macrophage Tumors

Anderson RC: Histiocytic medullary reticulosis with transient skin lesions. Br Med J 1:220, 1944.

Byrne GE, Rappoport H: Malignant histicylosis. Gann Monogr Cancer Res 15:145, 1973.

Cline MJ, Golde DW: A review and reevaluation of the histiocytic disorders. Am J Med 55:49, 1973.

Van der Volk P, Velde J, Jansen J, et al: Malignant lymphoma of true histiocytic origins: histiocytic sarcoma. Virchows Arch Pathol Anat 391:249, 1981.

Hodgkin's Disease

Aisenberg AC: Hodgkin's disease—prognosis, treatment, etiologic and immunologic considerations. N Engl J Med 270:508, 1964.

Carbone PP, Kaplan HS, Musshof K, Smithers DW, Tubiana M: Report of the committee on Hodgkin's disease staging. Cancer Res 31:1860, 1971.

Cassazza AR, Duvall CP, Carbone PP: Summary of infectious complications occurring in patients with Hodgkin's disease. Cancer Res 26:1290, 1966.

Clemmesen J: To the epidemiology of Hodgkin's lymphogranulomatosis. J Belg Radiol 3:1263, 1981.

Hodgkins T: On some morbid appearance of the absorbant glands and spleen. Med Chir Dig 17:68, 1832.

Hsu S-M, Yang K, Jaffe ES: Phenotypic expression of Hodgkin's and Reed–Sternberg cells in Hodgkin's disease. Am J Pathol 118:209, 1985.

Kadin ME: Possible origin of the Reed–Sternberg cells from an interdigitating reticulum cell. Cancer Treat Rep 66:601, 1982.

Kaplan HS: Hodgkin's disease and other human malignant lymphomas: advances and propects—G. H. A. Clowes Memorial Lecture. Cancer Res 36:3863, 1976.

Kaplan HS: Hodgkin's disease: biology, treatment, prognosis. Blood 57:813, 1981.

Peckham MJ, Cooper EH: Proliferation characteristics of the various classes of cells in Hodgkin's disease. Cancer 24:135, 1969.

Portlock CS, Robertson A, Turbow MM, Rosenberg SA: MOPP chemotherapy of advanced Hodgkin's disease: prognostic factors in 242 patients. Proc Am Assoc Cancer Res 17:248, 1976.

Rather LJ: Who discovered the pathognomonic giant cell of Hodgkin's disease? Bull NY Acad Med 48:943, 1972.

Reed DM: On the pathologic giant cell of Hodgkin's disease with especial reference to its relation to tuberculosis. Johns Hopkins Med J 10:133, 1902.

Ward PA, Berenberg JL: Defective regulation of inflammatory mediators in Hodgkin's disease. Supranormal levels of a chemotactic inhibitory factor. N Engl J Med 200:76, 1974.

Transplantation-Associated Lymphoma

Bieber CP, Heberling RL, Jamison SW, et al: Lymphoma in cardiac transplant recipients associated with the use of cyclosporin A, prednisone and antithymocyte globulin. *In* Pertillo DT (ed): Immune Deficiency and Cancer. New York, Plenum, 1985.

Cleary ML, Sklar J: Lymphoproliferative disorders in cardiac transplant recipients are multiclonal lymphomas. Lancet 2:489, 1984.

Penn I: Malignant lymphemas in transplant recipients. Transplant Pract 13:736, 1981.

Weintraub J, Warnke RA: Lymphomas in cardiac allotransplant recipients: clinical and histologic features and immunological phenotype. Transplant 33:347, 1982.

Treatment

See Chapters 18, 25, and 29.

DeVita VT Jr, Serpick A, Carbone PP: Combination chemotherapy in the treatment of advanced Hodgkin's disease. Ann Intern Med 73:881, 1970.

Gale RP, Foon KA: Chronic lymphocytic leukemia: recent advances in biology and treatment. Ann Intern Med 103:101, 1985.

Reilly RJ: Allogeneic bone marrow transplantation: current status and future directions. Blood 62:941, 1963.

Mathe G: Integration of modern data in WHO categorization of lympho-sarcomas: its value for prognosis, prediction, and therapeutic adaptation to prognosis. Biomedicine 26:377, 1977.

McGlave PB: The status of bone marrow transplantation for leukemia. Hosp Pract 20:97, 1985.

Petz CD, Blume KG (eds): Clinical Bone Marrow Transplantation. New York, Churchill Livingstone, 1983.

Ritz J, Pesando J, Sallan SE, et al: Serotherapy of acute lymphoblastic leukemia with monoclonal antibody. Blood 58:141, 1981.

Stevenson GT, Elliott EV, Stevenson FK: Idiotypic determinants on the surface immunoglobulin of neoplastic lymphocytes: a therapeutic target. Fed Proc 36:2268, 1977.

Stevenson GT, Stevenson FK: Treatment of lymphoid tumors with anti-idiotype antibodies. Springer Semin Immunopathol 6:99, 1983.

Thomas ED: The role of marrow transplantation in the eradication of malignant diseases. Cancer 49:1963, 1982.

Animal Models of Lymphomas

Biggs PNM: A discussion on the classification of the avian leukosis complex and fowl paralysis. Br Vet J 117:326, 1961.

Biggs PM: Marek's disease. *In* Kaplan AS (ed): The Herpes Viruses. New York, Academic Press, 1973, p557.

Else RN: Vaccinial immunity to Merek's disease in bursectomized chickens. Vet Rec 95:182, 1974.

Essex M: Immunity to leukemia, lymphoma and fibrosarcoma in cats: a case for immune surveillance. Contemp Top Immunobiol 6:71, 1977.

Green I, Forni G, Konen T, Hu C-P, Schwartz BD, Kask A, Shevach E: Immunological studies of the guinea pig L_2C leukemia. Fed Proc 36:2264, 1977.

Hudson L, Payne LN: An analysis of the T and B cells of Marek's disease lymphomas of the chicken. Nature 241:52, 1973.

Kaplan HS: On the natural history of murine leukemias. Presidential address. Cancer Res 27:1325, 1967.

Madel EM: History and further observations (1954–1976) of the L_2C leukemia in the guinea pig. Fed Proc 36:2249, 1977.

Mazerian K, Lee LF, Sharma JM: The role of herpes viruses in Marek's disease lymphoma of chickens. Prog Med Virol 22:123, 1976.

Morris JR, Jerome FN, Reinhart BS: Surgical bursectomy and the incidence of Marek's disease (MD) in domestic chickens. Poult Sci 48:1513, 1969.

Nazerian K: Marek's disease: a Herpes virus–induced malignant lymphoma of the chicken. *In* Klein G (ed): Viral Oncology, New York, Raven Press, 1980, p665.

Payne LN, Frazier JA, Powell PC: Pathogenesis of Marek's disease. Int Rev Exp Pathol 16:59, 1976.

Peterson RDA, Burmester BR, Fredrickson TN, Purchase HG, Good RA: Effect of bursectomy and thymectomy on the development of visceral lymphomatosis in the chicken. J Nat Cancer Inst 32:1143, 1964.

Potter M: Pathogenesis of plasmacytomas in mice. *In* Becker FF (ed): Cancer, Vol 1. New York, Plenum, 1975, p161.

Puchase HG: Prevention of Marek's disease: a review. Cancer Res 36:696, 1976.

Rouse BT, Wells RJH, Warner NL: Proportion of T and B lymphocytes in lesions of Marek's disease. Theoretic implications for pathogenesis. J Immunol 110:534, 1973.

Siccardi FJ, Burmester BR: The differential Diagnosis of Lymphoid

Leukoses and Marek's Disease. Bulletin 1412, Agric Res Sem USDA, 1970.

Zolla-Pazner S, Gilbert M, Fleit SA: Studies of antibody affinity in plasmacytoma-bearing mice: evidence for a maturational defect of B lymphocytes. Cell Immunol 62:149, 1981.

Etiology

Immunoregulation

Gatti RA, Good RA: Occurrence of malignancy in immunodeficiency disease: a review. Cancer 28:89, 1971.

Jarret WF, Mackey LJ: Neoplastic diseases of the hematopoietic and lymphoid tissues. Bull WHO 50:21, 1974.

Louie S, Schwartz RS: Immunodeficiency and the pathogenesis of lymphoma and leukemia. Semin Hematol 15:117, 1978.

Melief CJM, Schwartz RS: Immunocompetence and malignancy. In Becker FF (ed): Cancer, Vol 1. New York, Plenum, 1975, p121.

Yunis EJ, Ferndandes G, Greenberg LS: Tumor immunology: autoimmunity and aging. J Am Geriatr Soc 24:258, 1976.

Virus Infection

Hanna MG Jr, Rapp F (eds): Immunobiology of oncogenic viruses. Contemp Top Immunol 6:1, 1977.

Kaplan HS, Goodenow RS, Gartner S, Bieber MM: Biology and virology of the human malignant lymphomas. Cancer 43:1, 1979.

Chromosomal Translocations

Erikson J, ar-Rushdi A, Drwinga HL, Nowell PC, Croce CM: Transcriptional activation of the translocated c-myc oncogene in Burkitt lymphomas. Proc Nat Acad Sci USA 80:820, 1983.

Klein G: Specific chromosomal translocations and the genesis of B cell derived tumors in mice and men. Cell 32:311, 1983.

Nowell PC, Erickson J, Finan J, Emanuel B, Croce C: Chromosomal translocations, immunoglobulin genes and oncogenes in human B-cell tumors. Cancer Surv 3:531, 1984.

Rowley J: Biological implications of consistent chromosome rearrangements in leukemia and lymphoma. Cancer Res 44:3159, 1984.

Temin HM: Origin of retroviruses from cellular variable genetic elements. Cell 21:599, 1980.

Williams DL, Look AT, Melvin SL, et al: New chromosomal translocations correlate with specific immunophenotypes of childhood acute lymphobastic leukemia. Cell 36:101, 1984.

Yunis JJ, Oken MM, Theologides A, et al: Recurrent chromosonal defects are found in most patients with non-Hodgkin's lymphoma. Cancer Genet Cytogenet 13:17, 1984.

29 | Tumor Immunity

Cancer is not a single disease but a large number of diseases that are expressed as the abnormal and continued growth of cells of a given tissue. Instead of a steady state between the production and turnover of cells, cancer cells die at a slower rate than they are produced, leading to a progressive increase in the number of cancer cells and the mass of cancerous tissue. In some cases, growth occurs at only one site, whereas in others, the malignant cells seed to and grow at other sites (metastases). The events that lead to the development of cancer, as well as the factors that control it, are poorly understood. This chapter deals with the role of host immune mechanisms in the development and growth of cancer and the use of immune reactants for diagnosis and treatment of cancer.

Host–Tumor Relationships

One of the classic characteristics of a cancer is its apparent autonomy, that is, its ability to grow relatively independently of host controlling mechanisms. If a clone of cells arises with inappropriate markers or if cells with appropriate markers are put into an environment that will support growth but not limit the growth of the transplanted cell, unregulated cell growth may occur. On the other hand, tumor cells may express cell surface antigens that can be recognized as foreign by the immune system. The immune system may be able to prevent the emergence of tumors with "foreign" antigens (immune surveillance). A short history of observations leading to the demonstration of tumor immunity is given in Table 29-1.

The role of the immune system in controlling experimental tumor growth is illustrated by the nude mouse. Nude mice do not have a thymus and lack the ability to reject tissue grafts because of a defect in differentiation of T cells. Tumors of different species grow when transplanted into nude mice. Thus, the nude mouse lacks the mechanism to recognize the cells as foreign and limit their growth, and provides an environment that supports the growth of tumor cells of diverse origin.

725

Table 29-1. A Short History of Tumor Immunity

1898	Halsted	Lymphocytic infiltration of tumor and lymph node hyperplasia seen in cancer patients with good prognoses
1900	Ehrlich	Proposed tumor specific immunity
1906	Schone	Tumor immunity induced by fetal tissues in outbred mice
1908	Wade	Tumor grafts rejected in outbred animals, lymphocyte infiltration
1941	Gross	Tumor grafts rejected in partially inbred mice
1953	Foley	Tumor grafts rejected in fully inbred mice
1957	Prehn	Tumor-specific transplantation rejection in autochthonous immunized host (mice)

Tumor Immunity in Humans

There is substantial circumstantial evidence to support the conclusion that immune reactivity to tumors is important in humans (Table 29-2). However, definitive proof has not been obtained.

Table 29-2. Summary of Evidence for Tumor Immunity in Humans

Event	Comment
1. Spontaneous regression	Rare, usually tumors that could be controlled by developmental factors, or contain foreign antigens (paternal antigens in choriocarcinomas)
2. Regression of metastases after removal of primary	Rare, not necessarily immune mediated
3. Reappearance of metastases after long latent periods	Not necessarily immune mediated
4. Failure of circulating cells to form metastases	Most likely not immune mediated
5. Infiltration of tumors by mononuclear cells	Could be secondary effect, not always associated with tumor regression
6. High incidence of cancer in immunosuppressed, aged, or immunodeficient patients	Strong circumstantial evidence, but not proof
7. Depressed immune reactivity in cancer patients	Depressed immunity associated with debilitated state of patient, a secondary effect of cancer
8. Tumor antigens identified by in vitro assays on human cancers	In vitro assays not reliable indication of in vivo tumor rejection
9. Cancer patients may have delayed skin tests to cancer extracts	Significance of skin tests not clear
10. Immune complexes and glomerulonephritis are found in some cancer patients	Relationship of immune complexes to tumor resistance not documented

1. Spontaneous remissions of different human tumors have been recognized. Although many claims of spontaneous remission of human cancer do not hold up to critical review, Emerson, after an extensive survey, accepted 130 cases of spontaneous regression of malignant tumors. Of these, 10% were choriocarcinomas, in which paternal antigens foreign to the maternal host are expressed. Spontane-

ous regressions have been reported in about 15% of nodular lymphomas, a form of B cell cancer subject to control by other cells in the lymphocyte series.

2. Regression of metastases after removal of a primary tumor is a rare and complex phenomenon. One explanation is that removal of the primary tumor permits an immune response to tumor antigens to become focused on metastatic lesions. However, other complex phenomena involving the biology of the tumor and host factors, such as hormonal requirements for tumor growth being altered by removal of the primary tumor or dependence of the metastases on factors produced by the primary tumor, could be the explanation.

3. Reappearance of metastases after a long latent period is an example of tumor dormancy. It has been documented in experimental models that tumor cells may exist in a quiescent state for many years. Changes in blood supply, operative trauma, and other events are associated with tumor cells breaking out of the dormant state. This is often, but not always, related to an immunosuppressive event.

4. Failure of circulating tumor cells to form metastases has been well documented in both animal and human studies. During cancer surgery large numbers of tumor cells may be released into the circulation, yet later, metastases are not found. This can be explained by the inability of the tumor cells to escape successfully from the circulation and proliferate away from the primary site, clearing of tumor cells from the circulation by the reticuloendothelial system, or distribution of tumor cells to nonsupportive environments ("bad soil"). There is little or no evidence that immune mechanisms are involved.

5. Tumor tissue is often infiltrated by large numbers of lymphocytes, perhaps because of a cellular immunological reaction to tumor antigens. William Halsted, in 1898, described perivascular infiltration by lymphocytes and hyperplasia of draining lymph nodes in patients with large breast cancers that had a relatively prolonged course without metastases as compared with breast cancers without infiltrating lymphocytes. Although the significance of this observation remains controversial, there are many who have found that tumor infiltration by lymphocytes is associated with a good prognosis, as well as others who have not.

6. An increased incidence of cancer is found in patients with primary or secondary immune deficiency states. A tabulation of the occurrence of primary cancer in transplant patients during immunosuppressive therapy showed that the overall occurrence for all cancers was far greater (13/2000) than in the general population (8.2/100,000). However, immunosuppressed individuals have a prepon-

derance of lymphomas, which may reflect abnormalities in control of lymphoid cell proliferation rather than suppression of immunity per se or susceptibility to cancer in general.

7. Some cancer patients have decreased cell-mediated immune responses to a variety of antigens, and these patients appear to have more rapid tumor growth than cancer patients whose cell-mediated immunity is not decreased. In addition, cellular immune deficiency is more marked in patients with disseminated tumor growth or those who respond poorly to therapy. This may reflect the debilitated state of a terminal cancer patient, rather than a specific immune deficit.

8. Some human tumors have tumor antigens detectable by in vitro assays. Several human tumor-specific antigens have been identified by these assays (see below). Although reasonable data have been obtained in various animal systems that correlate cellular immune reactivity to ability of an animal to resist tumor challenge, the specificity of cellular tests for human tumors has been seriously questioned. One major problem has been the identification of natural killer cells. Thus, whereas lymphocytes from cancer patients may react with certain tumor target cells, similar cells from normal persons often react just as strongly. In addition, tumor cell in vitro lines have been used almost exclusively as target cells. These cell lines may not express the same antigenicity as the original tumor. Therefore, most of the data in which in vitro human tumor immunity was tested using cell lines must be reinterpreted. It may be necessary to perform all such tests using primary cultures of freshly obtained tumor target cells.

9. A tumor-bearing patient may produce a delayed hypersensitivity skin reaction against a membrane extract of his own tumor cells, but the significance of such a reaction is difficult to evaluate. In addition, immediate (2 minutes) skin reactions to tumor extracts preincubated with the patient's serum (Makari test) have been reported to be an indicator of the presence of tumors, but this has not been generally accepted.

10. Circulating immune complexes and glomerular immune complex disease, frequently subclinical, are found in about 10% of all cancer patients. In a few cases, the glomerular deposits of complexes have been demonstrated to contain tumor-associated antigen (carcinoembryonic antigen, CEA) or antibody to CEA. The relationship of these complexes to tumor resistance is not known, but suggests that an antibody to a tumor "antigen" is present.

The evidence is convincing that an immune response does occur to some human tumors and that this response may in rare cases be responsible for regression of inoperable primary tumors. However, clear-cut demonstrations of effective tumor resistance in humans due to an immune response to the tumor are exceptions to the general rule. At the present time tumor immunity in humans has limited application in treatment of human cancer.

Tumor Antigens

A number of antigenic changes may occur in tissues that undergo malignant change. These include the loss of antigenic specificities present in normal tissue, the addition of new antigenic specificities not present in normal tissue, the appearance of markers present in fetal or embryonic tissue but not present in normal adult tissue (oncodevelopmental products), and combinations of these (Fig. 29-1).

Figure 29-1. Some antigenic features of tumor cells. A number of changes in the cell surface of tumor cells have been noted, including loss or gain of histocompatibility antigen, loss or gain of cell surface carbohydrates, appearance of viral associated antigens (tumor-associated viral antigen (TAVA)), and tumor associated transplantation antigens common for tumors of the same histologic type (TATA). Also seen are tumor-specific transplantation antigens present on only one tumor (TSTA), antigens detected by only serological reactions that are unique for a given tumor (tumor-associated serological defined antigens), and markers shared by embryonic or developing tumors and tumors (oncodevelopmental antigens, ODA).

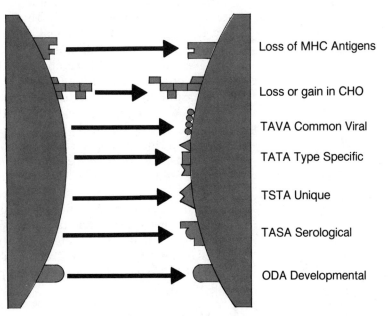

NORMAL CELL　　　　　TUMOR CELL

Loss of MHC Antigens

Loss or gain in CHO

TAVA Common Viral

TATA Type Specific

TSTA Unique

TASA Serological

ODA Developmental

A basic problem in the study of tumor immunity is the identification of new tumor-specific antigens not present in normal tissues. At least three types of tumor antigens have been identified: those found associated with chemically or physically induced tumors or with some spontaneous tumors of animals and man, virus-induced tumor antigens, and oncodevelopmental antigens (ODA).

Tumor-Specific Transplantation Antigens

The first type of tumor antigen has been identified by transplantation in experimental animals but has not yet been identified in human tumors. These antigens may be divided into two general classes: those that are specific for a given tumor, and those that are shared by two or more tumors, generally of a particular histologic type. A given tumor may have both unique and shared antigens. For diagnostic and therapeutic purposes in humans, antigenic specificities shared by a large number of tumors of a given class are potentially much more valuable than unique antigens. Detection of a shared antigen could be used as a screening test for tumors in different persons or for preventive immunization, whereas a unique antigen would not be detected by a common antigen screening test and would be effective as an immunogen only in the individual with that tumor. A tumor induced in a mouse by methylcholanthrene is usually antigenically different from every other tumor induced by methylcholanthrene. Indeed, two tumors induced in the same animal may be antigenically distinct. This demonstration of individually distinct antigenic specificities extends to other chemically induced tumors, including sarcomas induced by aromatic hydrocarbons, hepatomas induced by azo dyes, and mammary carcinomas induced by methylcholanthrene, as well as tumors induced by physical means such as implantation of cellophane films or millipore filters.

As early as 1910 it was observed that the serum of mice that had recovered from tumors inhibited tumor growth in other mice, sometimes causing regression and an apparent cure. Attempts were made to treat cancer with immunization methods similar to those that had proved successful with infectious diseases, and promising results were obtained in experimental animals. This raised hopes that tumor-specific immune reactions could cure cancer. However, it soon became apparent that the results obtained were not because of tumor-specific antigens, but because of histocompatibility antigens. In other words, normal tissue and tumor tissue from the tumor donor were rejected in a similar manner by the same recipient. Terms used to identify host–tumor relationships are the same as those used for tissue graft donor–recipient relationships (Table 29-3).

Table 29-3. Terminology of Host–Tumor Relationships

Same individual	Autochthonous
Genetically identical (twin, inbred strain)	Syngeneic
Different individual, same species	Allogeneic
Different species	Xenogeneic

The inability to demonstrate tumor-specific transplantation antigens (TSTA) led to a general loss of interest in tumor immunity until the development of inbred strains of mice. In 1943, Ludwig Gross transplanted tumors (sarcomas) induced by the chemical methylcholanthrene in inbred mice. He found that tumor nodules appeared after tumor cells were injected into the skin, grew for a few days, and then regressed. After regression, reinjection of cells from the same tumor did not produce a tumor nodule, demonstrating that the animals that had rejected the transplanted tumor were now resistant. Ten years later Foley followed up Gross' observations. He tested 6-methylcholanthrene–induced sarcomas of C3H/HE mouse origin. Immunization was accomplished by strangulation of the first or second transplant generation of tumor grafts. Following tumor regression, the animals were rechallenged with living cells, and the frequency of "takes" was compared with that in untreated controls. Resistance to challenge was noted when the mice were reinjected with the same tumor. Appropriate controls involving skin grafts and immunization with normal tissue ruled out the possibility that rejection was caused by antigens present in normal tissue and not specific for the tumor. In 1957, Prehn extended these observations by showing that tumor-specific immunity could be produced by allowing a tumor to grow and then removing it by surgical excision. Animals that had been immunized in this way could then reject the same transplantable tumor, even if greater numbers of tumor cells were injected. He also found that chemically induced tumors possessed individually specific tumor antigens; immunization of an animal to one chemically induced tumor did not protect it from growth of a different chemically induced tumor. These studies clearly demonstrated the presence of tumor-specific transplantation antigens in chemically induced transplantable tumors of mice.

Immune Response of Primary-Tumor–Bearing Host

The studies cited describe immunity to transplanted tumors. In 1960, it was shown that the primary-tumor–bearing animal can be immunized against its own autochthonous tumor. The term *autochthonous* is used to indicate the relationship between a tumor and the individual in which that tumor arose (primary host). Primary methylcholanthrene-induced sarcomas were excised from the autochthonous animal and maintained by passage in syngeneic recipients. Transplantation of the passaged tumor back to the autochthonous host resulted in rejection of the tumor 3–4 weeks later. Thus, an experimental animal may make an immune response to its own tumor and this response may be effective in controlling the growth of the tumor (autochthonous tumor resistance; Fig. 29-2). In some instances, the primary-tumor–bearing animal (autochthonous host) may have an immune response that can be demonstrated in vitro, but in spite of this response, the tumor grows progressively in vivo *(concomitant immunity)*.

The immunogenicity of a given tumor-specific antigen of an animal tumor depends on the nature of induction of the tumor. Tumors induced by large doses of carcinogens are generally more likely to express tumor-specific transplantation an-

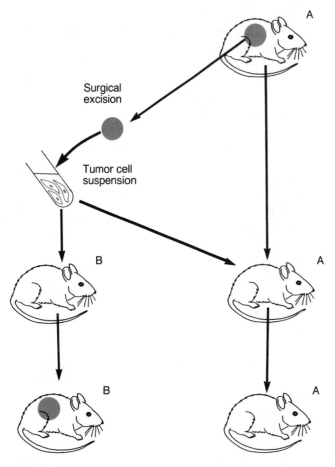
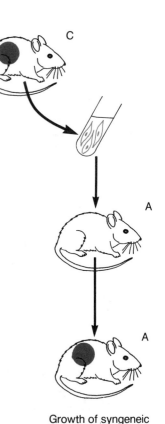

Surgical excision

Tumor cell suspension

Growth in normal syngeneic host

Resistance in autochthonous host

Growth of syngeneic tumor

Figure 29-2. Demonstration of specific rejection of an autochthonous tumor. A chemically induced primary tumor is removed surgically and a suspension of the tumor cells made. A dose of tumor cells that will grow in a normal syngeneic mouse of the same strain as that in which the tumor was induced is injected into the original primary-tumor– bearing animal (autochthonous host). This tumor does not grow in the autochthonous host (A); the autochthonous host has developed immune resistance to growth of his own tumor. The tumor will grow when injected with a normal recipient of the same strain (B). However, a second tumor arising in another individual of the same strain (C) will grow when injected into the host of the first tumor. Thus, the tumor resistance is specific for the first tumor and does not extend to other tumors (tumor-specific transplantation immunity). This type of experiment demonstrates that an individual can develop immunity to his own tumor.

tigens than tumors induced by smaller doses of carcinogens. In addition, tumors induced by "strong" carcinogens are more likely to be immunogeneic than tumors induced by "weak" carcinogens (Table 29-4). Individual tumor-specific antigens are more easily demonstrated on chemically induced tumors

Table 29-4. Immunogenicity of Rat Tumors

Origin	Common Antigens	TSTA	ODA
Viral	++++	++	+
Methylcholanthrene	+	+++	+
Diaminoazobenzene	+	+	+
Acetylaminofluorine	0	+	+
Spontaneous	0	+	+

TSTA, tumor specific transplantation antigens; ODA, oncodevelopmental antigens (serological); +, Degree of immunogenicity.

than on virally induced tumors because of the lack of viral (common) antigens. Spontaneous tumors of mice may lack tumor antigens or express them very weakly. Some tumor antigens may be identified only serologically; however, they do not necessarily induce a rejection reaction.

The nature of tumor-specific antigens remains unclear. Are these new molecules not present in normal tissues or rearrangements of normal cell surface structures? It is likely that most tumor antigens are not specific for tumors but may be present in small amounts in normal tissue. These are called *tumor-associated* antigens. For instance, protection against some syngeneic tumors may be induced by inoculation of recipient animals with normal tissues prior to tumor challenge.

Some tumor-specific antigens may represent altered histocompatibility structures. An inverse relationship was found between the expression of major histocompatibility complex (MHC) class I products and TSTA in mouse sarcomas, suggesting that TSTA and MHC antigen expression might involve a similar mechanism. Genetic analysis of hybrid cells has shown that MHC products and TSTA are controlled by different chromosomes. Different configurations or spatial arrangements of histocompatibility antigens may occur on tumor cells and be recognized as foreign by the immune system. New MHC antigens have been described on immune tumor cells after viral infections. In addition, infection of tumors with viruses leads to the appearance of virus-specific antigens as well as a marked increase in immunogenicity of nonviral tumor antigens (xenogenization). Thus tumor antigens may be entirely new structures, modifications of existing structures, or realignments of existing cell surface structures.

Attempts have been made to solubilize cell surface TSTA in order to isolate and characterize the tumor antigen. TSTA are protein or glycoprotein components of the cell wall, but the exact biochemical nature of tumor antigens is still not well known. Some soluble tumor-associated antigen extracts have been shown to possess antigenic activity, but the purity of such fractions is questionable. In other words, the tumor-antigen extract may be contaminated by a variety of nonantigenic or non-tumor-specific molecules extracted from the tumor cell surface.

Allogeneic Inhibition

Tumor cell growth may be controlled by nonimmunologically mediated processes involving interactions with other cell types that may recognize neoplastic cells. Normal nonimmune cells may inhibit the growth of tumor cells in vitro. As a rule, tumors arising in homozygous donors grow better when transplanted into syngeneic homozygous recipients than do the same tumors transplanted into semisyngeneic F_1 hybrid recipients. This phenomenon has been called *syngeneic preference* in reference to the parental syngeneic host, and *allogeneic inhibition* in reference to the F_1 hybrid host. F_1 hybrid recipients may also reject normal bone marrow grafts of parental origin, a phenomenon termed *hybrid resistance*. These phenomena are poorly understood but may represent nonimmunological surveillance mechanisms for eliminating incipient neoplastic cells. Some homozygous parental cells express antigens not expressed in the F_1, so that parental bone marrow or tumor cells may be recognized as foreign. These antigens may be preferentially expressed on certain cell types so that most parental organ grafts are accepted by the F_1 recipient, whereas certain other tissues are rejected.

Virus-Induced Tumor Antigens

In contrast to chemically induced or spontaneous cancers, virus-induced tumors share common antigens. These shared antigens may be products encoded by the viral genome or cellular products not expressed in the virus itself.

DNA Viruses

Each DNA virus induces unique nuclear and cell surface antigens. A given virus induces the expression of the same antigens regardless of the tissue origin or animal species. Although these antigens are coded for by the virus, they are distinct from virion antigens and are referred to as tumor-associated antigens. Virally induced tumors may also express other antigens coded for by the host genome (such as TSTA or ODA) as a result of host gene deregulation by the transforming event.

The association of DNA viruses with cell transformation and cancer in animals is well established and is linked to certain human tumors. For example, Epstein–Barr virus (EBV), one of the herpesviruses, is the cause of human infectious mononucleosis, and is also associated with (but not proved to be the etiologic agent of) Burkitt's lymphoma and nasopharyngeal carcinoma. Similarly, herpes simplex type 2 has been linked to human cervical carcinoma. In animals, herpesviruses have been shown to be oncogenic, as exemplified by Marek's lymphoma of chickens.

RNA Viruses

Tumors produced by RNA virus contain DNA that has been transcribed from the infected RNA by reverse transcriptase.

When the oncogenic RNA viruses (oncornaviruses) infect the host cell, a double-stranded circular DNA copy of the RNA genome is synthesized and inserted into the host cell genome during cell transformation. Tumor cells induced by oncornaviruses express antigens coded for by both the viral and host genomes. These include (1) the viral envelope antigens, mostly the envelope glycoprotein gp70, molecular weight approximately 70,000 (there is extensive immunological cross-reactivity among all gp70 determinants of murine oncornaviruses); (2) intrinsic viral proteins; and (3) cell surface antigens. While antibodies to gp70 will prevent infectivity, immunity against the neoplastic cell surface antigens is mainly responsible for the immunological rejection of the malignant cell. These cell surface antigens are distinct from the viral antigens and also from the H-2 histocompatibility antigens. The complexity of neoantigens expressed in virally induced tumors is illustrated by the Rous sarcoma system of hamsters: The antigens include virus envelope antigen (VEA), virus group-specific antigens (gs antigens), virus-coded nonviral proteins, cell-coded determinants activated by the virus, and oncodevelopmental antigens coded by cellular genes that are activated by virus-induced transformation.

A number of RNA retroviruses have been identified as having oncogene sequences by their ability to transfect cultured cells and effect changes in growth of the transfected cells (transformation). The tumors of many human cancers have been found to contain cDNA sequences similar to the transforming oncogenes. Normal mammalian DNA has also been found to contain such DNA sequences (protooncogenes) (Table 29-5). These oncogenes code for cellular products, particularly kinases, which are produced normally during devel-

Table 29-5. Chromosome Location of Human Protooncogenes

Protooncogene	Human Chromosome	Mouse Chromosome
c-src	20	2
c-myc	8 (band 24)	15
c-myb	6	10
c-fps/c-fes	15	2
c-mos	8	4
c-abl	9	2
c-Ha-ras-1	11	?
c-Ha-ras-2	X	?
c-Ki-ras-1	6	?
c-Ki-ras-2	12	?
c-sis	22	?
c-erb-A	17	?
c-erb-B	?	?
c-yes	?	?
c-fos	2	?
c-fms	5	?
c-raf-1	3	?

opment but which are also believed to contribute to the altered growth characteristics of transformed adult cells. Monoclonal antibodies have been produced to oncogene products of human tumors, but the applicability of such antibodies to diagnosis, therapy, or prevention remains to be determined. Chromosomal translocations may result in activation of protooncogenes in cancer cells.

Oncodevelopmental Antigens

Oncodevelopmental antigens (ODA) were identified by transplantation as early as 1906, when Schone found that tumor transplants that would kill normal mice would be rejected by mice that had been previously immunized with fetal tissue; immunization with adult tissue was ineffective. In the 1930s, humoral antibodies that cross-reacted with fetal and tumor tissue were reported. These studies were complicated by histocompatibility differences and are difficult to duplicate. General interest in oncodevelopmental antigens received little attention until the late 1960s, when antigens common to embryonic tissue and tumors were demonstrated in inbred strains by serologic cross-reactivity. In 1970, it was reported that lymph node cells from pregnant mice incubated in vitro with chemically induced syngeneic sarcoma cells caused death of the tumor cells. Although extensive experimental investigation of ODA followed, the significance of such antigens in regard to tumor immunogenicity remains undefined. The following general conclusions seem valid. Tumors and fetal tissue may share antigens that are different from TSTA. ODA are not specific for a given tumor but are shared by tumors of different histologic type and even of different species of origin. Immune products (antibody or sensitized cells) may be generated by immunization of adults with fetal tissue or by exposure to fetal antigen during pregnancy that reacts with tumors in vitro. However, no effect of this immunization on tumor incidence or growth has been consistently demonstrated. Animals that have in vitro immune reactivity to ODA may have resistance to tumor challenge, demonstrate no differences from nonimmune recipients, or have increased growth of transplanted tumors. In systems that have shown ODA by transplantation, immunogenicity is much more difficult to demonstrate than that to TSTA or viral tumor antigens. In humans, ODA have been tentatively identified by in vitro tests. However, there is little or no evidence that immunization to fetal antigens protects against cancer in humans. Only one study has shown that the course of cancer in multiparous women differs from that in nulliparous women. Previously pregnant women, after treatment for malignant melanoma, had slightly better survival rates than women with no previous pregnancies. Multiparous women have a higher incidence of carcinoma of the cervix but a lower incidence of carcinoma of the breast. These differences are not believed to be on the basis of immunity. A difference in the relative incidence of cancer in previously pregnant versus non-pregnant women on the basis of tumor immunity has not been reported.

Relevance to Humans of Animal Models of Tumor Immunity

The goal of the study of animal tumor models is to obtain insights into human disease. Studies on tumor immunity in animals have provided much provocative information. Animals do make both cellular and humoral immune responses to tumor antigens. The tumor antigens may be specific for a given tumor or shared by different tumors, usually of the same histologic type. Virus-induced experimental tumors have highly immunogenic antigens, which are shared by all tumors induced by a given virus (see below). Tumor-specific transplantation antigens are more easily demonstrated on chemically induced tumors because of the lack of viral antigens, but many chemically induced transplantable tumors are either very weakly antigenic (these tumor-specific antigens may not confer immunity) or nonantigenic. A sublethal dose of cells or inoculation of irradiated tumor cells may produce long-standing resistance against viral tumors, but resistance to chemically induced tumors is more difficult and, in many instances, impossible to induce by such techniques. Spontaneously occurring tumors in animals do not bear demonstrable tumor transplantation antigens. Since immune products may affect tumor growth in a variety of ways, preimmunization may result in increased tumor growth or decreased tumor growth or have no effect, depending on the nature of the tumor and the type of immune response stimulated.

From the animal models, one can predict that the immune response to tumors in man will be enormously varied and difficult to control. Some tumors would be expected to be highly antigenic and responsive to immunotherapeutic and immunoprophylactic procedures. Unfortunately, most human tumors seem to be more like the poorly or nonantigen chemically induced or spontaneously occurring tumors of animals. Thus, animal models of tumor-specific transplantation using highly antigenic tumors may have little relevance to human tumors. In addition, what is true for one tumor may not be true for the next. Even tumors of similar histologic type and growth pattern may provoke entirely different immune responses.

Mechanisms of Tumor Cell Destruction by the Immune System

In Vitro Exposure, in Vivo Transfer

One of the first successful demonstrations of the effect of immune cells on tumor growth was accomplished by mixing immune effector cells with tumor target cells in vitro, then injecting the mixture into a normal or irradiated syngeneic recipient (Winn assay) (Fig. 29-3). If growth of the transplanted tumor cells is inhibited by the in vitro pretreatment, it may be concluded that the tumor cells were adversely affected by the effector cells.

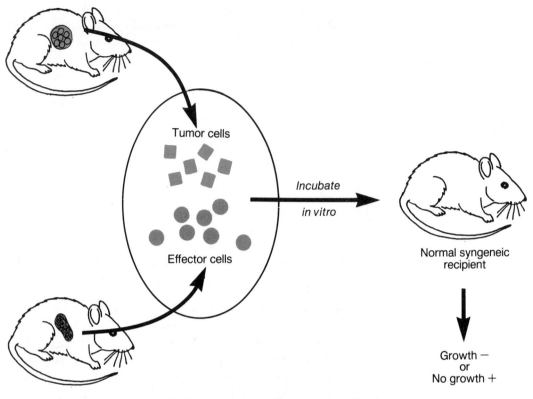

Figure 29-3. Winn assay. To determine the possible adverse or killing effect of lymphoid cells on a given tumor, the effector lymphoid cells are admixed in vitro with the tumor target cells and the mixture is transplanted into a normal syngeneic recipient. If growth of the tumor is inhibited in comparison with tumor cells alone or tumor cells treated with control (unsensitized) lymphoid cells, it may be concluded that tumor immunity exists in the tested lymphoid cells.

A partial listing of the methods used to demonstrate immune reactivity to tumors in vitro is given in Table 29-6. These

Table 29-6. Some in Vitro Assays for Human Antigens

Humoral	Cellular (CMI)
Immunodiffusion	Effect of immune cells on targets
Antibody binding	Reduction of cell number
Fluorescence	Cytotoxicity
Radiolabel	Vital dye uptake
Immunoperoxidase	Visual
Blocking of antibody binding	^{51}Cr release
Complement-dependent killing	Inhibition of metabolism
Complement fixation	Loss of cell adherence
C1 fixation and transfer	Cytostasis
Mixed hemadsorption	Colony inhibition
Cytostasis	In vitro incubation, in vivo growth (Winn assay)
Loss of cell adherence	Effect of targets on immune cells
Blocking of cellular reactions	Mixed lymphocyte–tumor reactions
Immune adherence	Macrophage migration inhibition (MIF)
ELISA	Leukocyte adherence inhibition

include almost every conceivable method of measuring the reaction of antibody or sensitized cells with antigens. Tests for humoral (circulating) immunoglobulin antibody to tumor antigens are hampered by the difficulty of obtaining soluble antigens from tumor cells and the lack of characterization of nonviral tumor-specific antigens. Both humoral and cellular reactions are usually measured by determining some effect of immune products on tumor target cells. The most frequently used assays measure target cell lysis (e.g., by ^{51}Cr release) as an endpoint.

In Vitro Tumor Cell Killing

Essentially, five general mechanisms for immune-mediated destruction of tumor cells have been identified. Studies of these in vitro mechanisms have resulted in new insights into how immune mechanisms might restrict the growth or kill tumor cells. However, the major in vivo mechanism for tumor cell killing is delayed hypersensitivity; the in vivo contribution of T killer cells, natural killer cells, and antibody-dependent cell-mediated cytotoxicity as defined by in vitro assays is not clear. For a more detailed description of the in vitro measurement of cell-mediated immunity see Chapter 8.

Complement-Mediated Lysis

Complement-mediated lysis occurs after activation by immunoglobulin (usually IgM) antibody to target cells. This mechanism may operate directly to produce lesions in the cell membrane or indirectly by opsonization of target cells. It is usually effective only on cells that are in suspension (i.e., leukemia) and not on cells in solid tissue. This mechanism has been demonstrated to be effective in certain animal models of leukemia.

Antibody-Dependent Cell-Mediated Cytotoxicity

Target cells are killed by effector cells that can react with antibody (usually IgG) via cell surface receptors for Fc. The effector cell types are heterogeneous and include polymorphonuclear leukocytes, macrophages, and lymphocytes. The lymphocytes involved usually have no distinguishing T or B cell surface markers. They have been called null cells or K (killer) cells. The Fc receptor for IgG is a common feature of antibody-dependent cell-mediated cytotoxic (ADCC) effector cells. Killing requires effector cell–target cell interaction accomplished by the antibody binding by its antigen recognition sites to the target cell and by its Fc to the effector cell. Lysis of the target cell by ADCC follows interaction with the killer cell. The mechanism of target cell destruction is not well understood and the in vivo significance remains unclear.

T Cell–Mediated Cytolysis (T Cytotoxic or T Killer Cells)

This type of killing requires the direct recognition of sensitized T cells with cell surface antigens of the target cell. The effector T cell can react with and lyse many target cells. The reaction of specific T cells with the target cell results in swelling of the target cell and eventual osmotic lysis. Lysis is frequently measured by the release of radiolabeled intracellular molecules (^{51}Cr release). The lysis is presumably caused by membrane alterations in the target cells. The lesion(s) have a morphological appearance similar to those produced by complement. It may be caused by reaction of the T cell with the target cell or by the release of soluble mediators (lymphotoxins) acting locally on the target cell.

Activated Macrophage Killing

The role of macrophages as scavengers that "clean up" injured cells is well known. Macrophages may be activated and attracted to inflammatory sites by mediators released from T_D lymphocytes (delayed hypersensitivity). However, nonspecific killing by macrophages has also been observed (activated macrophages). The mechanism of this type of killing involves the phagocytic activity of macrophages, through formation of oxygen radicals and activation of proteolytic enzymes.

Natural Killing/LAK

Lymphocytes from normal persons are just as reactive against some tumor cell lines as those from patients with tumors of the same or different histologic types. In normal unimmunized animals and humans, the presence of cells that have the capacity to kill certain tumor target cells may prevent development of cancers (see below). These are natural cytotoxic or natural killer (NK) cells. In addition, different populations of lymphocytes may be activated to kill tumor cells by interleukin 2. These are known as *lymphokine-activated killer* (LAK) cells.

In Vivo Tumor Killing: Delayed Hypersensitivity

The immune mechanism responsible for the rejection of solid tumors in experimental animals is the same as that responsible for homograft rejection. The mechanism is delayed hypersensitivity and is not reproducible in vitro. However, through the use of diffusion chambers (permeable to antibody and complement, but not permeable to cells), it has been demonstrated that antibody and complement may cause the death of some kinds of tumor cells. Lymphomas and leukemias are very sensitive to antibody in vivo and in vitro, whereas sarcoma and carcinoma cells are usually, but not always, resistant to the effect of antibody and complement. Thus, antibody-mediated cytotoxic reactions may be responsible for the death of tumor cells that grow primarily in suspension, and the delayed-type reaction responsible for the rejection of solid tumors.

Studies of transplantable tumors in animals have shown destruction of tumor cells in vivo by a two-step mechanism similar to other cell-mediated immune responses. Sensitized cells (T_D) are necessary to initiate the reaction with tumor cells, but macrophages accumulate at the site of the reaction with tumor cells and are responsible for the final tumor cell destruction. If macrophages are mixed with tumor cells, or if they are brought to the site of tumor cell inoculation by nonspecific means, tumor cell destruction may still occur. Thus, the mechanism of tumor cell killing in vivo is similar to that of the delayed skin reaction (see Chapter 19).

Immune Surveillance

If tumors have specific antigens that are recognizable by the autochthonous host, such antigens may be recognized by the host and stimulate an immune reaction that will eliminate developing cancer cells. A currently popular theory is that the immune system, in particular delayed hypersensitivity, provides an anticancer screening system (immune surveillance). Sir Frank Macfarlane Burnet postulated that if it were not for the graft rejection mechanism, vertebrates would die at an early stage of development from tumor growth. Potential malignant cells that develop new antigenic determinants are recognized as foreign by the immune system and are eliminated by a specific immune response. Burnet went on to suggest that the allograft rejection prevents tumors from being contagious; if allogeneic tissue were not rejected, the tumors of one person could easily grow in another, as occurs in nude mice.

Whereas there are considerable data that can be mustered in support of immune surveillance, there is enough conflicting evidence to suggest that immune surveillance operates either ineffectively or not at all. The existence of surveillance has been suggested experimentally by the increased incidence of virus-induced and chemically induced tumors in neonatally thymectomized animals, in antilymphocyte serum–treated animals, or after exposure of animals to whole body irradiation, and clinically by the more frequent appearance of cancer in individuals with depressed immune reactivity. Immunosuppressed patients are highly susceptible to tumors of the reticuloendothelial system, particularly B cell tumors. Therefore, it has been suggested that immunosuppression produces an effect on suppressor T cells so that control of lymphoid cell proliferation is deranged, leading to lymphoproliferative neoplasms because of overgrowth of B cell lines.

The findings in nude mice illustrate the difficulty in using an experimental system to confirm or deny such a hypothesis as immune surveillance. As discussed above, nude mice do not have functional T cells, are unable to reject foreign tissue grafts, and support the growth of allogeneic or even syngeneic tumors. In addition, the nude mouse is highly susceptible to virus-induced polyoma tumors. At first glance, these findings imply that the nude mouse proves the theory that the lack of an immune surveillance system leads to cancer. However, nude mice do not have an increased incidence of spontaneous tumors or increased susceptibility to chemical carcinogens. Therefore, at second glance, the lack of a T cell surveillance system does not appear to result in an increase in tumor development. On the other hand, nude mice do have active natural killer cells, perhaps even more than normal mice. Thus on third glance, it is possible that immune surveillance of tumors in nude mice may depend on the NK system. However, in mice deficient in NK activity, such as mice with the *beige* mutation, there is no increased susceptibility to chemically inducible tumors. These findings and the lack of an in vivo correlation between tumor development (either high or low) and NK activity in other models do not support a role for NK as a mechanism for immune surveillance.

Immune surveillance may be weakened by natural selection mechanisms. There is a clear difference in the vigorous immune response to many virus-induced tumors in animals as compared with little or no response to spontaneously arising human tumors. There appears to be a host selection for an immune mechanism favoring prompt rejection of virus-transformed cells along the lines of the response to other infectious agents (see Chapter 24). On the other hand there does not seem to be strong host selection for immune resistance to spontaneous tumors, presumably because most spontaneously occurring tumors arise after the host has passed the reproductive age. Thus immune surveillance may be effective against "strongly antigenic" tumors, but not against spontaneously developing tumors. In support of the above hypothesis is the observation that strongly antigenic virus-induced tumors of man are relatively rare compared with nonantigenic spontaneous tumors.

Failure of Immune Surveillance

If progressive growth of a tumor implies breakdown of an immune surveillance mechanism, then malignancy may represent a failure of the host's tumor immune defense. There are at least 12 explanations for the failure of the immune response in the tumor-bearing host (Table 29-7).

Nonantigenic Tumors

Clearly, if a given tumor does not have an antigen that can be recognized by the autochthonous host, an immune response to

Table 29-7. Factors Responsible for Failure of Immune Surveillance of Cancer

1. Lack of tumor antigen
2. Tumor antigen is not immunogenic
3. Immune tolerance to tumor antigen
4. Immunosuppression
5. Immune enhancement
6. Antigenic modulation of tumor antigen
7. Immunoselection of nonantigenic clones
8. Imbalance of tumor growth and immune response
9. Suppressor cells for tumor immunity
10. Growth of tumor in privileged site
11. Lack of self major histocompatibility complex recognition
12. Immunostimulation

the tumor will not take place. Most strong tumor antigens have been identified using virally or chemically induced tumors of animals. Such tumors are not comparable to "spontaneously occurring" human tumors. Spontaneous tumors in rodents frequently do not have demonstrable tumor antigens, and tumors that are induced with low doses of carcinogens are less immunogenic than those that are induced using higher doses. Antigenicity is not necessarily a constant feature of all tumors and, in some instances, tumor-specific antigens are undetectable even after extensive examination.

Nonimmunogenicity of Tumor Antigens in Primary (Autochthonous) Host

The tumor may contain an antigen that is recognized in another species, such as carcinoembryonic antigen, but is not immunogenic in the tumor-bearing animal. Most serologically defined tumor antigens are not able to induce an effective immune response in the autochthonous host.

Immune Tolerance

Increasing evidence shows that the primary host responds immunologically even in the face of tumor growth; this suggests that tolerance does not usually exist in the tumor-bearing animal. However, full tolerance was found to prevail in animal systems where an oncogenic virus was introduced into a fetal or newborn host capable of supporting virus proliferation and maturation. This included the RNA viruses such as mouse mammary tumor agent, murine leukemia agents of Gross, and other mouse leukemia agents. A role for tolerance in human cancer victims cannot be ruled out. (See Chapter 11.)

Immunosuppression

Increased tumor incidence has been observed in patients who have been treated with immunosuppressive drugs or who have congenital immunological deficiency disease. As stated above, tumors in immunosuppressed individuals frequently arise in the lymphoreticular system and do not necessarily imply a loss of immune surveillance in general, but may indicate an abnormality in control of lymphoid cell proliferation. Surveys have generally concluded that while patients with solid tumors may have normal ability to form antibodies, they often have an impaired delayed hypersensitivity. Even if impaired cellular immune mechanisms have no cause or effect relationship to the growth and/or development of the tumor, they have importance with respect to the problem of infectious diseases complicating cancer.

Immune Enhancement

The tumor-bearing animal may make an inappropriate immune response. Immune enhancement was described by Kaliss in 1956 as the progressive growth of normally rejected strain-specific tumors in recipients who had been pretreated either with antiserum directed against the tumor (passive enhancement) or with repeated injections of antigenic material of the tumor (active enhancement). Although first seen in allogeneic systems, enhancement has been demonstrated to occur in syngeneic transplantation models with methylcholanthrene-induced sarcomas, mammary adenocarcinomas derived from mice carrying mammary tumor virus, and possibly Moloney virus–induced lymphomas. Most of these later studies involved immunization of animals with tumor-derived materials in such a way as to induce the formation of humoral antibody, but not delayed hypersensitivity, a form of immune deviation. Transfer of tumors to such immunized recipients or to recipients injected with serum from immunized donors results in a more rapid growth than occurs in untreated tumor recipients. Growth of the tumor is enhanced in the presence of serum antibody, and such enhancement has been attributed to the presence of "blocking antibodies" (see Fig. 29-4).

Mechanisms of enhancement in relation to the immune response may be afferent, efferent, or central. Afferent inhibition implies that the recipient did not become immunized by graft antigens because the simultaneous presence of antibody prevents antigen from becoming available to immune responsive tissues. Central inhibition would occur if the host lymphoid cells failed to be stimulated, despite being presented with the antigen in a suitable immunogenic form. Efferent inhibition would apply if the recipient became immunized, but the response that resulted was ineffective against the tumor. It appears that enhancement is usually an efferent effect. In some instances, both cellular sensitivity and humoral factors are present in the autochthonous host, but a humoral factor blocks the colony-inhibiting effect of the sensitized cells (blocking factor). Although the term *blocking antibody* has been used to identify this factor, the antibody or immunoglobulin nature of the blocking factor has not been clearly established. It is possible that "blocking factor" is a complex of tumor antigen and antibody that inhibits the reaction of sensitized lymphocytes with antigen on the tumor cells, or it may be free antigen. In addition, a serum factor that can decrease the effects of blocking factor has been described and is called *unblocking factor*. Humoral factors may also cause enhanced tumor growth, either through physiological changes in the tumor cells or through stimulation of a substance produced by tumor cells that produces unresponsiveness in lymphoid cells.

Antigenic Modulation

Complete loss of antigenicity or a significant antigenic change with selective overgrowth of the changed variant is a possible mechanism of escape from immune rejection. Theoretically this escape mechanism is possible, but it has been difficult to demonstrate. Loss of the MHC antigens of one parental strain can be induced by passage of a tumor arising in an F_1 animal or in the other parental strain. Cell surface antigens of mouse

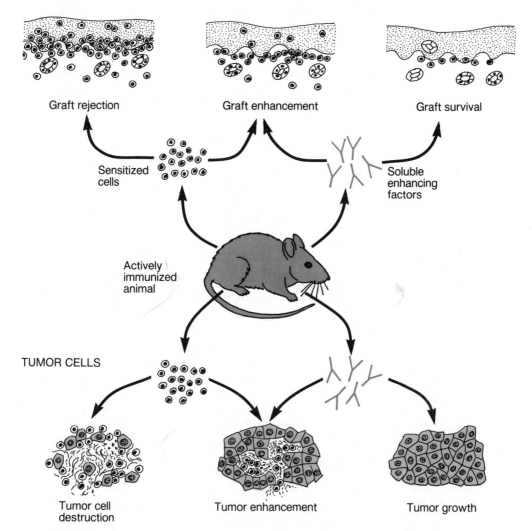

SKIN GRAFT

Graft rejection

Graft enhancement

Graft survival

Sensitized cells

Soluble enhancing factors

Actively immunized animal

TUMOR CELLS

Tumor cell destruction

Tumor enhancement

Tumor growth

Figure 29-4. Tumor enhancement: immune responses to tissue grafts and to tumors. An individual may produce two general types of immune reaction to tissue antigens: humoral antibody or delayed hypersensitivity. The eventual outcome of a tissue graft (survival or rejection) or a tumor graft (growth or rejection) depends upon the relative response. If delayed hypersensitivity is predomi-nant, then sensitized cells destroy the graft or kill the tumor cells. If humoral antibody is predominant, a foreign graft may survive and tumor cells grow. If a mixture of sensitized cells and humoral antibody is produced, the eventual out-come depends on their relative strengths. When at-tempts are made to manipulate the immune response of an individual to prolong graft survival or to promote tumor rejection, the possibility of inducing an effect opposite to that desired must be considered. Enhancing antibody is desirable for survival of a normal tissue graft, but is undesirable for growth of a malignant tumor. The effects of humoral enhanc-ing antibody may be mediated by antibody–antigen complexes in some situations.

leukemic cells, the TL antigen, may disappear after treatment of the cells with antiserum to the TL antigen but reappear after removal of the antiserum. A stable subline of a Moloney tumor that is resistant to specific antiserum to the parent tumor has been produced by incubating tumor cells in cytotoxic antiserum in the presence of complement and then inoculating these samples into preimmunized mice. These observations support the concept that tumor cells under immunological attack may be able to survive by not expressing the tumor-specific antigen to which the immune response is directed and thus thwarting immune surveillance.

Immunoselection of Nonantigenic Clones

Spontaneous tumors may produce successive clonal variants that replace each other as the tumor progresses. Each successful variant has greater autonomy and is less affected by restricting host mechanisms. In this manner the tumor may evolve, by natural selection, new clones with different antigens or nonantigenic clones that are not limited by host immune response.

Imbalance of Immunity and Tumor Mass

The ability of an immune response to protect against the continued growth of a tumor depends on the mass of the tumor that is being contained. Old and Boyse postulated that "sneaking through" of tumor cells might occur with a small number of tumor cells. In this situation, there may be insufficient antigenic stimulation to provide effective immunization until the tumor grows larger. At the higher cell number, antigenic stimulation is sufficient to provide effective immunization, which in turn prevents tumor growth. However, the presence of a large tumor mass may exhaust the supply of lymphocytes produced by the host (a form of desensitization). Most forms of immunotherapy effective in experimental animals may be overcome by a tumor of sufficient size. Immunotherapy is effective only for relatively small tumors or in preventing growth of small numbers of injected tumor cells.

Suppressor Cells

Specific suppressor cells may depress the effect of an immune response to a tumor antigen. Thus, an immune response to a tumor might result in the production not only of killer cells to the tumor but also of suppressor cells that protect the tumor by inhibiting the production of T killer cells.

Immune Privileged Site

A tumor may arise in an immunologically sheltered site, where surveillance functions play no role in antagonizing tumor development. Such a site is known to occur in the hamster cheek pouch. The hamster cheek pouch is frequently used to transplant tumors in a way that will avoid an immune reaction to the tumor. Propagation of human colonic tumors that produce CEA has been carried out using the hamster cheek pouch. It is possible that such sites may serve as a locus for the development of primary tumors that avoid immune surveillance until growth of the tumor cannot be reversed by the immune mechanism. However, a high incidence of tumors in similar sites in humans is not observed.

Lack of Self Recognition

It is possible that progression, a change in the growth potential of a given tumor, may be related to selection for cellular variants of a tumor with altered class I gene expression. The expression of MHC antigens, especially class I antigens, has been demonstrated to play an important role in the behavior of tumors in experimental models. In mice, some tumors having a TSTA, but lacking the self class I antigen H-2K, are resistant to T cell killing and readily grow when transplanted into normal syngeneic hosts. However, if these same tumors are transfected with DNA coding for the H-2K antigen and thereby induced to express the H-2K antigen, the tumors are then not transplantable. For these tumors, recognition of a TSTA in combination with self class I antigen may be needed for either induction or expression of tumor rejection (see Chapter 9). In other systems resistance to macrophage and/or natural killing may be correlated with a loss of class I antigen expression. In at least one instance of a virus-transformed cell line, low class I antigen expression may be reversed by interferon treatment. In other instances viral transfection or enhanced invasiveness of tumors is associated with increased class I antigen expression. Fibrosarcomas induced by ultraviolet (UV) irradiation tend to have increased class I antigen expression, express TSTA, and are rejected upon transplantation into syngeneic hosts. Yet UV-induced tumors grow progressively in the original UV-irradiated host. UV treatment induces suppressor components capable of specifically eliminating the T cell response against the autochthonous tumor. This suppressor effect is not demonstrable against chemically induced tumors. Thus alterations in self recognition may be important in the host–tumor immune relationship for some cancers. Yet many metastatic tumors do not have demonstrable alterations in the level or nature of the class I products expressed as compared with normal tissue.

Immunostimulation

A major premise of tumor immunology is that an immune response to a given tumor is a beneficial reaction, that is, that immune responses, particularly cellular, serve to limit or prevent tumor growth. However, Richard Prehn has argued that, in some instances, the lymphocytic infiltrate seen in tumors is actually required for early stages of tumor growth. In certain circumstances immune reactions stimulate tumor target cells rather than inhibit or kill them. This result is dependent on dose. Immune cells that kill tumor target cells in vitro when added at high killer cell–target cell ratios in vitro (100:1 is commonly used) may actually increase tumor cell growth when present in smaller relative numbers in vivo. Although the specificity of immunostimulation has been questioned, it must be considered that tumors could escape immune surveillance by immunostimulation at a critical point in their development and later become resistant to the specific inhibitory effects of immune cells.

Immunodiagnosis of Cancer

Pathologists recognize cancer tissue to be "less organized" and cancer cells to be "less differentiated" than normal tissue. During the last 20 years, there has been a growing appreciation that the morphological resemblance of cancer cells to embryonic or fetal cells is also reflected in the production of cellular macromolecules by cancer cells that are more typical of embryonic or fetal cells than of adult tissue (Fig. 29-5).

Many of these macromolecules are not only present in the cell or on the cell surface, but are also secreted into the body fluids. Measurement of these "oncodevelopmental markers" by the clinical laboratory has become increasingly important in the diagnosis of cancer. In addition, antibodies to cancer markers are being used to localize tumor tissue in vivo and to treat certain selected cancers. Some clinical applications of cancer markers are listed in Table 29-8.

Table 29-8. Some Clinical Applications of Cancer Markers

DIAGNOSIS

Serum concentration (monoclonal Ig, CEA, AFP, ectopic hormones)
Cell surface markers (homogenous surface Ig or T cell markers)
Tissue localization (CEA, other cellular markers)
Radioimmunoscintigraphy (CEA, AFP)

PROGNOSIS

Serial determination (CEA, AFP, ectopic hormones, Bence Jones protein, etc.)

THERAPY (EXPERIMENTAL)

Antibody, monoclonal antibodies (CEA, AFP, T cells, carbohydrate antigens)
Antibody–drug conjugate (ricin)
Radiolabeled antibody

CEA, carcinoembryonic antigen; AFP, α-fetoprotein.

Examples of different types of cancer markers are listed in Table 29-9. These are only a few examples of an increasingly recognized number of markers associated with cancer. In

Figure 29-5. Various oncodevelopmental markers are normally expressed at different stages of neonatal development and by proliferating tissues in the adult. The T-locus markers of the mouse and other differentiation antigens may be expressed on germinal cells and in the preimplantation embryo as well as in primitive teratocarcinomas. Oncogene products are expressed during development, and their role in cancer is under active investigation. Placental hormones, isoenzymes, and proteins may be expressed in adult tumors of testes, ovary, liver, and breast. Other markers such as α-fetoprotein and carcinoembryonic antigen are produced normally by developing liver or colonic mucosal cells, respectively, and are frequently expressed in tumors of these tissues, that is, hepatocellular carcinomas and adenocarcinomas of the colon, as well as other tumors of embryologically related tissues. Immunoglobulins and lymphocyte differentiation markers are found to be associated with lymphoproliferative tumors. Many surface glycoprotein and glycolipid carbohydrate differences are now being recognized using monoclonal antibodies. Gene rearrangements that occur normally during plasma cell development are used to identify clonality and B cell origin of "null" lymphoid tumors.

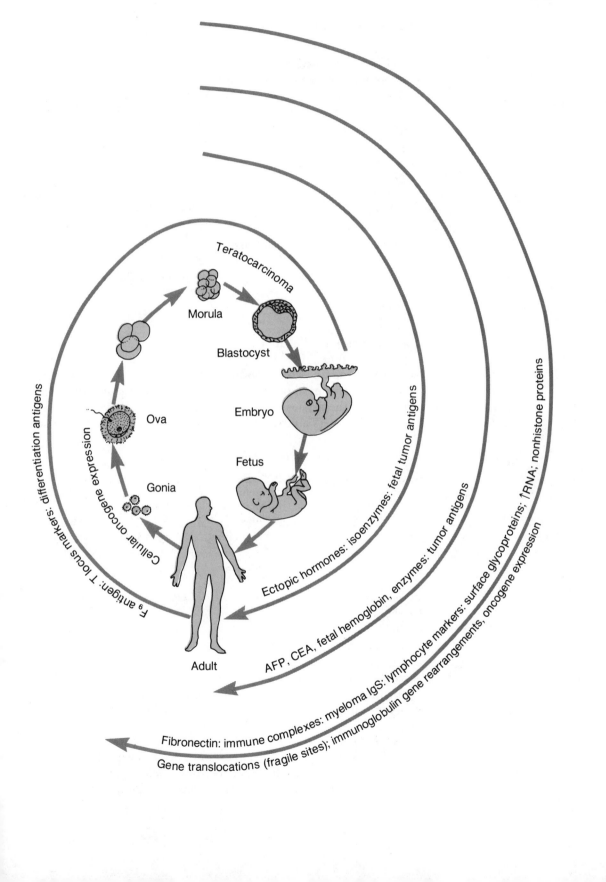

Teratocarcinoma

Morula

Blastocyst

Embryo

Fetus

Ova

Gonia

Adult

F₉ antigen: T locus markers: differentiation antigens

Cellular oncogene expression

Ectopic hormones: isoenzymes: fetal tumor antigens

AFP, CEA, fetal hemoglobin, enzymes: tumor antigens

Fibronectin: immune complexes: myeloma IgS: lymphocyte markers: surface glycoproteins; ↑RNA: nonhistone proteins

Gene translocations (fragile sites); immunoglobulin gene rearrangements, oncogene expression

Table 29-9. Types of Cancer Markers

Type	Example
Deletions of blood group markers	ABH
Exposure of backbone or blood group markers	Monosialoganglioside
Cell surface glycoproteins	Carcinoembryonic antigen
Secreted proteins	α-fetoprotein
Enzyme alterations	Glycosyltransferases
Isozymes	Alkaline phosphatase
Ectopic hormone	Human chorionic gonadotropin
Tumor antigens	Melanoma proteins identified by monoclonal antibodies
Cytoskeletal elements	Epidermal tumors (cytokeratin)
Immunoglobulin gene rearrangements	B cell tumors
Gene translocations	Lymphomas (Philadelphia chromosome)
Fragile sites	Leukemia

most, if not all, instances cancer markers are produced normally at some time during development, but are present in small or undetectable amounts in the adults. The adult tumors that produce these oncodevelopmental markers usually originate from the tissues that normally produce the markers during development (Table 29-10). For instance, tumors that arise from colonic mucosa are the most frequent producers of CEA, and the order of frequency of other cancers correlates with embryonic linkage relationships: stomach > lung > lymphoma.

Table 29-10. "Levels" of Expression of Oncodevelopmental Markers

	Production by Tumors			
Example	Normal Producing Tissue	Embryogenically Closely Related	Distantly Related	Different
Carcinoembryonic antigen	Colon	Stomach, pancreas, liver	Lung, breast	Lymphoma
α-Fetoprotein	Liver, yolk sac	Colon, stomach, pancreas	Lung	—
Serotonin	"Enteroendocrine" carcinoid	Adrenal	Oat cell lung	Epidermal lung
Chorionic gonadotropin	Placenta	Germinal tumors	Liver	Epidermal lung

Myeloma Proteins

The first cancer marker was recognized by Dr. H. Bence Jones in 1846 (see Chapter 28). Bence Jones protein was identified as a urinary precipitate that occurred upon heating at pH 4–6 the urine of a patient with "mollities ossium," a bone disease now known as multiple myeloma. It is remarkable that it took over 100 years from the first recognition of Bence Jones protein to identification of the chemical nature of this protein. It is now known that Bence Jones proteins are immunoglobulin light chains produced in excess by about half of patients with plasmacytomas, and are associated with the presence of monoclonal immunoglobulins in the serum. With application of immunoassays, the amount of Bence Jones protein found in urine or the amount of myeloma immunoglobulin in the serum may be used to follow the effects of therapy; the amount of these proteins in a given patient closely reflects the amount of myeloma tumor mass. This general principle also applies to other secreted tumor markers including hormones and serum enzymes.

Hormones and Enzymes

The extensive analysis of hormones, enzymes, and isozymes in cancer has clearly shown that cancers do not produce new or unique products. The hormones, enzymes or isozymes found are normally produced by the noncancerous tissue from which the cancer arises. However, the cancer may produce enzymes or hormones in different proportions or types than does the normal tissue, or cancers may produce isozymes normally produced by fetal or developing tissue and not by adult tissue.

Ectopic hormone production refers to the production of a hormone by a tumor that arises from an endocrine organ that usually does not produce that hormone (Table 29-11). How-

Table 29-11. Some Paraendocrine Syndromes Associated with Ectopic Hormone Production

Aberration	Hormone	Source
Hypercalcemia	PTH	Bronchogenic, pancreatic, and breast CA
Hypokalemia	ACTH	Apudomas
Diarrhea	VIP	Pancreatic CA, apudomas
Gynecomastia, precocious puberty	hCG	Pancreatic, gastric, and liver CA
Erythrocytosis	ERP	Lung and renal CA
Achromegaly	GH	Breast, lung, and stomach CA

PTH, parathyroid hormone; ACTH, adrenocorticotropic hormone; VIP, vasoactive intestinal polypeptide; hCG, human chorionic gonadotropin; ERP, erythropoietin; GH, growth hormone; CA, carcinoma.

ever, the tumor usually arises from a common lineage of cell types responsible for endocrine organ development. Symptoms related to excess ectopic production of a hormone are known as *paraendocrine syndromes.*

Enzyme levels in blood, with some notable exceptions, such as acid and alkaline phosphatase for prostatic cancer, are not diagnostic of cancer but may be elevated in cancer patients.

The enzyme content of hematopoietic cancer cells (leukemias and lymphomas) is helpful in determining the type of leukemia (Table 29-12).

Table 29-12. Enzymatic Reactions in Hematopathology

Enzyme	Common Use
Leukocyte alkaline phosphatase	Elevated in benign granulocytic proliferations, depressed in malignant granulocytic tumors
Acid phosphatase	Present in myeloid and monocytoid cells; T lymphocytes show particular pattern of acid phosphatase positivity
Chloroacetate esterase	Specific for granulocyte lineage
Myeloperoxidase	Specific for granulocyte lineage
Nonspecific esterase	Specific for cells of the monocyte series
Terminal deoxytransferase	Immature T and B lymphocytes

α-Fetoprotein

The modern era of cancer markers began with the discovery of α-fetoprotein by G. I. Abelev of the Soviet Union in 1963. He identified this protein in the sera of normal fetal mice and in the sera of adult mice with hepatocellular carcinoma, but not in normal adult mice. α-Fetoprotein (AFP) is an antigenically distinct serum protein with properties similar to those of albumin. It is found in high concentrations (up to 10 mg/ml) in fetal serum and in the serum of patients with hepatocellular or teratocarcinomas, but in low (< 10 ng/ml) concentrations in sera of adults. Elevations up to 500 ng/ml occur frequently in association with a variety of nonmalignant diseases, but elevations above this level are essentially diagnostic of an AFP-producing tumor (Table 29-13). Approximately half of the patients with

Table 29-13. Elevation of α-Fetoprotein in Patients with Various Diseases

Diagnosis	Percentage		
	> 10 μg/ml	> 320 μg/ml	> 400 μg/ml
Hepatocellular carcinoma	90	74	69
Other nongerminal carcinoma	20	1.5	0
Cirrhosis	34	1.4	0
Hepatitis	58	5	1
HBsAG[a] carriers	23	0	0

[a] HBsAg, hepatitis B surface antigen.

hepatocellular carcinoma may be diagnosed by such an elevation. Serial determinations of AFP may be used clinically to determine the effectiveness of therapy (Fig. 29-6). Failure of elevated serum AFP to return to normal after surgery is an indication that the tumor has not been completely removed or

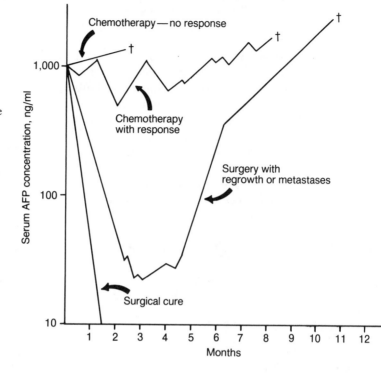

Figure 29-6. Representative responses of serum α-fetoprotein to therapy. Changes in serum concentration of α-fetoprotein correlate with growth of an α-fetoprotein–producing tumor and reflect the response to therapy.

that metastases are present. These patterns essentially hold true for other cancer markers found in the serum.

The amount of carbohydrate on AFP depends upon the level of glycosylating enzymes in fetal and tumor tissue. These enzymes differ in normal liver, yolk sac, and hepatocellular carcinomas. Differences in glycosylation of AFP can be measured by binding of AFP to the lectins concanavalin A (ConA) and lens culinaris lectin (LCA). Benign liver proliferation results in completely glycosylated AFP, which binds to LCA at a high percentage and to ConA at a low percentage. Hepatocellular carcinomas show heterogeneous binding patterns due to incomplete glycosylation, so that ratios of the percentage of AFP binding to ConA to the percentage binding to LCA are usually below 0.2 in cord serum and in patients with AFP elevations associated with benign liver disease (completely glycosylated), whereas in hepatocellular carcinomas ConA/LCA binding ratios are above 0.2 (incompletely glycosylated). ConA/LCA ratios are now being evaluated in regard to increasing the discrimination of serum AFP elevations in benign and malignant liver disease, as well as determining open spinal cord defects.

In animals exposed to chemical carcinogens, serum AFP elevations occur many months before cancer develops. The implication of this experimental observation in regard to identifying precancerous exposure of humans to chemical hepato-carcinogens remains undetermined.

Carcinoembryonic Antigen

Carcinoembryonic antigen is a cell surface glycoprotein that is normally produced by colonic epithelium and secreted in the intestine. In colonic and other cancers, alteration in the polarity of cells is associated with release of CEA in elevated levels into the blood. During development, CEA is produced by the fetal gastrointestinal tract; elevations of CEA associated with cancers in the adult reflect the developmental relationship to gastrointestinal tissue. CEA elevations also occur in association with nonmalignant diseases, so that elevated serum CEA can be used only as an adjunct to other diagnostic procedures (Table 29-14). In patients with colorectal cancer who have elevated

Table 29-14. Carcinoembryonic Antigen Concentrations in Human Sera

Type of Patient	Number of Patients Tested	Percentage			
		0–2.5 ng/ml	2.6–5.0 ng/ml	5.1–10 ng/ml	10 ng/ml
Healthy subjects					
Nonsmokers	892	97	3	0	0
Smokers	620	81	15	3	1
Colorectal carcinoma	544	28	23	14	35
Pulmonary carcinoma	181	24	25	25	26
Pancreatic carcinoma	55	9	31	25	35
Gastric carcinoma	79	39	32	10	19
Breast carcinoma	125	53	20	13	14
Other carcinoma	343	51	28	12	9
Benign breast disease	115	85	11	4	0
Severe alcoholic cirrhosis	120	29	44	25	2
Active ulcerative colitis	146	69	18	8	5
Pulmonary emphysema	49	43	37	16	4

Modified from Go V: Carcinoembryonic antigen. Cancer 37:562–566, 1976.

serum CEA the serum levels may be used to determine the effectiveness of therapy. Unfortunately, reelevation of CEA has not proven useful as an indication for "second-look" surgery. CEA levels in breast cancer become elevated when metastases occur, and serial CEA determinations are useful for determining effectiveness of chemotherapy, for determining prognosis, and to measure progression of the disease.

Radiolabeled antibodies to AFP and CEA have been used to localize clandestine tumors by radioimmunoscintigraphy. Labeled antibodies are injected into patients and localization of the label in tissues is determined by scanning the body for radioactivity. Accuracy of diagnosis has been improved by application of computer analysis to the photoscans. Primary cancers have been localized in 83% of colorectal cancer, and in 22% of patients cancer sites were located that no other detection method had found. In experimental systems, it has been shown that AFP is also taken up by some cancers in mice and that localization of selected tumors using radiolabeled AFP and scintigraphy is possible. Extension of this system to humans is under study.

Antibodies to CEA and AFP have also been used to treat tumors producing these markers in animals. So far the results, even when drugs such as daunomycin have been attached to the antibodies, have been equivocal. Trials in humans are not yet interpretable as being effective.

Mixed Markers

Since some tumors may produce more than one marker, the simultaneous measurement of more than one marker often provides information leading to a more precise diagnosis or prognosis than that using one marker alone. For instance, differentiation of germ cell tumor types can be accomplished on the basis of elevation of serum AFP or human chorionic gonadotropin (hCG) (Table 29-15). Similarly the significance of mea-

Table 29-15. hCG and AFP in Germ Cell Tumors

	hCG	AFP
Seminoma	−	−
Embryonal	+	+
Choriocarcinoma	+	−
Yolk sac	−	+
Teratoma	−	−

hCG, human chorionic gonadotropin; AFP, α-fetoprotein.

suring other mixtures of tumor markers, for instance CEA, AFP, tissue polypeptide antigen, and/or ectopic hormones, is being analyzed at several centers.

Other Tumor Markers

A number of other human tumor markers detected by antisera are listed in Table 29-16. Many of these have been tested and found lacking in their ability to diagnose or determine prognosis of cancer. Others such as melanoma-associated antigen have been chemically characterized but not applied systematically to the diagnosis of cancer. Pancreatic oncofetal antigen has shown promising preliminary evidence of being useful diagnostically and prognostically. Prostate antigen detected in tissue sections is useful in determining the origin of metastatic lesions.

Monoclonal Antibodies to Cancer Markers

The third era of cancer markers is now upon us. The development of monoclonal antibodies to "cancer antigens" is producing a new generation of "cancer markers." An example of the types of reactivity is illustrated by monoclonal antibodies to melanomas. Some monoclonal antibodies react only with the immunizing tumor; some with most melanomas, but not with other tumors; and some with most melanomas as well as many other cancers. Monoclonal antibodies to melanoma, neuro-

Table 29-16. Some Serologically Defined Human Tumor Markers

Name	Immunogen	Antiserum	Test Used	Tumor Tissue	Fetal Tissue
Oncofetal antigen	Colon CA, metastases	Rabbit	Diffusion, fluorescence	Many types	Epithelial, placenta
Carcinofetal ferritin	Fetal liver	Rabbit	Diffusion	Many	Liver
γ-Fetoprotein		Mammary CA patient	Diffusion	Many	Serum and some tissues
Fetal gut antigen	Fetal gut	Rabbit	Diffusion	GI CA (32%)	GI
Fetal sulfoglycoprotein	Gastric CA	Rabbit	Diffusion, fluorescence	CI CA	GI
Melanoma-associated antigen	Tumor	Rabbit	Precipitation, SDS–PAGE	Melanoma (240K), carcinoma (95K)	Melanocytes
Melanoma fetal antigen		Melanoma patients	Cytotoxicity	Melanomas	Skin, brain
Pancreatic cancer–associated antigen	Pancreatic CA–ascitic fluid	Rabbit	Diffusion, ELISA	Pancreas, stomach, others	Pancreas, stomach
Pancreatic oncofetal antigen	Fetal pancreas	Rabbit	Diffusion, rocket	Pancreas, others	Pancreas, others
Pregnancy-specific protein 1	Placenta extracts	Rabbit	Diffusion, ELISA	Trophoblastic germ cell	Pregnancy sera, etc.
Prostate antigen	Prostate	Rabbit	Diffusion	Prostate CA	Prostate (BPH)
Tissue polypeptide antigen	Tumors	Horse	Fluorescence, cytotoxicity	Various	Placenta, growing cells

CA, carcinoma; GI, gastrointestinal; SDS–PAGE, sodium dodecyl sulfate–polyacrylamide gel electrophoresis; ELISA, enzyme-linked immunoabsorbent assay; BPH, benign prostate hypertrophy.

blastoma, glioma, colorectal (CEA), liver (AFP), prostate (prostate specific antigen), lung, breast, and lymphoid tissue are being used to localize the respective antigen in tumor tissue by immunoperoxidase procedures. A monoclonal antibody to the major antigenic protein of melanomas is now being tested in therapeutic trials, as is a monoclonal antibody to T cells for selected T cell tumors (see Chapter 26). The selectivity of hybridoma techniques for producing monoclonal antibodies to tumor antigens could revolutionize the field of cancer markers in the next few years. Some human glycoprotein antigens identified by monoclonal antibodies now being actively studied are listed in Table 29-17. The results of this approach are awaited

Table 29-17. Some Human Glycoprotein "Cancer Antigens" Detected by Monoclonal Antibodies

Melanoma	240–250K	Melanomas, gliomas
	80, 94, 95, 97K	Melanomas, gliomas, normal
Glioma	20K	Gliomas, neuroblastomas
	S-100	Melanomas, gliomas
Breast	Milk globulin protein	CA, normal
	DF3 (290K)	Secretory cells
	MCF7	CA, normal
Pancreas	Dupan series (30, 70, 110, 200K)	Pancreatic, colon CA
Lung	600 series	Small cell CA, others
Prostate	αPro 3 (1200K)	Prostate, BPH, testicular
	αPro 13 (1400K)	Ductal
Kidney	S series (115, 120, 160K)	Renal, ovarian CA, normal kidney

K = 1000; CA, carcinoma; BPH, benign prostatic hypertrophy.

with great anticipation as many new monoclonal antibodies are produced and applications attempted.

Lymphoid Tumors

The application of monoclonal antibodies to lymphocyte differentiation antigens is changing the method of classification of lymphoid tumors. A brief description of monoclonal antibodies applied to diagnosis and therapy of lymphomas is presented in Chapter 28.

Cytoskeletal Elements

Monoclonal antibodies to cytoskeletal elements have been used to identify the cellular origin of cancers by immunohistochemistry (Table 29-18). Glial fibrillary acidic protein (GFAP) is

Table 29-18. Cytoskeletal Elements in Cancer

Element	Distribution	
	Normal	In Cancer
Prekeratin	Epithelial cells	Epithelial cancers
Glial fibrillary acidic protein	Astrocytes	Astrocytic tumors
Neurofilaments	Neural cells	Neuroblastomas, pheochromocytomas
Vimentin	Mesenchymal cells	Sarcomas, lymphomas
Desmin	Muscle	Myosarcomas

a major component of the intermediate filaments of astrocytes and appears to be useful for diagnosis of astrocyte neoplasms and mixed glial tumors as it is not found in epidermoid tumors, meningiomas, or other nonastrocytic brain tumors. Prekeratin, in the form of intermediate-sized filaments, is found exclusively in cells of epidermal origin and may be used immunohistochemically to identify cancer cells of epithelial origin. Neurofilament antigens are found in neuroblastomas and pheochromocytomas, vimentin in sarcomas and lymphomas.

Cell Surface Carbohydrates

Oligosaccharides on the surface of mammalian cells are attached to lipid (glycosphingolipid, GSL) or protein (glycoprotein, GP). The lipid or protein is hydrophobic and is located in the cell membrane, whereas the oligosaccharide is hydrophilic and extends from the cell surface, where it is readily accessible for reaction with antibody.

For GSL the terminal hydroxyl group of ceramide in the cell membrane is linked to glucose and additional monosaccharides are added by action of a series of membrane-bound glycosyltransferases, which join the anomeric carbon of one monosaccharide to one of the hydroxyl groups of another monosaccharide. In addition, carbohydrates may be removed by glycosidases, which cleave carbohydrates from glycoproteins after glycosylation. For GP the oligosaccharides are linked to membrane proteins through a glycosamine bond between *N*-acetylglucosamine and asparagine or between *N*-acetylgalactosamine and serine or threonine.

Of the more than 100 possible monosaccharides only 7 make up the oligosaccharides of the mammalian cell surface:

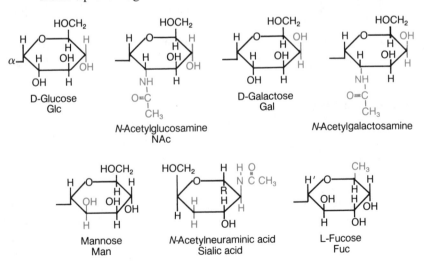

ity of cells. The composition and linkage of these polysaccharides provide numerous epitopes that may be recognized by monoclonal antibodies. Many "new" or tumor-related GSL and GP have been identified using monoclonal antibodies. The use of formalin-fixed tissue to screen for monoclonal antibody reactivity results in selection for monoclonal antibodies that react with carbohydrate antigens, since carbohydrates are preserved better than proteins after formalin fixation.

The appearance of "new" cell surface carbohydrates on cancer cells may be due to (1) the synthesis of different oligosaccharides by tumor cells, (2) the postsynthetic modification by glycolytic enzymes, or (3) the "unmasking" of cell surface carbohydrates by shedding or loss of masking cell surface material. The changes found in cell surface carbohydrates in tumor cells as compared to normal cells are usually secondary to changes in activity or levels of glycosylating enzymes or glycosidases in cancer cells. In the figures that follow the arrows indicate structural relations and do not necessarily imply synthetic pathways.

Neutral Glycolipids. Changes in triceramide expression in cancer cells were probably recognized as early as 1929 by Witebsky using conventional antisera (cytolipid H). Tumor associated changes in glycolipids occur in triceramide and in Forssman antigen expression. The triceramide antigen PK is not normally expressed in lymphoid or epithelial tissue, but may be found in human basophil leukemia and in many human colonic, gastric, and hepatic carcinomas. An abnormal triceramide, where the terminal saccharide is *N*-acetylgalactosamine, is found in some mouse tumors. Human tissues generally do not express Forssman antigen; however, many human cancers have detectable Forssman antigen (gastrointestinal tract, lung, etc).

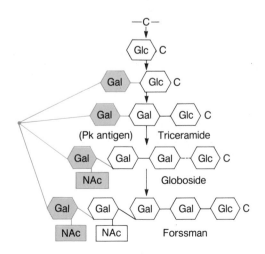

Blood Group Substances. The expression in cancers of oligo-saccharides that make up blood group substances is very complex.

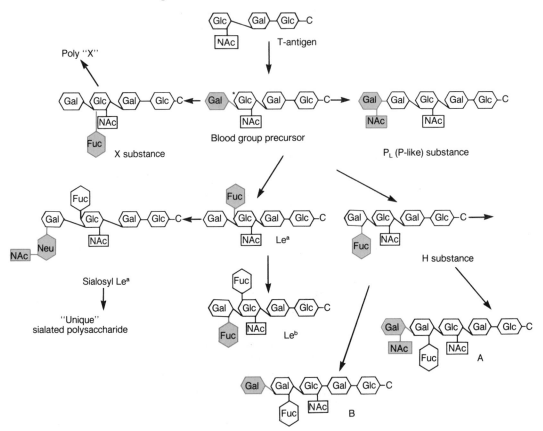

Three possibilities exist: (1) The expression of a normal blood group such as A or B blood group antigen in a tumor of a tissue that normally does not express that blood group, (2) the loss of expression of a blood group antigen in tissue that normally does express it, and (3) the appearance of an "abnormal" antigen or "new" antigens produced by addition of monosaccharides not normally found in the blood group pathway. Examples are T antigen, P-like substance, sialosyl Lea, X substance, poly X substance, and "unique sialylated mucin polysaccharide" as well as the presence of blood group precursor substance, group A or group B determinants, in tumor tissue derived from tissues that normally do not contain these determinants.

Gangliosides. Certain monoclonal antibodies identify GSL in the ganglioside series. These antibodies have a high degree of specificity for terminal sialic acid residues (NAcNeu). In addition, these particular "antigens" are found in fetal tissues and in tumors. Some of the first antigens in this series to be identified

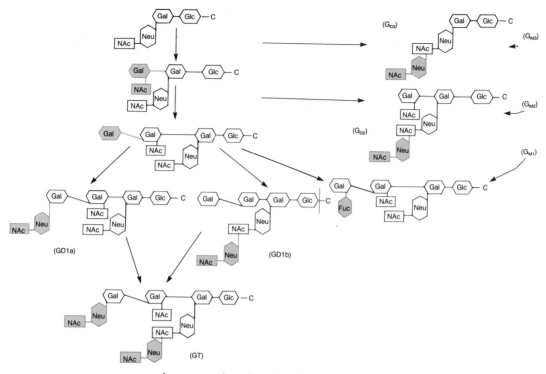

by monoclonal antibodies were in fact called OFAI-1 (GM2) and OFAI-2 (GD2) (OFA is an abbreviation for *oncofetal antigen*).

The expression of ganglioside as well as other oligosaccharide "antigens" on tumor cells generally falls into the category of "oncodevelopmental antigens." This expression is secondary to the "development" or presence of the glycosylating enzymes and glycosidases in developing, normal adult, and cancerous cells. GD3, GM1, and the terminal 4NAcNeu residue (Hanganitziu–Deicher antigen) have also been identified on cancer cells using monoclonal antibodies.

Cancer Markers of the Future

Chromosomal Translocations

In 1960 Nowell and Hungerford described the classic finding of a translocation of one arm of chromosome 22 to chromosome 9 (or 6) in the cells of patients with chronic granulocytic leukemia (CGL). The smaller chromosome 22 become known as the Philadelphia chromosome (Ph') and may be used as a marker for CGL cells. An acute blastic crisis in which a rapid increase in leukemic cells occurs in the peripheral blood may be predicted by an increase in the number of marrow cells containing Ph'. In Burkitt's lymphoma a portion of chromosome 8 containing the *myc* oncogene is translocated to chromosome 14 (or less often to 2 or 22). There are other tumors associated with detectable translocations (Table 29-19) and some investigators feel, with justification, that all tumors would contain some chromosomal abnormalities if we had the appropriate methodology to detect them.

Table 29-19. Some Abnormal Karyotypes in Neoplasms

Cancer	Chromosomal Abnormality
Chronic myelogenous leukemia	Philadelphia chromosome, 22 → 9 translocation
Meningioma	22 missing in 50%
Benign parotid tumor	3 → 8 translocation
Ovarian cystadenocarcinoma	6 → 14 translocation
Retinoblastoma	13 deletion
Wilm's tumor	11 deletion
Renal cell carcinoma	3 → 8 translocation
Burkitt's lymphoma	8 → 14 (or 2 or 22) translocation

Immunoglobulin Gene Rearrangements

The presence of immunoglobulin gene arrangements in lymphomas may give evidence of B cell lineage even if the tumor cells do not produce cytoplasmic or surface monoclonal Ig. Immunoglobulin gene rearrangements that result in splicing out of an intervening DNA sequence have been associated with maturation of B cells and the ability to produce Ig (see Chapter 10). However, some gene rearrangements are not associated with the capacity to synthesize Ig, but are still believed to be characteristic of B cells. Some non-Ig-producing null cell lymphomas demonstrate gene rearrangements, whereas others do not. The finding of Ig gene rearrangements in a null cell tumor indicates (1) that the cell line is monoclonal and therefore probably neoplastic, and (2) that the tumor is most likely of B cell origin. Studies on rearrangement of Ig genes and T cell receptor genes in T cell lymphomas are now underway (see Chapter 28).

Fragile Sites

Many cells from human cancers, when cultured in vitro in folic acid deficient medium, show "breaks" in the chromosomes when examined by high-resolution banding techniques. The location of these "fragile sites" appears to correlate with the type of malignancy. Although breaks are also found in normal chromosomes, these occur in a scattered fashion and in a smaller number of cells, whereas most cancer cells have a consistent site of breakage. Preliminary evidence suggests that cancer-associated fragile sites may also be found in normal cells of patients with cancer. A hypothesis now being tested is that "cancer-prone" individuals may also have such fragile sites.

Oncogenes

Confirmation of the prediction made in 1969 by Heubner and Todaro that genetic structures or rearrangements associated with cancer in animals (oncogenes) are also present in at least some human cancers raises the possibility of applying this property of cancer cells to diagnosis. Although there is already evidence that expression of oncogenes or gene rearrangements (which are well documented in leukemias) are not uniformly found in all cancers, the observations so far are promising. Perhaps cDNA probes for oncogenes (see Table 27-5), the ability of DNA from cancer cells to transform tissue culture cell in vitro, or restriction endonuclease analysis of transforming sequences activated in neoplastic cells might be applied to DNA derived from human tumors as a diagnostic procedure. This, of course, cannot be expected to occur in the near future.

In Summary
Cancer markers include secreted proteins, cell surface molecules, hormones, enzymes and isozymes, and cytoplasmic constituents. These are usually identified by heteroantisera, monoclonal antibodies, or biochemical properties. Cancer markers may be used for diagnosis, prognosis, or therapy. The most useful cancer markers are monoclonal immunoglobulins, α-fetoprotein, and carcinoembryonic antigen. Although the clinical applications of AFP and CEA have not fulfilled all the optimistic expectations that many predicted, these markers have achieved a place in cancer diagnosis and management. Many other cancer markers have not been nearly as useful, and the verdict has not yet been returned on several now being studied. Claims of a universal cancer marker have been made repeatedly, but have not been fulfilled. However, the availability of new hybridoma and immunoassay technology, such as enzyme-linked immunosorbent assays and flow cytometry, may justify a new wave of excitement. Identification of cancer markers by monoclonal antibodies offers an exciting opportunity not available with previous approaches. Recognition of abnormal expression of products produced normally by adult or fetal tissues appears to hold more promise in tumor diagnosis than identification of tumor specific markers. It is possible that molecular probes for human oncogenes or gene rearrangements might become a diagnostic approach in the future. A continued search for new tumor markers is more than justified by the tremendous potential for clinical applications.

Immunoprophylaxis of Cancer

The goal of many immunologists, some of whom were eminently successful in producing vaccines for infectious diseases, has been to produce a "cancer vaccine" that could prevent tumors in man. Popularization of a possible viral origin of cancer in man led to enthusiasm that a prophylactic tumor vaccine could be produced. This enthusiasm arises because tumors caused by viruses share common antigens. Proper immunization might produce an immune response that would prevent development of primary tumors caused by oncogenic viruses. Such vaccination has been effective in controlling virus-induced tumors of animals, such as Marek's disease of chickens and feline leukemia. However, although oncogenic viruses are widely disseminated in many animal species and presumably also in humans, there is little evidence for a common viral origin of most human tumors. Therefore, prophylactic immunization against human tumors will remain unfulfilled until a relatively common tumor human antigen can be identified, isolated, and tested for immunogenicity. The most likely possibilities now are in the virus-related tumors such as Burkitt's lymphoma (Epstein–Barr virus), adult T cell leukemia (HTLV-I), hepatitis B virus, and perhaps AIDS-related viruses.

Nonspecific prophylaxis may also prove feasible, but the effect of this type of prophylaxis is also subject to doubt. As described in detail below, certain agents serve to stimulate nonspecifically the reticuloendothelial system and, in particular, the phagocytic capacity of macrophages. One of the agents is bacillus Calmette–Guérin (BCG), a strain of *Myocobacterium bovis*. This is an attenuated organism that has been used as a vaccine for the prevention of human tuberculosis. It has been claimed that death from leukemia is half as common among BCG-vaccinated children as among nonvaccinated children. However, this exciting result has not been confirmed. Until clarified, this must be considered an isolated report.

Immunotherapy of Cancer

Immunotherapy of cancer is defined as any immune procedure that adversely affects the growth of an established tumor. Such immune procedures may be specific or nonspecific. Specific

Table 29-20. Immunotherapeutic Approaches to Human Cancer

Approach	Status
SPECIFIC	
Active	
Autologous tumor cells	Not effective
Autologous tumor extracts	Not effective
Passive Cellular	
Autologous lymphocytes	Not effective
Allogeneic lymphocytes	Some effect in bone marrow transplant recipients
Autologous stimulated lymphocytes	Clinical trials underway
Cytotoxic cell lines	Experimental
Transfer factor	Not effective
Immune RNA	Not effective
Passive Humoral	
Xenogenic antisera	Not effective
Monoclonal antibodies	Clinical trials underway
Anti-idiotypic antibody	Experimental, clinical trials underway
NONSPECIFIC	
BCG, *Corynebacterium parvum*	Clinical trials, limited effectiveness
Mycobacterial extracts	Experimental
Levamisole, polynucleotides	Experimental
DNCB	Established for selected skin cancers
Interferon	Clinical trials underway
Interleukin 2	Clinical trials underway
Tumor necrosis factor	Experimental

BCG, Bacillus Calmette–Guerin; DNCB, dinitrochlorobenzene.

immunotherapy involves the use of tumor-specific antigens for immunization, whereas nonspecific therapy involves procedures that increase the activity of the effector arm of the rejection response in a manner that does not involve the use of specific antigen (Table 29-20). Specific immunotherapy may be accomplished by active or passive immunization. Currently underway are clinical trials of specific passive immunotherapy using monoclonal antibodies and nonspecific immunotherapy using interferon and interleukin 2.

Active Immunization

Several requirements exist: the tumor must possess tumor-specific transplantation antigen(s) or tumor-associated antigen(s), the host must be able to recognize these antigens, there must be an effective means of immunizing the host against the tumor to produce an immune response that results in tumor cell destruction, and a small tumor mass must be treated because immune reactions cannot be expected to affect a large tumor. Autogenous human tumor vaccines using cells prepared from the tumor to be treated have generally been unsatisfactory. A variety of methods to accomplish immunization against the tumor have been attempted, including injection of living or killed tumor cells and coupling of cell extracts with chemical haptens or foreign proteins, in the hope that some postulated cancer specific antigen may be rendered more immunogenic. Attempts have also been made to immunize a patient with tumors from other patients. This therapy rests on the assumption that specific tumor antigens might be common to the cancers of other individuals. In humans, these approaches have been unsuccessful, but in animal models, where experimental conditions and time of immunization can be modified, some encouraging results have been observed. Caution must be exercised in attempts to immunize human patients actively, because the effects may be the opposite of those desired if blocking factors, tolerance, and/or suppressor cells are produced that might cause increased growth of the tumor.

Passive Immunization

Cellular

Requirements for passive immunization include a donor of serum or cells that recognize tumor antigens but not the recipient's normal tissue, and a donor immune response that is effective in destroying tumor cells. Tumor-bearing animals may be successfully treated with specifically sensitized lymphocytes against cancer tissue in selected model systems. However, the results of such procedures in humans have not been satisfactory. One major difficulty that is encountered in human passive immunotherapy is that of obtaining cells that react immunologically to tumors in numbers sufficient to effect an antitumor response, but not to normal tissues. Passive immunotherapy using large numbers of autologous cultured lymphocytes has been attempted, but the immune potential of such cells has not been documented and the results are equivocal. However, since immune cells may have marked specificity for tumor cells and be active against a small tumor load while chemotherapy and radiotherapy can destroy a large tumor load but are limited because of nonspecificity, the combination of passive immunotherapy with radiation or chemotherapy might prove effective in some instances. In addition, the use of autochthonous lymphoid cells nonspecifically activated in vitro is being attempted (see below). The use of transfer factor and "immune RNA" as a means of converting nonimmune lymphocytes to specifically reactive cells has not yielded positive results.

Cultured NK cells, T cells, or T cell lines with cytotoxic activity to cancer cells are now available because of the ability of cultured cells to respond to antigenic stimulation in vitro and to produce long-lived clones in the presence of T cell growth factors such as IL1. In addition, cytotoxic activity and proliferation may be induced in vitro by treatment of cultured lymphocytes with IL2 or lectins. The ability to obtain "activated" killer cells or cell lines from cultures of lymphocytes from a given patient permits passive specific immunotherapy using cells that will not be rejected or produce graft versus host disease (see below). Particularly noteworthy would be the ability to produce a cell line from a given patient that could be passively transferred back to the patient and induce regression of cancer. In experimental models it has been possible to achieve eradication of disseminated cancer by infusion of tumor-specific cultured T cell clones.

Humoral

Monoclonal Antibodies. Passive transfer of conventional antibodies has not been successful for treatment of human cancer. With the development of hybridoma techniques the possibility of application of monoclonal antibodies as a new specific mode of cancer therapy for treatment of human cancers arose. As described above, under Cancer Markers and in Chapter 28, many monoclonal antibodies to human tumor-associated antigens are now available and theoretically could be used to treat human cancers. In an experimental model of leukemia, monoclonal antibodies have significantly prolonged survival of tumor-bearing mice, and anecdotal cases have been reported of prolonged remissions of some B and T cell tumors in humans (see Chapter 28). However, so far the results of phase I and phase II clinical trials have been disappointing, but the conditions of these trials are not optimal to demonstrate therapeutic effectiveness. Problems limiting the application of monoclonal antibodies and possible approaches to circumvent these problems are listed in Table 29-21. These approaches are now being used in both experimental animal models and clinical trials. A

Table 29-21. Problems and Possible Solutions to Monoclonal Antibody Immunotherapy of Cancer in Man

Problem	Possible Solution
1. Tumors not antigenic	Use of immune enhancing mechanisms (adjuvants, carriers, etc.)
2. Tumor antigens present in normal tissue	Selection of monoclonal antibodies that selectively react with tumor tissue
3. Presence of circulating free tumor antigen	Increasing doses of antibody to "clear" antigen
4. Modulation of tumor antigen	Use of mixtures (cocktails) or different antibodies sequentially
5. Selection of nonexpressing clones	Use of mixtures (cocktails) or different antibodies sequentially
6. Immune response to foreign (mouse) monoclonal antibody	Use of human hybridomas to produce human monoclonal antibodies
7. Lack of cytotoxic effect of monoclonal antibody	Selection of cytotoxic monoclonal antibodies; conjugation of cytotoxic drugs to monoclonal antibodies

recommended strategy for production, testing, and application of monoclonal antibodies is given in Table 29-22.

Table 29-22. Strategy for Development of Monoclonal Antibodies for Use in Human Immunotherapy of Cancer

1. Identification of "antigen" in cancer tissue, not detectable or present in low amounts in normal tissue
2. Production of hybridoma cell line producing monoclonal antibodies to tumor antigen
3. Selection of monoclonal antibody that binds and kills tumor cells in vitro, not toxic to normal cells
4. Isolation and characterization of monoclonal antibody
5. Demonstration of tumor binding and cytotoxic effect in vivo (nude mice bearing transplantable tumor)
6. Evaluation in clinical trials (Phase I and II)

Development of a potential therapeutic monoclonal antibody requires thorough testing of the antibody in vitro and in animal model systems. The antibody should show relative specific binding to tumor cells and not normal cells and be able to kill tumor cells in vitro. It should localize and show some killing or growth retardation of tumor cells in animals. This latter effect is now tested by determining the effect of a monoclonal antibody on the growth of transplantable human cancers in nude mice. If a promising monoclonal antibody makes it through the steps in Table 29-22 and yet has no clearly demonstrable effect in clinical trials, further strategies to increase effectiveness include drug conjugation and use of mixtures of monoclonal antibodies. If a toxic drug is conjugated to a monoclonal antibody it is necessary to repeat steps 3–6 in Table

29-22. Of particular importance is to test whether or not the drug–antibody conjugate is more effective than drug alone, monoclonal antibody alone, or mixtures of drug and unconjugated monoclonal antibody. If mixtures of monoclonal antibodies are used, steps 3, 5, and 6 must be repeated. The expense in time and money of these approaches is enormous. Because of this it will be some time before it can be determined if definitive monoclonal antibody treatment of human cancer will become generally available. At the time of this writing no proven reproducible therapeutic reagent is available.

Anti-idiotypic Antibodies. Anti-idiotypic antibodies may also have a role in passive immunotherapy. Anti-idiotypic antibodies raised in rabbits to a mouse monoclonal antibody to human melanoma antigen p97 have been used to immunize mice to the idiotope. The immunized mice demonstrated delayed hypersensitivity when challenged with human melanoma cells. Similar anti-idiotypic antibodies have been induced in humans to antigens of human gastrointestinal tumors by inoculation with mouse monoclonal antibodies. The presence of similar anti-idiotypic antibodies in human sera is associated with long-term remissions in some patients. Thus it is possible that induction of an anti-idiotypic antibody with the internal image of the tumor antigen may be beneficial to the host. How this antibody could effect tumor growth remains unexplained.

Nonspecific Immunity

Nonspecific immunity was first recognized as an acquired cellular resistance to microbial infections in animals whose mononuclear phagocytes have an apparently increased capacity to destroy microorganisms. This capacity is established by inoculation of a variety of agents, including bacillus Calmette–Guérin (BCG), *Listeria monocytogenes, Corynebacterium parvum* endotoxin, pseudomonas vaccine, levamisole, mycobacterial extracts, and polynucleotides. For instance, an animal that has been inoculated with BCG develops an increased resistance to infection by unrelated organisms, which lasts for about 1 month. It has been postulated that such activation might also be operative against tumors.

Bacillus Calmette–Guérin

In experimental studies, stimulation with BCG of guinea pigs bearing transplantable hepatomas may result in complete destruction of the tumor. This response is most effective when BCG is injected directly into the tumor. Intradermal inoculation of the transplantable tumor results in local growth followed by metastases to the draining lymph node. After intralesional injection of BCG, there is not only total regression of the injected tumor but also regression of the growth in the lymph node. Both the tumor and the draining lymph node contain acid-fast bacilli and markedly increased numbers of macrophages. It is postulated that the tumor cells are destroyed because of the active host response to the injected BCG.

A number of studies in man suggest that in certain circumstances, inoculation of BCG may be effective in reducing tumor growth. BCG injected directly into melanoma nodules of patients with tuberculin sensitivity caused regression of some tumor nodules. Similar results have been obtained with metastatic breast tumors, basal cell tumors of the skin, and other solid tumor nodules. However, extensive clinical trials have not provided convincing evidence that BCG treatment is successful for noncutaneous tumors. There is no documented controlled study demonstrating that remission duration or survival in patients receiving BCG is longer than with other forms of therapy.

Other agents that may nonspecifically activate or potentiate a host response to a tumor include a variety of microorganisms such as *C. parvum* and subcellular fractions of BCG (see Chapter 27) as well as nonbacterial macromolecules (polynucleotides). However, the clinical efficacy of these agents has also not convincingly been demonstrated.

Dinitrochlorobenzene

Successful local therapy of tumors limited to the skin may be effected by elicitation of local contact dermatitis reactions to skin-sensitizing haptens such as dinitrochlorobenzene (DNCB). Edmund Klein has treated basal cell and squamous cell skin carcinomas by painting the skin lesions with contact sensitivity haptens such as DNCB, after the patients have been sensitized to DNCB. A delayed hypersensitivity reaction occurs to the sensitizing chemical, and the tumor tissue appears to be destroyed by the accumulation of macrophages that is stimulated by the reaction of sensitized lymphocytes to the DNCB. In persons sensitized systemically to this agent, skin painting of basal cell carcinomas with DNCB induces complete regression in approximately one-third of the treated lesions and partial regression in another third. Untreated lesions in patients with multiple basal cell carcinomas do not undergo regression at the time that other treated lesions are regressing. The mechanism of the selective DNCB-induced regression of basal cell carcinoma is not well understood. Presumably the tumor cells are more sensitive to delayed hypersensitivity reactions directed to DNCB than are normal epithelial cells. Such therapy is applicable only to cutaneous tumors and has little substantiated effect on noncutaneous tumors.

Lymphokines and Interleukins

A number of lymphokines have been shown to have antitumor effects in experimental systems (see Tables 27-2 and 27-3). The most important of these are interferon and interleukin 2. The use of interferon, interleukin 2, and other lymphokines and interleukins as therapeutic agents is discussed in Chapter 27.

Theoretically these agents have the potential to augment immune responses to tumor antigens. Interferons may have a direct cytostatic effect on cancer cells, activate NK cells, or increase specific immune responses to tumors. Interferon may also decrease NK activity. IL2 activates T cells and other killer cells. In experimental systems IL2-treated lymphoid cells may inhibit tumor growth in animals with transplanted tumors. Clinical trials of these agents are underway. Some beneficial effects of interferon in vivo have been reported for some lymphoid tumors, breast and renal carcinomas, and Kaposi's sarcomas. However, to date neither interferon nor IL2 has been convincingly demonstrated to have any effect superior to that of conventional cancer therapy, and they may have serious toxic side effects. Tumor necrosis factor (TNF) was originally found in the sera of mice infected with BCG and subsequently injected with bacterial lipopolysaccharide (endotoxin). Injection of sera from these mice into other mice sometimes causes necrosis of transplanted tumors. Human cell lines that produce TNF are now being used to clone the TNF gene and produce cloned TNF for possible human use.

Evaluation of Cancer Immunotherapy

The variable course of cancer as a disease makes therapeutic assessment extremely difficult. One of the major problems in the past has been the inclusion of a valid control group. Although there are many reports to the contrary and exceptional cases in which complete cure is documented, the effect of immunotherapy on many solid nonlymphoid tumors may be useful for individual patients, but is clinically unsatisfactory in most cases. The biological problems involved in evaluating the effects of therapy are even more complicated for immunotherapy than for chemotherapy. For instance, there are a number of mechanisms whereby an otherwise immunologically adequate individual is unable to make an effective response to a tumor (see Table 29-6). It is possible that by attempting to immunize a person to his own tumor, the physician may actually cause the tumor to grow more rapidly by influencing the immune response in such a way as to inhibit or block the rejection mechanism.

The possibility of successful immunotherapy of cancer has raised great excitement. The introduction of a new approach usually generates great expectations. In the past the enthusiasm of claims of success in the first clinical trials has been followed by the reality of little or no beneficial effect. It is hoped that the clinical trials now underway will give more promising results.

Summary

There is documented evidence in experimental animals and circumstantial observations in humans that tumors contain specific antigens and that immune responses to these antigens occur. The identification of cancer-associated markers in the serum of affected patients has resulted in diagnostic tests for a few human tumors (hepatoma, teratocarcinomas). Immune recognition of new tumor antigens may be important in preventing growth of newly mutated cancer cells (immune surveillance). Active or passive immunity to tumor antigens may restrict the growth of an established tumor under appropriate conditions, but a number of coexisting phenomena may interfere with this effect. Specific passive immunotherapy using monoclonal antibodies and nonspecific immune stimulation using interferon or IL2 are now being tested in clinical trials. Understanding and control of these phenomena may result in effective immunotherapy of cancer in humans.

References

Tumor Immunity

Berg JW: Morphologic evidence for immune response to breast cancer. Cancer 28:1453, 1971.

Black MM: Human breast cancer. A model for cancer immunology. Isr J Med Sci 9:284, 1973.

Catalona WJ: Commentary on the immunobiology of bladder cancer. J Urol 118:2, 1977.

Cudkowicz G, Bennett M: Peculiar immunobiology of bone marrow allografts. II. Rejection of parental grafts by resistant F_1 hybrid mice. J Exp Med 134:1513, 1971.

Emerson TC: Spontaneous regression of cancer. Ann NY Acad Sci 114:721, 1964.

Foley EJ: Attempts to induce immunity against mammary adenocarcinoma in inbred mice. Cancer Res 13:578, 1953.

Foley EJ: Antigenic properties of methylcholanthrene-induced tumors in mice of strain of origin. Cancer Res 134:853, 1953.

Gatti RA, Good RA: Occurrence of malignancy in immunodeficiency diseases: a literature review. Cancer 28:89, 1971.

Giovanella BC, Stehlin JS, Williams LJ: Hetero-transplantation of human malignant tumors in "nude" thymusless mice. II. Malignant tumors induced by injection of cell cultures derived from human solid tumors. J Nat Cancer Inst 52:921, 1974.

Green I, Cohen S, McCluskey RT (eds): Mechanisms of Tumor Immunity. New York, Wiley, 1977.

Gross L: Intradermal immunization of CSH mice against a sarcoma that originated in an animal of the same line. Cancer Res 3:326, 1943.

Haddow A: Immunology of the cancer cell. Br Med Bull 21:133, 1965.

Hattler B, Amos B: The immunology of cancer: tumor antigens and the responsiveness of the host. Monogr Surg Sci 3:1, 1966.

Hellstrom KE, Hellstrom I: Allogeneic inhibition of transplanted tumor cells. Prog Exp Tumor Res 9:40, 1967.

Hellstrom KE, Hellstrom I: Cellular immunity against tumor antigens. Adv Cancer Res 12:167, 1969.

Hersy P, Stone DE, Morgan G, McCarthy WH, Milton GW: Previous pregnancy as a protective factor against death from melanoma. Lancet 1:451, 1977.

Hewitt HB, Blake ER, Walder AS: A critique of the evidence for active host defense against cancer, based on personal studies of 27 murine tumors of spontaneous origin. Br J Cancer 33:241, 1976.

Kaplan BS, Klassen J, Gault MH: Glomerular injury in patients with neoplasia. Annu Rev Med 27:117, 1976.

Klein G: Experimental studies in tumor immunology. Fed Proc 23:1739, 1969.

Klein G: Immunological studies on a human tumor. Dilemmas of the experimentalist. Isr J Med Sci 7:111, 1971.

Klein G, Klein E: Immune surveillance against virus-induced tumors and nonrejectability of spontaneous tumors: contrasting consequences of host-versus-tumor evaluation. Proc Nat Acad Sci 74:2121, 1977.

Klein G, Sjogren HO, Klein E, Hellstrom KE: Demonstration of resistance against methycholanthrene-induced sarcomas in the primary autochthonous host. Cancer Res 20:1561, 1960.

Lewison EF: Conference on spontaneous regression of cancer. Nat Cancer Inst Monogr 44, 1976.

McKhann CF: Primary malignancy in patients undergoing immunosuppression for renal transplantation. Transplantation 8:209, 1969.

Mikulska ZB, Smith C, Alexander P: Evidence for an immunological reaction of the host directed against its own actively growing primary tumor. J Nat Cancer Inst 36:29, 1966.

Old LJ, Boyse EA: Immunology of experimental tumors. Annu Rev Med 15:167, 1964.

Outzen HC, Custer RP, Eaton GJ, Prehn RT: Spontaneous and induced tumor incidence in germfree nude mice. J Reticuloendothel Soc 17:1, 1975.

Prehn RT: Relationship of tumor immunogenicity to concentration of the oncogen. J Nat Cancer Inst 55:189, 1975.

Prehn RT, Main JM: Immunity to methycholanthrene induced sarcomas. J Nat Cancer Inst 18:769, 1957.

Schone G: Untersuchungen über Karzinomimmunität bei Mausen. Munch Med Wochenschr 53:2517, 1906.

Sell S: Tumor immunity: relevance of animal models to man. Hum Pathol 9:63, 1978.

Smith RT: Tumor specific immune mechanisms. N Engl J Med 278:1027,1268,1326, 1968.

Stutman O: Immunodepression and malignancy. Adv Cancer Res 22:261, 1975.

Stutman O: Natural antitumor resistance in immune deficient mice. *In* Sordat B (ed): Immune Deficient Animals. Basel, Karger, 1984, p30.

Svet-Moldavsky GS, Hamburg EA: Quantitative relationships in viral oncolysis and the possibility of artificial heterogenization of tumours. Nature 202:303, 1964.

Takeda K, Aiawa M, Kikuchi Y, Yamawaki S, Nakamura K: Tumor autoimmunity against methylcholanthrene-induced sarcomas of the rat. Gann 57:211, 1966.

Vose BM, Moore M: Human tumor infiltrating lymphocytes: a marker of host response. Semin Hematol 22:27, 1985.

Waldmann TA, Strober W, Blaese RM: Immunodeficiency disease and malignancy. Various immunologic deficiencies of man and the role of immune processes in the control of malignant disease. Ann Intern Med 77:605, 1972.

Tumor Antigens

Alexander P: Fetal antigens in cancer. Nature 235:137, 1972.

Baldwin RW: Tumor-specific antigens associated with chemically induced tumors. Rev Eur Etud Clin Biol 15:593, 1970.

Baldwin RW, Embleton MJ, Price MR, Vose BM: Embryonal antigen expression on experimental rat tumors. Transplant Rev 20:77, 1974.

Basombrio MA: Search for common antigenicities among twenty five sarcomas induced by methylcholanthrene. Cancer Res 20:2458, 1970.

Brawn RJ: Possible association of embryonal antigen(s) with seven primary 3-methylcholanthrene–induced murine sarcomas. Int J Cancer 6:245, 1970.

Chism SE, Wallis S, Burton RC, Warner NL: Analysis of murine onco-fetal antigens as tumor associated transplantation antigens. J Immunol 117:1870, 1976.

Comoglio PM, Forni G: Molecular basis of the immunogenicity of cell surface tumor antigens. Exp Cell Biol 44:150, 1976.

Davidsohn I, Louisa YN: Loss of isoantigens A, B, and H in carcinoma of the lung. J Pathol 57:307, 1969.

Goodenow RS, Vogel JM, Linsk RL: Histocompatibility antigens on immune tumors. Science 230:777, 1985.

Gorer PA: The antigenic structure of tumors. Adv Immunol 1:345, 1961.

Klein G: Tumor antigens. Annu Rev Microbiol 20:223, 1966.

Klein G: Tumor specific transplantation antigens—G.H.A. Clowes Memorial Lecture. Cancer Res 28:625, 1968.

Klein G, Klein E: Are methylcholanthrene-induced sarcoma-associated, rejection inducing (TSTA) antigens modified forms of H-2 or linked determinants? Int J Cancer 15:879, 1975.

Kobayashi H, Kodama T, Gotohda E: Xenogenization of Tumor Cells. Sapporo, Hokkaido University Medical Library Series, 1977.

Koldovsky P: Tumor specific transplantation antigen. *In* Rentchnick P (ed): Recent Results in Cancer Research, Vol 22. New York, Springer-Verlag, 1969.

Meltzer MS, Leonard EJ, Rapp HJ, Borsos T: Tumor-specific antigen solubilized by hypertonic potassium chloride. J Nat Cancer Inst 47:703, 1971.

Metzgar RS, Mohauakumar T, Bolognesi DP: Relationships between membrane antigens of human leukemia cells and oncogenic RNA virus structural components. J Exp Med 143:47, 1976.

Morton DL, Miller GF, Wood DA: Demonstration of tumor-specific immunity against antigens unrelated to the mammary tumor virus in spontaneous mammary adenocarcinomas. J Nat Cancer Inst 42:289, 1969.

Old LJ, Boyse EA, Geering G, Oettgen HF: Serologic approaches to the study of cancer in animals and in man. Cancer Res 28:1288, 1968.

Prehn RT: Tumor-specific antigens of nonviral tumors. Cancer Res 28:1326, 1968.

Stonehill EH, Bendich A: Retrogenetic expression: the reappearance of embryonal antigens in cancer cells. Nature 228:370, 1970.

Witebsky E: Zur serologischen Spezifität des Karzinomgewebes. Klin Wochenschr 9:58, 1930.

In Vitro Assays of Tumor Immunity

See Chapter 8.

Bloom BR, Glade PR (eds): In Vitro Methods in Cell-Mediated Immunity. New York, Academic Press, 1971.

Cerottini J-C, Brunner KT: Cell-mediated cytotoxicity, allograft rejection and tumor immunity. Adv Immunol 18:67–132, 1974.

Evans R, Alexander P: Role of macrophages in tumour immunity. I. Cooperation between macrophages and lymphoid cells in syngenetic tumour immunity. Immunology 63:615, 1972.

Hellstrom KE, Hellstrom I: Cellular immunity against tumor antigens. Adv Cancer Res 12:167, 1969.

Hellstrom KE, Hellstrom I: Lymphocyte-mediated cytotoxicity and blocking serum activity to tumor antigens. Adv Immunol 18:209, 1974.

Hellstrom KE, Moller G: Immunological and immunogenetic aspects of tumor transplantation. Prog Allergy 9:158, 1965.

Henkart PA: Mechanism of lymphocyte mediated cytotoxicity. Annu Rev Immunol 3:31, 1985.

Henney CS: Mechanisms of tumor cell destruction. *In* Green I, Cohen S, McCluskey RT (eds): Mechanisms of Tumor Immunity. New York, Wiley, 1977, p55.

Herberman RB: Cellular immunity to human tumor-associated antigens. Isr J Med Sci 9:300, 1973.

Herberman RB, Holden HT: Natural cell mediated immunity. Adv Cancer Res 27:305, 1978.

Keller R: Cytostatic elimination of syngeneic rat tumor cells in vitro by nonspecifically activated macrophage. J Exp Med 138:625, 1973.

Lundgren G, Collste L, Moller G: Cytotoxicity of human lymphocytes: antagonism between inducing processes. Nature 220:289, 1968.

Moller E: Antagonistic effects of humoral isoantibodies on the in vitro cytotoxicity of immune lymphoid cells. J Exp Med 122:11, 1965.

Pross HF, Baines MG: Spontaneous human lymphocyte medicated cytotoxicity against tumor target cells. VI. A brief review. Cancer Immunol Immunother 3:75, 1977.

Sjogren HO, Hellstrom I, Bansal SC, Warner GA, Hellstrom KE: Elution of "blocking factors" from human tumors, capable of abrogating tumor cell destruction by specifically immune lymphocytes. Int J Cancer 9:274, 1972.

Takasugi M, Koide Y, Akira D, Ramseyer A: Specificities in natural cell mediated cytotoxicity by the cross-competition assay. Int J Cancer 19:291, 1977.

Takasugi M, Mickey MR, Terasaki PI: Reactivity of lymphocytes from normal persons on cultured tumor cells. Cancer Res 33:2898, 1973.

Takasugi M, Mickey MR, Terasaki PI: Studies on specificity of cell mediated immunity to human tumors. J Nat Cancer Inst 53:1527, 1974.

Tumor Enhancement and Stimulation

Amos DB, Cohen I, Klein WS: Mechanisms of immunologic enhancement. Transplant Proc 2:68, 1970.

Bansal SC, Sjogren HO: Counteraction of the blocking of cell-mediated tumor immunity by inoculation of unblocking sera and splenectomy: immunotherapeutic effects on primary polyoma tumors in rats. Int J Cancer 9:490, 1972.

Hellstrom KE, Hellstrom I: Immunologic enhancement as studied by cell culture techniques. Annu Rev Microbiol 24:373, 1970.

Hellstrom KE, Hellstrom I: Evidence that tumor antigens enhance tumor growth in vivo by interactions with a radiosensitive (suppressor?) cell population. Proc Nat Acad Sci USA 75:436, 1978.

Ilfeld D, Carnaud C, Cotten IR, Tranin N: In vitro cytotoxicity and in vivo tumor enhancement induced by mouse spleen cells autosensitized in vitro. Int J Cancer 12:213, 1973.

Kaliss N: Immunological enhancement of tumor homografts in mice: a review. Cancer Res 18:992, 1958.

Kaliss N: Immunological enhancement. Int Rev Exp Pathol 8:241, 1969.

Kaliss N: Dynamics of immunologic enhancement. Transplant Proc 2:59, 1970.

Lamon EW: Stimulation of tumor cell growth in vitro: a critical evaluation of immunologic specificity. J Nat Cancer Inst 59:769, 1977.

Prehn RT: Immunostimulation of the lymphodependent phase of neoplastic growth. J Nat Cancer Inst 59:1043, 1977.

Immune Surveillance

Burnet FM: The concept of immunological surveillance. Prog Exp Tumor Res 13:1, 1970.

Fenyo EM, Klein E, Klein G, Sweich K: Selection of an immunoresistant Moloney lymphoma subline with decreased concentration of tumor-specific surface antigens. J Nat Cancer Inst 40:69, 1968.

Ioachim HL: The stromal reaction of tumors: an expression of immune surveillance. J Nat Cancer Inst 57:465, 1976.

Moller G, Moller E: The concept of immunological surveillance against neoplasia. Transplant Rev 28:3, 1976.

Prehn RT: Immunosurveillance, regeneration and oncogenesis. Prog Exp Tumor Res 14:1, 1970.

Rygaard J, Poulsen CO: The nude mouse vs the hypothesis of immunological surveillance. Transplant Rev 48:43, 1976.

Rygaard J, Poulsen CO: The mouse mutant nude does not develop spontaneous tumors. Acta Pathol Microbiol Scand (B) 82:99, 1974.

Schwartz RS: Another look at immunologic surveillance. N Engl J Med 293:181, 1975.

Stutman O: Tumor development after 3-methylcholanthrene in immunologically deficient athymic nude mice. Science 183:534, 1974.

Thomas L: Discussion. *In* Lawrence HS (ed): Cellular and Humoral Aspects of the Hypersensitive State. New York, Harper & Row, 1959.

Immunodiagnosis

Abelev GI: Production of embryonal serum α-globulin by hepatomas: review of experimental and clinical data. Cancer Res 28:1344, 1968.

Arnold A, Cossman J, Bakhshi A, et al: Immunoglobulin-gene rearrangements as unique clonal markers in human lymphoid neoplasms. N Engl J Med 309:1593, 1983.

Baylin JB: Ectopic production of hormones and other proteins by tumors. Hosp Pract 10:117, 1975.

Bence Jones H: Papers on chemical pathology, Lecture III. Lancet 2:269, 1847.

Carney DN, Marangos PJ, Ihde DC, Bunn PA Jr, Cohen MH, Minna JD, Gazdar AS: Serum neuron-specific enolase: a marker for disease extent and response to therapy of small cell lung cancer. Lancet 1:583, 1982.

Cooper D, Schermer A, Sun T-T: Classification of human epithelia and their neoplasms using monoclonal antibodies to keratins: strategies, application and limitations. Lab Invest 52:243, 1985.

Cooper GM: Cellular transforming genes. Science 217:801, 1982.

Elgort DA, Abelev GI, Levina DM, Marienbach EV, Martochkina GA, Laskina AV, Solovjeva EA: Immunoradioautography test for alpha fetoprotein in the differential diagnosis of germinogenic tumors of the testis and in the evaluation of the effectiveness of their treatment. Int J Cancer 11:586, 1973.

Fishman HW (ed): Oncodevelopmental Markers. New York, Academic Press, 1983.

Fukada M: Cell Surface glycoconjugates as onco-differentiation markers in hematopoietic cells. Biochim Biophys Acta 780:119, 1985.

Go VL: Carcinoembryonic antigen. Clinical application. Cancer 37:562, 1976.

Gold P, Freedman SO: Specific carcinoembryonic antigens of the human digestive system. J Exp Med 122:467, 1965.

Hakomori SI: Tumor associated carbohydrate antigens. Annu Rev Immunol 2:103, 1984.

Hansen HJ: Carcinoembryonic antigen (CEA) assay. Hum Pathol 5:139, 1974.

Klein G: Specific chromosomal translocations and genesis of B-cell derived tumors in mice and men. Cell 32:311, 1983.

Kupchick HZ, Zamcheck N, Savaris CA: Editorial: Immunologic studies of carcinoembryonic antigens: methodologic considerations and some clinical implications. J Nat Cancer Inst 51:1741, 1973.

Levy R, Miller RA: Tumor therapy with monoclonal antibodies. Fed Proc 42:2651, 1983.

Makari JG: The intradermal cancer test (ICT). J Am Geriatr Soc 17:755, 1969.

Moore TL, Kantrowitz PA, Zamcheck N: Carcinoembryonic antigen (CEA) in bowel diseases. JAMA 8:944, 1972.

Moss DW: Alkaline phosphatase isoenzymes. Clin Chem 28:2007, 1982.

Nakamura RM, Plow EF, Edgington TS: Current status of carcinoembryonic antigen (CEA) and CEA-S assays in the evaluation of neoplasm of the gastrointestinal tract. Am Clin Lab Sci 8:4, 1978.

Neville AM, Foster CS, Moshakis V, Gore M: Monoclonal antibodies and human tumor pathology. Hum Pathol 13:1067, 1982.

Nieburgs HE, Birkmayer GD, Klavins JV (eds): Human Tumor Markers: Biological Bases and Clinical Relevance. New York, Liss, 1982.

Niman HL, et al: Antipeptide antibodies detect oncogene-related proteins in urine. Proc Nat Acad Sci USA 82:7924, 1985.

Reisfeld R, Sell S: Monoclonal Antibodies and Cancer Therapy. New York, Liss, 1985.

Ruddon RW: Tumor markers in the recognition and management of poorly differentiated neoplasms and cancers of unknown primary. Semin Oncol 9:416, 1982.

Sell S: The biologic and diagnostic significance of oncodevelopmental gene products. *In* Waters H (ed): The Handbook of Cancer Immunology, Vol 3. New York, Garland, 1978, p1.

Sell S: Oncodevelopmental antigens. Cancer Biol Rev 1:215, 1980.

Sell S (ed): Cancer Markers: Developmental and Diagnostic Significance. Clifton, N.J., Humana Press, 1980.

Sell S, Becker FF: Guest editorial: alphafetoprotein. J Nat Cancer Inst 60:19, 1978.

Sell S, Reisfeld R (eds): Monoclonal Antibodies in Cancer. Clifton, N.J., Humana Press, 1985.

Sell S, Wahren B (eds): Human Cancer Markers. Clifton, N.J., Humana Press, 1982.

Tee DEH: Clinical evaluation of the Makari tumor skin test. Br J Cancer 28:187, 1973.

Thompson DM, Krupey J, Freedman SO, Gold P: The radioimmunoassay of circulating carcinoembryonic antigens of the human digestive system. Proc Nat Acad Sci USA 64:161, 1969.

Immunotherapy

Ascher MS, Gottlieb AA, Kirkpatrick CH (eds): Transfer Factor: Basic Properties and Clinical Application. New York, Academic Press, 1976.

Bast RC Jr, Zbar B, Borsos T, Rapp HJ: BCG and cancer. N Engl J Med 290:1413, 1458, 1974.

Biggs PM: Marek's disease — the disease and its prevention by vaccination. Br J Cancer 31:152, 1975.

Borsos I, Rapp H (eds): Conference on the use of BCG in therapy of cancer. Nat Cancer Inst Monogr 39, 1973.

Carswell EA, Old LJ, Kassel RL et al: An endotoxin induced serum factor that causes necrosis of tumors. Proc Nat Acad Sci USA 25:3660, 1975.

Davignon L, Lemonde P, Robillard P, Frappier A: BCG vaccination and leukemia mortality. Lancet 2:638, 1970.

Evans GA, Gorman LR, Ito Y, Weiser RS: Antitumor immunity in the Shope papilloma carcinoma complex in man. I. Papilloma regression induced by homologous and autologous tissue vaccine. J Nat Cancer Inst 29:277, 1962.

Fefer A: Adaptive tumor immunotherapy in mice as an adjunct to whole body irradiation and chemotherapy. A review. Isr J Med Sci 9:350, 1973.

Fink MA (ed): Immune RNA in Neoplasia. New York, Academic Press, 1976.

Friedman H, Southam C (eds): International conference on immuno-biology of cancer. Ann NY Acad Sci 276:1, 1976.

Golub SH: Immunological and therapeutic effects of interferon treatment of cancer patients. Clin Immunol Allergy 4:377, 1984.

Graham JB, Graham RM: Autogeneous vaccine in cancer patients. Surg Gynecol Obstet 114:1, 1962.

Herberman RB: Cancer immunology: innovative approaches to therapy. Hingham, Mass., Nijhoff, 1985.

Klein E: Immunotherapy of cutaneous and mucosal neoplasms. NY State J Med 68:900, 1968.

Klein E, Holterman OA, Helm F, et al: Topical therapy for cutaneous tumors. Transplant Proc 16:507, 1984.

Koprowski H, Herlyn D, Lubeck M, et al: Human anti-idiotype antibodies in cancer patients: is the moderation of the immune response beneficial for the patients? Prac Nat Acad Sci USA 81:216, 1984.

Lamoureaux G, Turcote R, Portelance V: BCG in Cancer Immunotherapy. New York, Grune & Stratton, 1976.

Levy R: Biologicals for cancer treatment: monoclonal antibodies. Hosp Pract 20:67, 1985.

Lewis WR, Kraemer KH, Klinger WG, Peck GL, Terry WD: Topical immunotherapy of basal cell carcinomas with dinitrochloro-benzene. Cancer Res 33:3036, 1973.

Mathe G, Amiel JL, Schwarzenbert L, Cattan A, Schneider M: Adaptive immunotherapy of acute leukemia: experimental and clinical results. Cancer Res 25:1525, 1965.

Meeker TC, Lowder J, Maloney DG, et al: A clinical trial of anti-idiotype therapy for B cell malignancy. Blood 65:1349, 1985.

Moeller G (ed): Antibody Carriers of Drugs and Toxins in Tumor Therapy. Immunol Rev 62, 1982.

Moore GE, Moore MB: Auto-inoculation of cultured lymphocytes in malignant melanoma. NY State J Med 69:460, 1969.

Morton DL: Immunotherapy of cancer, present status and future potential. Cancer 30:10, 1972.

Morton DL, Eilber FR, Holmes EC, Sparks FC, Ramming KP: Present status of BCG immunotherapy of malignant melanoma. Cancer Immunol Immunother 1:93, 1976.

Mule JJ, Ettinghausen SE, Spiess PJ, et al: Antitumor efficacy of lymphokine-activated killer cells and recombinant interleukin-2 in vivo: survival benefit and mechanisms of tumor escape in mice undergoing immunotherapy. Cancer Res 46:676, 1986.

Nadler SH, Moore GE: Immunotherapy of malignant disease. Arch Surg 99:376, 1969.

Nathanson L: Immunology and immunotherapy of human breast cancer. Cancer Immunol Immunother 2:209, 1977.

Oettgen HF: Immunotherapy of cancer. N Engl J Med 297:484, 1977.

Old LJ, Stockert E, Boyse EA, Kim JH: Antigenic modulation. Loss of TL antigen from cells exposed to TL antibody. Study of the phenomenon in vitro. J Exp Med 127:523, 1968.

Oldham RK: Biologics for cancer treatment: interferons. Hosp Pract 20:71, 1985.

Oldham RK, Smalley RV: Biologicals and biological response. *In* DeVita et al (eds): Modifiers in Cancer: Principles and Practice of Oncology. New York, Lippincott, 1985.

Prager MD: Immunologic stimulation with modified cancer cells. Biomedicine 18:261, 1973.

Prager MD: Specific cancer immunotherapy. Cancer Immunol Immunother 3:157, 1978.

Quesada JR, Reuben JR, Manning JT, et al: Alpha-interferon for induction of remission in hairy-cell leukemia. N Engl J Med 30:15, 1984.

Rapp HJ: Immunotherapy of cancer. *In* Anfinsen CB, Potter M, Schechter AN (eds): Current Research in Oncology. New York, Academic Press, 1972, p143.

Rosenberg S: Lymphokine-activated killer cells: a new approach to immunotherapy of cancer. J Nat Cancer Inst 75:595, 1985.

Rosenberg S, Lotze MT: Cancer immunotherapy using interleukin 2 and interleukin 2 activated lymphocytes. Annu Rev Immunol 4:681, 1986.

Southam CM, Friedman H (eds): International Conference on Immunotherapy of Cancer. Ann NY Acad Sci 277:1, 1976.

Stjensward J, Levin A: Delayed hypersensitivity-induced regression of human neoplasms. Cancer 28:638, 1971.

Stone HB, Curtis RM, Brewer JH: Can resistance to cancer be induced? Ann Surg 134:519, 1951.

Terry WD, Windhorst D (eds): Immunotherapy of cancer: present states of trials in man. *In* Progress in Cancer Research and Therapy, Vol 6. New York, Dover Press, 1978.

Tukey JW: Some thoughts on clinical trials. Especially problems of multiplicity. Science 198:679, 1977.

Vitetta ES, Krolick KA, et al: Immunotoxins: a new approach to cancer therapy. Science 219:644, 1983.

Vose BM: Activation of lymphocyte anti-tumor responses in man. Towards an understanding of effector cell heterogeneity? Cancer Immunol Immunother 17:73, 1984.

Williams AC, Klein E: Experiences with local chemotherapy and immunotherapy in premalignant and malignant skin lesions. Cancer 25:450, 1970.

Zbar B, Rapp HJ: Immunotherapy of guinea pig cancer with BCG. Cancer 34:1532, 1974.

Appendix A: Clinical Immunology

Immune tests are available for a large number of different diseases (Table A-1). These include not only antigen-specific reactions and general assays of immune competence, but also the use of immune reagents to measure the serum concentrations of biologically active agents such as hormones or enzymes and serum proteins such as α-fetoprotein. Most immune testing is done in vitro, although skin reactivity to specific antigens does have application in infectious disease and clinical allergy (atopic or anaphylactic reactions). Serological testing is applicable mainly to infectious diseases, autoallergies, hematology, and transplantation. A variety of serological and cellular tests are also applied to cancer diagnosis. The purpose of this appendix is to provide a listing of such tests. For more details on methods and application, the reader should consult the appropriate chapters of this text.

Table A-1. Clinical Immunologic Tests

A. SERUM PROTEINS; HUMORAL IMMUNITY

Major globulins	Serum electrophoresis	Immune deficiencies, myeloma
Serum Ig classes	Nephelometry, RID	Immune deficiencies, myeloma
Serum proteins	Immunoelectrophoresis, immune fixation, electrophoresis	Immune deficiencies, myeloma, others
Total complement	Hemolytic assay	Immune deficiencies, immune complex disorders
Serum complement components	Nephelometry, RID	Immune deficiencies, immune complex disorders
C1 esterase inhibitor	Nephelometry, inhibition of C1 activity	Angioedema
C breakdown products	RIA/ELISA	Acute inflammation

B. CELLULAR IMMUNITY

T cells

Total	SRBC rosettes	Immune deficiency
Mitogen response	PHA, Con A	Immune deficiency
Subclasses	Monoclonal antibody (cytofluorometry)	Immune deficiency, infectious disease
IL2 production	T cell line proliferation in vitro	Immune deficiency
MIF production	In vitro macrophage migration	Immune deficiency
T receptor gene rearrangement	cDNA binding on gels	Lymphoma

B cells

EAC rosettes	Microscopic observation	Immune deficiency
Surface Ig	Fluorescent flow cytometry	Immune deficiency
Subpopulations	MoAb (cytometry)	Lymphomas
Ig gene rearrangements	cDNA binding on gels	Lymphomas
SIg class clonality (or kappa/lambda ratio)	Fluorescence	Lymphomas, leukemia
Bence Jones protein	Solubility	Myeloma

Monocytes – macrophages

IL1 production	Growth of T cell lines in vitro	Immune deficiency
Bacterial killing	Cytotoxicity in vitro	Immune deficiency
Activation	Production of oxygen radicals	Immune deficiency

Neutrophils

Phagocytosis	Particle uptake	Immune deficiency

Digestion	Nitrobluetetrazolium induction	Immune deficiency
Bacterial killing	Bactericidal in vitro	Immune deficiency
Migration	Micropore filter in vitro	Immune deficiency
Total Cells	Complete blood count and differential	Infection, leukemia, immune deficiency
D. INFECTIOUS DISEASES (MICROBIOLOGY)		
Bacterial	Multiple (antibody titers)	Specific diagnosis
Mycobacterial	Immunofluorescence	Specific diagnosis
Parasites	Complement fixation, indirect hemagglutination	Specific diagnosis
Fungal	Complement fixation, double diffusion	Specific diagnosis
Virus	Immunofluorescence, ELISA, Western blot	Specific diagnosis
Rickettsia	Complement fixation	Specific diagnosis
Chlamydial	Immunofluorescence	Specific diagnosis
E. TRANSFUSION		
Blood group antigens	Type and cross-match (hemagglutination)	Donor selection
Platelet antigens	Flow cytometry	Donor selection
Ig Allotypes	Passive hemagglutination inhibition	Donor selection
AIDS antibody	ELISA, Western blot	Donor selection
Hepatitis antigen	ELISA, RIA	Donor selection
Fibrin split products	ELISA, RIA	Bleeding disorders
F. TRANSPLANTATION		
HLA (A–D) serologic antigens	Serologic cytotoxicity	Donor selection
HLA D cellular antigens	Mixed lymphocyte reaction	Donor selection
Lymphocyte killing	Cell mediated cytotoxicity, ADCC	Rejection activity
Antilymphocyte antibody	Serologic cytotoxicity	Donor activity
G. ALLERGIC REACTIONS		
Serum IgE	RIA, ELISA	Allergic predesposition
Allergen-specific IgE	RAST	Specific allergen
Basophil reactivity	Histamine release (fluorometry)	Specific allergen
Skin test	Wheal and flare	Specific allergen

(Continued on following page)

Table A-1. (Continued)

Schultz–Dale	Constriction of smooth muscle	Specific allergen
H. ANTIBODY-MEDIATED DISEASES		
1. Tissue antibodies		
Acetylcholine receptor Ab	Binding inhibition	Myasthenia gravis
Pancreatic islet cell Ab's	Tissue immunofluorescence	Type I diabetes mellites
Basement membrane Ab's	Tissue immunofluorescence	Goodpasture's syndrome
Mitochondrial Ab's	Tissue immunofluorescence	Primary biliary cirrhosis
TSH receptor Ab's	Tissue immunofluorescence	Graves' disease
2. Antinuclear antibodies: indirect SLE Sjögren's, polymyositides/dermatomyositides		
Anti-ssDNA	RIA or ELISA	Scleroderma, SLE, others
Anti-dsDNA	RIA or ELISA or crithea lucilade indirect immunofluorescence	SLE
Anti-Sm	Immunodiffusion or ELISA	SLE
Anti-RNP	Immunodiffusion or ELISA	SLE, MCTD, polymyositides, scleroderma
Antihistones	Immunodiffusion or ELISA	SLE, drug-induced LE
Anti-Scl 70	Immunodiffusion or ELISA	Scleroderma
Anticentromere	Indirect immunofluorescence	CREST syndrome
Anti-JO1	Immunodiffusion or ELISA	Polymyositis
Anti–Pn-Sc1 (Pn-1)	Immunodiffusion or ELISA	Polymyositis, scleroderma
Anti-Mi2	Immunodiffusion or ELISA	Dermatomyositis
3. Anticytoplasmic antibodies		
Ro(SS-A)	Immunodiffusion or ELISA	SLE, Sjögren's
La(SS-B)	Immunodiffusion or ELISA	SLE, Sjögren's
4. Other assays		
Rheumatoid factor	Latex agglutination, others	Rheumatoid arthritis
Immune complexes	RAJI cell binding; C1q binding; anti-Ig binding	Immune complex disease
I. CANCER		
1. Tumor immunity		
Antitumor antibodies	Binding to cells by indirect immunofluorescence or complement-mediated lysis	Reactivity to specific tumor
Cell-mediated cytotoxicity (CMC)	Direct (T-cell) natural killing antibody	Nonspecific and specific killing

	dependent	
Lymphocyte reactivity	Blast transformation	Tumor antigens
Blocking factors	Inhibition of CMC	Blocking of specific reaction
2. Tumor markers (serum)		
AFP	RIA, ELISA	Diagnosis, prognosis
CEA	RIA, ELISA	Diagnosis, prognosis
Prostate antigen	RIA, ELISA	Diagnosis, prognosis
CA 19-9	RIA, ELISA	Diagnosis, prognosis
Hormones[a]	RIA, ELISA	Diagnosis, prognosis
Myeloma proteins	Electrophoresis	Diagnosis
Isoenzymes	Electrophoresis	Diagnosis
Melanoma antigen	RIA	Diagnosis
3. Immune histology		
AFP	Immunofluorescence or immunoperoxidase	Tissue identification of cancer
CEA	Immunofluorescence or immunoperoxidase	Tissue identification of cancer
CA 19-9	Immunofluorescence or immunoperoxidase	Tissue identification of cancer
Cytokeratins	Immunofluorescence or immunoperoxidase	Tissue identification of cancer
Prostate antigen	Immunofluorescence or immunoperoxidase	Tissue identification of cancer
Hormones	Immunofluorescence or immunoperoxidase	Tissue identification of cancer
Isoenzymes	Immunofluorescence or immunoperoxidase	Tissue identification of cancer
Enzymes	Enzyme activity	Lymphoid tumors
Cell surface Ig expression	Immunoperoxidase	B cell tumors
Cell surface T cell markers	Immunoperoxidase	T cell tumors
4. Molecular biology		
Ig gene rearrangements	DNA binding on gels	B cell tumors
T cell receptor gene rearrangement	DNA binding on gels	T cell tumors

[a] Insulin, gastrin, renin–angiotensin, growth hormone, placental hormones, thyroid hormones, cortisol, estradiol, testosterone, and others.

Appendix B: Cluster Designations

Revised Nomenclature (Cluster Designations) for Human
Lymphocyte Markers Detected by Monoclonal Antibodies

Cluster Designation	Antibody
CD1	OKT6, anti-Leu-t, NA1/34
CD2	OKT11, anti-T11, anti-Leu-5, 9.6
CD3	OKT3, anti-T3, anti-Leu-4, UCHT-1
CD4	OKT4, anti-T4, anti-Leu-3
CD5	OKT1, anti-T1, anti-Leu-1, 10.2, T101
CD6	12.1, T411
CD7	Anti-Leu-9, 3A1, WT1, 4A
CD8	OKT5, OKT8, anti-T8, anti-Leu-2
CD9	BA-2, SJ-9A4, Du-ALL-1
CD10	J5, BA-3, anti-CALLA
CD11	Mol/OKM1, Mo5, OKM10, OKM9
CDw12	20.2
CDw13	DUHL60.4, MY7
CDw14	Mo2, MY4, MOP-15, FMC 17
CD15	FMC10, VIM-D5, 82H5, 1G10
CDw15	TG-1, FMC 13, 80H.3, DUHL 60.1, DUHL60.3
CD16	VEP13
CDw17	T5A7
CD19	Anti-B4
CD20	Anti-B1
CD21	Anti-B2
CD22	SHCL-1, HD6, HD39, 29-110
CD23	PL13, MNM6, Blast-2
CD24	BA-1
CD25	Anti-Tac

Anti-T9 and anti-Ti are not included in cluster designations.

Modified from Reinherz E, Haynes BF, Nadler LM, Bernstein ID (eds): Leukocyte Typing II
(3 vols). New York, Springer-Verlag, 1986.

Glossary

ABO blood groups. Major carbohydrate antigens on red blood cells responsible for transfusion reactions.

Absorption. Use of antibody or antigen to remove corresponding antigen or antibody from a mixture.

Acanthosis nigricans. Disease involving pigmentation, thickening of skin, and insulin-resistant diabetes associated with autoantibodies to insulin receptors.

Accessory cells. Monocytic, epithelial, or lymphocytic cells that cooperate with T or B cells in the induction of antibody formation or T cell sensitization; express class II MHC markers.

Acetylcholine receptors (AcChR). Binding sites for acetylcholine on muscle end plate of myoneuronal junction that serve to activate muscle contraction.

Acidophilic. Used to describe tissue having affinity for acidic dyes resulting in a red-to-pink color.

Acquired immunity. Protection that develops as a result of induction of an immune response.

Activation. Process of changing lymphoid cells (lymphocytes, macrophages) or proteins (complement, kinin, coagulation systems) from resting or inactive state to functionally active cells or effector molecules.

Activation factors. Proteins produced by activated cells or protein systems that serve to activate other cells.

Active immunity. Protection due to induction of an immune response by immunization or infection.

Acute phase substances. Nonantibody factors that appear in increased amounts in blood soon after induction of inflammation: α_2 macroglobulin, C-reactive protein, fibrinogen, α_1 antitrypsin, etc.

Adaptive differentiation. Process whereby thymocytes acquire

789

the ability to recognize class II major histocompatibility markers during maturation in the thymus to T helper/inducer cells.

Adaptive immunity. Specific acquired protection against infectious agents or product as a result of immunization.

Addison's disease. A metabolic disease caused by hypofunction of the adrenal cortex, due either to loss of adrenal tissue or to reduced levels of adrenal cortical stimulating hormone (ACTH).

Adenosine deaminase deficiency. Defect in purine metabolism resulting in severe combined immune deficiency.

Adjuvant. Material capable of enhancing an immune response.

Adjuvant disease. Lesions of synovia, colon, and skin produced by injection of complete Freund's adjuvant into rats.

Adoptive immunity. Transfer of state of immunity, using immune cells or serum, from an immune individual to an nonimmune individual.

Adoptive tolerance. Transfer of tolerance by cells from a tolerant individual to a normal individual.

Adult respiratory distress syndrome. Respiratory failure in adult humans caused by pulmonary edema secondary to increased vascular permeability.

Affinity. Strength of binding of antibody combining site (paratope) to antigenic determinant (epitope).

Agglutination. Joining together of visible antigenic particles or antigen-coated visible particles by reaction with antibody that can be visualized by the naked eye.

Aggretope. Postulated product resulting from combining of part of an antigen with class II MHC components of a processing macrophage that is recognized by the MHC–antigen receptor on T helper/inducer cells.

Agranulocytosis. Disease due to loss of or failure to produce polymorphonuclear leukocytes resulting in increased susceptibility to infection.

AIDS (acquired immunodeficiency syndrome). Severe immunodepression associated with human immunodeficiency virus (HIV) infection characterized by multiple opportunistic infections and death.

Aleutian mink disease. Virus-associated immune complex disease of mink. Findings include lymphadenopathy, hypergammaglobulinemia, glomerulonephritis, hepatitis, and arteritis.

Allele. One or more genes at the same chromosomal locus that control alternative different forms (phenotypes) of a particular inherited characteristic.

Allelic exclusion. The phenotypic expression of only one of the two allelic genes in cells containing two different allelic genes (heterozygous cells).

Allergen. Antigens that induce or evoke atopic or anaphylactic reactions.

Allergic bronchopulmonary aspergillosis. An infectious disease characterized by wheezing, fever, and asthmatic symptoms due to anaphylactic reactivity to aspergillus organisms in bronchi.

Allergic granulomatosis. A disease complex characterized by necrotizing vasculitis, extravascular granulomas, eosinophilic tissue infiltrates, and asthma (Churg–Strauss syndrome).

Allergy. Altered state of immune reactivity; usually used to refer to atopic/anaphylactic reactions.

Alloantigens. Antigens recognized by different individuals of the same species (see *allogeneic*).

Allogeneic. Used to describe genetically different phenotypes present in different individuals of the same species, such as human blood group antigens or immunoglobulin allotypes.

Allogeneic inhibition. Inhibition of growth of tumor or cell line by lymphocytes differing at the major histocompatibility complex.

Allograft. A tissue graft between two genetically different individuals of the same species.

Allotypes. Genetically different antigenic determinants on proteins of individuals of the same species (see *allogeneic*).

Alopecia areata. Loss of hair associated with autoantibodies to capillaries of hair follicles.

Alternative pathway of complement activation. Activation of complement involving factor B, factor D, properdin, and C3.

Alums. Compounds of aluminum or mineral salts used to precipitate proteins. When used as antigens, alum-precipitated proteins form a tissue deposit that has an adjuvant effect.

Amyloidosis. A disease with extracellular deposition of amorphous eosinophilic material due to accumulation of poorly catabolizable proteins: VL-dimers, protein P, protein AA.

Amyotropic lateral sclerosis. A disease of unknown origin characterized by destruction of anterior horn cells in the spinal cord and pyramidal cells in the cerebral cortex, believed to be due to a virus.

Anamnesis. Immune memory or secondary immune response.

Anaphylactoid reaction. A local or systemic reaction due to physical stimuli (heat, trauma, etc.) that mimics an anaphylactic reaction.

Anaphylatoxin. Activated complement components C3a and C5a, which cause increased vascular permeability.

Anaphylaxis. Immediate hypersensitivity reaction (wheal and flare, systemic anaphylaxis) due to release of mediators from mast cells sensitized by IgE antibody.

Anergy. Absence of skin test reactivity to common skin test antigens, due to secondary immune deficiency caused by overwhelming infection, cancer, etc.

Angioedema. Local areas of marked tissue swelling due to activation of complement in the absence of C1 esterase inhibition.

Angioimmunoblastic lymphadenopathy. Lymphoproliferative disease with polyclonal increase in B cells.

Anitschkow's myocytes. Large cardiac muscle cells with striated ("owl eye") nuclei, seen in the carditis of rheumatic fever (Aschoff bodies).

Antibody. Protein produced in response to immunization with antigens that specifically reacts with the antigen.

Antibody combining site (paratope). Area on antibody molecule that binds antigenic determinant (epitope); that part of an immunoglobulin antibody or T cell receptor that binds antigen.

Antibody-dependent cell-mediated cytotoxicity (ADCC). A form of lymphocyte-mediated target cell killing requiring immunoglobulin antibody reacting with the target cells and binding of K lymphocytes through Fc receptors.

Antigen. A substance that induces an immune response. A *complete* antigen both induces an immune response and reacts with the products of the response. An *incomplete* antigen (hapten) cannot induce an immune response by itself but can react with the products of an immune response. Incomplete antigens induce an immune response when complexed to a complete antigen (carrier).

Antigen binding capacity. A measurement of the ability of an antibody to bind antigen, based on the effects of dilution of the antibody (see Farr technique).

Antigen binding site (paratope). That part of an immunoglobulin antibody or T cell receptor that binds antigen.

Antigenic determinant (epitope). That area of an antigen that reacts with antibody or T cell receptors for antigen.

Antigenic modulation. Loss or change of expression of antigens on infectious organisms or tumor cells after exposure to specific antibody or sensitized cells.

Antihemophilic globulins. Blood clotting factors that replace missing components in patients with deficiencies in blood clotting components, usually factor VIII.

Antilymphocyte serum. Serum containing antibodies to lymphocytes used to produce immunosuppression, usually administered in the form of immunoglobulin (antilymphocyte globulin).

Antinuclear antibodies. Antibodies to DNA, RNA, and nucleoproteins found in sera of patients with rheumatoid (collagen) diseases, in particular SLE, scleroderma, and Sjögren's syndrome.

Antiserum. Component of blood without cells or coagulation factors that contains antibody.

Antitoxins. Antibodies that neutralize the effects of toxic products.

Aplasia. Failure to form; loss of a cell population due to failure of generation of cells.

Appendix. Gastrointestinal lymphoid organ located at junction of ileum and cecum.

Arthus reaction. Dermal vascular inflammation caused by immune complexes formed when antigen is injected into skin of an animal containing antibody to the antigen.

Aschoff body. Perivascular cellular reaction in myocardium of patients with rheumatic fever, characterized by mononuclear cells and Anitschkow myocytes.

Aspirin intolerance. Atopic symptoms (asthma, rhinitis, nasal polyps, etc.) caused by idiosyncratic reaction to aspirin.

Association constant (Ka value). Mathematical measure of affinity of binding between antigen and antibody.

Asthma. Difficulty in breathing due to bronchospasm caused by release of mediators from mast cells.

Ataxia–telangectasia. Severe combined immune deficiency associated with ataxic gait, oculocutaneous telangectasias, and ovarian dysgenesis.

Atopic dermatitis. Chronic phase of atopic skin reaction characterized by hyperkeratosis and spongiosis.

Atopic eczema. Weeping skin reaction associated with hay fever and asthma.

Atopy. "Strange" reaction; a term now used for genetic predisposition for anaphylactic reactions.

ATxBm. Designation for an adult thymectomized, irradiated mouse treated with a bone marrow transplant (B cell mouse).

Auer's colitis. Hemorrhagic necrotic inflammatory lesion of the colon caused by injection of antigen (albumin) into colonic cavity of rabbits with antibody to albumin (intestinal Arthus reaction).

Autoallergy. Production of disease or tissue lesion due to an immune reaction to self (endogenous) antigens.

Autoantibody. Antibody to self antigens.

Autoantigens. Substances that are recognized by autoantibodies.

Autochthonous. Arising in the same individual. Synonym: *autologous.*

Autogenous vaccines. Immunizing material made from cultured bacteria taken from an infected individual and injected back into the same individual.

Autograft. Tissue graft from one part of the body of an individual to another part of the body of the same individual.

Autoimmunity. A state of immunity to self antigens.

Autologous. Derived from self, as when: (1) source and recipient or grafted tissue is the same individual; (2) origin of immune response and source of antigen are from the same individual.

Autonomy. Independence — refers to growth characteristic of cancer cells; growth independent of controlling factors that apply to normal noncancerous cells.

Avidin – biotin technique. A system used to label antibodies or antigens, using the strong binding affinity of avidin and biotin.

Avidity. Strength of union between antibody or a receptor and antigen or a ligand.

Azotemia. Presence of nitrogenous waste products in blood, often secondary to renal failure.

B cell domain. Area of lymphoid organ containing high proportion of B cells.

B cell growth and differentiation factors. Substances that enhance B cell proliferation or development into plasma cells.

B cells (B lymphocytes). Lymphocytes that are precursors of plasma cells that produce antibody (term derived from *bursa-derived cells* that arise from the bursa of Fabricius in avian species).

B lymphocytes. See *B cells.*

B2 microglobulin. A peptide, MW 12,000, that is part of the class I major histocompatibility cell surface marker.

Bacillus Calmette – Guérin (BCG). Attenuated strain of *Mycobacterium tuberculosis* used to enhance macrophage activity as well as for prophylactic immunization against tuberculosis. Developed by two French microbiologists by prolonged culture on a glycerol – bile – potato medium.

Backcross. Breeding of a hybrid of two parental strains (F_1) with either one of the parental strains.

Bacteriolysin. An antibody or other substance that is capable of lysing bacteria.

Bacteriolysis. The process of disintegration of bacteria.

Bare lymphocyte syndrome. Combined immune deficiency associated with decreased expression of MHC markers on lymphoid cells.

Basophil. A polymorphonuclear leukocyte with granules containing acid glycoproteins that bind basic (blue) dyes. When released these glycoproteins mediate anaphylactic reactions.

Basophilic. Used to describe tissues having affinity for basic dyes resulting in a blue color.

Bb. A protein, MW 65,000, active in the alternative complement pathway.

BCG. See *bacillus Calmette–Guérin*.

Behcet's syndrome. Triad of oral and genital ulcers, vasculitis, and arthritis, believed to be immune complex mediated.

Bence Jones protein. Monoclonal immunoglobulin light chains found in the urine of patients with multiple myeloma or other paraprotein disorders; precipitated by heating acidified urine.

Benign monoclonal gammopathy. Elevated serum levels of a single immunoglobulin species in the absence of detectable disease.

Berylliosis. Chronic progressive granulomatous pulmonary disease due to sensitization to beryllium.

Beta cells. Endocrine cells in the islets of Langerhans that secrete insulin.

Beta-adrenergic system. System of cellular activation controlling extent of reaction of mast cells and smooth muscle. Stimulation of beta-adrenergic receptors decreases sensitivity to stimulation.

Binding site. Configuration of antibody or cell receptor that binds antigen or ligand.

Birbeck granules. Rod-shaped structures found in cytoplasm of Langerhans cells in the epidermis.

Bis Q. *trans*-3,3′-Bis[α-(trimethylammonia) methyl] azobenzene bromide, an acetylcholine agonist.

Blast cell. A large cell with dispersed chromatin and ribosome-rich cytoplasm usually in an active stage of the cell cycle prior to mitosis.

Blast transformation. Process of activating small lymphocytes to enter cell cycle and form blast cells.

Blocking antibody. Antibody capable of interfering with binding of another antibody (IgG blocking effects of IgE) or sensitized cells (antibody blocking cell-mediated graft rejection).

Blocking factors. Substances that inhibit induction or expression of an immune response.

Blood groups. Allogeneic antigenic differences on red blood cells responsible for transfusion reactions.

Bone marrow. Soft internal tissue in bones containing proliferating precursors of blood cells.

Booster. A dose of antigen given after primary immunization that induces a secondary response.

Bradykinin. A 9-amino-acid peptide, split from a larger serum α-globulin molecule by the enzyme kallikrein, that causes a slow, sustained contraction of smooth muscle.

Bruton's agammaglobulinema. X-linked defect in B cell differentiation resulting in B cell immunodeficiency.

Buffy coat. A thin white layer between red cells and plasma in blood that has been allowed to settle; contains white blood cells.

Bungarotoxin. Venom of Australian snake that binds to and blocks acetylcholine receptors, producing muscle weakness.

Burger's disease. Lymphocytic inflammation involving veins.

Burkitt's lymphoma. Tumor of B lymphocytes caused by Epstein–Barr virus.

Bursa equivalent. Postulated organ site of B-cell precursors in mammals (liver, GI tract, bone marrow, yolk sac).

Bursa of Fabricius. Lymphoid organ located in the cloaca of avian species from which B cells are derived.

Bursapoietin. Substance produced by epithelial cells of bursa of Fabricius that is responsible for B cell maturation.

C region. Constant region carboxyterminal portion of immunoglobulin H or L chains that is identical for a given class or subclass.

C1–C9. Designations used for components of classic complement sequence.

C3 convertase. $\overline{C42}$, activated enzyme of complement system that converts C3 to C3a and C3b.

C1 esterase inhibitor. A serum protein that inactivates activated C1, reducing levels of formation of C2b, which has a kinin-like activity causing edema.

C3 nephritogenic factor. Putative autoantibody to C3 that may be causative factor in hypocomplementemic glomerulonephritis.

Canine distemper virus. A virus producing an acute systemic disease in dogs that may be followed by a chronic demyelinating disease believed to be due to action of lymphocytes sensitized to myelin.

Caplan's syndrome. Lung involvement with rheumatoid nodules, a variant lesion of rheumatoid arthritis seen in individuals exposed to silica, such as hard coal miners.

Capping. Movement of surface molecules on a cell toward one pole, induced by cross-linking by mitogen, antibody, or antigen.

Carrier. An immunogenic molecule that when coupled to a nonimmunogenic incomplete antigen (hapten) renders the incomplete antigen immunogenic.

Caseous necrosis. Death of tissue resulting in a gross appearance that resembles cottage cheese (Latin *caseus,* cheese).

Castleman's disease. Giant lymph node hyperplasia; benign polyclonal hyperplasia of B cells with prominent vascular component.

CD (cluster designation). A term used to identify identical lymphoid cell markers detected by different monoclonal antibodies. For instance, CD4 refers to phenotypes of T lymphocytes identified by monoclonal antibodies: OKT4 and Leu-3. Replaces terms such as OK, Leu, T4, T8, etc.

Celiac disease. See *gluten-sensitive enteropathy.*

Cell-mediated immunity. Immune effects caused by sensitized lymphocytes or activated macrophages.

Cellular immunity. Immune state due to action of sensitized or activated lymphocytes or macrophages.

Cellular interstitial pneumonia. Inflammation of lung with mononuclear inflammatory cells in alveolar walls.

Central lymphoid organs. Lymphoid organs essential for development of lymphoid system, i.e., thymus, bone marrow, bursa of Fabricius.

CH_{50} unit. The amount of serum (dilution) required to lyse 50% of antibody-coated red blood cells in a standard assay for hemolytic complement.

Chancre immunity. Resistance to reinfection by *Treponema pallidum* that occurs 3 months after untreated syphilis infection.

Chediak–Higashi syndrome. Phagocytic dysfunction caused by a defect in microtubular function leading to deficiencies in phagosome–lysosome formation.

Chemotactic factor. Substance that attracts inflammatory cells.

Chemotaxis. Process by which cells are attracted by chemicals or factors.

Chimera. A mythical animal composed of body parts of different animal species (e.g., head of a lion on the body of a goat). Used to designate condition following bone marrow transplantation when blood cells of recipient are composed of a mixture of cells of donor and recipient.

Cholinergic urticaria. Edematous skin reaction caused by an abnormal response to acetylcholine associated with decreased cholinesterase activity.

Chorea. Involuntary twitching muscular movements found in association with acute rheumatic fever (St. Vitus' dance).

Chromium release assay. Measurement of cell death detected by release of intracellular radiolabeled chromium in vitro.

Chromosomal translocations. Rearrangement of DNA sequences from one chromosome to another; often associated with cancer.

Chronic active hepatitis. Progressive lymphocytic inflammatory disease of the liver.

Chronic granulomatous disease of children. Phagocytic disorder due to defect in production of oxygen radicals resulting in granulomatous lesions in multiple organs of the body and recurrent suppurative lymphadenitis in children.

Chronic mucocutaneous candidiasis. Persistent or recurrent infection of mucous membranes, nails, and skin by *Candida albicans* due to defect in specific cell-mediated immunity to *Candida*.

Churg–Strauss syndrome (allergic granulomatosis). A disease complex including necrotizing vasculitis, extravascular granulomas, eosinophilic tissue infiltrates, and asthma.

Circumsporate reaction. Precipitation reaction of antibody to malaria protozoa that extends from the tail of the organism.

Class I major histocompatibility markers. Tissue antigens responsible for graft rejection, encoded by HLA-A, B, and C loci in humans and H2K and D loci in mice.

Class II major histocompatibility markers. Tissue markers responsible for self recognition and graft rejection, encoded by HLA-D in humans and H2I region in mice.

Clonal restriction. Limitation of an immune response to expression by a few clones of reactive cells.

Clonal selection. Theory of antibody formation that the individual recognizes different antigens through many individual clones of cells. A given antigen selects those clones that react with that antigen and stimulates proliferation and differentiation of the clones.

Clone. A population of cells that arises from a single precursor cell.

Coagulation system. System of 12 proteins in serum that results in formation of fibrin that blocks bleeding from injured vessels.

Cogan's syndrome. Inflammation of the cornea (interstitial keratitis) and the ear causing nausea, vomiting, ringing, and vertigo, associated with collagen diseases or as a post-infectious episode.

Cold agglutinin disease. Hemolytic disease caused by IgM antibodies that require cold temperature to agglutinate cells.

Cold antibodies. Antibodies that are detectable at higher titers at 4°C than at 37°C (cryoglobulins).

Cold target inhibition. Assay in which addition of unlabeled target cells blocks antibody- or cell-mediated release of radioisotope from labeled target cells.

Collagen diseases. Group of diseases with common lesion of fibrinoid necrosis, also known as connective tissue or rheumatoid diseases.

Colony-stimulating factors. Substances that enhance the clonal growth of cells.

Common variable immunodeficiencies. Defects in immune responses that occur after apparently normal development; manifested as humoral, cellular, or combined deficiencies.

Competitive inhibition. Process in which one population of cells or molecules inhibits the reaction of antibody or cells with another population (e.g., cold target inhibition, radio-immunoassay).

Complement. A system of at least 13 serum proteins that are activated by enzymatic cleavages and aggregations to produce components with biological activity.

Complement fixation. A test for antibody–antigen reactions that depends on binding (consumption) of complement by antibody–antigen complexes.

Concanavalin A. A lectin derived from the jack bean that reacts with carbohydrate residues (mannosides) and stimulates mitosis of T cells.

Concomitant immunity. Resistance to infection or transplantable cancer growth in an individual who already has the infection or is bearing the cancer.

Constant regions. See *C regions.*

Contact allergy. Delayed type hypersensitivity caused by CTL invading epidermis; characterized by spongiosis, vesiculation, and pruritis.

Contact sensitivity. An epidermal cell-mediated immune reaction to chemicals placed on the skin.

Contrasuppressor cell. A subpopulation of T cells that inhibits the function of suppressor cells.

Coombs' test. In vitro agglutination test for nonagglutinating antibodies to red blood cells, employing anti-Ig. *Direct Coombs' test:* anti-Ig added to test red cells; agglutination indicates cells were coated with antibody. *Indirect*

Coombs' test: serum added to red cells, cells washed, and anti-Ig added; agglutination indicates serum contains antibody to red blood cells.

Cords of Billroth. Medullary cords of spleen.

Cortex. The outer parenchymal layer of an organ (*medulla* refers to inner part).

C-reactive protein. Serum protein, MW 105,000, that increases markedly during inflammation. It reacts with somatic C substance of *Streptococcus pneumoniae.*

CREST complex. Calcinosis, Raynaud's phenomena, esophageal dysmobility, sclerodactyly, telangectasia; a syndrome pattern observed with a chronic form of dermatomyositis.

Creutzfeldt–Jakob syndrome. Slow virus infection of brain characterized by membrane accumulations in brain cells.

Cross-matching. Test in which red blood cells and sera from two different individuals are mixed together to determine if the serum of either of the individuals contains factors (antibodies) that react with the red blood cells of the other.

Cross-reactivity. Reaction of antisera or sensitized cells with different antigens due to some shared antigenic determinants or shared structures within the determinant.

Cryoglobulinemia. Presence in serum of proteins that precipitate at cold temperatures, usually but not always monoclonal immunoglobulins.

Cutaneous basophil hypersensitivity. Form of delayed hypersensitivity characterized by infiltration of skin test site by basophils. (See *Jones–Mote reaction.*)

Cyclic adenosine monophosphate (cAMP). Adenosine 3′,5′-(hydrogen phosphate). Key intracellular regulator; derived from adenosine triphosphate by adenylcyclase; activates protein kinase C; functions as "second messenger" during activation of cells by hormones; increased levels in mast cells are associated with *decreased* responsiveness of mast cells to degranulation signals.

Cyclic guanosine monophosphate (cGMP). Guanosine cyclic 3′,5′-(hydrogen phosphate). An antagonist of cAMP, formed by conversion of guanosine triphosphate by guanylatecyclase; increased levels in mast cells are associated with *increased* responsiveness to degranulation signals.

Cyclophosphamide. An alkylating agent widely used as an immunosuppressive drug, particularly in organ transplant recipients.

Cyclosporine. A cyclic polypeptide of 11 amino acids widely used as an immunosuppressive drug, especially in organ transplant recipients (older term is *cyclosporin A*).

Cytolytic reaction. The effect of antibody or sensitized cells that results in lysis of a target cell.

Cytophilic antibody. Antibody that binds to the surface of effector cells through the Fc piece (e.g., IgE to mast cells, IgM to macrophages).

Cytotoxic T lymphocytes. Specifically sensitized T cells that are capable of killing target cells (also termed *T killer cells*).

D region. Segment of gene coding diversity region in the hypervariable region of immunoglobulin H chains.

Degranulation. Process of fusion of cytoplasmic granules of cells (mast cells, phagocytic cells) with cell membrane so that contents of the granules are released from the cell.

Delayed hypersensitivity. In vivo inflammatory reaction mediated by sensitized T cells (T_D cells). The classic skin reaction reaches a maximum 24–72 hours after injection of antigen.

Dendritic cells. Cells of macrophage lineage present in lymph nodes (follicular and interdigitating), spleen, other lymphoid organs, and skin (Langerhans cell) that bear class II MHC markers, have Fc receptors and can process antigen for an immune response.

Dermatitis herpetiformis. Skin disease featuring subepithelial bullae found in patients with gluten enteropathy. Findings include IgA and complement deposition in dermal microfibers.

Dermatitis venenata. See *contact dermatitis.*

Dermatographism. Immediate wheal and flare reaction produced by scratching the skin. The reaction is caused by the release of mediators from mast cells by physical stimulation (anaphylactoid reaction).

Dermatomyositis. A rheumatoid (collagen) disease characterized by skin rash and inflammation of muscles.

Dermatopathic lymphadenitis. Benign hyperplasia of lymph nodes secondary to infection or inflammation of the skin.

Desensitization. Production of a temporary loss of immune reactivity in a sensitized individual following administration of antigen, due to consumption of antibody or sensitized cells.

Diabetes mellitus. A group of diseases caused by abnormalities of glucose metabolism that results in high blood glucose levels and glycosuria.

Diapedesis. Passage of cells from small vessels into adjacent tissue due to constriction of endothelial cells.

Dick test. Lack of an inflammatory response in the skin to the scarlatina toxin of streptococci in individuals with neutralizing antibody.

Differentiation factors. Substances that induce maturation of cells.

DiGeorge syndrome. Failure of development of epithelial component of the thymus and parathyroids, leading to T cell immunodeficiency and disorders in Ca^{++} metabolism (neonatal tetany).

Dinitrochlorobenzene. Chemical hapten active in inducing contact dermatitis; effective as nonspecific immunotherapeutic agent for certain skin cancers.

Disulfide bonds. Chemical bonds between sulfhydryl-containing amino acids that bind together polypeptide chains.

Domains. (1) Segments of polypeptide chains that are folded together and stabilized by disulfide bonds. (2) Zones of lymphoid organs that contain high proportions of different lymphoid cell subpopulations.

Dopamine. A hormone produced by the adrenal gland that controls nerve function; loss of receptors for dopamine results in neurological diseases such as Parkinson's disease.

Double-diffusion test. Antibody–antigen precipitation reaction in agar or a similar gel in which antigen and antibody are allowed to diffuse toward one another and react at equivalence in the agar.

DPT. Diphtheria and tetanus toxoids combined with pertussis vaccine; used for routine childhood immunization.

Drug allergy. An immunopathologic reaction to a drug as a result of the drug acting as an antigen eliciting an immune response.

DTH. Delayed-type hypersensitivity.

Duncan's syndrome (X-linked lymphoproliferative syndrome). Lymphoproliferation and agammaglobulinemia associated with Epstein-Barr virus infection; susceptibility to infection is inherited as X-linked recessive.

Dysgammaglobulinemias. Abnormalities in production of immunoglobulin classes resulting in decreases in one or more Ig classes with normal or elevated levels of other Ig classes.

E antigen. An antigen of hepatitis B virus found in sera of patients with chronic active hepatitis.

E rosette. A lymphocyte surrounded by a cluster of red blood cells. Human T lymphocytes form E rosettes with sheep red blood cells.

EA. Erythrocyte coated with antibody; will be lysed if complement is added.

EAC rosette. A cluster of red cells sensitized with antibody and complement around lymphocytes that have cell surface receptors for complement (human B lymphocytes).

ECF-A. Eosinophil chemotactic factor: an acidic polypeptide, MW 500, that attracts eosinophils.

Ectoderm. Outer cellular layer of 3 cell layers of embryo. Gives rise to epidermis and neuronal tissue.

ecto-5′-*Nucleotidase deficiency.* Defect in purine metabolism leading to B cell immunodeficiencies.

Eczema. Weeping skin lesions associated with atopic reactions, characterized by erythema, papules, vesicles, and intense pruritus.

Eczematoid skin reaction. Erythematous, vesicular, pruritic skin reaction similar to eczema but not of atopic origin.

Edema. Swelling of tissue due to extravasation of fluid from intravascular space.

Effector cell. Cell capable of mediating a function.

Electroimmunodiffusion. A double-diffusion-in-gel technique in which antibody and antigen are pulled toward each other in an electric current.

Electrophoresis. Separation of molecules in an electrical field.

Elephantiasis. Lymphedema of extremities due to obstruction of lymphatics. Occurs as a complication of granulomatous reaction to filariasis.

ELISA (enzyme-linked immunosorbent assay). An immunoassay system employing enzyme bound to antibody or antigen.

Encephalitogenic peptide. Nonapeptide of myelin (Phe-Leu-Trp-Ala-Glu-Gly-Gln-Lys) that is smallest component that will induce experimental allergic encephalomyelitis.

End cell. A terminally differentiated cell, no longer capable of dividing.

Endocytosis. Process whereby material is taken into a cell.

Endoderm. Innermost of three cellular layers of embryo. Gives rise to gastrointestinal lining and some internal organs such as liver and pancreas.

Endogenous. Arising from within; autologous.

Endoplasmic reticulum. Membrane-like structure in cytoplasm of cells, in which proteins are synthesized or stored.

Endotoxins. Lipopolysaccharides derived from the cell wall of gram-negative bacteria that have pyrogenic, toxic, and stimulatory effects.

Enhancement. Prolonged survival of skin grafts or tumor grafts in individuals with humoral antibody, presumably due to blocking antibody.

Eosinophil. A polymorphonuclear leukocyte with granules that contain basic proteins believed to modulate inflammatory reactions and that stain red (acidophilic).

Eosinophilic granuloma. Subtype of tumor of macrophage lineage (histiocytosis X) containing eosinophils, found prominently in bones.

Epithelioid cells. Altered macrophages in granulomas that resemble epithelial cells morphologically.

Epitope. Antigenic determinant; the smallest structural area on an antigen that can be recognized by an antibody.

Epitype. A family of restricted epitopes; a set of epitopes.

Epstein–Barr virus. The virus that causes infectious mononucleosis and Burkitt's lymphoma in man.

Equilibrium dialysis. A technique used to measure the affinity of antibody–antigen binding, based on diffusion of unbound antigen across a dialysis membrane.

Equivalence. The ratio of antibody to antigen that gives the maximum precipitation in the quantitative precipitation reaction.

Erythema marginatum. Subcutaneous vasculitis due to immune complexes, found in association with rheumatic fever.

Erythema multiforme. Variable skin lesions due to subcutaneous vasculitis, associated with drugs and caused by immune complexes.

Erythema nodosum. Subcutaneous vasculitis involving small arteries, resulting in nodular lesions. The lesions are associated with infections and are caused by immune complexes.

Erythroblastosis fetalis. A disease of the human fetus caused by placental transfer of maternal antibodies to fetal red blood cells, resulting in destruction of fetal red blood cells and hyperplasia of blood-forming cells in the fetus.

Erythropoietin. Substance produced by the kidney that stimulates red blood cell production.

Exchange transfusion. Replacement of blood to remove toxic material, such as in kernicterus in infants with erythroblastosis fetalis.

Exhaustive differentiation. Processes whereby cells mature and die.

Exogenous. Arising from without; foreign.

Exon. Portion of a structural gene that is expressed in transcribed RNA.

Exotoxins. Diffusible toxic substances produced by microorganisms.

Experimental allergic encephalomyelitis. Autoimmune demyelinating disease induced in animals by immunization with myelin or myelin-derived antigens.

Extrinsic allergic alveolitis. Inflammation in the lung caused by immune (predominantly granulomatous) reaction to dusts, bacteria, mold, grain, or other inhaled antigens.

Exudation. Inflammation in which blood cells and fluid containing high-molecular-weight serum proteins are present in tissue.

F_1 hybrid. The first generation of a mating between two inbred strains.

Fab. The monovalent antigen-binding fragment of an IgG antibody molecule produced by digestion with papain.

$F(ab')_2$. The bivalent fragment of an IgG antibody molecule produced by digestion with pepsin.

FACS. Fluorescence-activated cell sorter.

Factor B (C3 proactivator). A component of the alternative pathway of complement activation that interacts with factor D.

Factor D. A serine esterase of the alternative pathway of complement activation that when activated cleaves factor B when the latter is complexed to C3b to form C3bB.

Farr technique. A primary binding assay for antibody activity employing radiolabeled antigen.

Fc. "Crystallizable fragment": the non-antigen-binding fragment of an immunoglobulin molecule produced after digestion with papain. When first recognized using rabbit IgG, this fragment formed crystals, but the Fc of most species does not crystallize.

Fc receptor. Structure on surface of some lymphocytes or other cells (mast cells, macrophages) that binds the Fc portion of immunoglobulin, usually when the Fc is aggregated, but not always.

Fd fragment. Part of the heavy chain of immunoglobulin that lies on the N-terminal side of the site of papain hydrolysis.

Fernandez reaction. Twenty-four-hour maximum delayed hypersensitivity reaction to lepromin, a skin test for leprosy.

Fibrinoid necrosis. Death of tissue that looks like fibrin microscopically, produced by enzymatic digestion of tissue by proteases released from neutrophils or deposition of fibrin in tissue.

Filariasis. Disease due to infection with filaria (e.g., *Wuchereria bancrofti);* takes different forms depending on type of immune effector mechanisms.

First set rejection. Tissue graft rejection that occurs when first graft to an unrelated donor is made. Rejection follows induction of immune reactivity, usually takes 12–14 days, and is mediated by delayed hypersensitivity.

Flocculation. Precipitation reaction of antibody and antigen in which the precipitate appears as flakes of insoluble protein, usually seen with horse antibody – toxin reactions.

Fluorescein. Yellow dye used to label antibody for fluorescence technique.

Fluorescence. Emission of light of a given wavelength by a substance activated by light of a different wavelength.

f-Met peptides. Tripeptides released by bacteria that are chemotactic for inflammatory cells (formyl-Met-Leu-Phe).

Follicle. Round-to-oval areas in lymphoid organs containing a high proportion of B cells.

Follicle-stimulating hormone. Substance produced in adrenal gland that induces formation of ovarian follicles and ovulation.

Follicular center cells. B cells in secondary follicles (germinal centers) representing different morphological stages of B cell cycle; similar morphology is seen in B cell tumors as homogeneous populations of lymphoma cells.

Food allergy. Diarrhea, vomiting, and nausea caused by anaphylactic reaction to allergens in food.

Forssman antigen. A common carbohydrate antigen on sheep cells, goat cells, human type A red cells, certain bacteria, etc. Antibody to Forssman antigen appears in patients who recover from infectious mononucleosis.

Fragile sites. Location of breaks in chromosomes of cancer or normal cells cultured in vitro in the presence of metabolic inhibitors.

Framework region. Sequences of amino acids in variable regions of H or L immunoglobulin chain other than hypervariable sequences.

Freemartin. Female twin of a male calf. These twins share a common placenta and exhibit mutual tolerance to each other's tissues as adults. Female twin is sterile.

Freund's adjuvant. A water-in-oil emulsion that enhances immune responses when antigen is included. Freund's complete adjuvant includes killed mycobacteria, Freund's incomplete adjuvant does not contain mycobacteria.

Gamma globulins. Serum proteins with least mobility to positive electrode during electrophoresis. Gamma globulins contain immunoglobulins and antibodies.

Gastrointestinal associated lymphoid tissue (GALT). Lymphoid organs located along the gastrointestinal tract: tonsils, Peyer's patches, appendix, and submucosal lymphocytes.

Gatekeeper effect. Role of IgE-mediated endothelial contraction in allowing blood components to enter extravascular tissue because of increased vascular permeability.

Gel diffusion. Technique of allowing antibodies and antigen to diffuse towards each other and react in gels.

Germinal center. A lymphoid follicle with a clear center and dense margin. A site of active proliferation of B cells.

Ghon complex. Healed granuloma or scar on pleural surface of the middle lobes of the lung and granulomas in the hilar lymph nodes; a consequence of healed primary tuberculosis.

Glial fibrillary acid protein (GFAP). Major protein component of the intermediate filaments of astrocytes; also identifiable in tumors arising from glial cells.

γ-Globulin. Obsolete term for immunoglobulin (e.g., γG for IgG).

Glomerulonephritis. Inflammation of glomeruli of the kidneys; often due to immune complexes deposited in glomeruli.

Gluten-sensitive enteropathy. A disease involving defective gastrointestinal absorption due to sensitivity to gluten. Associated with increased gastrointestinal IgA and dermatitis herpetiformis.

Gm. Allotypic marker on human IgG heavy chains.

Golgi apparatus. A collection of tubular cytoplasmic structures involved in rapid secretion of proteins.

Goodpasture's disease. A disease with pulmonary hemorrhage and glomerulonephritis caused by autoantibody that reacts with basement membrane of lung and kidney.

GP70. A protein antigen of MW 70,000 coded by viral oncogenes of mice.

Graft facilitation. Increased graft survival associated with IgG antibody (blocking antibody) and decreased cell-mediated immunity.

Graft rejection. Immune-mediated destruction of tissue transplanted from one individual to another.

Graft vs. host reactions. The systemic effects of reaction of transferred immunocompetent cells to the tissues of a histoincompatible host.

Granuloma. Tissue reaction of modified macrophages (epithelioid cells), lymphocytes, and fibroblasts to poorly degradable antigens.

Granulomatous hepatitis. Granulomatous inflammation of the liver.

Graves' disease (hyperthyroidism). Metabolic disease caused by hyperplasia of thyroid gland and increased secretion of thyroid hormone. May be associated with autoantibodies to thyroid-stimulating hormone receptors, long-acting thyroid stimulator (LATS).

Growth factors. Substances that stimulate or enhance the proliferation of cells.

Guillain–Barré neuritis. Chronic demyelinating disease of spinal cord and peripheral nerves believed to be due to autoimmunity to peripheral nerve myelin.

H chain (heavy chain). One pair of identical polypeptide chains of four-chain immunoglobulin molecules. The other pair of chains are the L (light) chains.

H substance. Core carbohydrate of ABO blood group system.

H1 receptors. Receptors for histamine on vascular smooth muscle cells that activate vasodilation.

H-2. The major histocompatibility complex of the mouse.

H2 receptors. Receptors on various tissue cells for histamine that activate asthma bronchial constriction, diarrhea (gastrointestinal constriction), and edema (endothelial constriction).

Hageman factor. Factor VII of the coagulation system. Activated Hageman factor initiates the intrinsic coagulation system as well as generation of inflammatory peptides.

Hairy cell leukemia. A leukemia of B cells with prominent cytoplasmic filopodia.

Hand-Schuller-Christian disease. Type of tumor of macrophage lineage (histiocytosis x) found predominantly in bone.

Hanganitziu–Deicher antigen. Altered ganglioside structure found in some human cancers (CD3, GM1, and terminal 4NAcNeu).

Haplotype. Phenotypic characteristics inherited through closely linked genes on one chromosome.

Hapten. An incomplete antigen. A hapten cannot induce an immune response unless complexed to a carrier. A hapten can react with immune products induced by a hapten–carrier immunogenic complex.

Hashimoto's disease. Inflammation of the thyroid gland characterized by lymphocyte infiltrate and lymphoid germinal centers, believed to be caused by autoimmunity to thyroid antigens.

Hassall's corpuscles. Whorls of epithelial cells in the medulla of the thymus believed to be the source of thymic hormones.

Hay fever. Seasonal allergic rhinitis; recurrent asthma, rhinitis, and conjunctivitis caused by atopic (IgE)-mediated reaction to environmental allergens, usually plant pollens, but also other airborne particles such as animal dander, insect parts, and house dust.

HBcAg. Hepatitis B core antigen.

HBsAg. Hepatitis B surface antigen.

H-chain disease. Presence of elevated levels of free H chains in serum. Usually caused by a type of multiple myeloma that produces heavy chains of Ig but not light chains.

Helper factor. Substance secreted by T helper cells or accessory cells that contributes to B cell activation.

Helper T cells. A subpopulation of T lymphocytes that cooperates with macrophages and B cells during induction of antibody formation.

Hemagglutinin. Antibody or substance that causes aggregation of red blood cells.

Hematologist. An individual who specializes in study and/or treatment of diseases of the blood and blood-forming system.

Hematuria. Blood in the urine; usually due to damage to glomerular basement membrane secondary to acute glomerulonephritis, but also found in other renal diseases.

Hemolysin. An antibody or substance capable of destroying red blood cells.

Hemolysis. Process of lysis of red blood cells.

Hemolytic anemia. A disease involving low numbers of circulating red blood cells due to destruction (lysis).

Hemolytic disease of the newborn (erythroblastosis fetalis). Destruction of red blood cells of a fetus due to placental transfer of antibody from the mother.

Hemophilia. A disease caused by a failure of blood to clot due to a deficiency in a blood clotting factor, e.g., factor VIII.

Henoch–Schönlein purpura. A clinical syndrome including hemorrhagic lesions in the skin, edema and hemorrhage in the gastrointestinal tract, and arthritis and glomerulonephritis associated with IgA deposits in glomeruli and dermal vessels.

Heparin. A glucoside antic██████████ ██iv█ liver and mast cells.

Herpes gestationis. A blistering █████ ██ch subepidermal bullae associated with pregnan██ ██tibody to dermal basement membrane.

Heteroclitic antibody. Antibody produced to one antigen that actually has a higher affinity to another antigen.

Heterocytotropic antibody. Antibody that has greater affinity to fix to mast cells of a different species than the species from which the antibody is derived; usually tested by ability to fix to skin, i.e., passive cutaneous anaphylaxis.

Heterologous. Used to describe: (1) a donor–host relationship between two different species (synonymous with *xenogeneic*); (2) a substance derived from a foreign source.

Heterophil antigen. An antigen found in different apparently unrelated organisms and/or tissues, usually carbohydrate.

Heymann nephritis. Experimental autoimmune inflammation of tubules of kidneys induced by immunization with renal tubular cells.

High endothelial postcapillary venules. Specialized vessels in lymphoid organs where circulating cells pass into parenchyma.

Hinge region. Amino acid segment between the first and second constant regions of the immunoglobulin heavy chain of IgG that permits bending of the molecule.

Histamine. A bioactive amine of MW 111 present in mast cells and platelets that causes immediate effects of anaphylactic and anaphylactoid reactions.

Histiocytes. Phagocytic cells of the macrophage series that are fixed in tissues.

Histiocytic lymphoma. Outdated term for large cell lymphomas, which are most commonly B cell tumors. *True histiocytic lymphoma* refers to lymphomas of macrophage lineage.

Histiocytosis X. Term used for tumors of macrophage lineage; includes Letterer–Siwe disease, Hand-Schuller-Christian disease, and eosinophilic granuloma of bone.

Histocompatibility. Relationship between tissues of different individuals; histocompatible organs or tissues will not evoke an immune rejection reaction.

Histocompatibility antigens. Antigens on cells responsible for tissue transplantation rejection.

HIV (human immunodeficiency virus). A term identifying the family of retroviruses that causes human acquired immunodeficiency syndrome (AIDS); replaces terms such as *AIDS-related retrovirus* and *HTLV-III*.

(wheal and flare reaction). Anaphylactic skin reaction mediated by histamine release from activated mast cells, characterized by edema, surrounding erythema, and pruritus.

HLA (human leukocyte antigen). The major histocompatibility complex genetic region of the human.

Hodgkin's disease. Type of lymphoid cancer believed to be of macrophage lineage, characterized by binucleated giant cells known as Reed–Sternberg cells.

Homocytotrophic antibody. An antibody that binds better to cells of animals of the same species than to cells of animals of different species from that of the antibody.

Homologous. Used to describe: (1) a substance derived from the same source; (2) a donor–host relationship within the same species (synonym: allogeneic).

Horror autotoxicus. A concept proposed by Paul Ehrlich in 1900 whereby individuals do not make an immune response to their own tissues.

Hot spots. Short amino acid sequences in the variable regions of H and L chains of immunoglobulin that appear together in the paratope (antigen binding site) of the folded antibody molecule. Also referred to as *hypervariable regions.*

HTLA. Human T lymphocyte antigen; obsolete term replaced by cluster designations (see Appendix B).

HTLV (human T cell leukemia virus). A generic name for viruses associated with human T cell leukemias. A subgroup of HTLV is now designated *HIV (human immunodeficiency virus).*

Human immunodeficiency virus (HIV). Retrovirus that infects human CD4 lymphocytes and causes acquired immunodeficiency syndrome (AIDS); formerly called *AIDS-related retrovirus, HTLV-III,* etc.

Humoral. Pertaining to blood or tissue fluid.

Humoral immunity. Immunity due to immunoglobulin antibody in blood or tissue.

Hybrid resistance. Resistance of F_1 to growth of transplantable tumors derived from either parental strain (see *allogeneic inhibition*).

Hybridoma. A transformed cell line formed by the fusion of two parental cell lines.

Hyperplasia. Reversible increase in the size of an organ due to an increase in the number of cells. Usually related to a physiological response to a stimulus.

Hypersensitivity. A state of increased reactivity or sensitiveness.

Hypersensitivity angiitis. A acute and chronic inflammation of small arteries and veins often, but not always, associated with drug use.

Hyperthyroidism. Metabolic disease due to hyperplasia of thyroid gland and increase secretion of thyroid hormone (see *Graves' disease*).

Hypervariable regions. See *hot spots.*

Hypocomplementemic glomerulonephritis. Chronic progressive glomerulonephritis associated with deposition of C3 in renal glomerular basement membrane (see *C3 nephritogenic factor*).

Hypocomplementemic vasculitic urticarial syndrome. Systemic inflammation featuring urticaria, leukoclastic vasculitis, and low serum complement levels.

Hypogammaglobulinemia of infancy. Transient delay in production of immunoglobulins during the first year or two of life, resulting in temporary immune deficiency.

Hyposensitization. Decreased responsiveness to antigens by anaphylactic or delayed hypersensitivity reactions due to presence of circulating IgG blocking antibody to the same antigen.

I region. That segment of the mouse major histocompatibility complex genome that controls immune responses and expression of Ia and Ie phenotypes; class II MHC region of the mouse.

Ia antigens. Cell surface markers controlled by the I region (a and e); class II MHC antigens of the mouse.

Iatrogenic. Used to describe diseases or lesions caused by treatment by a physician or other practitioner of the healing arts.

Idiopathic thrombocytopenic purpura. Hemorrhagic disease due to low platelets; often caused by autoantibodies to platelets.

Idiosyncrasy. Qualitatively abnormal response to normal doses of a drug.

Idiotope. An epitope on the V region of antibody molecules.

Idiotype. A set of unique antigenic determinants (idiotopes) on the V region of homologous or monoclonal antibodies.

Idiotype network. A series of idiotype–anti-idiotype reactions that is postulated to control production of idiotype-bearing antibody molecules or cells.

Idiotype vaccines. Immunizing material consisting of anti-idiotypic antibody molecules that mimic the epitope(s) of the original infecting organism.

Ig. Immunoglobulin.

IgA. Secretory immunoglobulin class, dimeric in secretions, monomeric in blood.

IgD. Immunoglobulin class on surface of B cells.

IgE. Immunoglobulin class that fixes to mast cells and is responsible for anaphylactic sensitivity.

IgG. Predominant serum immunoglobulin class in adults.

IgM. Pentameric immunoglobulin; first class of antibody produced to most antigens.

I-J. Postulated subsegment of mouse I region that codes for an antigen on suppressor cells and/or suppressor factors.

IL. See *interleukins*.

Immediate hypersensitivity. Inflammatory reaction that occurs within minutes of exposure to antigen (see *anaphylactic reactions*).

Immobilization test. An assay for antibody or factor that stops the motion of motile organisms.

Immune adherence. Binding of antibody–antigen complexes

or antibody-coated particles to primate erythrocytes, rabbit platelets, or white blood cells due to activation of C3 and formation of C3b.

Immune complex reactions. Tissue inflammation mediated by antibody–antigen complexes.

Immune deviation. Substitution or exchange of one immune effector mechanism for another (e.g., IgG antibody in preference to delayed hypersensitivity in lepromatous leprosy).

Immune elimination. Rapid clearance of an antigen from the circulation due to reaction with antibody and removal of immune complexes by the reticuloendothelial system.

Immune memory. Secondary response; property of more rapid and more intense immune response after the first exposure to an antigen (anamnesis).

Immune modulation. Change, usually loss, of cell surface markers on cells, usually tumor cells, exposed to antibody to the cell surface marker.

Immune paralysis. Inability to detect antibody to a nondegradable antigen due to repeated consumption of the antibody.

Immune surveillance. Postulated function of the immune system to prevent tumor cells from growing.

Immunity. State of protection from injury due to previous experience or special state of responsiveness.

Immunization. Process of inducing a state of immunity.

Immunoabsorption. Removal of an antigen by reaction with antibody or removal of a subset of antibodies by an antigen in a solid phase system or by precipitation.

Immunoblot (Western blot). Reaction of labeled antibodies with proteins absorbed on nitrocellulose paper.

Immunodeficiency. Defect in immune system resulting in decreased resistance to infection.

Immunodiffusion. Test for antibody–antigen reaction involving diffusion in gel precipitation.

Immunodominant epitope. That epitope on an antigen that best binds or absorbs the antibody made to that antigen.

Immunoelectrophoresis. A technique involving separation of proteins in an electric field followed by a precipitation reaction in gel with antibodies to the separated proteins.

Immunofluorescence. A histochemical technique employing fluorescence-labeled antibodies or antigens for localization in tissues or cell suspensions.

Immunogen. A complete antigen; an antigen that can induce an immune response and react with the antibodies elicited.

Immunogenic. Capable of inducing an immune response.

Immunoglobulin classes. Subfamily of immunoglobulins based on large differences in H-chain amino acid sequence: IgA, IgD, IgE, IgG, IgM (isotypes).

Immunoglobulin subclasses. Subpopulations of an Ig class based on more subtle structural or antigenic differences in the H chains than are class differences (e.g., IgG1, IgG2, IgG3, IgG4).

Immunoglobulin supergene family. Set of related genes coding for immunoglobulins and cell surface molecules (T cell receptor, MHC surface markers).

Immunoglobulins. A family of glycoprotein molecules having similar structure, to which antibodies belong.

Immunologically competent cell. A lymphocyte that has the ability to recognize and be activated by an antigen.

Immunologist. An individual who studies immunology.

Immunology. The study of immunity.

Immunopathology. The study of how immune mechanisms cause disease.

Immunotherapy. The use of immunization or immune products to modify disease.

Incomplete antibody. Antibody that binds antigen but does not precipitate or agglutinate the antigen.

Inducer cell. A subpopulation of T lymphocytes that cooperate with macrophages and precursor T cells during the generation of active T cell subpopulations (T suppressors, T CTL, etc.).

Inflammation. The process whereby blood proteins and cells enter tissue in response to infection or injury.

Inflammatory cell. Blood and tissue cells that take part in inflammation.

Inflammatory mediator. A substance involved in the inflammatory process.

Innate immunity. Protection from injury or infection that does not require immunization.

Innocent bystander. A cell that is destroyed by an immune effector mechanism that is specifically directed to a different cell population.

Instructive theory of antibody formation. An obsolete theory that antigen directs immune responsive cells to produce antibody of a given specificity by imposing a conformation on the antibody formed.

Interdigitating reticulum cells. A subclass of antigen-processing macrophages found in the paracortex of lymph nodes.

Interferons. A group of low-molecular-weight protein molecules, produced in virus-infected cells, that inhibit infection of noninfected cells.

Interleukin 1. A macrophage-derived substance, MW 15,000, that has multiple biologic properties including the ability to promote short-term growth of T cells (previously called *leukocyte activating factor*).

Interleukin 2. A substance, MW 35,000, derived from activated T helper cells that promotes growth of other activated T cells or B cells (previously called *T cell growth factor*).

Interleukin 3. MW-40,000 substance derived from activated T cells that stimulates proliferation of bone marrow cells.

Interleukin 4. A growth factor, MW 20,000, that stimulates resting T cells, B cells, and other lymphoid cells (previously called *B cell stimulating factor I*).

Interleukins. Substances produced by one mononuclear white cell population that act on other white cell populations.

Internal image. Epitope on an anti-idiotype antibody (Ab2) subpopulation that binds to the paratope of the antibody induced by the "foreign" antigen (Ab1).

Interstitial nephritis. Inflammation around tubules of kidney often associated with autoantibody to tubular basement membrane.

Intolerance. Increased sensitivity to normal doses of a drug.

Intrinsic factor. Substance produced by parental cells of gastric mucosa that enhances absorption of vitamin B12. Loss of intrinsic factor is responsible for the disease pernicious anemia.

Introns. Internal segments of a structural gene that are not transcribed into RNA.

InV. Allotype on κ light chains of humans.

Ir region. Genes in MHC that control immune responses (class II MHC).

Islets of Langerhans. Small collections of endocrine cells within the exocrine parenchyma of the pancreas; contain cells secreting insulin and other endocrine hormones.

Isohemagglutinins. Antibodies that react with antigens present on red blood cells of different individuals of the same species.

Isologous. Derived from the same species (see *allogeneic*).

Isotype. Antigens that define class or subclass specificity.

J chain. A polypeptide chain that joins individual four-chain immunoglobulin units to form polymeric immunoglobulins (IgA, IgM).

J region. That postulated portion of the mouse I region (class II MHC) that controls suppression.

Jarisch–Herxheimer reaction. Systemic febrile reaction associated with skin rash, lymphadenopathy, and headache following penicillin treatment of syphilis, believed to be caused by release of toxic substances from *Treponema pallidum*.

Job's syndrome. Phagocytic dysfunction due to deficiencies in glutathione reductase and glucose-6-phosphatase; inherited as autosomal recessive.

Jones–Mote reaction. Delayed skin reaction to protein antigens characterized by dermal infiltration by basophils (see *cutaneous basophil hypersensitivity*).

K and D regions. Class I MHC genomic regions of the mouse.

Kallikrein (kininogenase). Activated by cleavage of prekallikrein in tissue fluids, kallikrein acts on kininogen to produce kinin.

Kaposi's sarcoma. Tumors of blood vessels originally described as relatively benign subcutaneous growths in lower extremities of elderly people; more aggressive systemic distribution in visceral organs is seen in patients with AIDS.

Kappa (κ) chains. One of two major types of immunoglobulin light chains.

Kawasaki's syndrome. Mucocutaneous lymph node syndrome; includes vasculitis (particularly of coronary arteries), conjunctivitis, skin rash, edema, and lymphadenopathy.

Kernicterus. A condition, due to high levels of red blood cell breakdown products in infants with erythroblastosis fetalis, that causes discoloration of the skin and neurological dysfunction.

Killer cells (K cells). Lymphocytes that mediate antibody-dependent cell-mediated cytotoxicity (ADCC).

Kinin system. A humoral amplification system for inflammation, involving activation of substrate protein molecules to active polypeptides by enzymatic cleavage.

Kinins. Inflammatory peptides formed by action of kallikrein on kininogen.

Koch phenomenon. The classic delayed hypersensitivity skin reaction to tuberculin in guinea pigs following infection with *Mycobacteria tuberculosis*.

Kupffer cells. Fixed mononuclear phagocytic cells in the sinusoids of the liver.

Kuru. A slow virus disease characterized by membrane accumulation in brain cells. The virus is transmitted from brains of infected individuals through lesions in the skin of food handlers during preparation for ritual cannibalism by certain native tribes of New Guinea.

L chain (light chain). A polypeptide chain of MW 22,000 present in all immunoglobulin molecules in two forms, κ and λ. Each four-chain Ig molecule has either two κ or two λ light chains.

Lacteals. Small lymphatic vessels that drain intestinal villi.

Lambda (λ) chain. One of two major types of immunoglobulin light chains.

Lamina propria. Thin layer of connective tissue supporting the epithelium of the gastrointestinal tract.

Langerhans cells. Antigen-processing, class II MHC marker–positive monocytic dendritic cells in the epithelial layer of the skin.

Large granular lymphocytes. Lymphocytes in the NK/K series with large cytoplasmic lysosomes.

LATS. Long-acting thyroid stimulator; an anti-thyroid cell antibody to the thyroid-stimulating hormone receptor that stimulates thyroid hormone production.

L2C leukemia. Transplantable B cell tumor of guinea pigs.

LE cell. An outdated diagnostic test detecting antinuclear antibody in sera of individuals with SLE. The LE cell is a polymorphonuclear neutrophil that has phagocytosed a lymphocyte nucleus oposonized by antinuclear antibodies.

LE factor. Antinuclear antibodies found in serum of patients with systemic lupus erythematosus; responsible for formation of the LE cell.

Lectin. A substance derived from a plant that binds to and sometimes is mitogenic for lymphocytes. Some lectins also bind red blood cells.

Lepromin. Skin test antigen used to test for cell-mediated immunity in leprosy.

Lesch–Nyhan syndrome. Hypoxanthine–guanosine phosphoribosyl deficiency resulting in neurological impairment and B cell immune deficiency.

Letterer–Siewe disease. Type of tumor of macrophage lineage (histiocytosis X) that occurs prominently in skin, lymph nodes, and spleen.

Leukemia. Literally "white blood"; term used for malignant proliferation of circulating white blood cells. Usually arises in bone marrow and results in large numbers of circulating white blood cells, giving blood a white color.

Leukoclastic vasculitis. Histologic description of inflammation of vessels by fragmented polymorphonuclear neutrophils, most often an immune complex–mediated lesion.

Leukocyte. White blood cell.

Leukopenia. Low number of white blood cells in the blood.

Leukotrienes. Metabolic products of arachidonic acid, some of which have inflammatory properties.

Levamisole. An antihelminthic drug that may potentiate immune responses or effector mechanisms.

Lichenification. Thickening of skin caused by chronic inflammation (severe hyperkeratosis).

Ligand. A molecule that binds to another molecule (receptor).

Light chain. See *L chain.*

Linkage disequilibrium. The tendency for a set of genetically determined characteristics to be inherited together in a given population.

Lipopolysaccharides. Substances produced by gram-negative bacteria that may have pyrogenic, inflammatory, or mitogenic effects. (See *endotoxins.*)

Low responder mice. Inbred mice who produce a low, usually IgM-only, antibody response to antigens that induce normal responses in other strains of mice. Low responsiveness is controlled by the class II MHC region.

L3T4. A mouse lymphocyte marker defined by a monoclonal antibody that identifies T helper/inducer cells.

Lupus erythematosus. A disease complex featuring vasculitis, arthritis, glomerulonephritis, and skin and other lesions included in the collagen disease group; associated with autoantibodies to DNA, RNA, and nuclear proteins.

Ly antigens. T-lymphocyte antigens of mice (see *Lyt*).

Lymph. Fluid in lymphatic system.

Lymph node. Organ of lymphoid system that filters lymphatics. Major site of immune responses.

Lymphatics. Vessels that collect interstitial fluid and deliver it back to the bloodstream.

Lymphocytes. Small cells with round nuclei containing densely packed chromatin. Many different subpopulations may be identified.

Lymphocytic choriomeningitis. Inflammatory brain lesion of mice caused by delayed hypersensitivity reaction to viral antigens on infected brain cells (LCM virus).

Lymphoid organs. Organs of the body that contain dense populations of lymphocytes (thymus, spleen, lymph nodes, GALT, etc).

Lymphoid system. Lymphatics and lymphoid organs.

Lymphokine-activated cytotoxic cells (LAC). A population of killer cells activated by lymphokines (IL2, interferon).

Lymphokines. Soluble substances, produced and secreted by lymphocytes, that act on other cells.

Lymphoma. Malignant tumor (cancer) of lymphoid tissue.

Lymphorrhages. Foci of lymphocytic inflammation in muscle, seen in myasthenia gravis and other muscle diseases.

Lymphotoxin. A lymphokine that lyses selected target cell lines.

Lysosomes. Granules that contain hydrolytic enzymes; present in many cells, but prominent in neutrophils and macrophages.

Lysozyme (muraminidase). A cationic low-molecular-weight enzyme present in tears and other secretions that digests the mucopeptides of bacterial cell walls.

Lyt1, Lyt2, Lyt3. A set of surface antigens defining subpopulations of mouse T cells. Lyt1 is associated with helper T cells, Lyt2 and Lyt3 with suppressor T cells. In practice the helper phenotype is now defined by a monoclonal antibody that detects a marker termed *L3T4*.

M protein. (1) Monoclonal immunoglobulin found in myelomas. (2) Type-specific cell surface antigens of group A β-hemolytic streptococci.

Macroglobulins. Glycoproteins of MW greater than 200,000.

Macrophage. Large bone marrow–derived phagocytic cells in the monocyte series that function as accessory cells in induction of immune response and as effector cells in inflammatory responses.

Macrophage activation factor. A lymphokine that increases the phagocytic activity of macrophages.

Macrophage chemotactic factor. A lymphokine that attracts macrophages.

Macrophage migration test. In vitro test for cellular immunity that depends on ability of antigen to induce formation of a lymphokine that inhibits migration of macrophages on agar.

Major histocompatibility complex. The set of genes that code for histocompatibility and related markers.

Makari test. Immediate skin reaction to autochthonous tumor extracts preincubated with patient's serum; of dubious significance.

Malaria. Febrile hemolytic disease caused by infection with protozoan parasites that infect red blood cells.

Mantle. Tightly packed zone of lymphocytes that surround a germinal center.

Marek's disease. A herpesvirus-induced lymphoproliferative disease of chickens that may include demyelination; believed to be due to autosensitized lymphocytes.

Marginal zone. Outer layer of lymphoid follicles of spleen containing loosely packed T and B cells and capillary network involved in lymphocyte circulation.

Margination. Attachment of blood cells to endothelium of vessels during inflammation.

Mast cell. A polymorphonuclear cell with large cytoplasmic granules containing basophilic mediators of anaphylaxis, related to blood basophil.

Masugi nephritis. Experimental glomerulonephritis produced by passive transfer of antibody to glomerular antigens.

Medulla. Central portion of parenchyma of an organ. *Cortex* refers to outer layer of parenchyma.

Medullary cord. Area of medulla of lymph node separating lymphatic sinusoids.

Megakaryocyte. Large multinuclear giant cells in bone marrow from which portions of membrane-bound cytoplasm break off to form blood platelets.

Memory cell. Hypothetical immune competent cell that has ability to recognize and respond more vigorously to antigen because of previous exposure (immunization).

Mesoderm. The middle layer of the three cellular layers of the developing embryo. This layer of cells gives rise to connective tissue and blood cells.

Microglia. Phagocytic cells in the central nervous system.

Migration inhibitory factor. A lymphokine that inhibits the movement of macrophages.

Mikulicz's syndrome. Lymphocytic inflammation of the parotid gland; a variant of Sjögren's syndrome.

Minor histocompatibility antigens. Cell surface molecules not coded in the major histocompatibility complex that contribute to tissue graft rejection.

Mitochondria. Cellular organelles where metabolism takes place.

Mitogen. Substance that activates resting cells to transform into blast cells, synthesize DNA, and divide.

Mitsuda reaction. Late-appearing (2–4 weeks) subcutaneous granulomatous reaction to lepromin indicating granulomatous sensitization in leprosy.

Mixed connective tissue disease. Disease complex characterized by features of different collagen diseases. May be an early form of progressive systemic sclerosis.

Monoclonal antibody. A homogeneous antibody population produced by a clone of antibody-forming cells.

Monocyte. Cells in the macrophage series found in the blood and lymph.

Monokine. Generic term for biologically active factors produced by macrophages (monocytes).

Monomer. A single polypeptide chain. Basic components of Ig molecules are four monomers: two H chains and two L chains.

Mononuclear cells. Cells in the leukocyte lineage with rounded single nuclei (i.e., lymphocytes and macrophages in contrast to polymorphonuclear cells).

Mouse hepatitis virus (MHV). DNA virus that produces hepatitis and encephalitis in mice. MHV infects oligodendrocytes and produces demyelination that does not require involvement of immune cells.

Multiple myeloma. A neoplasm (cancer) of plasma cells.

Multiple sclerosis. Chronic remitting demyelinating disease believed to be caused by cell-mediated immunity to myelin.

Muramyl dipeptide. Peptidoglycan extract of mycobacterial cell walls used to replace mycobacteria in complete Freund's adjuvant.

Myasthenia gravis. A disease of muscle weakness due to a loss of acetylcholine receptors on muscle caused by autoantibodies to acetylcholine receptors.

Myeloblast, myelocyte. Immature precursor cells in the polymorphonuclear leukocyte series.

Myeloma protein. A homogeneous immunoglobulin molecule or part of an Ig molecule produced by cells of a tumor of plasma cells (see *multiple myeloma*).

Myeloperoxidase. Major enzyme in the granules of phagocytic cells that catalyzes peroxidation.

Nasal polyps. Grape-like masses of mucous inflammatory reaction in the mucosa of the nasal cavity occurring in individuals with hay fever.

Natural antibody. Antibody present in the serum of an individual with no known previous contact with the homologous antigen with which the antibody reacts.

Natural killer cells (NK cells). Lymphocytes present in nonimmunized normal individuals that are cytotoxic for a variety of target cell lines.

Natural selection. A theory of antibody formation in which antigen selects immunocompetent cells that already have the ability to recognize and react with the antigen.

NBT test (nitroblue tetrazolium reduction test). A test to determine the activity of the hexomonophosphate shunt in phagocytic cells.

Necrosis. Death of tissue.

Neoantigens. New antigens that appear on cells during development or in tumors.

Nephelometry. An assay that measures the turbidity or cloudiness of a suspension.

Nephritogenic. Substances that cause inflammation of the kidney, such as streptococcal M protein and C3 nephritogenic factor.

Nephron. Functional unit of kidney including the glomerulus and tubule system.

Nephrotic syndrome. Proteinuria and edema seen secondary to kidney disease.

Network theory. A theory that immune responses are controlled by a series (network) of anti-idiotypic reactants.

Neutralization. Process by which an antibody inactivates a toxin or activity of an infectious agent (e.g., virus neutralization).

Neutrophil. A polymorphonuclear cell whose granules stain neither strongly acidophilic nor strongly basophilic.

New Zealand black mice. An inbred strain of mice produced in New Zealand that spontaneously develop autoantibodies and autoimmune diseases.

Nezelof's syndrome. Dysplasia of thymus inherited as an autosomal recessive character causing T cell immunodeficiency.

Non-Hodgkin's lymphoma. Cancers of lymphoid cells that are not Hodgkin's disease; includes T cell, B cell, and null lymphomas.

Nonsteroidal anti-inflammatory drugs (NAID). Agents that inhibit generation of arachidonic acid metabolites (mainly cycloxygenase inhibitors) and thus inhibit inflammation.

Nude (athymic) mice. A hairless mouse strain that congenitally lacks a thymus and T cell function.

Null cells. Lymphocytes with no defining cell surface markers (i.e., neither T nor B cell phenotype).

Nylon wool. A substance that binds mouse T cells; used in fractionation of T and B cells.

NZB mice. See *New Zealand black mice.*

Old tuberculin. Extract of tissues or cultures containing tubercle bacillus antigens used for tuberculin skin tests.

Oligoclonal response. Immune response restricted to a small number of individual clones resulting in limited number of immunoglobulin bands in agarose electrophoresis.

Oncodevelopmental markers (antigens). Markers found in fetal tissues and in cancers of adults, but not found (or found in very low amounts) in normal adult tissue.

Ontogeny. The process of development of an individual from conception to maturity.

Opsonization. The process of enhancing phagocytosis (e.g., by aggregated antibody or activated complement).

Original antigenic sin. The tendency of an individual, when challenged with a cross-reacting antigen, to produce antibody specific to an antigen to which he was previously exposed, even though the cross-reacting antigen may not contain some of the epitopes that are recognized by the antibodies.

Osteoclast-activating factor. A lymphokine that promotes resorption of bone by activating osteoclasts.

Ouchterlony technique. Double diffusion in agar; antibody–antigen precipitation occurring in gel when antigen and antibody diffuse toward each other, react, and form a precipitate.

Oudin tube. Single diffusion in agar. Antigen in solution is placed over agar containing antibody in a capillary tube. Antigen diffuses into agar and forms a precipitin band at equivalence.

OZ. Allotypic markers on human λ chains.

Pannus. Chronic progressive granulation tissue reaction that causes joint destruction in rheumatoid arthritis.

PAP (peroxidase–antiperoxidase technique). An enzyme labeling technique employing complexes of antibody and peroxidase and anti-immunoglobulin to bind the PAP complex to antibodies to tissue antigens.

Papain. Proteolytic enzyme from papaw plant used to hydrolyze immunoglobulin.

Paracortex. T-lymphocyte domain between and beneath follicles in cortex of lymph node; thymus-dependent area.

Paraendocrine syndromes. Clinical symptoms caused by production of hormones by tumors.

Paratope. Antigen (epitope) binding site of antibody.

Paroxysmal cold hemoglobinuria. Production of dark urine after exposure to cold, due to reaction of antibody to red blood cells requiring cold temperature; lysis occurs upon warming and fixation of complement.

Passenger lymphocytes. Lymphocytes present in solid tissue grafts that may contribute significantly to induction of tissue graft rejection by being immunogenic for histocompatibility antigens.

Passive Arthus reaction. Inflammatory vasculitis induced in a skin site of a normal individual previously injected with serum containing IgG antibody.

Passive cutaneous anaphylaxis (Prausnitz–Kustner test). Skin test eliciting wheal and flare reaction by injection of allergen into a skin site of a nonreactive individual that has been pretreated by injection of serum containing skin-fixing antibody (IgE) to the allergen.

Passive immunity. Immunity conferred by transfer of immune products (antisera or sensitized cells) from an immune donor to a nonimmune recipient.

Passive leukocyte-sensitizing activity. Ability of serum from an allergic individual to sensitize leukocytes (mast cells) of a normal individual to release histamine upon exposure to allergen.

Passive transfer. Transfer of immunity from an immunized individual to a nonimmune individual by serum or cells.

Pathologist. An individual who studies disease.

Paul–Bunnell test. Agglutination of sheep red blood cells by serum of patients with infectious mononucleosis; due to reaction to Forssman antigen on sheep cells.

Pemphigoid. A blistering skin disease with subepidermal bullae and autoantibodies to dermal basement membrane.

Pemphigus. A blistering skin disease with intraepithelial bullae and autoantibody to epithelial cells.

Pepsin. Gastric enzyme used to hydrolyze immunoglobulin.

Pernicious anemia. A disease in which low number of red blood cells is caused by a block in metabolism due to a vitamin B_{12} deficiency; often secondary to a lack of a factor necessary for B_{12} absorption known as *intrinsic factor.*

Peyer's patch. Submucosal gastrointestinal lymphoid tissue containing follicles and diffuse lymphoid areas.

Phacoanaphylactic endophthalmitis. Chronic inflammation of the lens of the eye following acute injury of the lens, believed to be caused by autoimmunity to lens proteins.

Phagocytic dysfunction. Defect in ability of phagocytic cells (neutrophils and/or macrophages) to ingest organisms or digest ingested organisms, leading to immune deficiencies.

Phagocytic index. An in vivo measurement of clearance of foreign particles.

Phagocytosis. Engulfment of particles by cells.

Phagolysosome. A membrane-limited cytoplasmic vesicle formed by fusion of a phagosome and a lysosome.

Phagosome. A membrane-limited vesicle containing phagocytosed material.

Pharyngeal pouch. Embryonal organ in the neck that contributes epithelial cells to thymus, parathyroids, and other tissues.

Phenotype. Characteristic of a given cell or individual that reflects which genetically determined properties are expressed.

Philadelphia chromosome. Translocation of one arm of chromosome 22 to chromosome 9 (or 6) in cells of human chronic granulocytic leukemia.

Photoallergy. Anaphylactoid reaction occuring upon exposure to light.

Phylogeny. The evolutionary history of a given species.

Phytohemagglutinin (PHA). Lectin derived from red kidney bean that agglutinates red blood cells and is mitogenic for lymphocytes.

Phytomitogens. Glycoproteins derived from plants that stimulate blast transformation of lymphocytes.

Piecemeal necrosis. Individual cellular necrosis of liver cells surrounded by lymphocytes in chronic active hepatitis.

Plaque-forming cells. Cells producing antibody to antigens on red blood cells suspended in agar that results in a clear zone of cell lysis in the agar.

Plasma. Fluid component of uncoagulated blood after cells are removed.

Plasma cell. Mature cells of the B cell series that synthesize and secrete immunoglobulin. These cells have small nuclei and prominent cytoplasm filled with endoplasmic reticulum.

Plasmapheresis. Removal of plasma components from the circulation of an individual with replacement of cells and plasma substitutes.

Plasminogen activator. Enzyme that converts plasminogen to plasmin.

Platelets. Small cytoplasmic fragments in blood, responsible for activation of coagulation.

Poison ivy. A plant, *Rhus toxicodendron*, that contains a hapten, urushiol, which is a potent inducer and elicitor of contact dermatitis.

Pokeweed mitogen (PWM). A lectin extracted from the plant *Phytolacca americana* that is mitogenic for lymphocytes and stimulates differentiation of human B cells.

Polyarteritis nodosa. Systemic vasculitis involving medium-sized arteries, most likely caused by immune complex reactions in blood vessels.

Polyarthritis. Inflammation of multiple joints; frequently seen in rheumatic fever, SLE, and other rheumatoid diseases.

Polyclonal. Derived from many clones.

Polyclonal activation. Stimulation of a number of different clones of cells (lymphocytes) resulting in a heterogenous immune response.

Polymers. Molecules made up of more than one repeating unit.

Polymorphonuclear cells. Leukocytes (white blood cells) with lobulated nuclei; these cells take part in inflammatory reactions. Major subpopulations are neutrophils, eosinophils, and basophils.

Polymyositis. Inflammation of muscles often associated with rheumatoid diseases, particularly dermatomyositis.

Polynucleotides. Chains of double-stranded DNA; have adjuvant effects when injected with antigen.

Postcapillary venules. Small vessels through which blood flows after capillaries before reaching veins; often the site of migration of inflammatory cells into tissue during inflammation.

Postinfectious encephalomyelitis. Autoimmune demyelination mediated by delayed hypersensitivity to myelin that follows a virus infection.

Postinfectious iridocyclitis. Inflammation of the iris and ciliary body of the eye following a virus or bacterial infection; believed to be caused by an autoimmune reaction.

Poststreptococcal glomerulonephritis. Inflammation of the glomeruli of the kidney that follows infection with group A β-hemolytic streptococci.

Prausnitz–Küstner test. See *passive cutaneous anaphylaxis.*

Pre-B cells. Immature cells in the B cell lineage with cytoplasmic μ chains but no surface Ig.

Precipitation. Formation of insoluble complexes from a mixture of soluble antigen and soluble antibody, producing a macromolecular hydrophobic complex that precipitates from solution.

Primary follicles. Tightly packed aggregates of small lymphocytes in cortex of lymph node and white pulp of spleen. Site of B cells that develop into germinal centers.

Primary response. First immune response to an immunogen not previously recognized; predominantly IgM antibody.

Private specificity. Epitope defined by a single allele and expressed only when the allele is active.

Privileged sites. Places in the body where the immune system cannot function; a place where infectious organisms or tumor cells may grow by avoiding immune effector mechanisms.

Progressive multifocal leukoencephalopathy. A disease characterized by focal destruction of brain cells with little or no associated inflammation that occurs in immunosuppressed individuals with latent virus infection (measles).

Progressive systemic sclerosis (scleroderma). A rheumatoid (collagen) disease characterized by thickening (scarring) of dermis of skin and submucosal connective tissue.

Properdin system. A group of serum proteins (factor B, factor D, properdin, and C3) that interact to activate complement through the alternative pathway.

Prostaglandins. Aliphatic acids derived from arachidonic acid metabolism that have a variety of biological activities including increasing vascular permeability, causing smooth muscle contraction, and decreasing the threshold for pain. Originally identified in prostatic fluids.

Protein A. Protein extracted from cell wall of *Staphylococcus aureus* that binds the Fc of most IgG molecules.

Protein AA. A protein of MW 8,500 found in amyloid deposits.

Protein kinase C. A cytoplasmic enzyme activated by Ca^{++} that is involved in activation of different cell types.

Protein P. A pentameric protein of MW 23,000 found in amyloid deposits.

Proteinuria. Presence of protein in the urine, usually due to damage to glomerular basement membrane; a finding consistant with acute glomerulonephritis.

Prothymocyte. A postulated thymocyte precursor that arises in the bone marrow and circulates to the thymus.

Protooncogenes. Oncogene sequences present in normal mammalian DNA.

Prozone. Suboptimal precipitation or agglutination that occurs in antibody excess.

Pseudoallergic reaction. Clinical state that mimics allergic reaction but is not caused by immune mechanism (anaphylactoid reaction).

Pseudolymphomatous lymphadenitis. Reversible hyperplasia of lymphoid organs, resembling lymphoma.

Psoriasis. A skin disease with abnormal keratinization and autoantibody to keratin.

Public specificity. Antigenic specificity coded by more than one allele of an alloantigenic system.

Purified protein derivative. Extract of proteins from cultures of tubercle bacilli used for tuberculin skin tests.

Purine nucleotide phosphorylase deficiency. Defect in purine metabolism leading to a T cell immunodeficiency.

Purpura. Purple spots on skin due to bleeding into the skin. *Palpable purpura* applies to raised firm purple spots due to inflammation of vessels in the skin.

Pyrogens. Substances released from white blood cells, bacteria, or tissue that cause fever.

Qa locus. Genetic subregion between H2D and TL of the MHC region in mice that encodes the Qa antigen found on T cells.

Quelling test. The swelling of the capsules of pneumococci exposed to antibodies to pneumococci.

Radioallergosorbent test (RAST). Measurement of IgE antibody by binding serum antibody to specific insoluble antigen; the nonbound IgE is washed off and the IgE bound is detected by binding of radiolabeled anti-IgE.

Radioimmunoassay. A competitive inhibition assay in which an unknown amount of antigen competes with radiolabeled antigen binding to antibody.

Radioimmunoscintigraphy. Localization of tumors or other lesions using radiolabeled antibodies and radioactivity scanning after injection in vivo.

RAJI cell test. A test for immune complexes by binding to the cells of a lymphoblast line (RAJI) that has receptors for immune complexes.

RANA (rheumatoid arthritis–associated nuclear antigen). An antigen found in lymphoid cell lines immortalized by Epstein–Barr virus that reacts with sera of patients with rheumatoid arthritis.

RAST. See *radioallergosorbent test.*

Reagin. Originally used for the complement-fixing antisyphilis antibody detected by the Wassermann reaction with cardiolipin; now used synonymously with *skin-fixing antibody* (IgE).

Recombinant vaccines. Immunizing material made by synthesis of proteins using cloned complementary DNA.

Red pulp. Area of cords of Billroth and sinusoids of spleen.

Reed–Sternberg cells. Binucleated giant cells with prominent nucleoli characteristic of Hodgkin's disease.

Regional enteritis. Chronic segmental lymphocytic and granulomatous inflammation of the gastrointestinal tract.

Respiratory disease viruses. Group of viruses, including influenza, paramyxoviruses, rhinoviruses, pneumoviruses, enteroviruses, colonaviruses, and mastadenoviruses, that cause respiratory tract infections of man.

Reticular dysgenesis. Congenital absence of precursors of blood cells resulting in abortion or stillbirth.

Reticuloendothelial system. A composite of the phagocytic cells of the body, primarily the sinusoidal cells of the liver (Kupffer cells), spleen, and lymph nodes.

Reticulum cell sarcoma. Outdated term for large cell lymphoma.

Rheumatic fever. An acute systemic inflammatory disease following group A streptococcal infections.

Rheumatoid factor. Anti-immunoglobulin autoantibody (usually IgM) directed against denatured or allotypic determinants usually on IgG; present in sera of patients with rheumatoid arthritis and other connective tissue diseases.

Rheumatoid nodules. Characteristic granulomatous lesions with central necrosis surrounded by a palisade of mononuclear cells seen in tissues of patients with rheumatoid diseases, particularly rheumatoid arthritis.

Ribosome. A subcellular cytoplasmic organelle that serves as a site for amino acid incorporation during synthesis of proteins.

Rocket electrophoresis. A technique to measure antigens by electrophoresing antigen into an agar layer containing antibody, resulting in a rocket-like pattern of precipitation in agar.

Rosai–Dorfman disease. Sinus histiocytosis with massive lymphadenopathy; a benign hyperplasia of lymph nodes with massive increase in macrophages in sinusoids.

Rosette. A central cell (usually a lymphocyte) surrounded by cells of another type (usually red blood cells); used as a way to detect cell surface receptors or antigens.

Round cells. Mononuclear cells; tissue cells with round or oval nuclei; usually lymphocytes and monocytes.

Russell body. A fully mature plasma cell with large immunoglobulin-containing cytoplasmic granules made up of swollen endoplasmic reticulum.

S region. Chromosomal region of mouse MHC complex that codes for a serum β-globulin.

S value (Svedberg unit). Sedimentation coefficient obtained by ultracentrifugation of a protein.

Sabin vaccine. Attenuated live polio virus used for prophylactic immunization.

Salk vaccine. Formalin-killed polio virus used for prophylactic immunization.

Sarcoidosis. Systemic granulomatous disease of unknown etiology, prominently affecting the lung.

Schick test. A skin test for neutralizing antibody to diphtheria toxin. The test is positive if the characteristic 5–6-hour inflammatory reaction to toxin does not occur after injection of toxin.

Schistosomiasis. Disease due to infection with *Schistosoma* organisms; usually manifested as granulomatous reactions in tissues.

Schultz–Dale reaction. In vitro assay for anaphylactic reactivity employing contraction of smooth muscle sensitized by IgE antibody upon exposure to antigen.

SCID (severe combined immune deficiencies). A group of diseases in which there is essentially an absence of both humoral and cellular immune responses; may be congenital or acquired.

Scleroderma. A rheumatoid (collagen) disease characterized by thickening of skin and submucosal connective tissue (progressive systemic sclerosis).

Second set rejection. Rejection of tissue graft that occurs when the recipient has already rejected a graft from the same histocompatible donor or has been immunized to donor antigens. Second set rejection occurs more rapidly than first set rejection because immunity has already been induced.

Secondary follicle. See *germinal center.*

Secondary immune deficiencies. Defects in immune function due to administration of drugs, infections, or cancer or other diseases.

Secondary response. The more rapid and intense immune response that occurs upon rechallenge of a previously immunized individual with antigen.

Secretory IgA. IgA dimers prominently found in external secretions.

Secretory piece (T piece). A molecule of MW 70,000 produced by epithelial cells and found in secretory immunoglobulins.

Selective theory. A theory of antibody formation in which antigen selects cells that have cell receptors for the antigen and stimulates them to proliferate and differentiate.

Sensitized cell. An immunologically reactive cell induced by exposure to specific antigen.

Serologically defined (SD) antigens. Antigens of the MHC detected by antibodies; originally class I, now both class I and II.

Serotonin (5-hydroxytryptamine). A catecholamine of MW 176 present in mast cells and platelets that contributes to anaphylactic reactions.

Serum. Fluid component of coagulated blood; serum differs from plasma in that serum does not contain fibrinogen.

Serum sickness. A systemic vasculitis, glomerulonephritis, and arthritis due to intravascular immune complex formation following injection of foreign antigen (serum).

Sezary syndrome. Malignant lymphoma of T helper cells; occurs prominently in the skin.

Shock organ. A term used to identify the tissue exhibiting an atopic or anaphylactic reaction.

Shwartzman reaction. (1) Disseminated intravascular coagulation produced in an animal with blockade of the reticuloendothelial system by injection of endotoxin (systemic). (2) Local inflammatory reaction caused by thrombus formation at skin sites injected with two doses of endotoxin 24 hours apart (localized).

Sicca complex. Dryness of the mouth and lack of tearing due to lymphoid inflammation in Sjögren's syndrome.

Side chain theory. A theory of antibody formation, proposed in

1896 by Paul Ehrlich, that first postulated cell surface receptors for antigens.

Side effect. Normal but undesired effect of a drug, such as infections occurring following immunosuppression of organ transplant recipients.

Single radial diffusion. An in vitro gel diffusion test in which antigen placed in a hole in agar diffuses into agar containing antibody, forming a ring of precipitation.

Sjögren's syndrome. Chronic destructive mononuclear-cell inflammation of salivary and tear glands, believed to be caused by autoimmunity to glandular epithelium.

Skin-fixing antibody. Antibody (usually IgE) that remains in skin after local passive transfer (passive cutaneous anaphylaxis). Synonym: *reagin.*

Skin reactive factor. A lymphokine that produces a mild inflammatory reaction when injected into the skin.

Skin-sensitizing antibody. Antibody (usually IgE) that fixes to mast cells in skin. Synonym: *reagin.*

Slow virus infections. Viral infections that have a protracted course characterized by membrane accumulations in brain cells, e.g., kuru, Creutzfeldt–Jakob disease.

Slow-reacting substance A. An acidic lipoprotein of MW 400, derived from arachidonic acid, that has a prolonged constrictive effect on smooth muscle.

"Sneaking through." Ability of low numbers of inoculated transplantable tumor cells to grow, whereas larger doses induce tumor immunity and do not grow.

Somatic mutation. Acquisition of genetic variability that occurs within a given individual after conception.

Spleen. Lymphoid organ that filters circulating blood. Located in left side of abdominal cavity.

Split tolerance. State in which one form of immune response (e.g., antibody) to an antigen is active, while another form (delayed hypersensitivity) is not active.

Spongiosis. Intraepithelial edema.

Spontaneous remission. Rarely occurring reversal of progressive growth of cancer.

Sprue. See *gluten-sensitive enteropathy.*

St. Vitus' dance (chorea). Involuntary twitching muscular movements found in association with acute rheumatic fever.

Staphylococcal protein A. Protein extracted from staphylococci that binds the Fc of most immunoglobulins and is mitogenic for some lymphocytes.

Stem cell. A multipotential precursor cell that may give rise to different functionally and phenotypically differentiated cell types.

Steric hindrance. Physical interference with binding of one ligand by another ligand already bound to a receptor site.

Streptococcal M protein. Nephritogenic factor produced by group A β-hemolytic streptococci.

Strongyloides hyperinfection. Autoinfection of tissues by invasive larvae of *S. stercoralis* in immunosuppressed individuals with intestinal *Strongyloides*.

Subacute sclerosing panencephalitis. A progressive destructive brain disease caused by slow replication of defective viruses.

Sultzberger–Chase phenomenon. Abrogation of delayed hypersensitivity to simple chemicals by oral feeding.

Suppressor cell. A subset of cells that suppress immune responses; usually a T cell subpopulation, but other cell types may also suppress.

Suppressor factor(s). Substances produced by suppressor cells that down-regulate immune responses.

Swiss type agammaglobulinemia. Severe combined immune deficiency disease inherited as autosomal recessive trait.

Switch region. Segment of amino acids at the junction of variable and constant regions of H or L Ig chains coded for by D and J genes.

Sympathetic ophthalmia. Inflammation of the uvea of the previously undamaged eye of an individual following injury to the other eye of the same person.

Sympathetic tuning. "Rebound" hyperresponsiveness to sympathetic stimulation following parasympathetic stimulation.

Syngeneic. Used to describe the relationship between genetically identical individuals of the same species (i.e., identical twins, inbred strains of mice).

Syngeneic preference. Preferential growth of tumors when transplanted to recipients with identical histocompatibility markers.

Synthetic vaccines. Immunizing material for infectious disease made by artificial means, such as by peptide synthesis or from cloned DNA.

T1–T12. Designations for T cell developmental phenotypes detected by monoclonal antibodies (obsolete terms; see Appendix B).

T cell domain. Zones of lymphoid organs predominantly occupied by T cells.

T lymphocyte (T cell). A thymus-derived lymphocyte.

TAC. Transferrin receptor on activated lymphocytes detected by monoclonal antibodies.

Takayasu's arteritis. Mononuclear inflammation of large arteries and aorta.

Terminal deoxynucleotidyl transferase (TdT). An enzyme found in immature lymphocytes, but not in mature lymphocytes; also found in leukemias and lymphoma cells.

Tetanus. A spastic muscular disease caused by action of an endoneurotoxin of *Clostridium tetani.*

Theiler's virus myelitis. Inflammatory demyelination of spinal cord of mice believed to be a postinfectious immune complication of a virus infection.

Thrombocytopenia. A condition of bleeding caused by low numbers of platelets in the blood.

Thrombotic thrombocytopenic purpura. Hemorrhagic disease of unknown etiology with low levels of blood platelets and widespread thrombotic lesions.

Thy 1 + dendritic cells. Intraepithelial cells in mouse epidermis of T cell lineage. Human equivalent not yet identified.

Thy (theta). Antigens present on mouse thymocytes and most mouse T cells.

Thymectomy. Removal of the thymus.

Thymic alymphoplasia. Severe combined immune deficiency inherited as X-linked recessive trait.

Thymic hormones. Substances produced by thymic epithelium that induce differentiation of thymocytes.

Thymic nurse cells. Large epithelial cells in thymus believed to effect maturation of thymic lymphocytes.

Thymocytes. Lymphocytes in the thymus.

Thymoma. Tumor of thymic epithelial cells, usually accompanied by benign proliferation of thymic lymphocytes.

Thymopoietin (thymin). A thymic hormone of MW 7,000.

Thymosin. A thymic hormone of MW 12,000.

Thymus. A central lymphoid organ that is the site of differentiation of T cells.

Thymus-dependent antigens. Immunogens that require T cell cooperation to induce an antibody response.

Thymus-dependent areas (TDA). Zones of lymphoid organs that do not develop in neonatally thymectomized animals; zones that contain a high proportion of T cells in lymphoid organs of normal animals.

Thymus-independent antigens. Immunogens that do not require T cell cooperation for induction of antibody formation.

Tingible bodies. Macrophages containing phagocytosed debris found in lymphoid organs, particularly in areas of the dome of the appendix and in germinal centers of lymph nodes, tonsils, and spleen.

Tissue-fixed macrophages. See *histiocytes.*

TL (thymic–leukemia antigen). A membrane antigen found on thymocytes of TL+ mice that is lost during maturation of T cells but reappears in leukemia.

Tolerance. Active state of unresponsiveness to a given immunogen; immune responses to other immunogens are normal.

Tolerogen. An antigen that induces tolerance.

Tonsils. Gastrointestinal lymphoid organs located at the junction of the oral cavity and the pharynx.

TORCH. Wasting syndrome associated with neonatal infection with *t*oxoplasmosis, *r*ubella, *c*ytomegalovirus, *h*erpes simplex, or *o*ther agents.

Total lymphoid irradiation (TLI). Irradiation of lymphoid organs with protection of other organs, used in treatment of lymphomas and to induce immunosuppression.

Toxin. A substance that produces deleterious effects.

Toxoids. Altered forms of toxins that are immunogenic but not toxic.

Transfer factor. A dialyzable extract of immune lymphocytes that is capable of adoptively transferring delayed hypersensitivity to a specific antigen (e.g., tuberculin) to nonsensitized humans.

Transfusion reaction. Hemolysis in vivo due to reaction of preformed antibodies to passively transferred red blood cells.

Transudation. Passage of fluid, electrolytes, and low-molecular-weight proteins from intravascular to extravascular tissue during mild or early inflammation.

TSF. Suppressor T factor.

Tuberculin type hypersensitivity. Term used in the past for delayed type hypersensitivity, as reaction to tubercular antigens was prototypical of DTH.

Tumor enhancement. Accelerated growth of transplanted tumor due to presence of blocking antibody that reduces expression of cell-mediated immunity to the tumor.

Tumor-associated antigen. Serologically or cellularly (in vitro) identifiable antigen found in tumors, but undetectable or found in very low levels in normal adult tissue.

Tumor-specific antigen (TSA). An antigen found on cancer cells, but not on normal cells. TSAs have been demonstrated in mice by transplantation rejection *(tumor-specific transplantation rejection).* Such antigens have not been convincingly demonstrated in man.

Tumor-specific transplantation antigens. Antigens responsible for immune rejection of tumors transplanted within histocompatible (syngeneic) animals.

Type I reactions. Synonymous with *anaphylactic reactions.*

Type II reactions. Synonymous with *cytotoxic reactions.*

Type III reactions. Synonymous with *immune complex reactions.*

Type IV reactions. Synonymous with *delayed hypersensitivity reactions.*

Ubiquitin. A polypeptide of MW 8,451 found in many organisms that induces both T and B cell differention and is related to the lymphocyte homing receptor on high endothelial venules.

Uremia. Increased uric acid in blood, usually due to chronic renal failure.

Urticaria. Large wheal and flare reactions (cutaneous anaphylaxis).

V region. Variable region of N-terminal portion of immunoglobulin H and L chains.

Vaccination. Immunization for prevention of infectious diseases; originally used for administration of vaccinia virus to induce immunity to smallpox.

Vaccinia. A relative of the smallpox virus (variola) formerly used to induce immunity to smallpox (vaccination). The origin of vaccinia is now obscure, but it is believed to have been derived from cowpox.

Valence (of antibody). The number of epitopes with which one antibody can combine. The valence of most antibodies is 2. IgM may have a valence up to 10; IgA has different valences depending on degree of polymerization.

van der Waals force. A weak force of attraction between all molecules that is active only at very short distances.

Variable region. See *V region.*

Variolation. Immunization procedure for smallpox (variola) using eschars taken from an individual with a mild form of smallpox.

Vasoactive intestinal polypeptide. A 28-amino-acid polypeptide present in mast cells, neutrophils, and nerves that induces vasodilation and potentiates edema produced by bradykinin and C5a des-Arg.

Vasoconstriction. Contraction of precapillary arterioles leading to decreased blood flow.

Vasodilation. Dilation of precapillary arterioles leading to increased blood flow through capillaries.

Vesiculation. Formation of small fluid-filled spaces (sterile abscesses) within epidermal layers, characteristic of contact dermatitis.

Viral interference. State of resistance to infection by one virus in cells already infected by another virus.

Vitiligo. Loss of pigmentation of skin associated with autoantibodies to melanocytes.

Waldeyer's ring. Lymphoid tissue of tonsils and adenoids located around junction of pharynx and oral cavity.

Warm antibody disease. Hemolytic anemia due to IgG autoantibody to red blood cells that is more readily detectable at 37°C than at 4°C (see *paroxysmal cold hemoglobinuria*).

Wassermann reagin. Antibody to cardiolipin originally described as a diagnostic serologic test for syphilis.

Wasting disease (runt disease). A chronic fatal illness associated with weight loss and lymphoid atrophy in (1) neonatally thymectomized mice, (2) late stages of a graft vs. host reaction, and (3) immune deficiency diseases, including AIDS.

Wegener's granulomatosis. Triad of granulomatous arteritis, glomerulonephritis, and necrotizing sinusitis.

Weil–Felix reaction. Diagnostic test: agglutination of *Proteus* X bacteria by the sera of patients with typhus.

Western blot. Localization of antigens present in nitrocellulose paper using labeled antibodies after transfer of antigens from separation media.

Wheal and flare. A skin reaction due to histamine release initiated by trauma or cutaneous anaphylaxis, characterized by central raised edema (wheal) surrounded by a rim of erythema (flare).

White blood cells. Polymorphonuclear leukocytes, lymphocytes, and monocytes in peripheral blood.

White graft rejection. Acute necrosis of tissue graft caused by injection of antibody into a graft site or presence of preformed circulating antibody at the time of grafting.

White pulp. Areas of splenic parenchyma surrounding penicilli arterioles containing high numbers of lymphocytes.

Widal reaction. Bacterial agglutination (by antibody) reaction used in diagnosis of enteric infections by *Salmonella*.

Winn assay. Test of ability of lymphoid cell populations to inhibit in vivo growth of transplantable tumors after preincubation of lymphoid cells and tumor cells in vitro.

Wiskott–Aldrich syndrome. Severe combined immunodeficiency inherited as an x-linked recessive characterized by thrombocytopenia and increased IgA and IgE levels.

Xenogeneic. Denotes a relationship between two members of different species.

Xenograft. A tissue or organ graft between members of two different species.

Zirconium granuloma. Dermal granuloma in axillary areas due to sensitization to zirconium in solid deodorants.

Zollinger–Ellison syndrome. Gastric ulceration produced by increased gastric acid secretion secondary to increased gastrin production.

Zymosan. Preparation of cell wall of yeast that can activate the alternative pathway of complement.

Index